Double Contrast Gastrointestinal Radiology

THIRD EDITION

Marc S. Levine, M.D.

Professor of Radiology
University of Pennsylvania School of Medicine
Chief, Section of Gastrointestinal Radiology
University of Pennsylvania Medical Center
Philadelphia, Pennsylvania

Stephen E. Rubesin, M.D.

Professor of Radiology
University of Pennsylvania School of Medicine
Section of Gastrointestinal Radiology
University of Pennsylvania Medical Center
Philadelphia, Pennsylvania

Igor Laufer, M.D.

Professor of Radiology
University of Pennsylvania School of Medicine
Section of Gastrointestinal Radiology
Associate Chair, Education
University of Pennsylvania Medical Center
Philadelphia, Pennsylvania

W.B. SAUNDERS COMPANY

A Division of Harcourt Brace & Company

Philadelphia   London   Toronto   Montreal   Sydney   Tokyo

W.B. SAUNDERS COMPANY

A Division of Harcourt Brace & Company

The Curtis Center
Independence Square West
Philadelphia, Pennsylvania 19106

Library of Congress Cataloging-in-Publication Data

Levine, Marc S.
    Double contrast gastrointestinal radiology / Marc S. Levine,
Stephen E. Rubesin, Igor Laufer. — 3rd ed.
        p.   cm.
    Includes bibliographical references and index.
    ISBN 0-7216-8211-1
    1. Gastrointestinal system—Radiography.   2. Radiography, Double-
contrast.   3. Gastrointestinal system—Diseases—Diagnosis.
I. Rubesin, Stephen E.   II. Laufer, Igor.   III. Title.
    [DNLM: 1. Gastrointestinal System—radiography.   2. Contrast
Media.   WI 141 L373d 2000]
RC804.R6L38   2000
616.3'30757—dc21
DNLM/DLC
                                                                    99-29019

DOUBLE CONTRAST GASTROINTESTINAL RADIOLOGY   ISBN 0-7216-8211-1

Printed in the United States of America

Last digit is the print number: 9   8   7   6   5   4   3   2   1

Contributors

Clive I. Bartram, F.R.C.P., F.R.C.S., F.R.C.R.

Honorary Senior Lecturer, Imperial College School of Medicine, South Kensington, London; Consultant Radiologist, St. Mark's Hospital, Northwick Park, Harrow, United Kingdom

Hans Herlinger, M.D., F.R.C.R.

Professor of Radiology (Emeritus), University of Pennsylvania School of Medicine, Philadelphia, Pennsylvania; Honorary Consultant, St. James's Hospital, Department of Radiology—Leeds, University of Leeds, England

Herbert Y. Kressel, M.D.

Miriam H. Stoneman Professor of Radiology, Harvard Medical School; President and Chief Executive Officer, Beth Israel Deaconess Medical Center, Boston, Massachusetts

Giles Stevenson, B.M., B.Ch., F.R.C.P., F.R.C.R.

Professor Emeritus, McMaster University, Hamilton, Ontario; Medical Director, Diagnostician, Sudbury, Ontario, Canada

Akiyoshi Yamada, M.D.

Emeritus Professor, Institute of Gastroenterology, Tokyo Women's Medical University, Tokyo, Japan

Preface

Eight years have passed since the publication of the second edition of *Double Contrast Gastrointestinal Radiology*. During this time, dramatic changes have occurred in barium imaging of the gastrointestinal (GI) tract. With the continued AIDS epidemic, we have made considerable strides in our ability to diagnose AIDS-related GI infections, including giant esophageal ulcers caused directly by HIV itself. In the upper GI tract, *Helicobacter pylori* has been recognized as a major cause of gastritis, peptic ulcer disease, gastric carcinoma, and even gastric lymphoma (known as mucosa-associated lymphoid tissue, or MALT, lymphoma). *H. pylori* infection of the stomach may be manifested on double-contrast studies by a spectacular form of polypoid gastritis, whereas MALT lymphoma may be associated with distinctive mucosal abnormalities, enabling detection of this early, curable form of gastric lymphoma on barium studies. In the colon, the double-contrast barium enema has emerged as a safe, inexpensive alternative to colonoscopy for colorectal cancer screening. In fact, the American Cancer Society has endorsed a new set of clinical guidelines that include double contrast barium enema examinations at 5- or 10-year intervals as a screening option for average-risk people over the age of 50. As a result, the demand for double-contrast barium enemas could increase dramatically as we enter the next millennium. Finally, barium radiology has been revitalized by the development and refinement of digital GI imaging, which allows us to acquire images electronically and to interpret them at a workstation in the new space-age era of GI radiology.

For all of these reasons, it is time for the third edition of *Double Contrast Gastrointestinal Radiology*. For this edition, we have taken on a co-author, Stephen Rubesin, our long-time colleague in the GI radiology section at the University of Pennsylvania Medical Center. Steve not only updated his extraordinary chapter on the pharynx but also undertook a major revision of the chapters on the colon and has included a wealth of new illustrations. We are fortunate that Steve has assumed the responsibilities of co-authorship with the same passion and energy we have come to expect from him in our years together in GI radiology.

The reader will notice additional changes in the third edition. In order to produce a more compact text, we have omitted several chapters from the second edition, consolidating this material in other chapters. We also have changed the format of the book, using a more streamlined style for the text and images. As always, our goal has been to present the material in an economical yet aesthetically pleasing fashion.

The third edition of *Double Contrast Gastrointestinal Radiology* is intended not only for residents and students learning the art of double contrast imaging but also for practicing radiologists needing to hone their skills for performing and interpreting these studies. We have continued to place emphasis on the description and ample illustration of the most common conditions encountered in the luminal GI tract. We believe that the third edition builds on the tradition of its predecessors as a new, updated primer on double contrast gastrointestinal radiology for young and experienced enthusiasts of double contrast imaging alike.

Marc S. Levine, M.D.
Igor Laufer, M.D.

Contents

Introduction

MARC S. LEVINE
IGOR LAUFER

GENERAL COMMENTS

The status of barium studies of the gastrointestinal tract is no longer as secure as it was in previous generations. Some of the diagnostic burden has been allocated to newer diagnostic modalities such as ultrasonography and computed tomography. In addition, diagnostic endoscopy has gained a major role in the diagnosis of gastrointestinal diseases. Thus barium studies no longer clearly represent the first choice for gastrointestinal diagnosis.[1] In view of the increasing competition for the diagnostic dollar, it is vital that radiologists emphasize the value of double contrast studies for the diagnosis of early or minimal disease.

The detection of early or minimal disease requires the ultimate in radiologic technique and a thorough familiarity with normal appearances and their variations. For this reason, the emphasis in this book will be on technical details, on normal appearances and their variations, and on the early manifestations of the multitude of neoplastic and inflammatory lesions that affect the gastrointestinal tract.

There are three basic components of barium contrast studies in the gastrointestinal tract: (1) barium-filled views with compression, (2) mucosal relief, and (3) double contrast. Figure 1–1 illustrates these three components in the examination of the colon. The ideal examination technique would utilize each of these components to best advantage. In practice, however, this is not feasible because optimal results in the various phases of the examination require different types of barium suspensions and radiographic technique. The examiner must therefore choose an approach to gastrointestinal contrast studies that emphasizes one or two of the basic components, realizing that other components of the examination may be compromised by this approach.

Many authors have shown that a combination of techniques produces the best achievable results.[2–4] Nevertheless, double contrast images allow detection of the smallest and most subtle lesions.

CONVENTIONAL BARIUM STUDIES
Principles

The most prevalent approach to barium contrast studies of the gastrointestinal tract in the Western world still emphasizes barium-filled views with compression and mucosal relief views. We refer to these as "conventional barium studies." Because of the need to penetrate the opacity of the barium column, these films are exposed at a relatively high kVp. Mucosal relief films are obtained with the organ collapsed either after the administration of a small volume of barium, as in the stomach, or after evacuation of the barium, as in the colon. Even here, there must be a compromise in the choice of barium suspension, since a low-density barium chosen for its suitability for barium-filled compression studies will not give the optimal coating for mucosal relief views. "Air contrast" views are frequently obtained to supplement the information obtained during the earlier phases of the examination. In

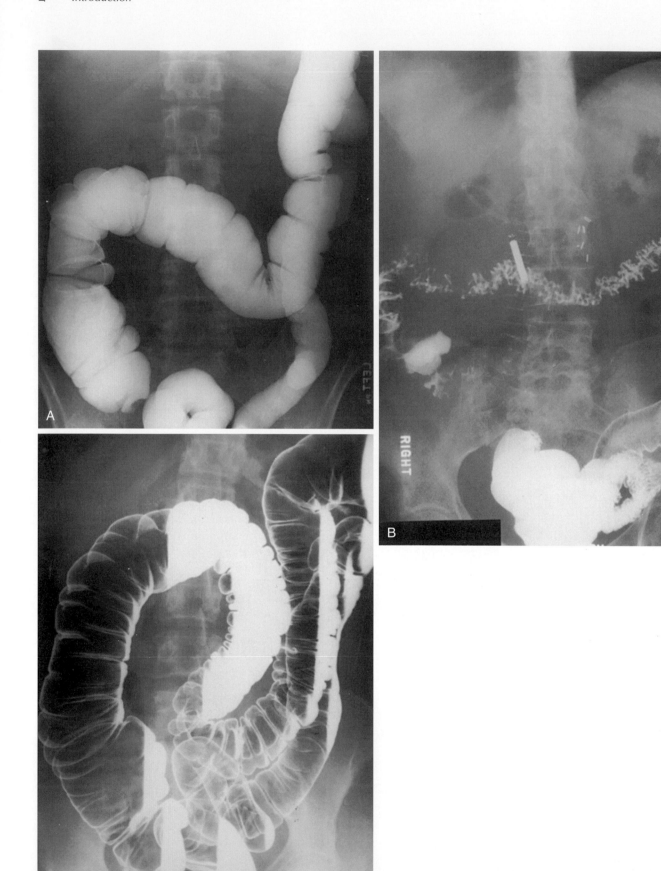

FIGURE 1–1. The three basic elements in barium examinations illustrated in the examination of the colon are barium filling *(A)*, mucosal relief *(B)*, and double contrast *(C)*.

the upper gastrointestinal study the volume of gas that happens to be in the stomach is used, and adequate distention of the antrum and duodenum can occasionally be obtained. However, the quality of mucosal coating is seldom high, and there is rarely sufficient distention for an adequate study of the body and fundus of the stomach. In the colon, double contrast views are frequently obtained by insufflation of air after the patient has evacuated the barium. This type of "secondary air contrast study" has many deficiencies. The type of barium used for the single contrast enema does not produce adequate mucosal coating. The degree of evacuation is variable, and the volume of residual barium is therefore also variable. The time interval during which the patient is evacuating the barium may result in flocculation or flaking of the barium coating. In addition, there is frequently flooding of the small bowel, which obscures the sigmoid colon.

Drawbacks

It is clear that the accuracy of the type of examination just described depends primarily on the quality of the barium-filled and mucosal relief films. Several major problems are encountered when using the conventional barium technique:

1. To obtain greater distention of the organ, it is necessary to increase the volume of barium. Increasing distention therefore results in increasing opacity, which can obscure lesions that are not caught in profile. This problem also applies to the examination of segments of the gastrointestinal tract with a wide caliber, such as the gastric fundus or the right colon.
2. Areas of the gastrointestinal tract that are not accessible for palpation cannot be examined optimally. This generally includes areas such as the gastric fundus, the colonic flexures, and the rectum. This problem also exists in any patient in whom effective compression cannot be applied, either because of obesity, anatomic abnormalities, or local tenderness.
3. In the colon, high-quality mucosal relief films are not obtained reproducibly. The degree of evacuation is variable. In some patients, virtually all the barium is evacuated, leaving no mucosal relief, whereas in others very little barium is evacuated, and again no mucosal relief is seen. Even when the mucosal relief is well seen in one part of the colon, it is usually not possible to map the state of the mucosa thoroughly throughout the entire colon. This is particularly important in the assessment of patients with inflammatory bowel disease and in the differentiation between ulcerative and granulomatous colitis.
4. Single contrast technique depends heavily on diagnostic fluoroscopy. It relies on the keenness of the fluoroscopist's powers of observation in detecting

lesions, and in many cases, diagnostic conclusions are based on fluoroscopic impressions. This may not pose a problem if the fluoroscopist is extremely skilled and experienced. However, it is often difficult or impossible to obtain an intelligent second opinion, as the critical information may have been acquired at fluoroscopy. This poses a particular problem in departments in which many studies are performed by residents and trainees whose fluoroscopic skills are not fully developed.

Diagnostic Accuracy

Despite these theoretical deficiencies, conventional barium studies were thought to be reasonably accurate in the past. This is understandable, as radiologic errors were usually found only at surgery or autopsy when advanced lesions missed by radiologic study would have been discovered. Nevertheless, it seems reasonable to assume that smaller lesions may have been missed in many patients who did not come to surgery or autopsy. The development of fiberoptic endoscopy has provided a valuable tool with which to evaluate the accuracy of these contrast studies in a way that was not previously possible. Endoscopic experience has shown that the majority of small lesions and even a disturbing number of large lesions are missed by conventional barium studies.

Upper Gastrointestinal Tract

Several endoscopic studies have assessed the accuracy of conventional barium examinations of the stomach and duodenum.[5-9] The results are summarized in Table 1–1. Radiologic errors were found in an average of 29% of patients coming to endoscopy. In 22%, the radiologic error was a false-negative error in which a significant lesion was not detected. For the purpose of these statistics, mucosal inflammation and erosions were not included as significant lesions. In an additional 7% of patients, a lesion diagnosed radiographically could not be confirmed by endoscopy. It is likely that in some of these cases the radiologic diagnosis was correct, and the lesion may have been overlooked at endoscopy. In most cases, however,

TABLE **1–1.** *Radiologic Error Rates With Conventional Barium Study*

Series	No. Patients	False Negative (%)	False Positive (%)	Total (%)
Laufer et al.[5]	175	11	11	22
Cotton[6]	518	27	6	33
Papp[7]	85	18	6	24
Dellipiani[8]	137	19	5	24
Barnes et al.[9]	50	14	4	18
TOTAL	965	22	7	29

From Laufer, I.: Assessment of the accuracy of double contrast gastroduodenal radiology. Gastroenterology *71:*874, 1976, with permission.

the endoscopic diagnosis was probably accurate. The major causes of false-negative errors are failure to recognize an abnormality on the film and the small size of some of the lesions.[10] Most false-positive diagnoses are due to contour deformities or to prominent mucosal folds that are mistaken for or simulate pathologic lesions.[5] It seems to us that many of these errors can be avoided by using a technique that makes gross pathology more obvious, allows for detection of smaller lesions, and results in better gastric distention and effacement of normal mucosal folds.

Colon

Colonoscopy has had a dramatic effect on our approach to colonic polyps. A major fringe benefit of the development of colonoscopy has been the opportunity to assess the accuracy of radiologic examination of the colon, particularly with respect to polyp detection but also with respect to inflammatory bowel disease. Several studies have found that 40% to 50% of all colonic polyps are missed on the conventional barium enema.[11,12] These results are particularly important because of the increasing evidence that many colonic carcinomas arise in preexisting adenomas.[13]

Of course, it is difficult to distinguish between errors due to imperfect performance or interpretation and errors due to inherent limitations of technique.[14] Nevertheless, it seems safe to suggest that the conventional barium enema has definite limitations in the examination of segments not accessible to palpation, such as the rectum and the colonic flexures; in the differentiation of extraneous material from true pathologic findings; and in the detection of the early changes in inflammatory bowel disease, such as mucosal granularity in ulcerative colitis and aphthoid ulcers in Crohn's disease.[15,16]

DOUBLE CONTRAST STUDIES

The accumulated evidence regarding the deficiencies of these conventional barium studies led many radiologists to reconsider their gastrointestinal radiologic techniques. This search renewed interest in the development of double contrast techniques, either for routine use or for supplementation of the standard examination. In response to this renewed interest, new barium suspensions and other accessories were developed to make possible an efficient, high-quality double contrast examination on a routine basis.[17–21] With increasing use of these techniques, many new and confusing radiologic appearances have been seen. In this respect, fiberoptic endoscopy has been an invaluable tool for clarifying the nature and significance of these findings and for sharpening interpretative skills.

Advantages

Double contrast diagnosis depends primarily on gaseous distention and mucosal coating with a thin layer of high-density barium. In theory, many of the deficiencies associated with the conventional barium study can be overcome:

1. Increasing distention is obtained without increasing opacity and therefore without loss of surface detail. As a result, the wide caliber portions of the gastrointestinal tract are easily examined.
2. Segments of the gastrointestinal tract that are inaccessible to palpation are easily examined.
3. Excellent mucosal detail is achieved routinely.
4. Diagnostic fluoroscopy is minimized. The emphasis is instead placed on a series of routine radiographs obtained in standard projections. Fluoroscopy is used primarily for determining the correct volume of contrast media for positioning and timing spot films. Of course, if an abnormality is detected at fluoroscopy, additional views are obtained.

Another advantage of the double contrast technique is that it becomes much easier to distinguish between true pathology and extraneous material. This distinction is made by the use of gravity and horizontal beam films. The extraneous material almost always flows to the dependent segment with barium, leaving the air-filled segments clean. Even on double contrast images obtained with the patient recumbent, it is possible to differentiate filling defects on the elevated wall from those on the dependent wall (see Chapter 2). Thus, any filling defect on the elevated wall is almost certainly a true polyp because extraneous material would be expected only on the dependent wall. Because of these factors, it has frequently been possible to find small polypoid lesions in the colon even in the presence of extensive fecal residue.

Because of the interest in surface detail, the radiographic exposures in a double contrast study are considerably lighter and can be exposed at a lower kV than the single contrast study. As a result, it is usually possible to obtain high-quality spot films even when using equipment capable of very low mA and kV output. The exposures are shorter and there is less scatter because there is no need to penetrate the opaque barium column.

Historical Development
Double Contrast Enema

The history of gastrointestinal radiology has recently been reviewed by Margulis and Eisenberg.[22,23] The principles of double contrast technique were first applied to the colon in 1923 by Fischer in Germany and subsequently by Weber at the Mayo Clinic. Major advances in the understanding, performance, and interpretation of these studies were contributed by Welin in Malmö, Sweden, where over 70,000 such examinations have been performed.[24] Despite its high polyp detection rate and exquisite demonstration of minute mucosal abnormalities in neoplastic and inflammatory disease, the technique did not become popular in North America. It is likely that many radiologists tried the double contrast technique but could not reproduce the results obtained by Welin. This is probably the result of failure to obtain the same degree of colonic cleansing and failure to appreciate the need for specific types of barium suspensions, different diagnostic maneuvers, and variations in the appearance of various pathologic lesions on double contrast images.

In the 1960s, the message of the double contrast enema was taken up by the late Roscoe Miller, who was largely responsible for the development of new apparatus, barium suspensions, and accessories.[25,26] These developments led to renewed interest in the double contrast technique by making it possible to perform efficient double contrast studies of high quality. Several surveys have confirmed the continuing increase in double contrast examinations of the colon at the expense of the single contrast study.[27,28]

Upper Gastrointestinal Tract

The potential value of the double contrast technique as an alternative to the palpation method was recognized by Hampton in 1937.[29] Utilizing swallowed air and a barium suspension of creamy consistency, he showed examples of duodenal ulcers and a prepyloric carcinoma. Schatzki and Gary described the importance of en face views with air contrast for diagnosis of gastric ulcers.[30] In 1952, Ruzicka and Rigler described a method for double contrast examination of the stomach that required nasogastric intubation.[31] Unfortunately, the quality of the coating was not optimal because of the barium suspensions available at that time.

In about 1950, a group of gastroenterologists in Japan, under the leadership of Professor Hikoo Shirakabe, studied the pathologic morphology of intestinal tuberculosis on double contrast examinations of the colon. This work led to the development of a double contrast technique for examination of the stomach.[32] Initial interest was in the demonstration of gastric ulcers, particularly linear ulcers that had not been demonstrated on conventional studies. This experience led to further refinements of the technique for the radiologic diagnosis of early gastric cancer.[33] Double contrast examination became standard in Japan during the 1960s, and spectacular results were achieved in both mass screening programs and the evaluation of symptomatic patients. As a result, patients with early gastric ulcer have had 5-year survival rates of greater than 90%.[34]

The Japanese work initially attracted little interest in the West because of the emphasis on early gastric cancer, a disease with a much lower incidence in the West. In the late 1960s and early 1970s, several modifications of the Japanese technique were described.[35,36] The quality of mucosal coating in these early radiographs was suboptimal because of the poor effervescent agents available and the relatively poor coating produced by the barium suspensions at that time. In the early 1970s, more attention was directed to technical details of the examination and in particular to the quality of the barium preparations. This led to the development of new barium suspensions specifically designed to produce high-quality double contrast examinations of the stomach.[21] Several investigators then reported that subtle pathologic lesions that had not been seen before were now being diagnosed. These included superficial gastric erosions,[37,38] linear ulcers,[39,40] and ulcer scars.[40,41] A report by Quizlbash and coworkers[42] suggested that an increased incidence of early gastric cancer in their hospital could be attributed at least in part to the institution of double contrast examination of the stomach.

Diagnostic Accuracy
Colon

Several studies have shown that the double contrast enema can be highly accurate for the detection of polypoid lesions greater than 5 mm in diameter. Ninety percent or more of such polyps are detected on high-quality double contrast enema examinations.[43] This type of study has also been shown to be accurate in demonstrating the visual mucosal abnormalities in patients with inflammatory bowel disease.[15,44]

Upper Gastrointestinal Tract

A number of investigators have compared the radiologic diagnoses using double contrast technique with endoscopic findings. In these series the double contrast method has been found to be more than 90% accurate.[40,45,46] More recently, the double contrast upper gastrointestinal study has been shown to have a sensitivity of greater than 95% in the diagnosis of both esophageal and gastric cancer.[47,48] With increasing confidence in the radiologic diagnosis, the endoscopic examination can be reserved for those patients in whom the radiologic study is equivocal or demonstrates a lesion requiring histologic confirmation.

Drawbacks

Despite the advantages of increased resolution with double contrast studies, there are a number of significant drawbacks. For the practicing radiologist, the method represents a commitment of time and energy to learn new techniques. It requires a revised concept of the relative roles of fluoroscopy and radiography in gastrointestinal diagnosis. It also requires a reorientation for interpreting the films because much more emphasis is placed on the en face appearance of lesions than on their appearance in profile. The examiner may discover that old familiar pathology may have different appearances and that self-retraining is necessary to find the more subtle lesions that are diagnosable by these techniques.

It is likely that double contrast examinations are slightly more time-consuming than conventional barium studies. This is particularly true during the early stages when the examiner is becoming familiar with these techniques. However, if one considers the increased yield and the fewer number of repeat examinations, we believe that the extra time is more than justified.

The technical quality of a double contrast study is highly dependent on the materials used and in particular on the quality of the barium suspension. Thus, the radiologist must constantly monitor the quality of barium preparations and must be willing to try new products that might improve the quality of the study.

A high-quality double contrast study can provide aesthetic pleasure approaching that of a work of art. However, a poor study, whether the fault of the examiner, the patient, or both, may be not only useless but also misleading.[49] In fact, it is probably true that a poor-quality double contrast examination is more dangerous than a poor-quality single contrast examination. The use of double contrast techniques therefore requires a commitment to the development of technical excellence.

STATE OF THE ART: SINGLE VERSUS DOUBLE CONTRAST

Although the volume of barium studies decreased by 25% to 30% during the 1980s,[50] double contrast examinations represent greater than 40% of all barium studies being performed.[51] In fact, the absolute number of double contrast examinations actually increased over this period.

It must be re-emphasized that the term "double contrast examination" refers to an examination relying primarily on double contrast images but also incorporating the elements of single contrast and, where possible, mucosal relief. In the majority of studies, this type of double contrast examination has been shown to be clearly superior to the type of examination relying primarily on single contrast. The difficulty of comparing statistics regarding the diagnostic accuracy of these two types of studies has been described by Gelfand and Ott.[52] Nevertheless, in their own work, Gelfand and coworkers also found that the double contrast views are the single most informative part of the examination.[3] We believe that there is strong feeling in the general medical community that single contrast studies, as they have been performed, cannot compete effectively with the results achieved by endoscopy.[52–54] At the same time, evidence is increasing that the double contrast examination can be competitive, particularly in this era of cost-containment.[55–57]

CONCLUSION

We feel certain that the radiologist who spends the time and effort to master these techniques will be rewarded by gastrointestinal studies of increased diagnostic value and, in many cases, of great aesthetic quality. Our experience suggests that this combination stimulates interest in gastrointestinal radiology not only for the radiologist but also for students, technologists, and referring physicians. This can only result in greater diagnostic accuracy and an enhanced appreciation of the role of radiology in the diagnosis of gastrointestinal disorders.

REFERENCES

1. Op den Orth, J.O: Use of barium in evaluation of disorders of the upper gastrointestinal tract: Current status. Radiology *173*:601, 1989.
2. Montagne, J.P., Moss, A.A., and Margulis, A.R.: Double-blind study of single and double contrast upper gastrointestinal examinations using endoscopy as a control. AJR Am. J. Roentgenol. *130*:1041, 1978.
3. Gelfand, D.W., Chen, Y.M., and Ott, D.J.: Multiphasic examinations of the stomach: Efficacy of individual techniques and combinations of techniques in detecting 153 lesions. Radiology *162*:829, 1987.
4. Dekker, W., and Op den Orth, J.O.: Biphasic radiologic examination and endoscopy of the upper gastrointestinal tract. J. Clin. Gastroenterol. *10*(4):461, 1988.
5. Laufer, I., Mullens, J.E., and Hamilton, J.: The diagnostic accuracy of barium studies of the stomach and duodenum—correlation with endoscopy. Radiology *115*:569, 1975.
6. Cotton, P.B.: Fiberoptic endoscopy and the barium meal—results and implications. Br. Med. J. *2*:161, 1973.
7. Papp, J.P.: Endoscopic experience in 100 consecutive cases with the Olympus GIF endoscope. Am. J. Gastroenterol. *60*:466, 1973.
8. Dellipiani, A.W.: Experience with duodenofiberscopes. Scott. Med. J. *19*:7, 1974.
9. Barnes, R.J., Gear, M.W.L., and Nicol, A.: Study of dyspepsia in a general practice as assessed by endoscopy and radiology. Br. Med. J. *4*:214, 1974.
10. Gelfand, D.W., Ott, D.J., and Tritico, R.: Causes of error in gastrointestinal radiology. Gastrointest. Radiol. *5*:91, 1980.
11. Wolff, W.I., Shinya, H., Geffen, A., et al.: Comparison of colonoscopy and the contrast enema in five hundred patients with colorectal disease. Am. J. Surg. *129*:181, 1975.
12. Thoeni, J.F., and Menuck, L.: Comparison of barium enema and colonoscopy in the detection of small colonic polyps. Radiology *124*:631, 1977.
13. Lane, N., and Fenoglio, C.M.: The adenoma-carcinoma sequence in the stomach and colon. 1. Observations on the adenoma as precursor to ordinary large bowel carcinoma. Gastrointest. Radiol. *1*:111, 1976.
14. Kelvin, F.M., Gardiner, R., Vos, W., et al.: Colorectal carcinoma missed on double contrast barium enema study: A problem in perception. AJR Am. J. Roentgenol. *137*:307, 1981.
15. Laufer, I.: Air contrast studies of the colon in inflammatory bowel disease. CRC Crit. Rev. Diagn. Imaging *9*:421, 1977.
16. Laufer, I., and Costopoulos, L.: Early lesions of Crohn's disease. AJR Am. J. Roentgenol. *130*:307, 1978.
17. Miller, R.E.: Barium enema examination with large bore tubing and drainage. Radiology *82*:905, 1964.
18. Gelfand, D.W., and Hachiya, J.: The double contrast examination of the stomach using gas-producing granules and tablets. Radiology *93*:1381, 1969.
19. Miller, R.E., Chernish, S.M., Skucas, J., et al.: Hypotonic roentgenography with glucagon. AJR Am. J. Roentgenol. *121*:264, 1974.
20. Laufer, I.: A simple method for routine double-contrast study of the upper gastrointestinal tract. Radiology *117*:513, 1975.
21. Gelfand, D.W.: High density, low viscosity barium for fine mucosal detail on double-contrast upper gastrointestinal examinations. AJR Am. J. Roentgenol. *130*:831, 1978.
22. Margulis, A.R., and Eisenberg, R.L.: Gastrointestinal radiology from the time of Walter B. Cannon to the 21st century. Radiology *178*:297, 1991.
23. Eisenberg, R.L., and Margulis, A.R.: Brief history of gastrointestinal radiology. Radiographics *11*:121, 1991.
24. Welin, S.: Results of the Malmö technique of colon examination. JAMA *199*:369, 1967.
25. Miller, R.E.: Examination of the colon. Curr. Probl. Radiol. *5*(2):3, 1975.
26. Miller, R.E.: Recipes for gastrointestinal examinations. AJR Am. J. Roentgenol. *137*:1285, 1981.
27. Semelka, R.C., and MacEwan, D.W.: Changes in diagnostic investigation and improved detection of colon cancer, Manitoba 1964–1984. J. Can. Assoc. Radiol. *38*:251, 1987.
28. Thoeni, R.F., and Margulis, A.R.: The state of radiographic technique in the examination of the colon: A survey in 1987. Radiology *167*:7, 1988.
29. Hampton, A.O.: A safe method for the roentgen demonstration of bleeding duodenal ulcers. AJR Am. J. Roentgenol. *38*:565, 1937.

30. Schatzki, R., and Gary, J.E.: Face-on demonstration of ulcers in the upper stomach in a dependent position. AJR Am. J. Roentgenol. *79:*722, 1958.
31. Ruzicka, F.F., and Rigler, L.G.: Inflation of the stomach with double contrast: Roentgen study. JAMA *145:*696, 1951.
32. Shirakabe, H.: Double Contrast Studies of the Stomach. Stuttgart, Georg-Thieme Verlag, 1972.
33. Shirakabe, H., Ichikawa, H., Kumakura, K., et al.: Atlas of X-Ray Diagnosis of Early Gastric Cancer. Philadelphia, J. B. Lippincott, 1966.
34. Yamada, E., Nagazato, H., Koite, A., et al.: Surgical results of early gastric cancer. Int. Surg. *59:*7, 1974.
35. Obata, W.G.: A double-contrast technique for examination of the stomach using barium sulfate with simethicone. AJR Am. J. Roentgenol. *115:*275, 1972.
36. Scott-Harden, W.G.: Radiological investigation of peptic ulcer. Br. J. Hosp. Med. *10:*149, 1973.
37. Laufer, I., Hamilton, J., and Mullens, J.E.: Demonstration of superficial gastric erosions by double contrast radiology. Gastroenterology *68:*387, 1975.
38. Poplack, W., Paul, R.E., Goldsmith, M., et al.: Demonstration of erosive gastritis by the double contrast technique. Radiology *117:*519, 1975.
39. Poplack, W., Paul, R.E., Goldsmith, M., et al.: Linear and rod-shaped peptic ulcers. Radiology *122:*317, 1977.
40. Laufer, I.: Assessment of the accuracy of double contrast gastroduodenal radiology. Gastroenterology *71:*874, 1976.
41. Gelfand, D.W.: The Japanese-style double contrast examination of the stomach. Gastrointest. Radiol. *1:*7, 1976.
42. Quizlbash, A., Harnorine, C., and Castelli, M.: Early gastric carcinoma: Value of combined use of endoscopy, air contrast x-ray films, cytology and multiple biopsy specimens. Arch. Pathol. *101:*610, 1977.
43. Laufer, I., Smith, N.C.W., and Mullens, J.E.: The radiological demonstration of colorectal polyps undetected by endoscopy. Gastroenterology *70:*167, 1976.
44. Simpkins, K.C., and Stevenson, G.W.: The modified Malmö double-contrast enema in colitis: An assessment of its accuracy in reflecting sigmoidoscopic findings. Br. J. Radiol. *45:*486, 1972.
45. Moule, E.B., Cochrane, K.M., Sokhi, G.S., et al.: A comparative study of the diagnostic value of upper gastrointestinal endoscopy and radiology. Gut *16:*411, 1975.
46. Herlinger, H., Glanville, J.N., and Kreel, L.: An evaluation of the double contrast barium meal (DCBM) against endoscopy. Clin. Radiol. *28:*307, 1977.
47. Levine, M.S., Chu, P., Furth, E.E., et al.: Carcinoma of the esophagus and esophagogastric junction: Sensitivity of radiographic diagnosis. AJR Am. J. Roentgenol. *168:*1423, 1997.
48. Low, V.H.S., Levine, M.S., Rubesin, S.E., et al.: Diagnosis of gastric carcinoma: Sensitivity of double-contrast barium studies. AJR Am. J. Roentgenol. *162:*329, 1994.
49. Hartzell, H.V.: To err with air. JAMA *187:*455, 1964.
50. Gelfand, D.W., Ott, D.J., and Chen, Y.M.: Decreasing numbers of gastrointestinal studies: Report of data from 69 radiologic practices. AJR Am. J. Roentgenol. *148:*1133, 1987.
51. Ominsky, S.H., and Margulis, A.R.: Radiographic examination of the upper gastrointestinal tract. Radiology *139:*11, 1981.
52. Gelfand, D.W., and Ott, D.J.: Single- vs. double-contrast gastrointestinal studies: Critical analysis of reported statistics. AJR Am. J. Roentgenol. *137:*523, 1981.
53. Tedesco, F.J., Griffin, J.W. Jr., Crisp, W.L., and Anthony, H.F. Jr.: "Skinny" upper gastrointestinal endoscopy—the initial diagnostic tool: A prospective comparison of upper gastrointestinal endoscopy and radiology. J. Clin. Gastroenterol. *2:*27, 1980.
54. Martin, T.R., Vennes, J.A., Silvis, S.E., and Ansel, H.J.: A comparison of upper gastrointestinal endoscopy and radiography. J. Clin. Gastroenterol. *2:*21, 1980.
55. Young, J.W., Ginthner, T.P., and Keramati, B.: The competitive barium meal. Clin Radiol. *36:*43, 1985.
56. Levine, M.S., and Laufer, I.: The upper gastrointestinal series at a crossroads. AJR Am. J. Roentgenol. *161:*1131, 1993.
57. Levine, M.S.: Role of the double-contrast upper gastrointestinal series in the 1990s. Gastroenterol. Clin. North Am. *24:*289, 1995.

2

Principles of Double Contrast Diagnosis

IGOR LAUFER
HERBERT Y. KRESSEL

INTRODUCTION

Why Double Contrast?

Despite the data outlined in Chapter 1 regarding the consistent superiority of double contrast techniques throughout the gastrointestinal tract, many radiologists have chosen not to change their gastrointestinal techniques. Perhaps the most convincing argument for switching to double contrast is illustrated in Figure 2–1. The example is that of a conventional Styrofoam cup examined by single contrast in which no "lesions" are seen. With double contrast technique, a complete ring of artificial erosions is seen both en face and in profile. Even in retrospect, none of these lesions can be recognized in the barium-filled cup. This example illustrates the number of lesions that may be present and obscured by barium and yet are clearly demonstrated by double contrast.

Orientation

Successful application of double contrast techniques in gastrointestinal radiology requires the development of skill both in the performance and in the interpretation of these studies. The transition from single contrast to double contrast radiology requires more than a minor adjustment in technique. Indeed, the double contrast approach requires a major reorientation to the performance and interpretation of gastrointestinal studies.

The purpose of this chapter is to outline general principles in the performance and interpretation of double contrast examinations. When properly performed, they make it possible to provide a precise translation from the radiographic abnormalities to the gross pathology and, in many cases, to the microscopic pathology. Some of these principles are illustrated in vitro using Styrofoam cups and simulated pathologic lesions. This work was performed by Dr. Miriam C. Green during a student elective in our department. In addition, examples and illustrations are drawn from the entire gastrointestinal tract to stress the general applicability of these principles. Their specific applications are discussed in detail in the appropriate chapters. We would also like to stress the causes of potential error in the use of double contrast techniques and to suggest some approaches whereby some of these errors can be avoided.

DIFFERENCES BETWEEN SINGLE AND DOUBLE CONTRAST STUDIES

To understand the double contrast approach to gastrointestinal radiology, it is important to clarify the basic differences between single and double contrast studies. The single contrast study concentrates on examination of the contour and lumen of the gastrointestinal tract.[1] Its most important component is the fluoroscopic study, whereby the volume of barium is monitored, graded compression is applied, and in most cases a diagnostic impression is reached during fluoroscopy. The purpose of multiple radiographs is to provide complementary views of the same lesion or the same surface. In general we expect to see a lesions on all or most radiographs that incorporate the area in question. We are generally content to identify an abnormality and suggest its pathologic nature. We are usually not interested in precise three-dimensional reconstruction or localization, and in particular we are rarely concerned with differentiation between the dependent and the nondependent surfaces.

By comparison, the double contrast examination is concerned primarily with delineation of mucosal detail and secondarily with abnormalities of the contour and lumen. Fluoroscopy is used primarily for monitoring of the volume of contrast materials and for accurate localization and timing of spot images. Diagnostic fluoroscopy is minimized. The mainstay of diagnosis is careful examination of multiple radiographs. The multiple radiographs taken in different projections are additive rather than complementary, since each film presents a certain proportion of the mucosal surface for diagnostic evaluation, while the remainder of the mucosal surface is obscured by the high-density barium. Thus the total examination requires the interpolation and integration of the information obtained from the multiple radiographs.[2] It is not surprising that some lesions may be visible on only one or two of a dozen or more images.

The adequacy of the double contrast study is judged by the en face appearance of the mucosal surface and not by the visibility of the contour of the bowel. Similarly, diagnostic interpretation is based largely on an analysis of the en face appearance of the mucosal surface. Accurate interpretation of these radiographic findings depends on a clear understanding of the differing appearances of structures and lesions on the dependent and nondependent surfaces. This understanding allows for an accurate translation from radiographic abnormalities to pathologic condition. It also allows for an appreciation of the limitations of each radiograph and suggests maneuvers for demonstrating suspected lesions in greater detail.

Finally, these techniques present a variety of artifactual appearances. [3] These are discussed in general terms and are also illustrated in specific chapters in conjunction with the types of pathology they may simulate.

COMPONENTS OF THE DOUBLE CONTRAST EXAMINATION

Patient Preparation

Adequate cleansing of the mucosal surface throughout the gastrointestinal tract is of obvious importance in preparing the patient for double contrast examination, so that the barium coating will provide an accurate reflection of the mucosal surface. Residual debris obscures the mucosal surface, and residual fluid results in dilution of

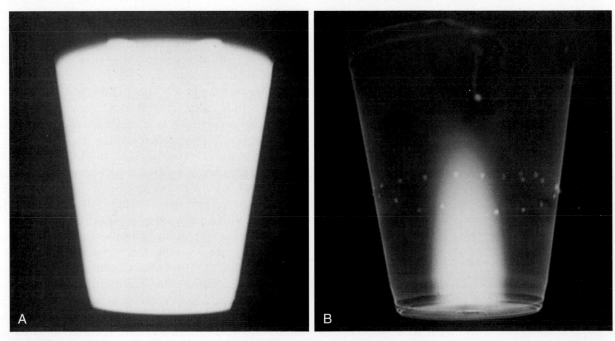

FIGURE 2–1. The advantage of double contrast. *A,* The Styrofoam cup is examined by single contrast. No lesion is seen. *B,* With double contrast, a ring of "erosions" is clearly seen both en face and in profile.

the barium suspension, producing poor mucosal coating and artifacts because of patchy coating (Fig. 2–2).

Mucosal Coating
High-Density Barium

Relatively little is known about the ingredients and additives in the various commercial barium suspensions.[4,5] In particular, the physical and chemical properties that produce good mucosal coating are unknown. One would expect the ideal barium suspension for double contrast studies to have low viscosity and high density. However, there are other important factors, such as the resistance of a suspension to acid, mucin, or alkali. Because of these many factors, there is no single barium suspension that produces good results throughout the gastrointestinal tract. As a result, in our barium kitchen we have a "menu" from which we choose a barium suspension best suited for the examination being performed. In general terms, the upper gastrointestinal study requires a high-density (200% to 250% w/v), low-viscosity barium suspension, whereas the colon examination gives best results with an intermediate-density (85% to 100% w/v), higher-viscosity suspension. The requirements for the small bowel examination are still different (see Chapter 11).

The important point is that barium cannot be considered a homogeneous product with differences only in concentration, flavoring, and coloring. There are variations in viscosity, as well as other differences related to the addition of unspecified ingredients, that may affect the stability of the suspension and the quality of mucosal coat-

ing. Therefore, the radiologist interested in performing double contrast examinations must be familiar with the properties of these suspensions and must be able to choose a product appropriate to the specific study being performed.

Criteria for Good Mucosal Coating

When there is good mucosal coating, the mucosal surface has a uniform grayness that fades at the edge to blend with the continuous smooth white line at the periphery, representing the profile view of the mucosa. The coating must be continuous, with no artifacts resulting from patchy coating. In the stomach, demonstration of the areae gastricae pattern serves as an additional criterion for good coating.[6] A similar surface pattern, the innominate grooves, may be seen in the colon, but with much less frequency (Fig. 2–3).[7]

Poor mucosal coating can be recognized by a lack of grayness in the en face appearance of the mucosa, with contrast provided only by the gas. The profile view of the mucosa may show thin, irregular, or interrupted coating (see Fig. 2–2). This type of coating may be the result of incorrect choice of barium or of improper preparation of the barium suspension or of fluid, acid, or mucus within the bowel. In the colon such poor coating, with flaking of the barium suspension, may be seen on postevacuation films.

In the presence of poor or patchy coating, lesions are easily missed[8] (Fig. 2–4A). Therefore in such cases the barium bolus must be washed across the area of poor coating until adequate coating is achieved (Fig. 2–4B).

Distention

Gaseous distention is produced by different means throughout the gastrointestinal tract. The common goal is to separate the surfaces of the viscus and to efface the mucosal folds. In some areas, such as the gastric fundus, this is difficult to achieve, but at least the mucosal folds should be straightened.

It is easy to appreciate that inadequate gaseous distention may hide lesions (Fig. 2–5). However, it may not be so obvious that overdistention may also obscure lesions (Fig. 2–6). Figure 2–7 shows that varying degrees of distention give different information about the lesion. With overdistention, an area of rigidity is accentuated, whereas with partial collapse, the appearance of the mucosal surface may be appreciated more readily. This is particularly true in lesions with a submucosal component. Therefore, when evaluating a complex or subtle lesion, it is important to use the concept of varying degrees of distention and to examine the lesion with overdistention, adequate distention, and partial collapse. One can then synthesize the information obtained from each of these views to come to a final conclusion regarding the nature and extent of the lesion. This concept is illustrated in Figure 2–8 in a patient with adenocarcinoma of the distal esophagus in Barrett's epithelium. The double contrast film, with the esophagus

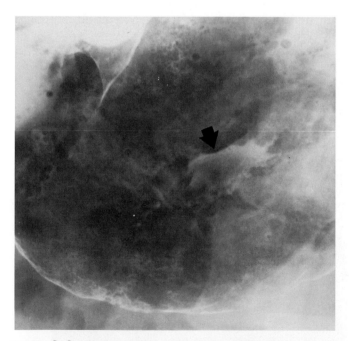

FIGURE 2–2. Patchy coating simulating an ulcer. The poor coating is due to fluid and debris within the stomach. This has resulted in an irregular collection on the posterior wall resembling an ulcer *(arrow)*. A repeat study with good mucosal coating showed no abnormality.

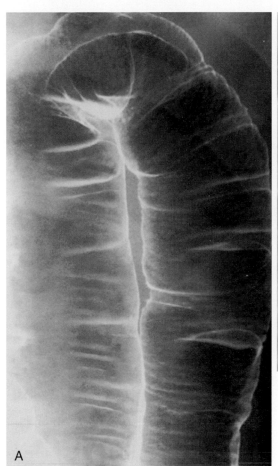

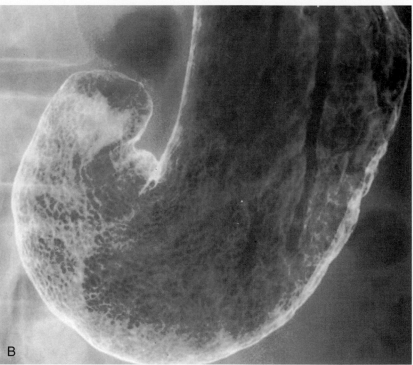

FIGURE 2–3. Normal surface patterns. *A,* The innominate lines and pits representing the surface pattern of the colon. *B,* The areae gastricae. The fine reticular appearance of the normal surface pattern of the stomach is seen particularly in the gastric antrum.

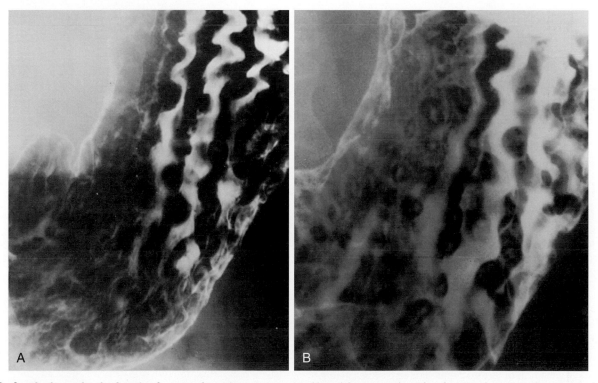

FIGURE 2–4. The hazards of suboptimal mucosal coating. *A,* A supine film of the stomach with suboptimal coating shows only thickening of the gastric rugal folds. *B,* With improvement in mucosal coating, a diffuse erosive gastritis becomes obvious.

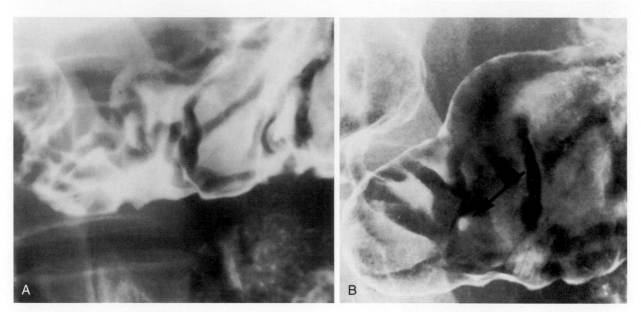

FIGURE 2–5. The hazards of underdistention. *A,* Film of the gastric antrum collapsed shows only prominent folds and no definite ulcer can be identified. *B,* With adequate distention, a small ulcer *(arrow)* becomes obvious with its radiating folds. (*B,* From Laufer, I., et al.: The diagnostic accuracy of barium studies of the stomach and duodenum—correlation with endoscopy. Radiology *115:*569–573, 1975, with permission.)

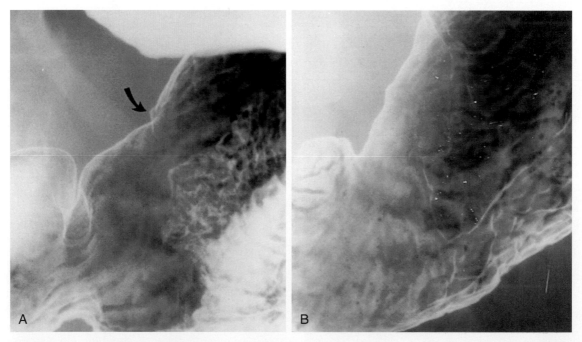

FIGURE 2–6. Risks of overdistention. *A,* With moderate distention, a small ulcer crater is seen along the lesser curve of the stomach *(arrow).* *B,* With overdistention, the ulcer becomes unrecognizable.

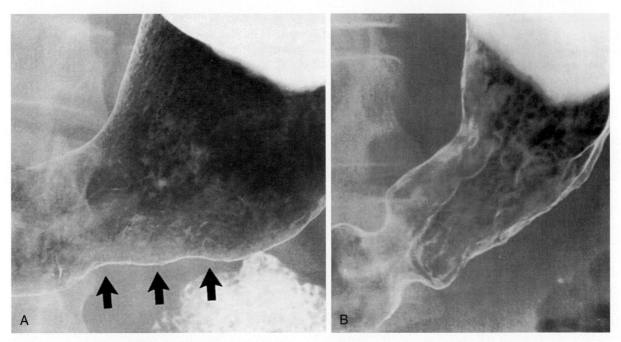

FIGURE 2–7. Value of varying degrees of distention. *A,* With the stomach overdistended, the rigidity along the greater curvature is clearly seen *(arrows). B,* With the stomach partially collapsed, the nodularity of the mucosal surface is more easily appreciated but the area of rigidity is not as evident. These findings were due to a scirrhous carcinoma of the stomach.

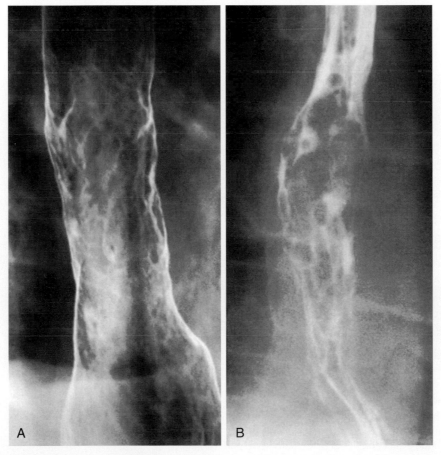

FIGURE 2–8. Adenocarcinoma of Barrett's esophagus. *A,* The double contrast view shows ulceration and slight rigidity of the contour. *B,* The mucosal relief film shows the polypoid nature of the lesion.

well distended, shows slight rigidity, abnormality of the contour, and areas of ulceration (Fig. 2–8*A*). With the esophagus collapsed, the polypoid nature of the lesion is more clearly shown (Fig. 2–8*B*). Thus we cannot say that either one of the films is better than the other. Rather, the combination of the two gives us the most information about the nature and extent of the lesion.

Projection

For each examination, attempts should be made to keep the number of films to a minimum. The minimum number of films is that required to show each area free of overlapping loops of bowel. A series of maneuvers must therefore be designed to optimize mucosal coating and to yield the required spot images. The purpose of these maneuvers is to optimize mucosal coating by removing mucus and debris from the mucosal surface. The more frequent the washing, the better the mucosal coating. The maneuvers should also be designed to avoid loss of contrast material and to avoid overlapping loops of bowel until spot images of any given segment have been obtained. If there are overlapping loops, additional views in different obliquities are required (Fig. 2–9). The procedure must be executed quickly to prevent both overlap and deterioration in the quality of coating.

Compression

The compression study is not as critical in the double contrast study as it is in the single contrast study. Nevertheless, in some cases a lesion may be seen only on the compression images, whereas in others it may be appreciated and defined more easily with compression (Fig. 2–10). Therefore it must be emphasized that compression is a routine and indispensable component of the complete double contrast examination.

Relaxant Drugs

There is no doubt that the use of relaxant drugs results in a higher-quality double contrast examination. In the examination of the colon it has the additional advantage of decreasing patient discomfort.[9,10] However, the use of an injectable drug presents a slight nuisance and delay in the examination and an increase in cost. With the use of glucagon there are few side effects. Some patients become nauseous or vomit within minutes of a rapid infusion or within 1 to 3 hours after a slow infusion of 1 mg glucagon.[11] There is also the remote possibility of a hypersensitivity reaction.[12] However, glucagon in the upper gastrointestinal tract may delay filling of the duodenum, which may prolong the examination. It must be appreciated that the various organs differ in their sensitivity to glucagon. The upper gastrointestinal tract is very sensitive to glucagon in doses as low as 0.05 mg, whereas in the colon we believe that a dose of at least 1 mg is required to be effective.[13]

Occasionally we require a relaxant drug for the examination of the esophagus. For this purpose we use propantheline bromide (Pro-Banthine), 15 to 30 mg intravenously, since glucagon is ineffective in abolishing esophageal peristalsis.[14]

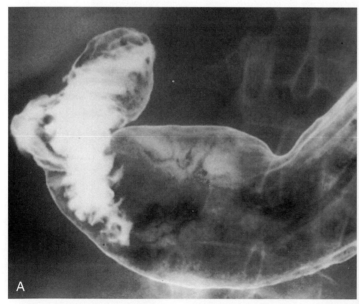
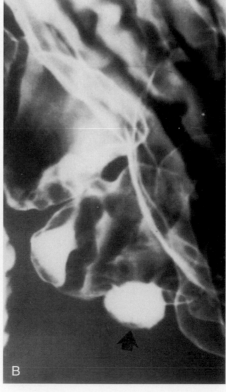

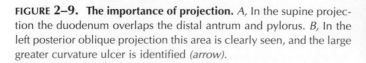
FIGURE 2–9. **The importance of projection.** *A,* In the supine projection the duodenum overlaps the distal antrum and pylorus. *B,* In the left posterior oblique projection this area is clearly seen, and the large greater curvature ulcer is identified *(arrow)*.

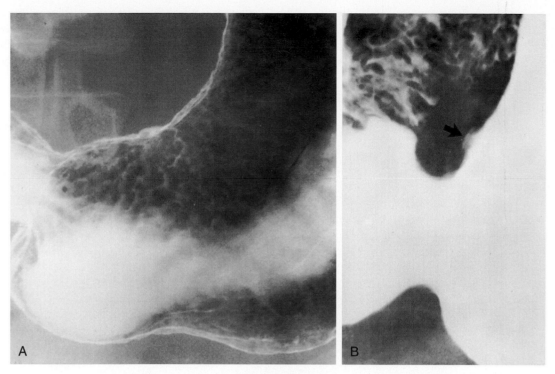

FIGURE 2–10. The importance of compression. *A,* The double contrast film shows a course areae gastricae pattern along the lesser curvature. An ulcer crater is difficult to recognize. *B,* Barium filling with compression shows a small ulcer crater *(arrow)* in this area.

Radiographic Technique

Attention to radiographic technical details is of utmost importance because surface detail can easily be obscured by faulty technique.

For the demonstration of surface detail a low kV would be desirable. However, this lengthens the exposure and may result in a film that shows too much contrast, such that a small area of the film is well exposed, while the rest is poorly exposed. The exposure is particularly sensitive to the position of the phototimer cell. We have used approximately 105 kV for our films to shorten the exposure and to provide greater latitude. The rare earth screens with 400-speed film screen combinations seem to provide the optimal combination of radiographic detail and short exposure. Digital fluoroscopy with the possibility of image processing allows for further optimization of the image.

Endoscopic and Pathologic Correlation

With the use of double contrast techniques many unfamiliar appearances will be encountered. We have relied heavily on endoscopic and pathologic correlation for clarification of the nature and significance of new radiologic findings.[15,16] It is important for the radiologist to actually see the specimen or to look through the endoscope to appreciate the mucosal surface, rather than to rely on a written report. By recognizing the normal appearances and their variations throughout the gastrointestinal tract and the gross pathologic appearances of various types of surface abnormalities, the radiologist will come to appreciate the limitations and confidence limits of endoscopic and pathologic diagnosis. With the development of technical and interpretative skills, the radiologist can help the endoscopist and the pathologist to appreciate more subtle anatomic and pathologic details. We consider constant endoscopic and pathologic correlation an indispensable tool in the development of technical and interpretative skills in gastrointestinal radiology.

ESSENTIALS OF INTERPRETATION

Elements of the Double Contrast Image

In general terms, there are three elements contributing to each double contrast image: the dependent surface, the nondependent surface, and the barium pool (Fig. 2–11). The specific surface that is in the dependent or nondependent position is determined by the position of the patient. The barium pool will be found in the most dependent segments.

Dependent Surface

The dependent surface is covered by a barium pool of varying depth. Under ideal conditions, there will be just enough barium to outline protrusions without covering over and obscuring shallow lesions. If the dependent surface has any undulations, barium will collect in puddles

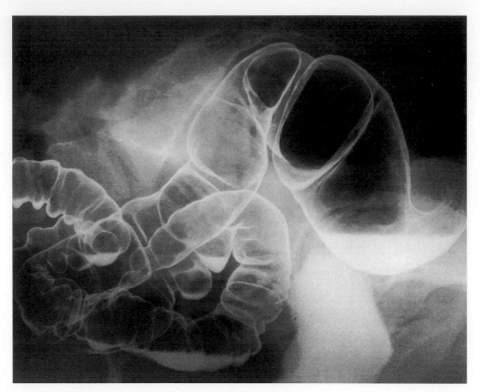

FIGURE 2–11. Components of the double contrast image. Cross-table lateral view of the rectum and sigmoid with the patient prone. Dependent and nondependent surfaces can be identified. There are barium pools on the anterior wall of the distal rectum and sigmoid in addition to smaller barium puddles throughout the sigmoid colon.

or pools within the valleys between the hills. The barium pool is discussed in detail later in this chapter.

Nondependent Surface

The nondependent surface has a thinner coating of barium because all the free barium falls off into the dependent surface. Thus, there is no barium pool or puddle on the nondependent surface, only a thin coating of barium.

Anterior Versus Posterior Wall Structures

Because of the differences in barium coating of the dependent and nondependent surfaces, anatomic structures on the anterior and posterior walls have different appearances. These differences are illustrated diagrammatically in Figure 2–12. Assuming that the patient is in the supine position, the posterior surface is dependent and the anterior surface is nondependent. A rugal fold on the posterior wall of the stomach appears as a radiolucent defect in the barium pool on the posterior wall. However, a rugal fold on the anterior wall appears as parallel white lines, as the x-ray beam is attenuated by barium coating on the sides of the fold. Thus the anterior wall fold is "etched in white." On the supine radiograph in Figure 2–13 it is possible to distinguish between posterior wall and anterior wall folds. Similar reasoning applies to any protrusion, whether it is a normal fold or a polypoid

lesion. On the dependent surface it appears as a radiolucent filling defect, whereas on the nondependent surface the margin of the lesion is etched in white (Fig. 2–14).

Stalactite Phenomenon

With these high-density barium suspensions, drops of barium are frequently seen hanging from protrusions on the nondependent surface (Fig. 2–15A). This has been termed the "stalactite phenomenon" by Op den Orth and Ploem.[17] An appreciation of the differences between dependent and nondependent wall structures makes it easy to recognize these stalactites and to differentiate them from ulcers. They are always seen in relation to a protrusion on the nondependent surface, and therefore they could not possibly represent ulcers. Furthermore, the presence of the stalactite indicates a protrusion on the nondependent surface. This may be either a normal fold (Fig. 2–15B) or a polypoid lesion (Fig. 2–15C). In some cases, the stalactite may be the first and only clue to the presence of a protruded lesion on the nondependent surface. Additional films can then be obtained that will confirm the presence of the lesion.[18]

Basic Roentgen Pathology

Two basic types of pathologic processes are encountered in the gastrointestinal tract: protruded lesions, such as polyps, inflammatory swellings, or malignant tumors,

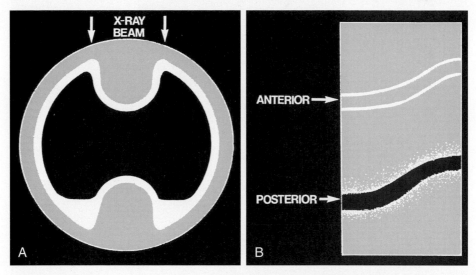

FIGURE 2–12. *A* and *B,* Diagrammatic representation of the appearances of a rugal fold on the anterior and posterior walls of the stomach.

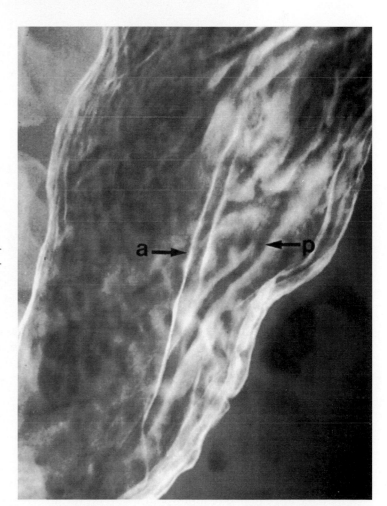

FIGURE 2–13. Supine view double contrast radiograph, showing the distinction between anterior *(a)* and posterior *(p)* wall rugal folds.

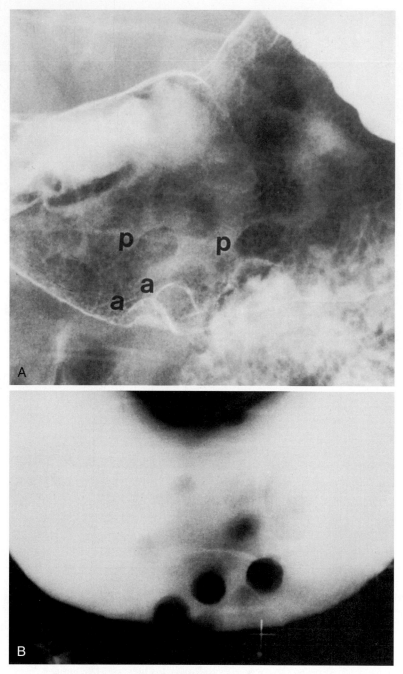

FIGURE 2–14. Anterior and posterior wall polyps. *A,* On the supine view double contrast radiograph, the anterior wall polyps *(a)* are etched in white, whereas the posterior wall polyps *(p)* are seen as radiolucent filling defects. *B,* The compression study shows the polyps to good advantage, but it is not possible to distinguish between the anterior and posterior wall lesions.

and depressed lesions, such as ulcers and diverticula. The basic roentgen manifestations of these types of lesions are similar throughout the gastrointestinal tract.

Protruded Lesions

The basic appearance of a polypoid lesion on the anterior or posterior wall has been described earlier. A polyp on the dependent surface appears as a radiolucent filling defect, whereas a polyp on the nondependent surface is "etched in white" (Fig. 2–14). This distinction is clearly

seen in a Styrofoam cup with "polyps" on both the anterior and posterior walls (Fig. 2–16). Several additional features of polypoid lesions are frequently seen. The "bowler hat sign" indicates that the filling defect forms an acute angle with the bowel wall.[19] This sign is illustrated and explained diagrammatically in Figure 2–17. It consists basically of a ring, representing the barium in the angle between the polyp and the bowel wall, and a curvilinear density, representing the dome of the polyp. When the two densities are caught at a particular oblique angle, the bowler hat sign is

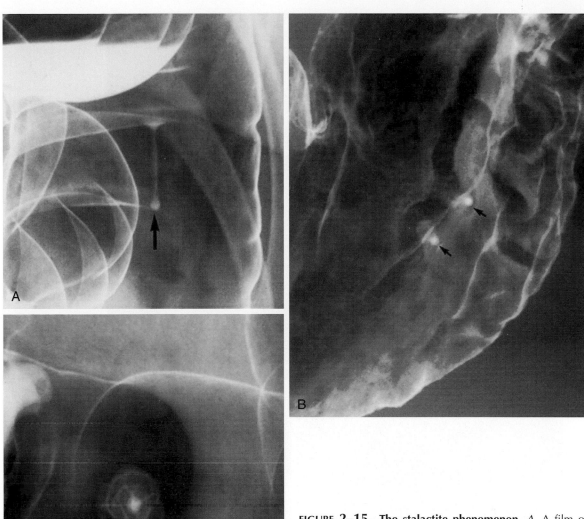

FIGURE 2–15. The stalactite phenomenon. *A,* A film of the colon in the upright position shows a long droplet of barium *(arrow)* hanging from a haustral fold. *B,* Two stalactites *(arrows)* hanging from a rugal fold on the anterior wall. *C,* Sigmoid polyp with a stalactite. A polypoid lesion is seen in the sigmoid colon. The lesion is etched in white and is therefore on the nondependent surface. The central density represents a hanging droplet or stalactite.

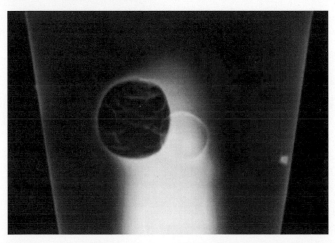

FIGURE 2–16. Styrofoam cup with "polyps" on the dependent and nondependent surfaces. The large filling defect represents a polyp on the dependent surface, whereas the polyp on the nondependent surface is etched in white.

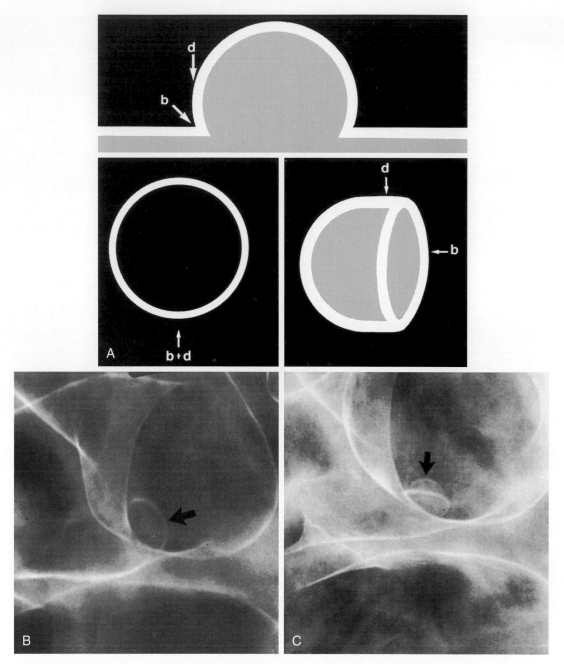

FIGURE 2–17. The bowler hat sign. *A,* Diagrammatic representation of the bowler hat sign showing the base *(b)* and the dome *(d). B,* With the dome of the polyp and its base overlapping, a ring shadow is produced. *C,* A typical bowler hat sign is produced when a sigmoid polyp is viewed obliquely.

produced. At other angles differing appearances are produced, and when the lesion is seen en face, only a single ring shadow is visible (see Fig. 2–17).

Although the bowler hat sign was originally described as a sign of a polypoid lesion, Tobin and Young pointed out that in most cases, the bowler hat sign is due to a diverticulum.[20] Miller and coworkers showed clearly in a model and in clinical studies that the distinction between a polyp and a diverticulum could be made using the axis of the bowler hat.[21] When the bowler hat faces toward the

axis of the bowel, it is a polyp. When the bowler hat faces away from the axis of the bowel, it represents a diverticulum (Fig. 2–18).

Ament and Alfidi have explored some aspects of the radiologic appearance of sessile polyps using a phantom.[22] They showed that basal indentation is simply a reflection of the proportion of the circumference of the bowel that is covered by the polyp. The larger the lesion, the more likely the base is to be seen in profile as a basal indentation. Therefore, the relationship to basal indenta-

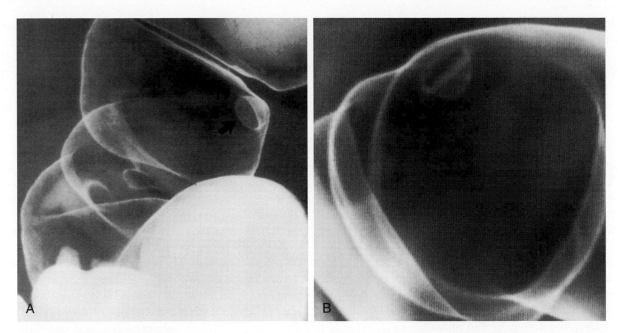

FIGURE 2–18. Bowler hat: diverticulum or polyp? *A,* When the dome of the hat points away from the axis of the bowel, it is a diverticulum. *B,* When the dome of the hat points toward the lumen of the bowel, it is a polyp.

tion to carcinoma is related only to the size of the lesion. Ament and Alfidi also described the "figure 8" sign as a variation of the basal indentation.

The demonstration that a filling defect has a stalk is also conclusive proof that it is a true polypoid lesion. The stalk may be seen in profile, but it may also be seen end-on through the head of the polyp, producing the "Mexican hat sign"[19] (Fig. 2–19). The bowler hat and the Mexican hat signs are helpful in the distinction between true polyps and extraneous material. In addition, if a protruding lesion can be demonstrated to be on the nondependent surface either because it is etched in white or be-

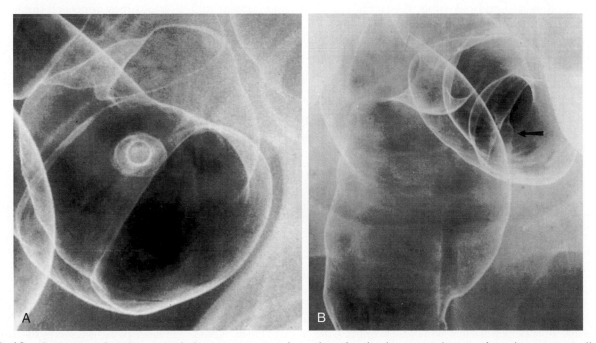

FIGURE 2–19. The Mexican hat sign. *A,* With the patient supine, the pedunculated polyp is seen hanging from the anterior wall. The central ring represents the stalk seen end-on, whereas the outer ring represents the head of the polyp. *B,* With the patient in the upright position, the polyp and its stalk are clearly seen *(arrow).*

cause it is associated with a stalactite, it almost certainly represents a true polypoid lesion because extraneous material would usually be expected only on the dependent surface. However, in some cases fecal residue may be adherent to the nondependent surface and cannot be differentiated from a true polyp.

The appearance of protrusion is determined not only by the lesion's location but also by its shape, and in particular by the configuration of its margins. Figure 2–20 illustrates diagrammatically various types of polypoid lesions. Lesion A is a protruded lesion with gradually tapered margins. When it is located on the dependent surface, it is seen as a radiolucent filling defect. However, it appears to be smaller than it really is because the peripheral parts of the lesion are obscured by the barium pool. If this lesion with gradually tapered margins is located on the nondependent surface, it may be invisible because there is no edge for the x-ray beam to catch tangentially. A stalactite may be hanging down from the tip of this lesion, which may be the only clue to its presence on the nondependent surface.[18] Lesions such as this are best demonstrated by turning the patient over so that the lesion is situated on the dependent surface. In addition, a protruded lesion may be demonstrated by compression; that is, a lesion may be compressed into the barium pool and then seen as a filling defect.

Lesion B is a flat, plaquelike lesion. When situated on the dependent surface, it may be covered over and rendered invisible by the barium pool. As the barium pool is thinned out, the lesion may appear. When the barium pool disappears completely, the lesion may again be invisible. Lesions such as this are, in fact, best demonstrated with a very shallow barium pool using "flow technique."[23] With this technique, the barium pool flows around or across lesions on the dependent surface, and spot films should be exposed when the lesion is seen to best advantage. When such a lesion is on the nondependent surface,

it is faintly etched in white. The density of the etching depends on the thickness of the lesion. If the lesion is flat enough, the etching may be so faint as to be invisible. In addition, if there is a significant barium pool on the opposite wall, it may obscure the etching of this lesion.

Lesion C has one abrupt margin and one tapered margin. In cases in which the lesion is on the nondependent surface, only the portion of the lesion with an abrupt margin can be seen. Therefore the lesion may be manifested only as a line or semicircle (Fig. 2–21).

Lesion D is a plaquelike lesion located on a curved surface (Fig. 2–22). Medially, the margin of the lesion can be seen, but laterally, only the normal bowel wall can be seen. On single contrast studies, such colonic tumors are recognized either as filling defects in the barium pool or as contour defects. Therefore those unaccustomed to interpreting double contrast radiographs may have difficulty recognizing such a lesion. It is important to realize that polypoid lesions may appear on double contrast studies as abnormal lines seen only en face, as well as the traditional filling defect or contour defect.

Annular lesions can be recognized as contour defects on double contrast studies, just as on the single contrast examination. In addition, they can be recognized end-on when seen through overlapping loops of bowel (Fig. 2–23). The irregularity and nodularity of the lumen are clearly apparent and can be confirmed by the appropriate oblique projection.

Submucosal lesions (Fig. 2–24) form a right angle with the bowel wall and stretch the overlying mucosa. Therefore they have a very smooth surface in profile and very sharp margins en face. In addition, mucosal folds may appear to fade out as they approach the lesion (Fig. 2–24C).

Extrinsic masses (Fig. 2–25) may be seen in profile or en face as an ill-defined radiolucency. When such a mass is viewed in an oblique projection, only a white line rep-

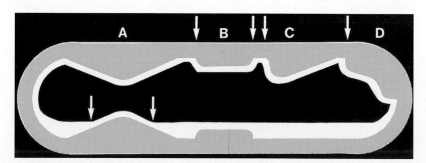

FIGURE 2–20. Diagrammatic representation of the effect of the shape of the polyp on its roentgen appearance. A polypoid lesion with sloping edges on the nondependent surface *(A)* will probably not be seen on the radiograph in the supine position because no edge will be visible tangentially. A similar lesion on the dependent surface may be detected, although it may appear to be smaller than its true size because the peripheral portion of the lesion may be obscured by barium. A flat plaquelike lesion on the nondependent surface *(B)* will produce a very fine white etching that may be difficult to detect. A similar lesion on the dependent surface may be obscured by the barium pool, but will be seen if the barium pool is thinned out. A polypoid lesion with a sloping margin *(C)* may be seen as only a single line representing the nonsloping edge. See Figure 2–21. A plaquelike lesion on a curved surface *(D)*. Only the edge of the lesion tangential to the x-ray beam will be seen. See Figure 2–22.

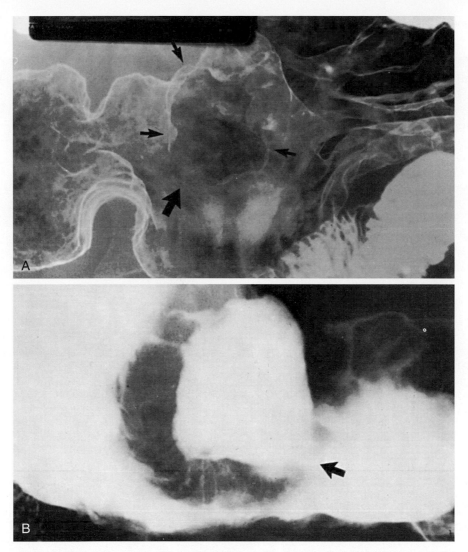

FIGURE 2–21. Ulcerated, plaquelike carcinoma on the anterior wall. A, The supine view double contrast radiograph shows an irregular ring density representing the ulcerated mass on the anterior wall *(small arrows).* The distal margin of the lesion is ill defined *(large arrow)* because of its sloping margin. B, A film taken with patient in prone position shows the large ulcer, filled with barium, and the core of tumor tissue surrounding it except at its distal edge *(arrow),* where the tumor mass becomes less prominent.

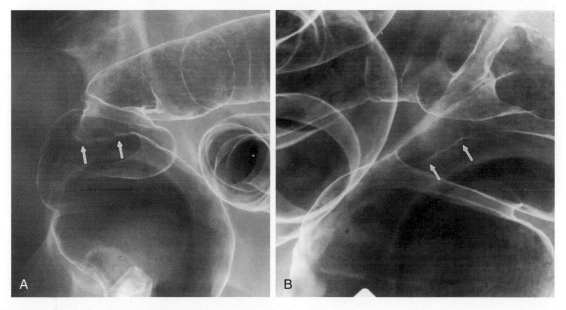

FIGURE 2–22. Plaquelike lesion on a curved surface. A, An oblique film of the rectum shows a linear density *(arrows)* adjacent to the normal bowel wall. This is the subtle manifestation of a plaquelike carcinoma on a curved surface. B, The presence of the plaquelike carcinoma is confirmed in the lateral projection.

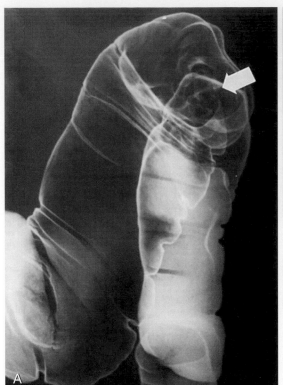

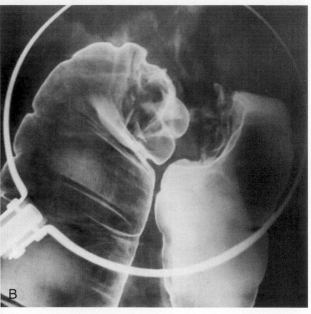

FIGURE 2–23. Annular carcinoma seen en face and in profile. *A,* The irregularity of the lumen seen end-on *(arrow)* is the result of an annular carcinoma. *B,* Carcinoma is confirmed on the appropriate oblique projection.

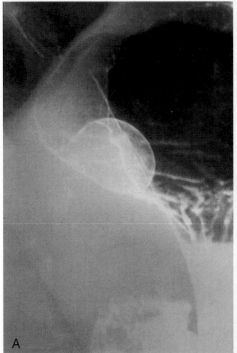

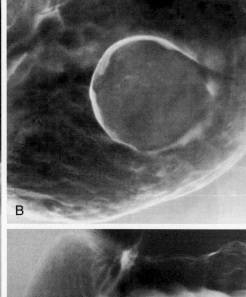

FIGURE 2–24. Typical submucosal lesion. *A,* The profile view shows the right angle formed by the mass and the gastric wall and the smooth mucosal surface. *B,* En face view shows the very abrupt, well-defined edge of the tumor. *C,* Another projection shows mucosal folds fading out at the edge of the lesion.

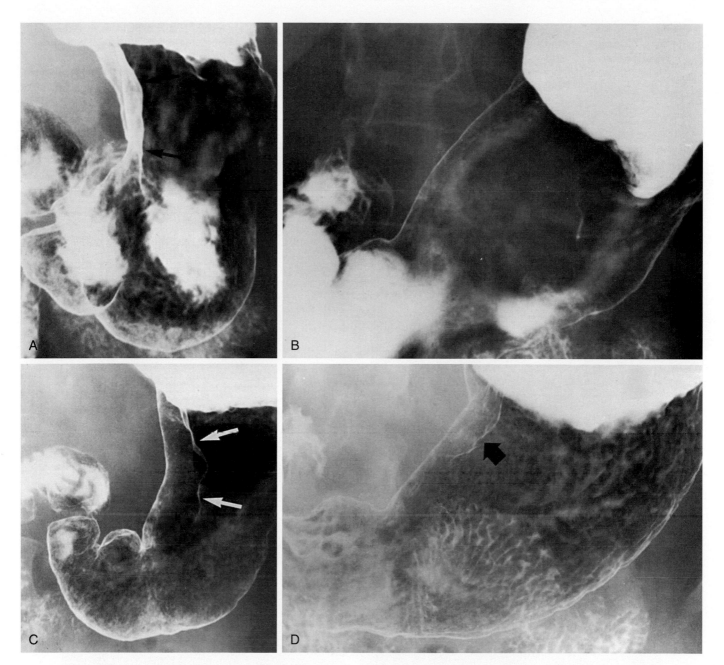

FIGURE 2–25. Extrinsic mass due to carcinoma of the pancreas. *A,* Lateral view, showing extrinsic compression on the posterior wall of the stomach *(arrows). B,* Frontal view, showing an ill-defined radiolucency caused by the retrogastric mass. *C,* Oblique projection, showing a curving line representing the edge of the retrogastric mass *(arrows). D,* In another patient a prominent impression owing to an enlarged caudate lobe of the liver *(arrow)* is seen. The appearance simulates an intramural gastric lesion.

resenting one edge of the extrinsic mass may be seen (Fig. 2–25*C*). Because of the marked gastric distention, the stomach may appear to surround an extrinsic mass, which may simulate an intramural lesion[24] (Fig. 2–25*D*).

Depressed Lesions

Depressed lesions are lesions that extend beyond the mucosal surface, most typically ulcers or diverticula. A depressed lesion on a dependent surface is easily recognized by the familiar barium collection or niche (Fig. 2–26*A*). If there are associated radiating folds, these also

will have the characteristics of dependent wall structures; that is, they will be seen as radiolucent filling defects (Fig. 2–26*B*). When an ulcer is situated on a nondependent surface, the barium empties out, leaving the sides and base of the ulcer coated with barium. The resulting radiographic appearance is a ring shadow that can be considered to be an empty crater (Fig. 2–27). Radiating folds associated with such a lesion are etched in white.

Therefore the appearance of a ring shadow may cause diagnostic confusion. It may represent either a depressed or protruded lesion on the nondependent surface. In ad-

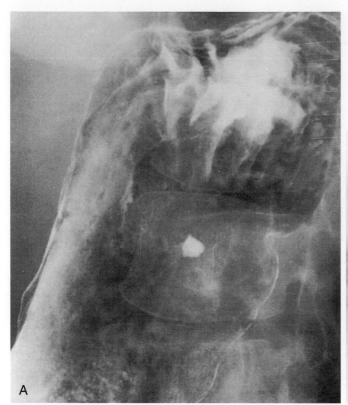

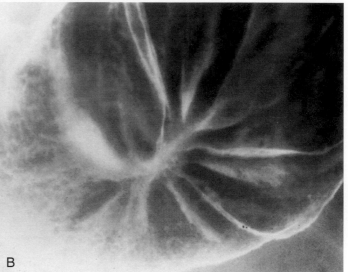

FIGURE 2–26. Depressed lesions on the dependent surface. *A,* Film of the stomach in the right posterior oblique (RPO) projection shows a typical high lesser curve ulcer en face. *B,* In another patient, prominent radiating folds are seen on the posterior wall in relationship to a healing posterior wall ulcer.

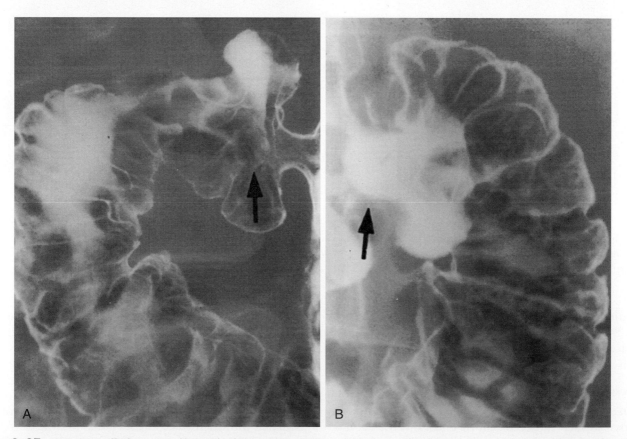

FIGURE 2–27. Anterior wall ulcer. *A,* A film in the left posterior oblique (LPO) projection shows a ring shadow in a deformed duodenal cap *(arrow).* *B,* With patient in prone position, the ring shadow fills with barium *(arrow),* indicating an anterior wall duodenal ulcer.

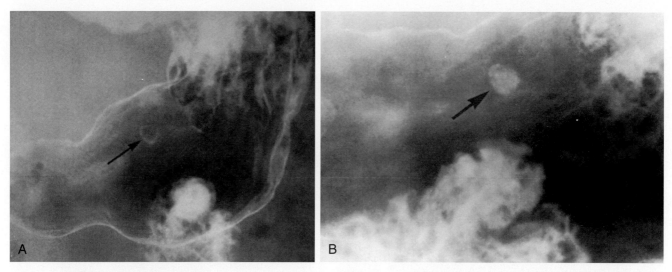

FIGURE 2–28. Ring shadow due to an ulcer. *A,* A shallow posterior wall ulcer with an empty crater. The ring shadow is the result of coating of the sides of the ulcer crater. Note that the ring shadow has a sharp outer border and fades to the inside. (From Laufer, I.: Simple method for routine double contrast study of the upper gastrointestinal tract. Radiology *117:*513–518, 1975, with permission.) *B,* With further manipulation of the barium pool, the ulcer crater can be filled with barium *(arrow).*

dition, either type of lesion may produce a ring shadow when it is situated on the dependent surface and when there is absolutely no barium pool. A careful analysis of the radiographs can usually reveal whether the ring shadow is due to a protrusion or a depression. A depressed lesion has a sharp outer border and fades to the inside (Fig. 2–28), whereas a protruded lesion has a sharp inner border and fades to the outside[19] (Fig. 2–29).

A ring shadow may also be caused by several types of depressed lesions, such as an empty diverticulum (Fig. 2–30A) or an empty ulcer crater on either the dependent (Fig. 2–28A) or nondependent surface (Fig. 2–30B). It may also be the result of a filling defect, such as a blood

clot within an ulcer crater (Fig. 2–31). For further evaluation of a ring shadow the patient can be turned to demonstrate the lesion in profile. Attempts should also be made to wash the lesion with barium to demonstrate its appearance in the barium pool.

Occasionally a double ring shadow may be seen and usually indicates a lesion on the nondependent surface. It may indicate an ulcer or diverticulum, with the inner ring representing the neck and the outer ring the base (Fig. 2–32), or it may indicate an ulcerated protruded lesion, with the inner ring representing the ulcer and the outer ring representing the edge of the protrusion (see Fig. 2–36).

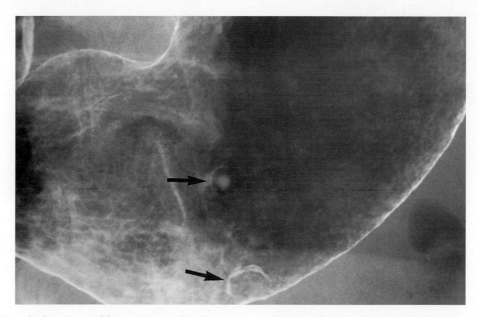

FIGURE 2–29. Ring shadows caused by anterior wall polyps *(arrows).* The central polyp also exhibits the stalactite phenomenon.

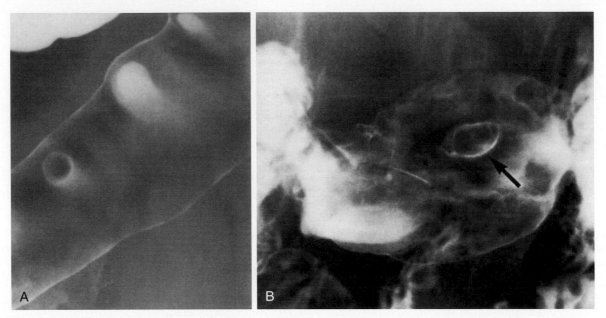

FIGURE 2–30. Other causes of ring shadows. *A,* An empty diverticulum. *B,* Anterior wall duodenal ulcer. With patient in supine position, a ring shadow is seen in the center of the duodenal cap *(arrow).* This could be filled only in the prone position, indicating that it is an ulcer on the anterior wall.

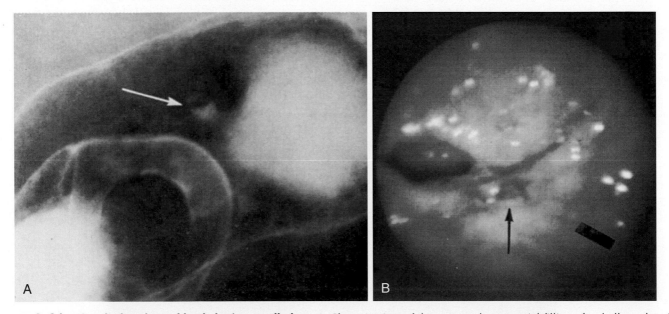

FIGURE 2–31. Ring shadow due to blood clot in a small ulcer. *A,* Close-up view of the antrum shows partial filling of a shallow ulcer in the distal antrum with a radiolucency representing the blood clot *(arrow). B,* The endoscopic photograph shows the blood clot *(arrow)* adherent to the base of the ulcer. (From Laufer, I., Hamilton, J., and Mullens, J.E.: Demonstration of superficial gastric erosions by double contrast radiography. *Gastroenterology 68:*387, 1975, with permission.)

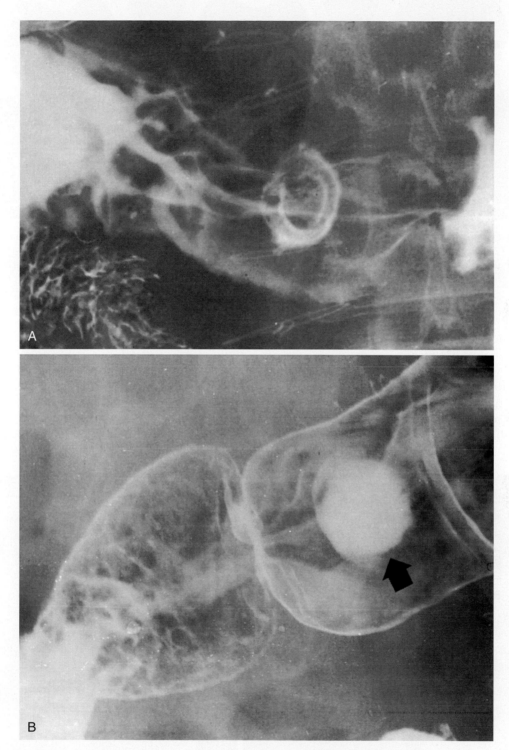

FIGURE 2–32. Double ring shadow due to an ulcer. *A,* With the patient in the prone position a double ring is seen. The inner ring represents the neck of the ulcer, whereas the outer ring represents the outer margins of the ulcer crater, where it is wider in diameter. *B,* The corresponding film with the patient in the supine position confirms that the ulcer crater is on the posterior wall *(arrow).*

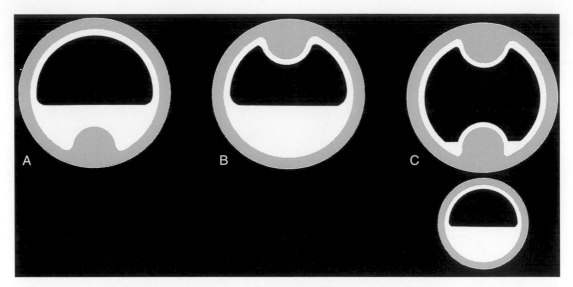

FIGURE 2–33. Diagrammatic representation of the hazards of the barium pool. *A,* Barium pool obscures the lesion on the dependent surface. See Figure 2–35. *B,* The barium pool obscures the fine white etching of the lesion on the nondependent surface. See Figure 2–36. *C,* The barium pool in the overlapping loop of bowel may obscure a lesion on either the dependent or the nondependent surface. See Figure 2–9.

The Barium Pool

The barium pool is the bolus of free barium that is not adherent to the mucosal surface. The major portion of the bolus, which we shall call the barium pool, is found in the most dependent segments of the bowel. In addition, small "puddles" may be found in any segment where minor depressions are located. The barium pool is of critical importance because it is used to wash and coat the mucosal surface and to fill any depressed lesions. It can also be used to demonstrate posterior wall protrusions more clearly. Indeed, the entire double contrast examination rests on skillful manipulation of the barium pool. Nevertheless, the barium pool can lead to serious error in several different ways (Fig. 2–33). A dependent wall protrusion may not be seen because it is covered over by the barium pool (Fig. 2–34). However, even a small barium

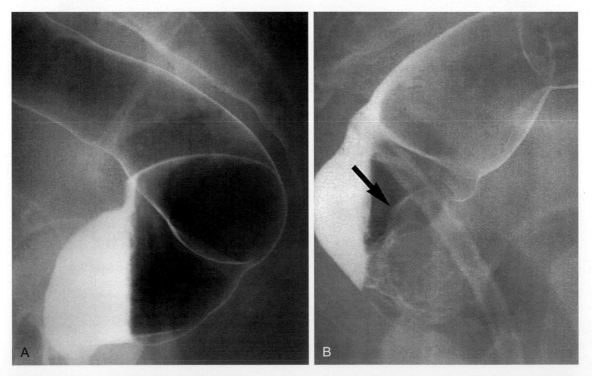

FIGURE 2–34. Dependent wall lesion obscured by barium. *A,* The patient is prone. The barium pool on the anterior wall of the rectum obscures a large polypoid tumor. *B,* With the patient supine, the barium pool has shifted to the posterior wall and the polypoid tumor is clearly seen *(arrow).*

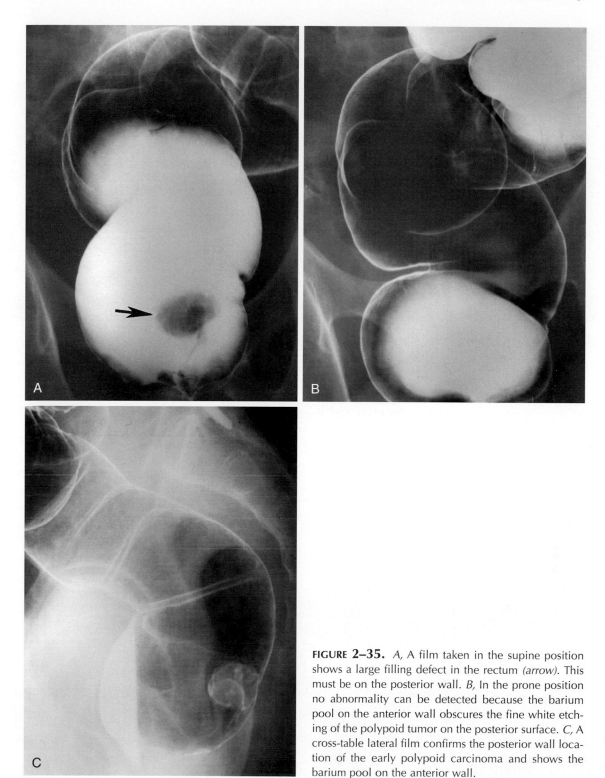

FIGURE 2–35. *A,* A film taken in the supine position shows a large filling defect in the rectum *(arrow).* This must be on the posterior wall. *B,* In the prone position no abnormality can be detected because the barium pool on the anterior wall obscures the fine white etching of the polypoid tumor on the posterior surface. *C,* A cross-table lateral film confirms the posterior wall location of the early polypoid carcinoma and shows the barium pool on the anterior wall.

puddle may obscure or veil the fine white etching of a relatively large polypoid lesion on the nondependent surface. This principle is illustrated in Figure 2–35. In the supine position a large polypoid tumor on the posterior wall of the rectum is clearly seen as a filling defect in the barium pool on the posterior wall (Fig. 2–35*A*). With the patient in the prone position the lesion is now on the nondependent surface and should be etched in white (Fig. 2–35*B*). However, the delicate etching of this poly-

poid lesion is entirely obscured by the barium pool on the anterior wall. A lateral view confirms the posterior wall location of this lesion and shows the barium pool (Fig. 2–35*C*).

In addition, a barium pool may collect in an overlapping structure and obscure a pathologic lesion (see Fig. 2–9). Some of the problems associated with the barium pool can be avoided by compression, as illustrated in Figures 2–36 and 2–37. A lesion on the nondependent sur-

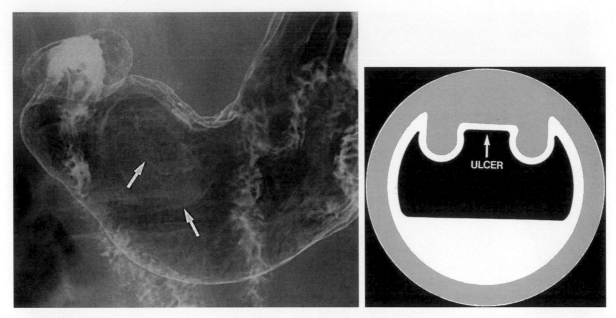

FIGURE 2–36. Value of compression in anterior wall lesions. The plaquelike lesion on the anterior wall and the central ulcer are faintly seen.

face may be seen only faintly (Fig. 2–36). However, with compression it is immersed in the barium pool and is clearly seen as a radiolucent filling defect (Fig. 2–37).

Thus a barium pool or puddle may be either a blessing or a curse. It improves mucosal coating; it may fill an ulcer crater on the dependent surface; and it helps to demonstrate dependent wall protrusions. On the other hand, it can obscure lesions on both the dependent and nondependent surfaces. This concept is illustrated in Figure 2–38. With the Styrofoam cup coated and all the free barium poured off, two rows of "polyps" can be iden-

tified, one on the dependent surface and one on the nondependent surface (Fig. 2–38A). With the addition of 10 ml of high-density barium, the polyps on the nondependent surface are entirely obscured (Fig. 2–38B), and with 40 ml of barium, both the dependent and nondependent wall polyps become invisible (Fig. 2–38C). This shows clearly the hazards of the barium pool and the importance of thinning out this barium pool. An understanding of the potential value and hazards of the barium pool is an important step in mastering double contrast techniques.

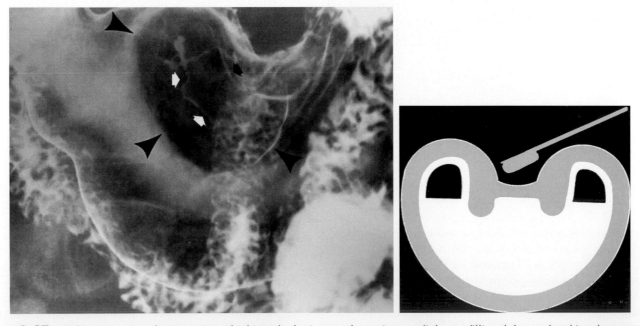

FIGURE 2–37. With compression the tumor is pushed into the barium pool, causing a radiolucent filling defect and making the tumor *(arrowheads)* and the ulcer *(small arrows)* more apparent.

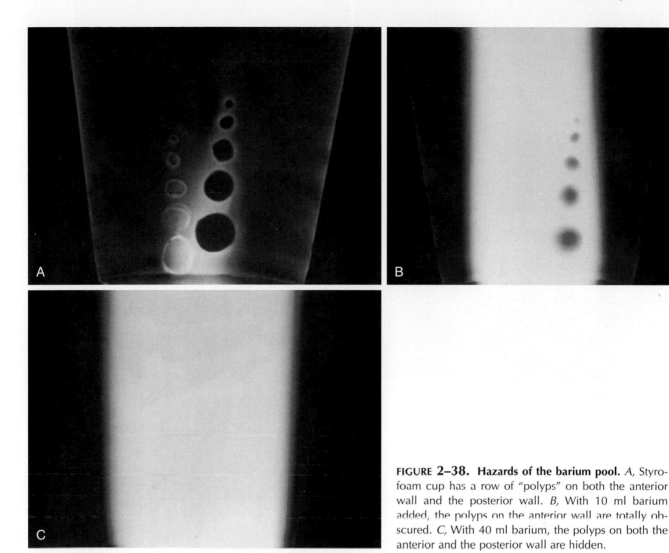

FIGURE 2–38. Hazards of the barium pool. *A,* Styrofoam cup has a row of "polyps" on both the anterior wall and the posterior wall. *B,* With 10 ml barium added, the polyps on the anterior wall are totally obscured. *C,* With 40 ml barium, the polyps on both the anterior and the posterior wall are hidden.

ARTIFACTS

In addition to becoming familiar with a new array of normal and pathologic appearances, the radiologist starting to use double contrast techniques must also learn to recognize a variety of artifacts that may be peculiar to double contrast techniques.[3] The causes of these artifacts are listed in Table 2–1. Many artifacts can be attributed to the high viscosity of the barium suspension and to the variations in mucosal coating. Some of these artifacts, such as patchy coating (see Fig. 2–2) and the stalactite phenomenon (see Fig. 2–15), have already been mentioned. Some barium suspensions may cause precipitation or flaking, which may simulate diffuse mucosal ulceration (Fig. 2–39). In many cases these artifacts can be avoided by the choice of an appropriate barium suspension. However, in some patients with excessive fluid and debris they may be unavoidable. Cho and colleagues[25] described a peculiar artifactual appearance in the esophagus simulating an intraluminal diverticulum. This artifact is caused by the interaction of barium with debris and mucus in the esophagus.

In some patients there is insufficient gas to separate the anterior and posterior walls. The area of contact between the anterior and posterior walls may produce an irregular outline that may simulate an ulcer or polypoid lesion[8] (Fig. 2–40). With further distention of the area, the artifact disappears. We have termed this a "kissing" artifact.

TABLE 2–1. *Causes of Double Contrast Artifacts*

Barium-Related	See-Through Effect	Extraneous or Foreign Material
High viscosity—stalactite phenomenon[17]	Normal anatomic structures	Gas bubbles
Patchy coating	Calcified structures	Effervescent agent
Precipitation and flaking	Contrast-filled structures	Adherent fecal material
"Kissing" artifact		Others—mineral oil, Telepaque
Pseudointraluminal diverticulum[25]		

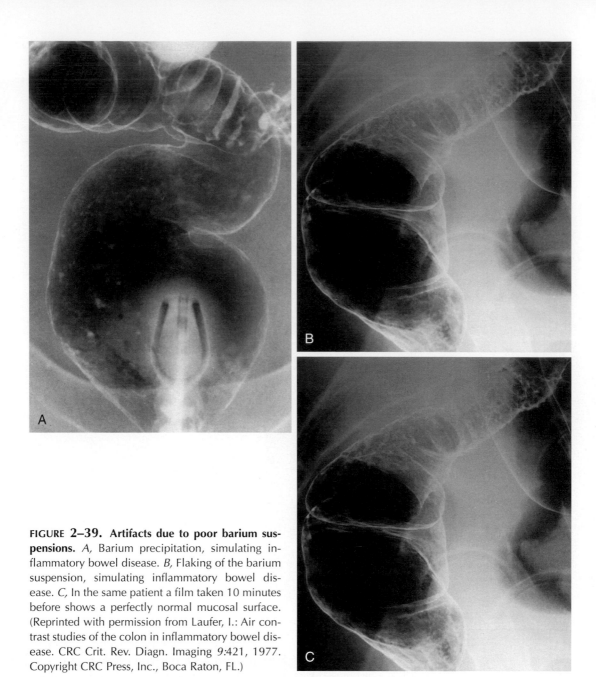

FIGURE 2–39. Artifacts due to poor barium suspensions. *A,* Barium precipitation, simulating inflammatory bowel disease. *B,* Flaking of the barium suspension, simulating inflammatory bowel disease. *C,* In the same patient a film taken 10 minutes before shows a perfectly normal mucosal surface. (Reprinted with permission from Laufer, I.: Air contrast studies of the colon in inflammatory bowel disease. CRC Crit. Rev. Diagn. Imaging *9:*421, 1977. Copyright CRC Press, Inc., Boca Raton, FL.)

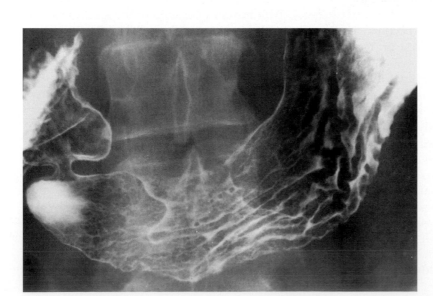

FIGURE 2–40. Kissing artifact in the antrum due to adherence of the anterior and posterior walls of the stomach as it crosses in front of the aorta.

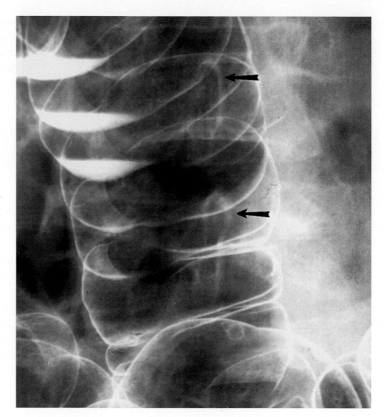

FIGURE **2–41. See-through artifacts.** Spinous processes *(arrows)* seen through the gas-filled colon may simulate polypoid lesions.

The segment of the gastrointestinal tract outlined by double contrast becomes transparent. Therefore opacities overlying any segment can be clearly seen and may simulate an intrinsic lesion. These opacities may be normal skeletal structures (Fig. 2–41); calcified structures, such as lymph nodes, uterine fibroids, or phleboliths; or contrast-filled structures, such as diverticula or lymph nodes.

Extraneous material in the lumen must be differentiated from polypoid lesions in both single and double contrast techniques. However, with double contrast techniques there are additional artifacts, such as gas bubbles and undissolved effervescent pills or granules (Fig. 2–42), that must be recognized.

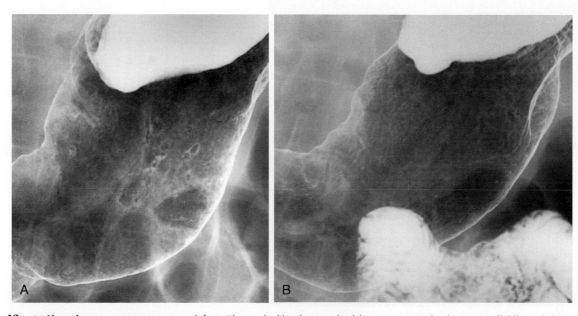

FIGURE **2–42. Artifact due to extraneous material.** *A,* The early film from a double contrast study shows small filling defects in the stomach due to undissolved effervescent agent. *B,* A later film shows that the filling defects are no longer present.

TABLE 2–2. *Pathologic Conditions That May Be Simulated by Artifacts*

Diffuse Superficial Ulceration	Discrete Ulceration	Polypoid Lesion
Barium precipitation	Colonic or duodenal diverticulum	See-through effect
Flaking	Patchy coating	Extraneous material
Debris	Stalactite phenomenon	"Kissing" artifact
	"Kissing" artifact	
	Pseudointraluminal diverticulum	

Table 2–2 lists the various types of pathologic conditions that may be simulated b y artifacts. Some of these artifacts are discussed in further detail in the specific chapters under the lesion they simulate.

SUMMARY

The use of double contrast techniques requires an understanding of the basic differences in approach between single and double contrast studies of the gastrointestinal tract. The transition from one approach to the other demands a major reorientation to the performance and interpretation of gastrointestinal radiologic studies. It also requires an understanding of the elements that combine to form the double contrast image—the dependent wall, the nondependent wall, and the barium pool. Great attention must be paid to the quality of mucosal coating as a criterion of the adequacy of the study. Materials such as barium suspensions, which are designed for double contrast studies, must be used. Although gaseous distention is generally desirable, it is important to understand the value of varying the degree of distention to best demonstrate certain types of lesions. Management of the barium pool is a critical aspect of double contrast technique. The examiner must be aware of the importance of the barium pool and of its potential hazards.

Interpretation of these studies requires a clear understanding of the difference in appearance between structures and lesions on the dependent and nondependent walls. The examiner should aim at a precise translation from the radiologic findings to the gross pathologic features of the lesion. Accurate interpretation requires a basic analysis of the lines, points, and shadows on the film. Endoscopic and pathologic correlation should be viewed as an extension of the radiologic examination whereby the radiologist can improve the quality of his or her studies and the precision of interpretation.

Figures 2–43 to 2–52 illustrate additional examples of the application of these principles to the performance and interpretation of double contrast studies.

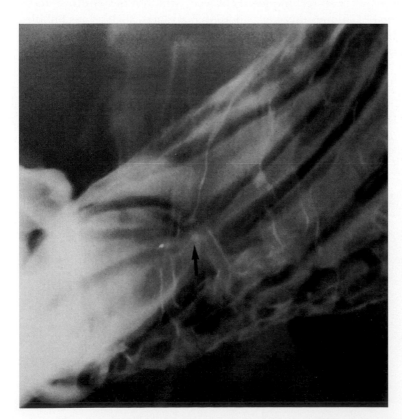

FIGURE 2–43. Separation of anterior and posterior wall folds. On the supine film of the stomach, the normal anterior wall folds are seen etched in white and running transversely. The posterior wall folds are seen as radiolucent filling defects with an area of convergence toward a very small ulcer *(arrow)*. Thus the separate analysis of anterior and posterior walls allows for correct diagnosis of small posterior wall ulcer with converging folds.

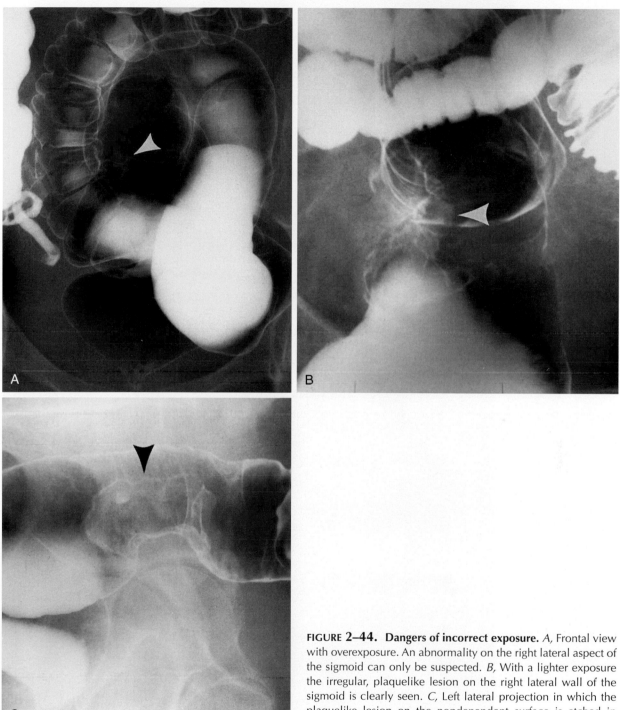

FIGURE 2–44. Dangers of incorrect exposure. *A,* Frontal view with overexposure. An abnormality on the right lateral aspect of the sigmoid can only be suspected. *B,* With a lighter exposure the irregular, plaquelike lesion on the right lateral wall of the sigmoid is clearly seen. *C,* Left lateral projection in which the plaquelike lesion on the nondependent surface is etched in white.

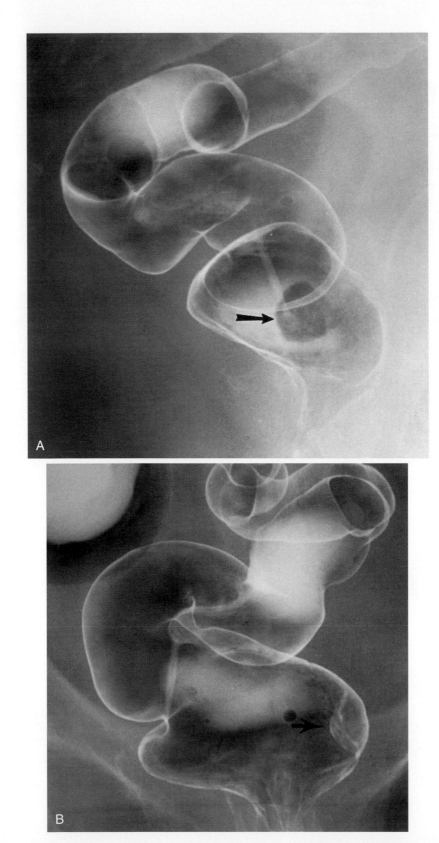

FIGURE 2–45. *A,* Left lateral view of the rectum shows a rounded filling defect in the barium pool. Therefore the polypoid lesion must be on the dependent surface (i.e., the left lateral wall of the rectum). *B,* This is confirmed in the frontal projection.

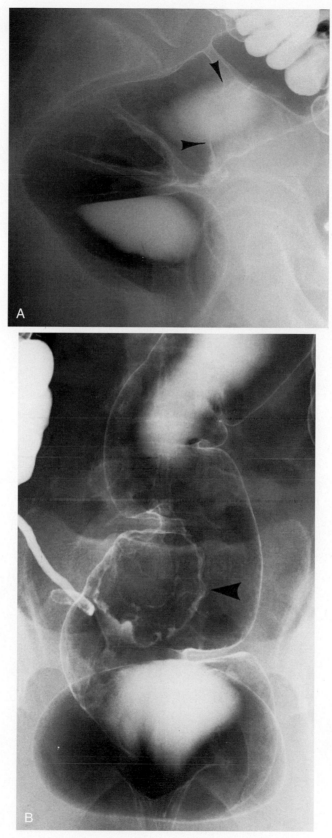

FIGURE 2–46. *A,* In the left lateral projection the fine white etching *(arrowheads)* is almost obscured by a small barium puddle. Because of the etched outline of the lesion, it must be on the nondependent (right lateral) wall. *B,* The location of the lesion is confirmed on the frontal projection, which shows an ulcerated mass on the right lateral wall of the rectosigmoid *(arrowhead).*

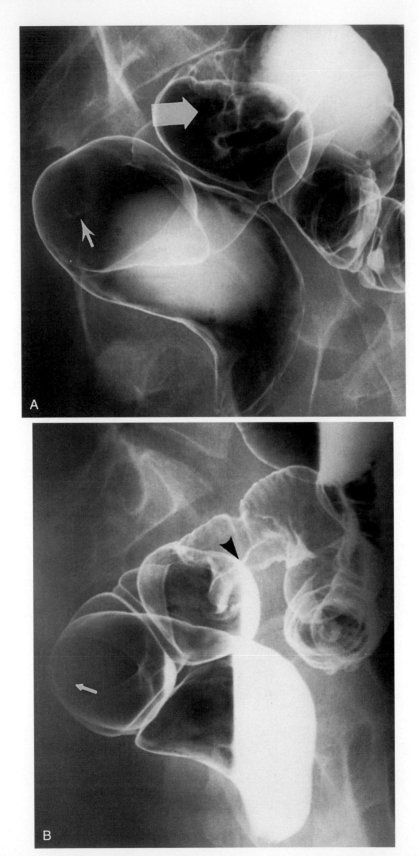

FIGURE 2–47.   *A,* Oblique view of the rectosigmoid is suggestive of an abnormality at the rectosigmoid junction. The abnormality is seen through overlapping loops of bowel *(large arrow).* There is also a small polypoid lesion in the rectum *(small arrow). B,* Lateral view shows more clearly a plaquelike lesion at the rectosigmoid junction *(black arrowhead)* due to carcinoma. The small polyp on the posterior wall of the rectum *(white arrow)* is faintly seen.

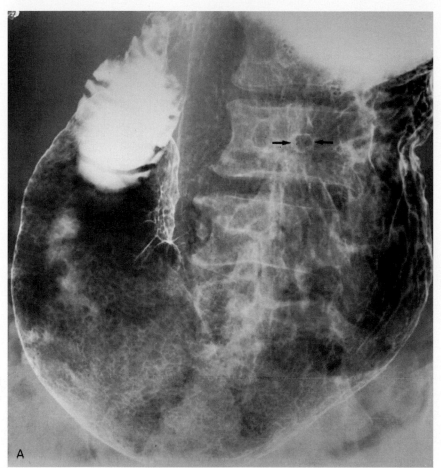

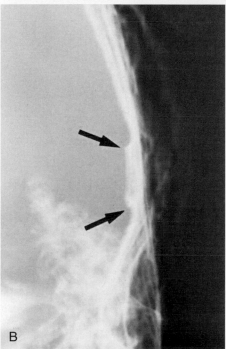

FIGURE 2–48. *A,* Double contrast view of the stomach in RPO projection. A ring shadow *(arrows)* is seen on the dependent surface (i.e., the lesser curvature). Because this represents an empty crater, the ulcer is probably very shallow. *B,* Tangential view confirms presence of broad, shallow crater *(arrows).* (Courtesy of Hans Herlinger, M.D., Philadelphia, Pennsylvania.)

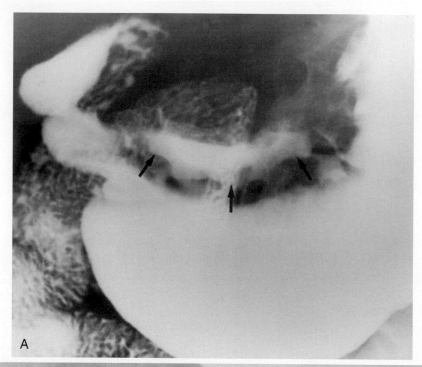

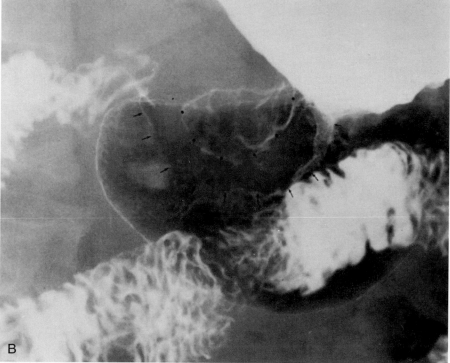

FIGURE 2–49. Carman's meniscus sign seen on conventional study and with double contrast. *A,* Conventional view of the lesser curvature ulcer *(arrows)* and the surrounding rim of tumor tissue. *B,* The double contrast view shows the rim of tumor tissue *(arrows)* and the outline of the ulcer *(dots).* Note the absence of the areae gastricae over the tumor tissue. (Courtesy of Hans Herlinger, M.D., Philadelphia, Pennsylvania.)

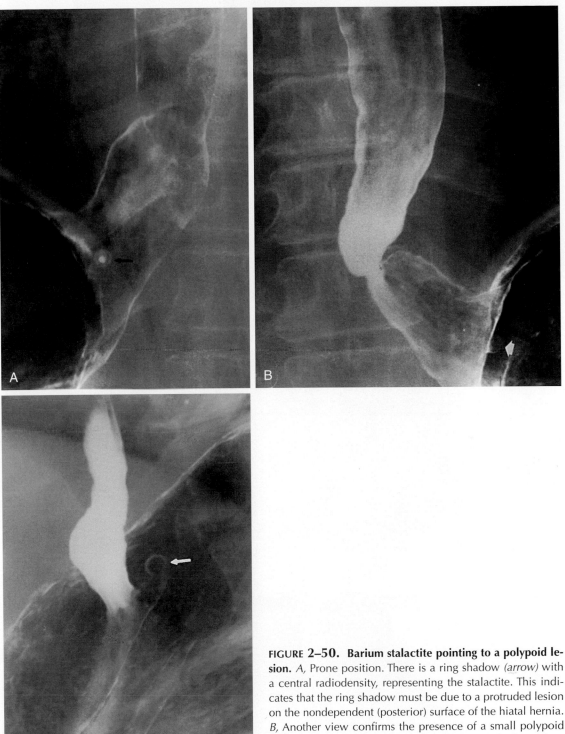

FIGURE 2–50. Barium stalactite pointing to a polypoid lesion. *A,* Prone position. There is a ring shadow *(arrow)* with a central radiodensity, representing the stalactite. This indicates that the ring shadow must be due to a protruded lesion on the nondependent (posterior) surface of the hiatal hernia. *B,* Another view confirms the presence of a small polypoid lesion *(arrow)*. *C,* Steep RPO projection, with the hiatal hernia reduced back into the stomach. The polypoid lesion is seen to lie posteriorly *(arrow)*.

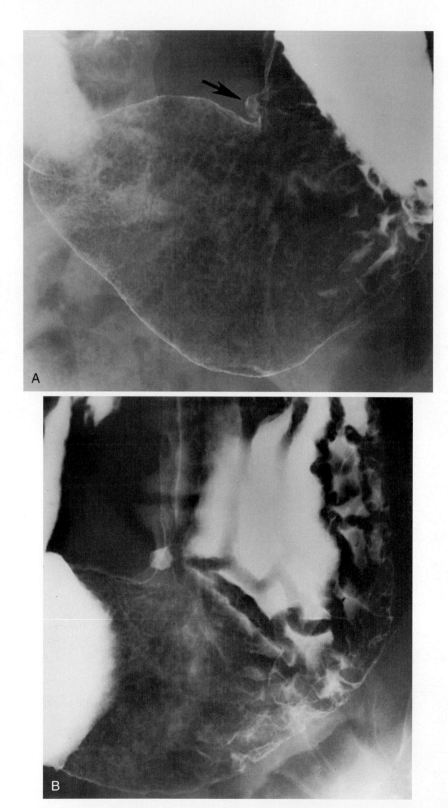

FIGURE 2–51. The value of flow technique for demonstration of posterior wall structures. *A,* Supine view double contrast radiograph shows a lesser curvature ulcer *(arrow).* The surrounding folds are not well seen. *B,* In a slight RPO projection the ulcer crater is filled with barium, and the surrounding mucosal folds are seen much more clearly.

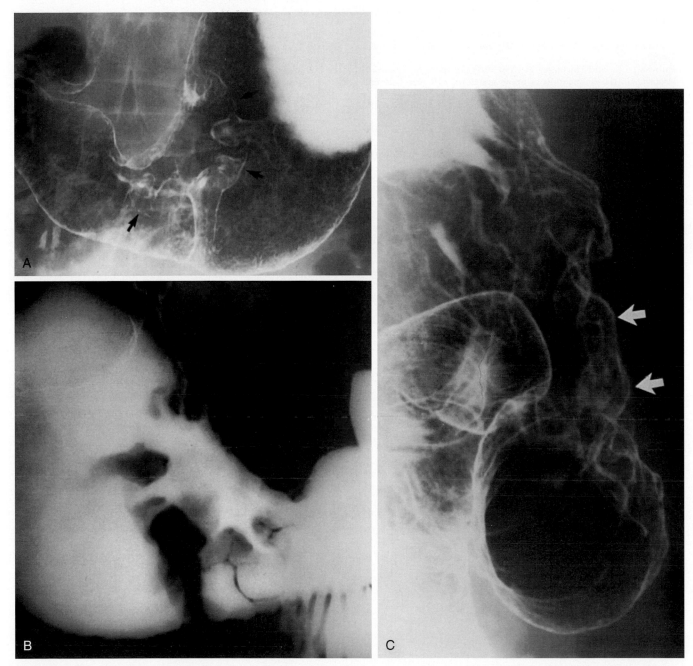

FIGURE 2–52. Analysis of a complex case. *A,* The supine film shows the edge of a lesion etched in white *(arrows).* Radiating folds are also etched in white. The tips of the folds are clubbed and stalactites are hanging down from the folds. This film suggests that an anterior wall lesion is associated with ulceration and clubbing of the radiating folds. *B,* The prone film confirms the presence of a large ulcer with a rim of tumor tissue. The radiating folds are now seen as filling defects. *C,* The left lateral film confirms the presence of a large mass on the anterior wall with a large central ulcer *(arrows).* These findings were due to an excavated adenocarcinoma of the anterior wall of the stomach.

REFERENCES

1. James, W.B.: Double contrast radiology in the gastrointestinal tract. Clin. Gastroenterol. *7*:397, 1978.
2. Ichikawa, H.: What is double contrast radiography? *In* Shirakabe, H. (ed.): Double Contrast Studies of the Stomach. Stuttgart, Georg Thieme Verlag, 1972, pp. 4–6.
3. Gohel, V.K., Kressel, H.Y., and Laufer, I.: Double contrast artifacts. Gastrointest. Radiol. *3*:139, 1978.
4. Skucas, J.: Gastrointestinal agents. *In* Skucas, J. (ed.): Radiographic Contrast Agents, ed. 2. Rockville, MD, Aspen Publishers, 1989, pp. 10–82.
5. Rubesin, S.E., and Herlinger, H.; The effect of barium suspension viscosity on the delineation of areae gastricae. AJR Am. J. Roentgenol. *146*:35, 1986.
6. Mackintosh, C.E., and Kreel, L.: Anatomy and radiology of the areae gastricae. Gut *18*:855, 1977.
7. Matsuura, K., Nakata, H., Takeda, N., et al.: Innominate lines of the colon. Radiology *123*:581, 1977.
8. Laufer, I.: A simple method for routine double contrast study of the upper gastrointestinal tract. Radiology *117*:513, 1975.
9. Miller, R.E., Chernish, S.M., Skucas, J., et al.: Hypotonic roentgenography with glucagon. AJR Am. J. Roentgenol. *121*:264, 1974.
10. Meeroff, J.G., Jorgens, J., and Isenberg, J.I.: The effect of glucagon on barium enema examination. Radiology *115*:5, 1975.
11. Chernish, S.M., and Maglinte, D.D.: Glucagon: Common untoward reactions—review and recommendations. Radiology *117*:145, 1990.
12. Gelfand, D.W., Sowers, J.C., DePonte, K.A., et al.: Anaphylactic and allergic reactions during double-contrast studies: Is glucagon or barium suspension the allergen? AJR Am. J. Roentgenol. *144*:405, 1985.
13. Feczko, P.J., Simms, S.M., Lorio, J., and Halpert, R.: Gastroduodenal response to low-dose glucagon. AJR Am. J. Roentgenol. *140*:935, 1983.
14. Hogan, W.J., Dodds, W.J., Hoke, S.E., et al.: The effect of glucagon on esophageal motor function. Gastroenterology *69*:160, 1975.
15. Laufer, I., Mullens, J.E., and Hamilton, J.: The diagnostic accuracy of barium studies of the stomach and duodenum—correlation with endoscopy. Radiology *115*:569, 1975.
16. Laufer, I., Mullens, J.E., and Hamilton, J.: Correlation of endoscopy and double contrast radiography in the early stages of ulcerative and granulomatous colitis. Radiology *118*:1, 1976.
17. Op den Orth, J.O., and Ploem, S.: The stalactite phenomenon in double contrast studies of the stomach. Radiology *117*:523, 1975.
18. Aronchick, J., Laufer, I., and Glick, S.: Barium stalactites: Observations on their nature and significance. Radiology *149*:588, 1983.
19. Youker, J.E., and Welin, S.: Differentiation of true polypoid tumors of the colon from extraneous material: A new roentgen sign. Radiology *84*:610, 1965.
20. Tobin, K.D., and Young, J.W.R.: The bowler hat: A valid sign of colonic polyps? Gastrointest. Radiol. *12*:250, 1987.
21. Miller, W.T., Jr., Levine, M.S., Rubesin, S.E., and Laufer, I.: Bowlerhat sign: A simple principle for differentiating polyps from diverticula. Radiology *173*:615, 1989.
22. Ament, A.E., and Alfidi, R.J.: Sessile polyps: Analysis of radiographic projections with the aid of a double-contrast phantom. AJR Am. J. Roentgenol. *139*:111, 1982.
23. Kikuchi, Y., Levine, M.S., Laufer, I., et al.: Value of flow technique for double-contrast examination of the stomach. AJR Am. J. Roentgenol. *147*:1183, 1986.
24. Battle, W.M., Laufer, I., Moldofsky, P.J., et al.: Anomalous liver lobulation as a cause of perigastric masses. Am. J. Dig. Dis. *24*:65, 1979.
25. Cho, S.R., Henry, D.A., Shaw, C.I., et al.: Vanishing intraluminal diverticulum of the esophagus. Gastrointest. Radiol. *7*:315, 1982.

3

Upper Gastrointestinal Tract: Technical Aspects

MARC S. LEVINE
IGOR LAUFER

BASIC REQUIREMENTS
Gaseous Distention
Mucosal Coating
Hypotonia
Attention to Technical Details
Maneuvers

THE ROUTINE EXAMINATION
Patient Preparation
Materials
Procedure
Variations

PROBLEMS AND PITFALLS
Esophagus
Stomach
Duodenum

DIGITAL FLUOROSCOPIC IMAGING
Performance
Interpretation

BASIC REQUIREMENTS

The routine double contrast upper gastrointestinal examination should be performed as a biphasic study with double contrast and single contrast views of the esophagus, stomach, and duodenum to optimize the diagnostic yield of the procedure. In the double contrast portion of the study, a series of maneuvers is required to achieve adequate gaseous distention while a thin layer of high-density barium is spread on the mucosa. The effects of gravity are utilized to manipulate the barium pool so that each portion of the upper gastrointestinal tract is visualized en face and in profile. The double contrast study is facilitated by the routine use of hypotonic agents. The examination is then completed by obtaining prone or upright (or both) single contrast views of the esophagus, stomach, and duodenum with low-density barium and varying degrees of compression.

It should be emphasized that double contrast views permit a more detailed assessment of the appearance of the mucosa en face than conventional single contrast techniques. The basic elements of the double contrast examination are (1) gaseous distention, (2) mucosal coating, (3) hypotonia, (4) attention to technical details, and (5) a routine set of maneuvers for performing the study. These are discussed separately in the following sections.

Gaseous Distention

Gaseous distention is required to efface normal folds so that the overlying mucosa can be adequately visualized. If distention is inadequate, prominent folds may obscure small lesions, and barium trapped between folds may simulate ulcers. At the same time, overdistention may impair mucosal coating or obliterate abnormal folds, such as those radiating toward an ulcer or ulcer scar. Similarly, varices may be effaced or even obliterated by overdistention. Thus, it is critical to obtain the proper degree of gaseous distention (i.e., just enough to efface normal folds without interfering with mucosal coating).

A variety of methods can be used to introduce gas into the stomach and duodenum. The ideal method for distending these structures is nasogastric intubation. However, intubation techniques would meet with considerable patient resistance if applied on a routine basis. Instead, the simplest method for introducing gas is to have the patient swallow effervescent granules, powder, or tablets that rapidly release 300 to 400 ml of carbon dioxide on contact with fluid in the stomach.[1-3] Unfortunately, bubble formation may occur as an undesirable artifact as gas is liberated in the esophagus or stomach. Because of this problem, most effervescent agents contain simethicone, an antifoaming agent that disperses bubbles.[3] We prefer to chase the granules with 10 ml of water before giving barium. This appears to promote more rapid release of carbon dioxide without trapping bubbles in the barium.[4]

While the stomach and duodenum are readily distended by effervescent agents, the patient must gulp the high-density barium suspension as quickly as possible to achieve adequate gaseous distention of the esophagus. With rapid swallowing, the peristaltic sequence is interrupted, and the esophagus becomes hypotonic. As the patient gulps the high-density barium, swallowed air also distends the esophagus, contributing further to the double contrast effect. Nevertheless, some elderly or debilitated patients may be able to take only small sips of barium, so that adequate distention of the esophagus cannot always be achieved.

Mucosal Coating

Adequate mucosal coating is obtained by washing a high-density barium suspension over the mucosa. The quality of mucosal coating depends on a variety of factors, including the properties of the barium suspension, the volume of barium and gas, the frequency of washing, and the amount of fluid or secretions in the stomach. In general, a larger volume of barium results in better mucosal coating. If there is too much barium, however, only a small portion of the mucosa can be seen in double contrast. Optimal coating is achieved by turning the patient through 360 degrees to wash the barium suspension across all surfaces of the stomach. However, the quality of mucosal coating tends to deteriorate rapidly during the fluoroscopic examination, so that repeated turning of the patient is required to manipulate the barium pool and obtain a fresh coating before each exposure. In the absence of good mucosal coating, small or even large lesions may be missed. Uneven coating may also simulate lesions (see Fig. 5–13).

Because mucosal coating depends on the physical and chemical properties of the barium suspension, the choice of barium directly affects the quality of the double contrast examination.[4–7] In general, the best results are obtained with a high-density barium (250% w/v) of intermediate viscosity.[8] Adequate mucosal coating is usually present when a thin, uniform white line is observed along the contour of the stomach. The quality of coating can also be judged on the basis of whether an areae gastricae pattern is visible in the stomach. With standard barium suspensions, the areae gastricae can be detected in about 70% of patients.[9] However, visualization of these structures depends on many factors, including the amount and viscosity of mucus in the stomach, so that failure to demonstrate an areae gastricae pattern does not necessarily indicate that coating is inadequate.

Excess fluid or secretions in the stomach also impair mucosal coating. Patients with gastric outlet obstruction, gastroparesis, or hypersecretory states are more likely to have excess fluid. In such cases, the properties of the barium suspension become even more important, as some suspensions precipitate rapidly on contact with acid in the stomach and others are more resistant to acid.[6] When excessive fluid is present, the patient may be given additional high-density barium and rotated several times to wash the barium across the stomach and improve the coating. If adequate coating is still not achieved, the stomach can be filled with a low-density barium suspension for a conventional single contrast study, or the examination can be repeated at a later date after fluid is aspirated from the stomach with a nasogastric tube.

Hypotonia

A variety of hypotonic agents can be used to facilitate the double contrast examination. In the past, propantheline bromide (Pro-Banthine) was used to induce gastric hypotonia,[10] but because of its anticholinergic side effects, this drug has been largely supplanted by glucagon. A standard dose of 0.1 mg of glucagon administered intravenously produces adequate gastric hypotonia within 45 seconds of the injection in most patients.[11,12] As a result, it is possible to obtain better double contrast views of the antrum and body of the stomach in a relaxed, hypotonic state. Glucagon also tends to contract the pylorus and delay gastric emptying, so that the stomach can be visualized in double contrast before it is obscured by overlapping loops of barium-filled duodenum or small bowel. Because glucagon delays filling of the duodenum, however, the examination may be prolonged in some patients.

Glucagon is an extremely safe drug that has virtually no side effects, except for the remote possibility of a hypersensitivity reaction.[11,12] However, some patients may have nausea or vomiting if the drug is injected too rapidly.[13] There is also the occasional patient who has a vasovagal reaction to the sight of the needle. The only contraindications to the use of glucagon are pheochromocytoma; insulinoma; brittle, insulin-dependent diabetes; and a history of allergy to glucagon.

In the evaluation of known gastric lesions (e.g., healing of gastric ulcers), larger doses of glucagon (usually 1 mg) should be given intravenously to achieve greater levels of gastric hypotonia for a more detailed examination. In patients who have undergone partial gastrectomy, a large dose of intravenous glucagon should also be given to prevent rapid spillage of barium through the gastroenterostomy into the proximal small bowel (see Chapter 7). To obtain a more detailed examination of the duodenum, 0.5 to 1 mg of glucagon should be given intravenously only after barium has entered the duodenum. This "tubeless" hypotonic duodenogram is a valuable technique for evaluating known or suspected lesions in or around the duodenum (see Chapter 9).

Although glucagon is a useful hypotonic agent for the stomach and duodenum, it has no effect on esophageal peristalsis and does not produce better double contrast views of the esophagus. However, it has been shown that glucagon relaxes the lower esophageal sphincter[14] and therefore increases the frequency of spontaneous gastroesophageal reflux.[15] Alternately, propantheline may be given intravenously in doses of 20 to 30 mg to paralyze the esophagus. This drug is particularly helpful for visualizing esophageal varices.[16] However, as indicated earlier, propantheline is rarely used because of its many side effects.

Buscopan (hyoscine N-butyl bromide) is another anticholinergic agent that is frequently used in double contrast examinations.[2] This drug produces effective but transient hypotonia of the esophagus, stomach, and duodenum. It has the additional advantage of relaxing the pylorus, so that excellent double contrast views of the duodenum can be obtained. Buscopan appears to be free of the major side effects of propantheline, although blurred vision is still a common complaint. It should also be recognized that Buscopan markedly prolongs small bowel transit time, so that a small bowel study becomes impractical in these patients. Buscopan is a popular hypotonic agent in Europe but is not available in the United States.

Attention to Technical Details

Meticulous attention to technical details is required to achieve consistently high-quality double contrast studies.[4] The preparation of the barium is critical. The suspension is prepared by adding a precise amount of water (usually 65 to 70 ml) measured in a syringe or graduated cylinder to a cup of powdered, high-density barium.[9] This results in a 250% w/v barium suspension that is ideal for double contrast studies of the upper gastrointestinal tract. Most high-density barium settles quickly from the suspension, so that the cup of barium must be vigorously stirred or shaken immediately before starting the examination. We prefer to expose our spot films at about 110 kVp, although lower kVp can be used with the rare earth intensifying screens. The density settings on the phototimer should generally be lower than those used on conventional barium studies to avoid washing out the surface detail of the mucosa.

Maneuvers

A standard set of maneuvers is required to achieve adequate mucosal coating of all surfaces of the esophagus, stomach, and duodenum and to produce unobscured double contrast views of each area.[17] The examination must be performed quickly, since overlapping loops of barium-filled small bowel may impair visualization of the stomach and duodenum. The major purpose of fluoroscopy is to determine the volume of barium and gas, to assess mucosal coating, and to ensure accurate positioning and timing of spot films. Because careful fluoroscopic positioning of the patient is required, the routine double contrast study consists only of fluoroscopic spot films. In general, overhead radiographs have not been found to contribute additional information to the study.[18] However, we do obtain overhead films when a surgical lesion is encountered or when a large extrinsic mass is seen displacing the esophagus, stomach, or duodenum.

Flow technique refers to the fluoroscopic observation of the flow of barium across the dependent wall of the stomach to provide a barium pool of varying thickness.[19] By turning the patient one way or the other, barium can be made to flow "uphill" from the antrum into the fundus or "downhill" from the fundus into the antrum. It is an ideal technique for detecting relatively subtle lesions in the stomach as barium flows around small protrusions or fills small ulcers on the dependent surface (see Chapter 7).[19]

Although it is important to develop a standard routine for performing the fluoroscopic examination, additional maneuvers or spot films may be required if an abnormality is suspected at fluoroscopy. When the double contrast portion of the study has been completed, prone views of the esophagus and prone or upright compression views of the stomach and duodenum should be obtained with a low-density barium suspension to supplement the double contrast examination. These views are particularly important for showing small polypoid lesions or ulcers on the anterior wall of the stomach and duodenum (see Chapters 7 to 9).

THE ROUTINE EXAMINATION

Our routine procedure for examining the upper gastrointestinal tract is described in the following section. Of course, this routine can be altered as dictated by the indications for the examination or by findings during the examination.

Patient Preparation

Retained fluid in the stomach may significantly interfere with the quality of mucosal coating. Patients are therefore instructed to fast overnight before undergoing the examination to minimize the amount of fluid or secretions in the stomach. They should also be discouraged from smoking on the day of the examination because cigarette smoke increases gastric secretions and therefore compromises mucosal coating in the stomach and duodenum.[20,21] Finally, antacids or other medications that coat the mucosal surface of the stomach should not be taken until the examination has been completed. For obvious reasons, patients with insulin-dependent diabetes should have their study done early in the day and should not receive their insulin injections until they are free to eat after the examination.

Materials

1. Barium: E-Z-HD (E-Z-EM Co., Westbury, NY).
2. Effervescent agent: E-Z Gas or Baros (E-Z-EM Co.).
3. Glucagon: 0.1 mg of glucagon diluted to 0.25 ml with sterile water in a tuberculin syringe with a 25-gauge needle.

Procedure

Our routine technique is designed to evaluate the upper gastrointestinal tract with the greatest economy in patient movement and film utilization while still obtaining a thorough examination.[17] It is important to be aware that each spot film is taken after patient turning has provided a fresh coating of barium on the mucosal surface being studied.

1. A standard dose of 0.1 mg of glucagon is given intravenously.
2. The patient swallows one packet of effervescent granules or "fizzies" followed by 10 ml of water. The patient is instructed to swallow repeatedly to avoid belching.
3. The patient rapidly gulps a cup of high-density barium (120 ml) as one 3-on-1 or two 2-on-1 left posterior oblique (LPO) spot films are obtained in rapid sequence to visualize the entire esophagus (Fig. 3–1A). (All radiographic projections are indicated with respect to the tabletop.)
4. The table is brought to the horizontal position with the patient's back to the tabletop.
5. The patient is turned to the right through a 360-degree circle back to the supine position. If mucosal coating is adequate, a frontal spot film of the stomach is obtained for a double contrast view of the antrum and body (Fig. 3–1B), since barium pools in the fundus in the supine position.
6. The patient is turned through another 360-degree rotation, and a spot film of the antrum and body of the stomach is obtained in the LPO projection (Fig. 3–1C).
7. The patient is turned to the right lateral position for a double contrast view of the gastric cardia and fundus (Fig. 3–1D). This view also permits visualization of the retrogastric area.
8. "Uphill" flow technique is performed by turning the patient onto the back and then slowly to the LPO position. Four-on-one spot films are deliberately taken while the posterior wall of the body and antrum are covered by a thin layer of barium (Fig. 3–1E). Downhill flow technique is performed by slowly turning the patient to the right posterior oblique (RPO) position and obtaining 4-on-1 spot films of the high lesser curvature and gastric cardia in a steep RPO and right lateral position.
9. With the table semiupright, the patient is turned to the RPO position for a double contrast view of the upper body and lesser curvature of the stomach (Fig. 3–1F). The gastric cardia can also be studied in more detail in this position.
10. By this time, barium usually has emptied into the duodenum. With the table semiupright or horizontal, the patient is turned to the LPO position for 4-on-1 or 2-on-1 spot films of the duodenal bulb and descending duodenum in double contrast (Fig. 3–1G).
11. The table is lowered to the horizontal position, and the patient drinks a low-density barium suspension in the prone right anterior oblique (RAO) position. The patient is initially instructed to take single swallows of barium, so that esophageal peristalsis can be evaluated. A single 3-on-1 or two 2-on-1 spot films of the esophagus are then obtained during continuous drinking to permit optimal distention of the distal esophagus and gastroesophageal junction (Fig. 3–1H).
12. With the patient in the prone or prone RAO position, 4-on-1 spot films of the gastric antrum and body and duodenal bulb are obtained with varying degrees of compression using an inflatable balloon or other prone compression device positioned beneath the patient's abdomen (Fig. 3–1I).
13. The patient is turned to the left side and then onto the back, so that barium pools in the gastric fundus. The gastroesophageal junction is then monitored fluoroscopically as the patient is turned slowly to the right to elicit spontaneous gastroesophageal reflux. A straight-leg-raising maneuver or Valsalva maneuver can also be performed to provoke reflux.
14. The table is fully elevated with the patient in the right lateral position. This maneuver tends to keep barium in the antrum and duodenum, so that upright 4-on-1 spot films of these areas can be obtained with graded compression. An upright film of the gastric fundus can also be obtained in the LPO projection (Fig. 3–1J).

The filming sequence and purpose of each radiograph are summarized in Table 3–1. With some experi-

TABLE **3–1.** *Summary of Filming Sequence for Biphasic Examination of Upper Gastrointestinal Tract*

View	No. of Films	Purpose
Upright LPO	1 (3-on-1)	Double contrast, esophagus
Supine	1 (3-on-1)	Double contrast, antrum and body
LPO	1 (3-on-1)	Double contrast, antrum and body
Right lateral	1 (3-on-1)	Double contrast, cardia and fundus; retrogastric area
Flow technique	1 (4-on-1)	Posterior wall of antrum and body
Semiupright RPO	1 (3-on-1)	Double contrast, upper body, fundus, and cardia
Semiupright or recumbent LPO	1 (4-on-1)	Double contrast, duodenum
Prone RAO	1 (3-on-1)	Single contrast, esophagus and gastroesophageal junction
Prone compression	1 (4-on-1)	Single contrast, stomach and duodenum
Upright compression	1 (4-on-1)	Single contrast, stomach and duodenum
Upright LPO	1 (3-on-1)	Double contrast, fundus

LPO, Left posterior oblique; RPO, right posterior oblique; RAO, right anterior oblique.

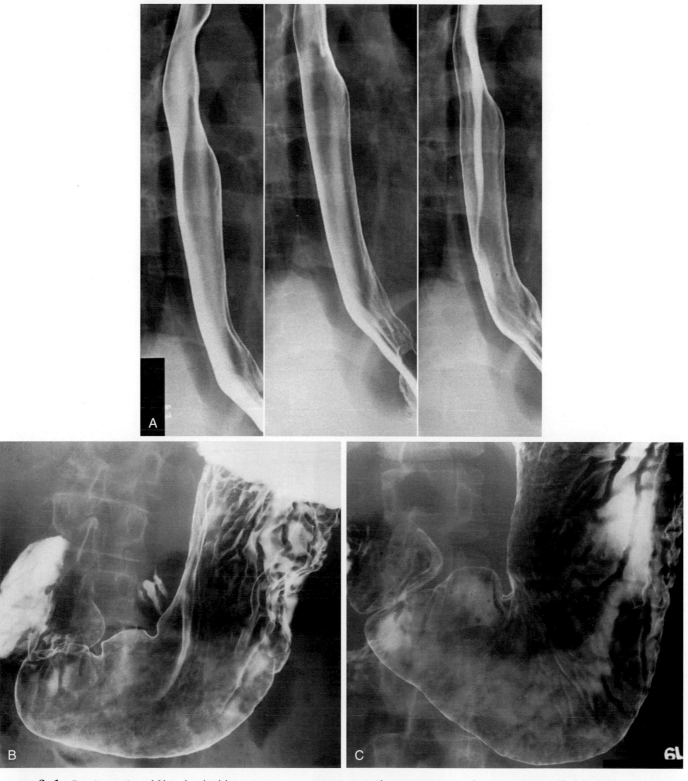

FIGURE 3–1. Routine series of films for double contrast upper gastrointestinal examination. *A,* Three-on-one upright LPO views of esophagus. (From Levine, M.S.: Radiology of the Esophagus. Philadelphia, W.B. Saunders, 1989, p. 5, with permission.) *B,* Supine view of gastric antrum and body. *C,* LPO view of gastric antrum and body. *Figure continued on following pages*

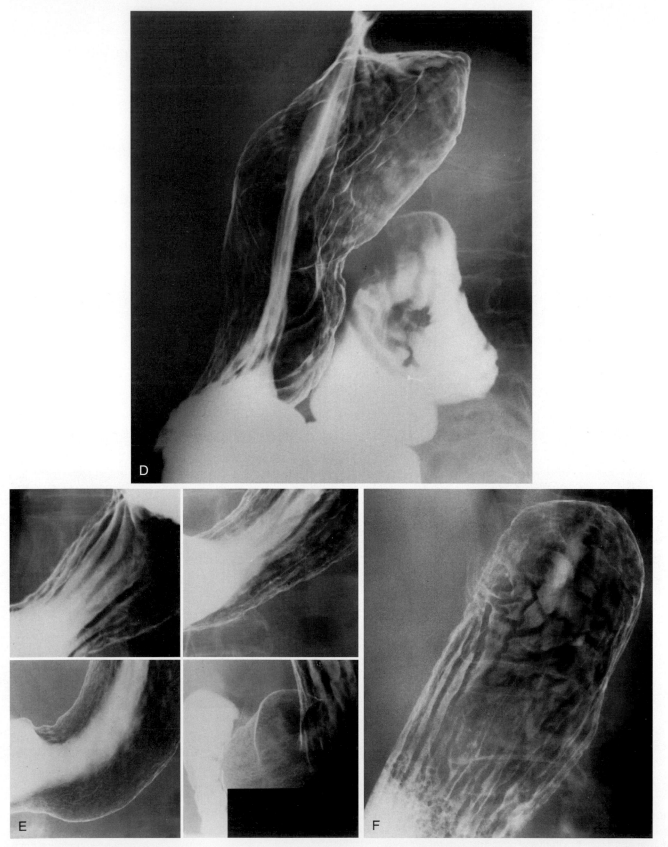

FIGURE 3–1 *Continued* *D,* Right lateral view of gastric cardia and fundus. *E,* Flow technique with 4-on-1 spot films showing thin barium pool on posterior wall of stomach. *F,* Semiupright RPO view of high lesser curvature, upper body, and fundus.

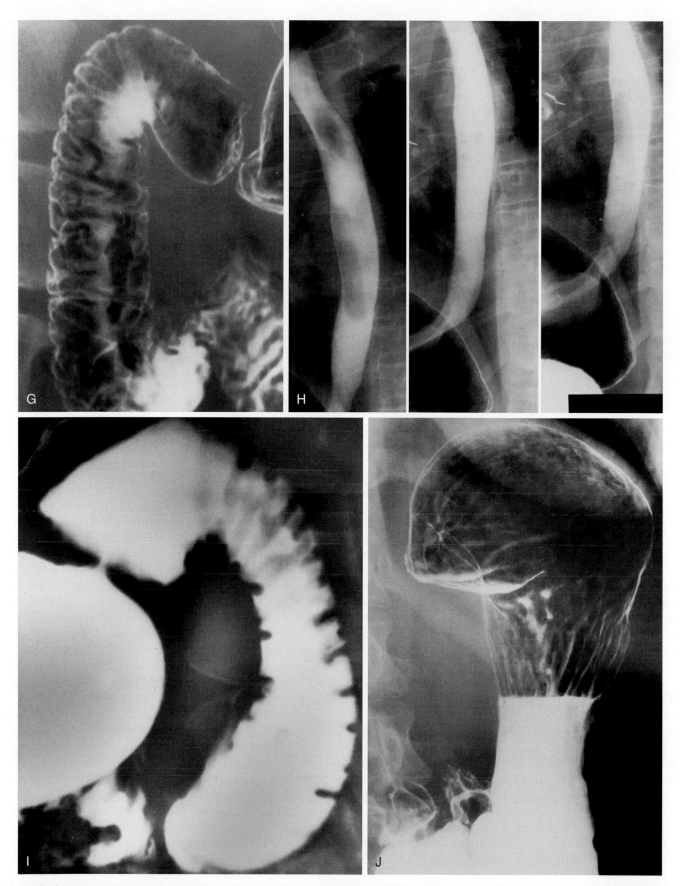

FIGURE 3–1 *Continued*   *G,* LPO view of duodenum. *H,* Three-on-one prone RAO views of barium-filled esophagus. *I,* Prone RAO view of barium-filled duodenum. *J,* Upright, slightly LPO view of gastric fundus. (From Laufer, I.: A simple method for routine double contrast study of the upper gastrointestinal tract. Radiology *117:*513, 1975, with permission.)

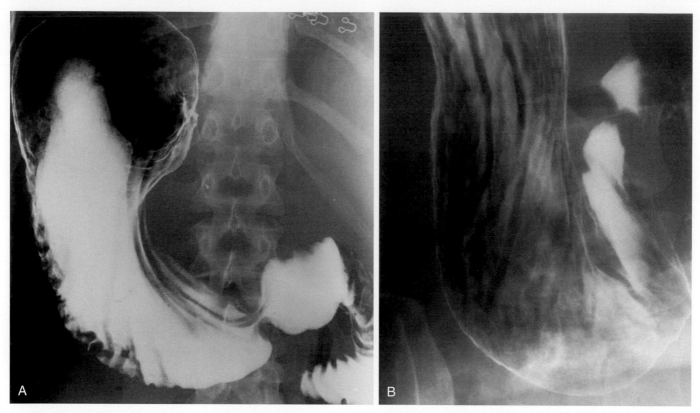

FIGURE 3–2. Double contrast examination of the anterior wall. *A,* Prone view shows barium outlining rugal folds on anterior gastric wall. *B,* Double contrast view of anterior wall of antrum and body in prone LAO projection with table tilted 20 to 30 degrees head down.

ence, it should be possible to complete the examination in 3 to 4 minutes of fluoroscopy time and about 10 minutes of room time. When a lesion is suspected at fluoroscopy, the barium study should be tailored to demonstrate the lesion en face and in profile with both single and double contrast techniques. Ultimately, each radiologist should develop a set routine for performing the examination. Although individual maneuvers or filming sequences may vary, the end result should be a thorough and efficient evaluation of all surfaces of the upper gastrointestinal tract.

Variations

If the initial 360-degree rotation of the patient fails to produce adequate mucosal coating in the stomach, the patient may be rotated one or more additional turns before obtaining a film. Although some barium may spill into the duodenum during this maneuver, 360-degree rotation of the patient permits optimal coating of all mucosal surfaces of the stomach by high-density barium. If the patient cannot be rotated 360 degrees because of age, debilitation, or other reasons, a gentle rocking maneuver can be performed to achieve adequate mucosal coating in most cases.

Many lesions on the anterior wall of the stomach can be shown by the combination of supine double contrast

and prone compression radiographs. Although routine double contrast views of the anterior wall do not appear to be warranted, a more detailed double contrast study of the anterior wall may be performed on patients who have equivocal findings on the initial examination or in whom there is a high index of suspicion of a gastric lesion.[22] These views are obtained by placing the patient in the prone position, so that barium pools on the anterior wall of the stomach, outlining the rugal folds (Fig. 3–2A). The table is then tilted head down while the patient is turned to the prone left anterior oblique (LAO) position, allowing barium to drain into the fundus. This maneuver leaves only a thin residual layer of high-density barium on the anterior wall of the antrum and body, so that excellent double contrast views of this region can be obtained (Fig. 3–2B). The head of the table is then elevated for double contrast views of the anterior wall of the upper body and fundus (Fig. 3–2C). A profile view of the anterior wall can also be obtained by turning the patient to the left lateral position (Fig. 3–2D). This particular view often permits visualization of the duodenum through the gas-filled stomach. Finally, the anterior wall may be demonstrated by a supine cross-table horizontal beam view of the stomach.

Anterior wall views of the duodenum may also be helpful in some patients. Starting in the LPO position for dou-

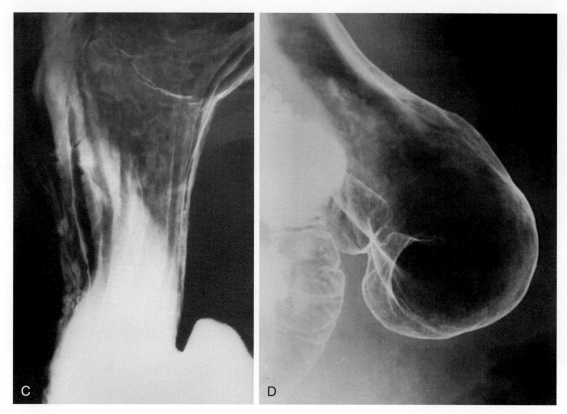

FIGURE 3 2 *Continued* *C,* Double contrast view of anterior wall of upper body with head of table elevated. *D,* Profile view of anterior wall of antrum in left lateral projection.

ble contrast views of the duodenum, the patient is turned to the left side and then to the prone position. This causes barium to coat the anterior wall of the duodenum while gas is trapped in the descending duodenum. An inflatable balloon or pad may be used to displace the barium-filled antrum if it overlaps the duodenum. This maneuver permits recognition of the minor duodenal papilla (an anterior wall structure) as well as anterior wall lesions that may not be demonstrated on the routine study.

Additional variations in technique are described elsewhere for the evaluation of the postoperative stomach[23,24] (see Chapter 7).

PROBLEMS AND PITFALLS
Esophagus

Technical factors related to the amount of barium and gas in the esophagus may greatly affect the quality of the double contrast study. Because double contrast radiographs of the esophagus are obtained with the patient in an upright position, pooling of barium in the distal esophagus may obscure mucosal detail. As barium enters the stomach, a residual layer of high-density barium in the esophagus may also obscure the mucosa. When this "flow artifact" is observed at fluoroscopy, additional views obtained moments later should better delineate mucosal

lesions as the layer of residual high-density barium on the mucosa thins out[25] (see Fig. 5–16). At the same time, esophageal peristalsis causes the esophagus to collapse almost immediately after passage of the barium bolus into the stomach. The fluoroscopist therefore must time the exposures to capture the esophagus during the relatively brief period of optimal distention and coating. With some experience, it is possible to obtain satisfactory double contrast views of the esophagus in 75% to 85% of patients.[26,27]

When esophageal disease is believed to be present, the cup of high-density barium may be split into two portions for a more detailed double contrast study. By having the patient drink half of the barium in the typical LPO projection and half in the RPO projection, protruded or depressed lesions in the esophagus may be evaluated both en face and in profile. Alternatively, a tube esophagram may be performed when the routine double contrast study is inconclusive[28] (see Chapter 5).

Whereas mucosal disease is best evaluated with double contrast technique, abnormalities of the longitudinal folds are better seen on mucosal relief views of the collapsed or partially collapsed esophagus. Esophageal varices may be effaced or even obliterated by esophageal distention, so that mucosal relief views are particularly important when varices are suspected.[29] Various types of

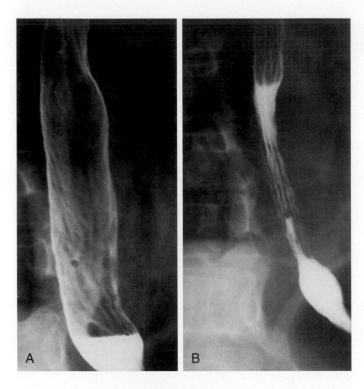

FIGURE 3–3. Reflux esophagitis with abnormal folds on collapsed view. *A,* Note slight nodularity of mucosa in lower third of esophagus. *B,* Mucosal relief view of collapsed esophagus shows irregular, crenulated longitudinal folds due to esophagitis.

esophagitis may also be recognized by the presence of thickened, irregular, or crenulated longitudinal folds in the collapsed esophagus (Fig. 3–3).

When a ring or stricture is suspected in the distal esophagus, particular emphasis should be placed on prone single contrast views of the esophagus during con-

tinuous drinking of a low-density barium suspension to produce better distention of the distal esophagus and gastroesophageal junction. Schatzki rings or peptic strictures that are not visible on double contrast radiographs may be detected when the esophagus is optimally distended by this technique[30,31] (Fig. 3–4).

FIGURE 3–4. Importance of prone single contrast views for demonstrating lower esophageal rings. *A,* Upright double contrast view of esophagus shows no evidence of lower esophageal ring. However, note pooling of barium in distal esophagus with suboptimal distention of this region. *B,* Prone single contrast view from same examination shows hiatal hernia with unequivocal Schatzki ring *(arrows)* above hernia.

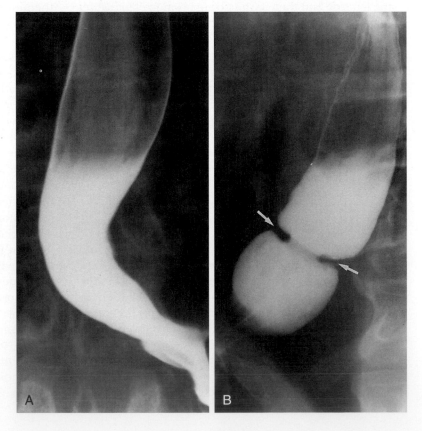

Stomach

The proper volume of barium and gas is required for optimal double contrast views of the stomach. Although a single 120-ml cup of high-density barium is usually adequate for this purpose, barium occasionally may empty rapidly from the stomach despite intravenous administration of glucagon. In such cases, additional barium may be given to the patient in a recumbent LPO position to obtain better mucosal coating. Similarly, if the patient belches during the examination, an additional packet or half packet of effervescent agent may be required to produce adequate gaseous distention. Conversely, the patient may be asked to belch if the stomach is overdistended with gas, since overdistention may efface abnormal folds associated with ulcers or ulcer scars.

In patients who are relatively unresponsive to glucagon, rapid emptying of barium into the duodenum may cause portions of the stomach to be obscured by overlapping loops of barium-filled duodenum or small bowel. This overlap may particularly impair visualization of the distal antrum. If it is a frequent problem, the first part of the double contrast study may be modified so that the table is returned to the horizontal position with the patient facing the table immediately after swallowing the high-density barium suspension. The patient then may be turned from the prone position onto the left side and back to obtain unobscured double contrast views of the distal antrum before barium spills into the duodenum. The usual routine then may be followed for the rest of the examination.

In patients who are unusually sensitive to glucagon, gastric hypotonia may significantly delay spillage of barium into the duodenum, prolonging the examination. When this problem is encountered, the patient may be asked to wait outside the examining room for 10 or 15 minutes until the glucagon effect has subsided. Because another study can be performed while the patient is waiting, the fluoroscopy schedule need not be delayed by a glucagon-sensitive person.

Duodenum

After the duodenum has filled with high-density barium, adequate double contrast views of the duodenal bulb and descending duodenum usually can be obtained by placing the patient in a recumbent or semiupright LPO position to distend the bulb with gas. If, however, the bulb is inadequately distended with gas or obscured by barium, the table may be elevated further (even to a fully upright position). This maneuver causes barium to pool in the antrum or descending duodenum and air to rise into the duodenal bulb, which tends to assume a vertical configuration, so that adequate double contrast views of the bulb can be obtained. If the duodenal bulb is located in a posterior position, the patient may also be turned to the left lateral or even the prone LAO position to achieve adequate gaseous distention of the bulb and descending duodenum (Fig. 3–5). If, despite these maneuvers, satisfactory double contrast views of the duodenum cannot be obtained, the fluoroscopist should proceed to the single contrast portion of the study rather than prolong the

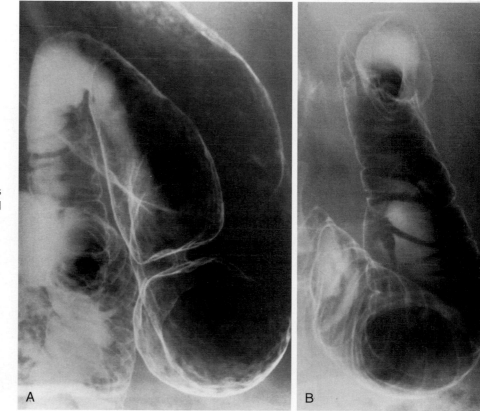

FIGURE 3–5. Double contrast views of duodenum in left lateral *(A)* and prone LAO *(B)* positions.

A

B

double contrast examination because it usually is possible to obtain adequate prone or upright compression views of the duodenum. After these compression films have been taken, the table may be lowered with the patient in the LPO position. Gas is often seen to percolate from the antrum into the duodenum during this maneuver, providing a final opportunity for double contrast views of the bulb.

DIGITAL FLUOROSCOPIC IMAGING

Performance

Digital fluoroscopic equipment has increasingly been used for gastrointestinal imaging studies, including double contrast upper gastrointestinal examinations.[32] Digital imaging systems require an image intensifier, digital image processor, and high-resolution monitor.[33–35] These systems provide much faster data acquisition and transmission than conventional film-screen radiography equipment and the capability for instant image display as well as image postprocessing to optimize interpretation. Digital gastrointestinal equipment also produces lower radiation doses per exposure than conventional fluoroscopic equipment,[35–37] but this advantage may be offset by the tendency to take an increased number of exposures. Finally, the shorter exposure times with digital equipment decrease image blurring because of motion artifact, a feature that is particularly useful for imaging the esophagus.

When double contrast upper gastrointestinal studies are performed with digital fluoroscopic equipment, rapid image acquisition provides the fluoroscopist a larger window of opportunity for taking exposures that show the pertinent findings. This window of opportunity becomes especially critical when obtaining double contrast views of the esophagus because of the relatively brief period of optimal esophageal coating and distention.

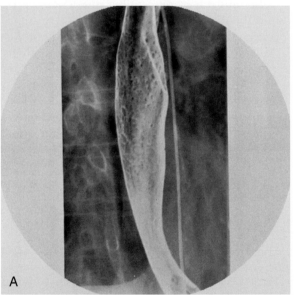

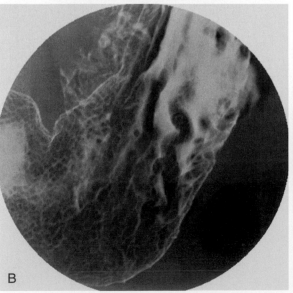

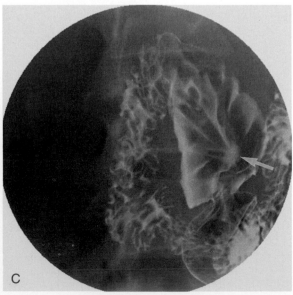

FIGURE 3–6. Demonstration of subtle abnormalities with digital spot images of upper gastrointestinal tract. *A, Candida* esophagitis with multiple tiny plaques. *B, H. pylori* gastritis with enlarged areae gastricae and thickened folds in gastric body. *C,* Duodenal ulcer *(arrow)* with radiating folds. (*A, B,* and *C* from Levine, M.S., and Laufer, I.: The gastrointestinal tract: Do's and don'ts of digital imaging. Radiology *207:*311, 1998, with permission.)

Digital equipment also allows for greater quality control of the study. Every digital exposure is captured on the monitor as a "frozen" image until fluoroscopy is resumed. The radiologist therefore has the opportunity to review each image on the monitor to determine whether the fluoroscopic findings have been adequately shown. If any questionable or uncertain findings are encountered, additional images can immediately be obtained for a more definitive diagnosis.

The major limitation of digital fluoroscopic equipment is a lower spatial resolution than conventional radiographic equipment because of the limited number of pixels.[33,38] Despite lower spatial resolution, recent studies indicate that the diagnostic capability of digital equipment is comparable to that of conventional equipment for gastrointestinal imaging.[35,39] In our experience, digital images can readily depict subtle mucosal abnormalities such as the nodules, plaques, or ulcers in esophagitis (Fig. 3–6*A*), abnormal areae gastricae in *Helicobacter pylori* gastritis (Fig. 3–6*B*), and small gastric or duodenal ulcers (Fig. 3–6*C*).[32] Thus digital imaging systems are capable of providing the clarity and resolution needed to achieve high-quality double contrast upper gastrointestinal examinations.

Interpretation

Interpretation of digitally performed double contrast upper gastrointestinal examinations should be performed at a computer workstation that allows rapid and convenient display of images.[40] Ideally, this workstation should be integrated with picture archiving and communications systems (PACS). At most workstations, the radiologist can review the images with nearly the same clarity and resolution as on the original monitor. A major reason for viewing and interpreting digital studies at the workstation is that such a format allows for postprocessing of the images.[32–35] Such parameters as the brightness, contrast, and magnification of the image can be altered in gradual increments to highlight or accentuate various findings. Although some effort is required to become adept at manipulating images at the workstation, a relatively small investment of time and energy allows us to maximize the diagnostic capability of this technology.

After the upper gastrointestinal study has been interpreted, the workstation can be used to annotate findings of interest and also to indicate in text form the final radiologic diagnosis. The images can then be transferred to optical disks or, ideally, a digital archives or "jukebox" for long-term storage and rapid retrieval. Paper prints containing representative images can also be generated for the referring physicians to show the pertinent findings described in the radiologic reports. Because the images are stored electronically without generating hard copies (excluding overhead films), this approach produces a considerable cost savings over time that helps offset the higher initial cost of the digital equipment.

REFERENCES

1. Laufer, I.: A simple method for routine double contrast study of the upper gastrointestinal tract. Radiology *117*:513, 1975.
2. Hunt, J.H., and Anderson, I.F.: Double contrast upper gastrointestinal studies. Clin. Radiol. *27*:87, 1976.
3. Koehler, R.E., Weyman, P.J., Stanley, R.J., et al.: Evaluation of three effervescent agents for double-contrast upper gastrointestinal radiography. Gastrointest. Radiol. *6*:111, 1981.
4. Miller, R.E.: Recipes for gastrointestinal examinations. AJR Am. J. Roentgenol. *137*:1285, 1981.
5. Cumberland, D.C.: Optimum viscosity of barium suspension for use in the double contrast barium meal. Gastrointest. Radiol. *2*:169, 1977.
6. Roberts, G.M., Roberts, E.E., Davies, R.L., et al.: Observations on the behaviour of barium sulfate suspensions in gastric secretion. Br. J. Radiol. *50*:468, 1977.
7. Kormano, M., Makela, P., and Rossi, I.: Visualization of the areae gastricae in a double contrast examination—dependence on the contrast medium. Fortschr. Rontgenstr. *128*:52, 1978.
8. Gelfand, D.W.: High density, low viscosity barium for fine mucosal detail on double-contrast upper gastrointestinal examinations. AJR Am. J. Roentgenol. *130*:831, 1978.
9. Rubesin, S.E., and Herlinger, H.: The effect of barium suspension viscosity on the delineation of areae gastricae. AJR Am. J. Roentgenol. *146*:35, 1986.
10. Merlo, R.B., Stone, M., Baugus, P., et al.: The use of Pro-Banthine to induce gastrointestinal hypotonia. Radiology *127*:61, 1978.
11. Miller, R.E., Chernish, S.M., Greenman, G.F., et al.: Gastrointestinal response to minute doses of glucagon. Radiology *143*:317, 1982.
12. Maglinte, D.D.T., Caudill, L.D., Krol, K.L., et al.: The minimum effective dose of glucagon in upper gastrointestinal radiography. Gastrointest. Radiol. *7*:119, 1982.
13. Chernish, S.M., Maglinte, D.D.T.: Glucagon: Common untoward reactions—review and recommendations. Radiology *177*:145, 1990.
14. Hogan, W.J., Dodds, W.J., Hoke, S.E., et al.: Effect of glucagon on esophageal motor function. Gastroenterology *69*:160, 1975.
15. Haggar, A.M., Feczko, P.J., Halpert, R.D., et al.: Spontaneous gastroesophageal reflux during double contrast upper gastrointestinal radiography with glucagon. Gastrointest. Radiol. *7*:319, 1982.
16. Dalinka, M.K., Smith, E.H., Wolfe, R.D., et al.: Pharmacologically enhanced visualization of esophageal varices by Pro-Banthine. Radiology *102*:281, 1972.
17. Levine, M.S., Rubesin, S.E., Herlinger, H., et al.: Double-contrast upper gastrointestinal examination: Technique and interpretation. Radiology *168*:593, 1988.
18. Bova, J.G., Friedman, A.C., Hudson, T., et al.: Radiographs obtained during upper gastrointestinal fluoroscopy: Adequacy and comparison to postfluoroscopy images. Radiology *147*:875, 1983.
19. Kikuchi, Y., Levine, M.S., Laufer, I., et al.: Value of flow technique for double-contrast examination of the stomach. AJR Am. J. Roentgenol. *147*:1183, 1986.
20. Thoeni, R.F., and Goldberg, H.I.: The influence of smoking on coating of the gastric mucosa during double contrast examination of the stomach (abstract). Invest. Radiol. *15*:388, 1980.
21. Rose, C., Somers, S., Mather, D.G., et al.: Cigarette smoking and duodenal coating with barium. J. Can. Assoc. Radiol. *33*:77, 1982.
22. Goldsmith, M.R., Paul, R.E., Poplack, W.E., et al.: Evaluation of routine double-contrast views of the anterior wall of the stomach. AJR Am. J. Roentgenol. *126*:1159, 1976.
23. Gold, R.P., and Seaman, W.B.: The primary double-contrast examination of the postoperative stomach. Radiology *124*:297, 1977.
24. Gohel, V.K., and Laufer, I.: Double-contrast examination of the postoperative stomach. Radiology *129*:601, 1978.
25. Maglinte, D.D.T., Lappas, J.C., Chernish, S.M., et al.: Flow artifacts in double-contrast esophagography. Radiology *157*:535, 1985.
26. Balfe, D.M., Koehler, R.E., Weyman, P.J., et al.: Routine air-contrast esophagography during upper gastrointestinal examinations. Radiology *139*:739, 1981.
27. Maglinte, D.D.T., Schultheis, T.E., Krol, K.L., et al.: Survey of the esophagus during the upper gastrointestinal examination in 500 patients. Radiology *147*:65, 1983.
28. Levine, M.S., Kressel, H.Y., Laufer, I., et al.: The tube esophagram: A technique for obtaining a detailed double-contrast examination of the esophagus. AJR Am. J. Roentgenol. *142*:293, 1984.

29. Nelson, S.W.: The roentgenologic diagnosis of esophageal varices. AJR Am. J. Roentgenol. *77:*599, 1957.

30. Chen, Y.M., Ott, D.J., Gelfand, D.W., et al.: Multiphasic examination of the esophagogastric region for strictures, rings, and hiatal hernia: Evaluation of the individual techniques. Gastrointest. Radiol. *10:*311, 1985.

31. Ott, D.J., Chen, Y.M., Wu, W.C., et al.: Radiographic and endoscopic sensitivity in detecting lower esophageal mucosal ring. AJR Am. J. Roentgenol. *147:*261, 1986.

32. Levine, M.S., and Laufer, I.: The gastrointestinal tract: Do's and don'ts of digital imaging. Radiology *207:*311, 1998.

33. Feczko, P.J., Ackerman, L.V., Kastan, D.J., et al.: Digital radiography of the gastrointestinal tract. Gastrointest. Radiol. *13:*191, 1988.

34. Steiner, E., Hahn, P.F., Taaffe, J., et al.: Digital videofluorography for direct digital spot filming of gastrointestinal studies. Gastrointest. Radiol. *14:*193, 1989.

35. Takahasi, M., Ueno, S., and Yoshimatsu, S.: Gastrointestinal examinations with digital radiography. RadioGraphics *12:*969, 1992.

36. Martin, C.J., and Hunter, S.: Reduction of patient doses from barium meal and barium enema examinations through changes in equipment factors. Br. J. Radiol. *67:*1196, 1994.

37. Broadhead, D.A., Chapple, C.L., and Faulkner, K. The impact of digital imaging on patient doses during barium studies. Br. J. Radiol. *68:*992, 1995.

38. Kastan, D.J., Ackerman, L.V., and Feczko, P.J.: Digital gastrointestinal imaging: The effect of pixel size on detection of subtle mucosal abnormalities. Radiology *162:*853, 1987.

39. Barkhof, F., David, E., and de Geest, F.: Comparison of film-screen combinations and digital fluorography in gastrointestinal barium examinations in a clinical setting. Eur. J. Radiol. *22:*232, 1996.

40. Arenson, R.L., Chakraborty, D.P., Seshadri, S.B., et al.: The digital imaging workstation. Radiology *176:*303, 1990.

4

Pharynx

STEPHEN E. RUBESIN

The pharynx serves as the gateway to the gastrointestinal tract and as the crossroads of speech, respiration, and swallowing. During swallowing, the pharynx channels the bolus to enter the gastrointestinal tract and not the airway. During respiration, the pharynx actively maintains an open passage from the nasopharynx to the laryngeal aditus. During speech, the pharynx acts as a resonator, changing size and shape to alter sounds. The pharynx also participates in other activities, such as yawning, gagging, choking, and vomiting.

Pharyngeal disorders are common and may be manifested by swallowing, speech, or respiratory symptoms. Aspiration pneumonia, often due to pharyngeal dysmotility, is a frequent cause of increased morbidity and mortality. Approximately 8000 to 10,000 people die of choking yearly,[1] and 4% of malignant neoplasms in men are head and neck tumors.[1]

This chapter serves as an introduction to the complicated world of the pharynx. Because this textbook focuses on double contrast radiology, this chapter emphasizes normal double contrast anatomy and structural abnormalities of the pharynx. However, the radiologist should remember that most disorders of the pharynx are motility disorders. Although double contrast studies can demonstrate structural correlates of functional disorders,

high-resolution videofluoroscopy or cineradiography must be performed to evaluate pharyngeal function. Helpful references concerning performance and interpretation of pharyngeal motility studies are cited in the following discussions.[2–10]

NORMAL APPEARANCES

A detailed knowledge of the complex anatomy of the pharynx is necessary for interpretation of the double contrast pharyngogram.[11–14] The major landmarks that can be identified radiographically include the soft palate, the base of the tongue, the valleculae, the epiglottis, and the piriform sinuses (Fig. 4–1).

The pharynx is arbitrarily divided into three parts: the nasopharynx, the oropharynx, and the hypopharynx (Fig. 4–2). The nasopharynx is a respiratory tract structure and is excluded from the digestive tract by the soft palate. The oropharynx relates to the oral cavity and base of the tongue and extends from the soft palate to its arbitrary division from the hypopharynx at the level of the hyoid bone. Some anatomists regard the oropharynx as being divided from the hypopharynx by the pharyngoepiglottic fold (Fig. 4–3), a mucosal fold overlying the stylopharyngeus.[11] The

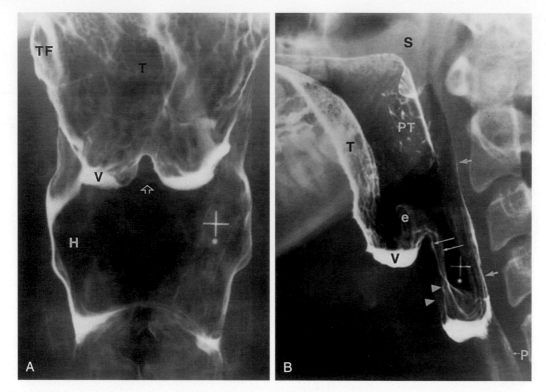

FIGURE 4–1. Normal pharynx. The frontal *(A)* and lateral *(B)* views of the pharynx are shown. On the frontal view, the contours of the tonsillar fossa (TF), valleculae (V), and hypopharynx (H) are demonstrated. The en face view of the surface of the base of the tongue (T) is seen. The median glossoepiglottic fold *(open arrow in A)* crosses from tongue base to epiglottis, dividing the retroglottic space into the two cup-shaped valleculae (right vallecula identified with V). On the lateral view, the soft palate (S), palatine tonsil (PT), base of the tongue (T), valleculae (V), epiglottic tip (e), aryepiglottic folds *(long arrows)*, and posterior pharyngeal wall *(short arrows)* are well imaged. The anterior walls of the piriform sinus are identified *(arrowheads)*. The pharyngoesophageal segment (P) is collapsed. (Reprinted with permission from Rubesin, S.E., and Glick, S.N.: The tailored double-contrast pharyngogram. Crit. Rev. Diagn. Imaging *28*:133, 1988. Copyright CRC Press, Inc., Boca Raton, FL.)

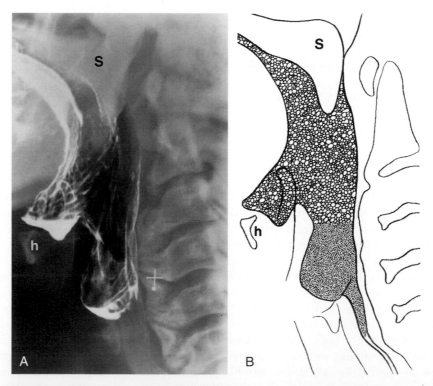

FIGURE 4–2. Divisions of the pharynx. The pharynx is arbitrarily divided into three parts: the nasopharynx, the oropharynx *(bubble pattern)*, and the hypopharynx *(granular pattern)*. The division between the nasopharynx and the oropharynx is the soft palate (S); the division between the oropharynx and the hypopharynx is either the level of the hyoid bone (h) or the pharyngoepiglottic fold (see Fig. 4–3). (From Rubesin, S.E., Jessurun, J., Robertson, D., et al.: Lines of the pharynx. RadioGraphics *7*:217, 1987, with permission.)

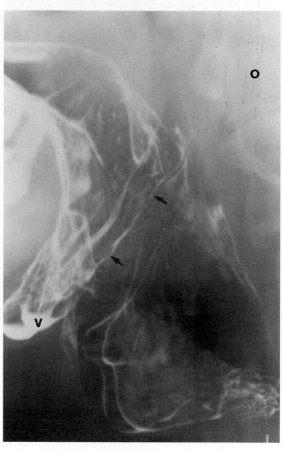

FIGURE 4–3. The pharyngoepiglottic fold *(arrows)* overlies the stylopharyngeus, which runs from the styloid process into the lateral wall of the pharynx. The pharyngoepiglottic fold is seen coursing obliquely across the pharynx from approximately the level of the odontoid (O) process to the junction of the base of the vallecula (V) and epiglottis. The pharyngoepiglottic fold is the mucosal dividing line between the oropharynx and hypopharynx. (Reprinted with permission from Rubesin, S.E., and Glick, S.N.: The tailored double-contrast pharyngogram. Crit. Rev. Diagn. Imaging *28*:133, 1988. Copyright CRC Press, Inc., Boca Raton, FL.)

hypopharynx extends from the level of the hyoid bone to the lower portion of the cricopharyngeus at the inferior margin of the cricoid cartilage. These divisions are arbitrary because the soft palate and hyoid bone change position with phonation, swallowing, and respiration.

The pharynx is primarily a skeletal muscular tube extending 12 to 14 cm from the skull base to the lower border of the cricoid cartilage. The pharynx is confined posteriorly by the cervical spine and laterally by the muscles of the neck. The shape of the pharynx is determined by underlying musculature, impinging cartilages (Fig. 4–4), the supporting skeleton, and the hyoid sling—the suspensory apparatus of the pharynx.[14] The pharyngeal portion of the digestive tract (oropharynx and hypopharynx) has four openings: superiorly, the velopharyngeal portal between the nasopharynx and the oropharynx; anteriorly, the opening to the oral cavity; anteriorly, the laryngeal aditus; and inferiorly, the opening into the esophagus.

The tapered epiglottic tip rises above the valleculae. The valleculae are paired cup-shaped spaces behind the tongue created by the median glossoepiglottic fold, which joins the mid-epiglottis to the base of the tongue. The aryepiglottic folds form the upper lateral margins of the epiglottis, connecting the epiglottic tip with the mucosa overlying the muscular process of the paired arytenoid cartilages.

The shape of the lower hypopharynx is created by posterior protrusion of the larynx into the lower hypopharynx, forming two lateral channels in the anterior

hypopharynx—the piriform sinuses. The lowermost hypopharynx and its junction with the esophagus—the pharyngoesophageal segment—are constricted by mass effect of the cricoid cartilage and tonic contraction of the cricopharyngeus muscle.

The muscular tube of the pharynx is divided into two layers: the outer circular (constrictor) layer and the inner longitudinal layer. The constrictor layer forms a ring that is incomplete anteriorly. It functions to push the bolus out of the pharynx. The major folds of mucosa (the palatoglossal, palatopharyngeal, and salpingopharyngeal folds) are determined by the inner longitudinal muscle layer (Fig. 4–5; see Fig. 4–3).[14] Anteriorly, the median glossoepiglottic fold (see Fig. 4–4) and the aryepiglottic folds are created by the median glossoepiglottic ligament and the paired aryepiglottic muscles, respectively.

The double contrast appearance and landmarks of the pharynx, to a large extent, depend on the mucosa resting on the inner longitudinal muscle layer. Numerous transverse and longitudinal lines give the pharynx a striated appearance on double contrast radiographs (Fig. 4–6). Longitudinal lines reflect mucosa closely apposed to the longitudinally striated inner muscle layer (Fig. 4–6). Transverse folds overlying the muscular processes of the arytenoid cartilages and cricoid cartilage (Fig. 4–7) reflect the redundant mucosa overlying these structures.[14] Numerous round nodules on the vertical surface of the base of the tongue reflect the variable lymphoid tissue in the lingual tonsil (Fig. 4–8).[15]

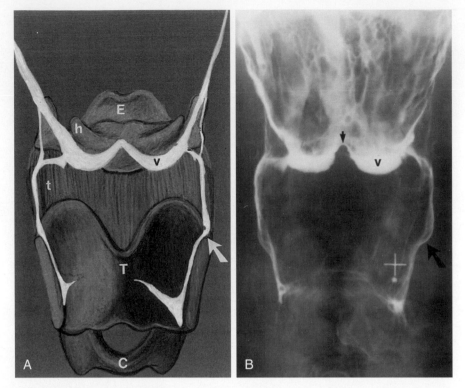

FIGURE 4–4. Relationship of laryngeal cartilages to pharynx. The laryngeal cartilages and hyoid bone (h) are shown in *A* in relationship to a frontal view of the barium coated pharynx in *B*. The epiglottic tip (E) lies above the valleculae (v). The thyrohyoid membrane (t) connects the hyoid bone (h) to the thyroid cartilage (T). The lower hypopharynx is confined laterally by the ala of the thyroid cartilage. The cricoid cartilage (c) supports the anterior wall of the pharyngoesophageal segment. The junction of the ala of the thyroid cartilage and the thyrohyoid membrane *(white arrow)* is seen as a notch in the lateral wall of the hypopharynx *(large black arrow)*. The median glossoepiglottic fold is seen *(small arrow)*. (From Rubesin, S.E., Jessurun, J., Robertson, D., et al.: Lines of the pharynx. RadioGraphics *7*:217, 1987, with permission.)

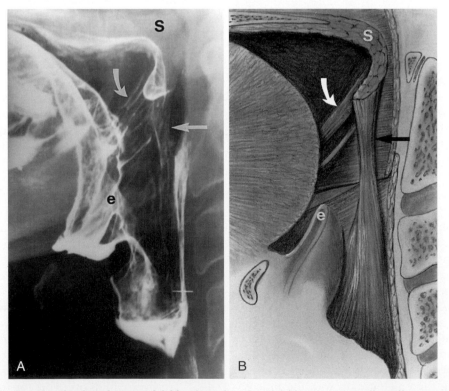

FIGURE 4–5. The palatoglossal and palatopharyngeal folds. The palatoglossal fold (anterior tonsillar pillar) *(curved arrow in A)* is formed by the palatoglossus *(curved arrow in B)* and extends from the mid–soft palate (S) to the junction of the middle and posterior third of the tongue. The palatopharyngeal fold (posterior tonsillar pillar) *(straight white arrow)* overlies the palatopharyngeus *(straight black arrow)*. This muscle extends from the middle portion of the soft palate (S) to the lateral and posterior pharyngeal walls and is the major intrinsic elevator of the pharynx. e, Epiglottic tip. (From Rubesin, S.E., Jessurun, J., Robertson, D., et al.: Lines of the pharynx. RadioGraphics *7*:217, 1987, with permission.)

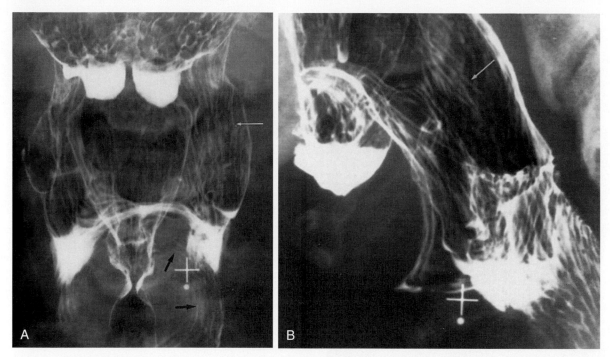

FIGURE 4–6. The squamous mucosa of the pharynx is closely apposed to the innermost layer of muscle. Laterally and posteriorly, the squamous mucosa is separated from the inner longitudinal layer of skeletal muscle by only a thin tunica propria. As a result, longitudinal striations *(white arrow)* appear on images obtained from double contrast pharyngography. Transverse folds *(black arrows)* along the anterior wall of the hypopharynx reflect redundant mucosa overlying the mobile muscular processes of the arytenoid cartilages and the cricoid cartilage. (Reprinted with permission from Rubesin, S.E., and Glick, S.N.: The tailored double-contrast pharyngogram. Crit. Rev. Diagn. Imaging *28*:133, 1988. Copyright CRC Press, Inc., Boca Raton, FL.)

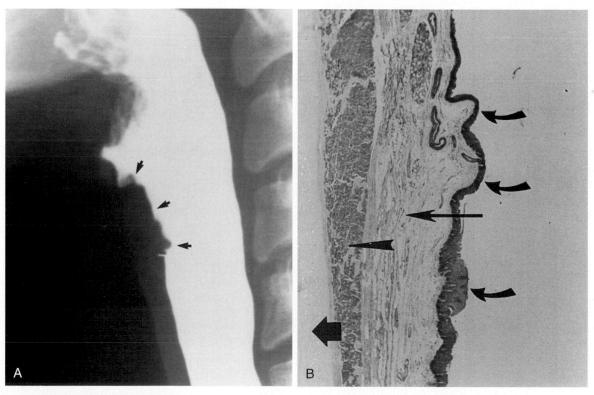

FIGURE 4–7. Redundant folds in the postcricoid region. *A,* During swallowing, redundant mucosa along the anterior wall of the pharyngoesophageal segment is seen as an undulating or plaquelike contour *(arrows)* that changes size and shape with passage of the bolus. *B,* this photomicrograph of the postcricoid mucosa shows undulation of the squamous epithelium *(curved arrows)* above abundant submucosa *(long arrow).* The cricoarytenoid muscle *(arrowhead)* lies anterior to the cricoid cartilage *(large arrow).* As long as prominent postcricoid folds seen on barium studies change size and shape, they are due to redundant mucosa and submucosa in this region. If prominent postcricoid folds do not change size or shape or are semiannular or circumferential in distribution, endoscopy should be performed to rule out a neoplastic or inflammatory stricture. (*A* and *B* from Rubesin, S.E., Jessurun, J., Robertson, D., et al.: Lines of the pharynx. RadioGraphics *7*:217, 1987, with permission.)

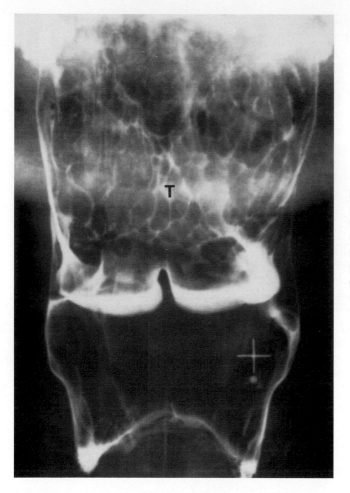

FIGURE 4–8. Lymphoid tissue at the base of the tongue. Normal lymphoid tissue lies at the base of the tongue (T) and appears on the frontal view as numerous round and ovoid lines that are approximately 2 to 4 mm in size. There is no definite criterion identifying normal variant lymphoid tissue versus lingual tonsil lymphoid hyperplasia. (Reprinted with permission from Rubesin, S.E., and Glick, S.N.: The tailored double-contrast pharyngogram. Crit. Rev. Diagn. Imaging *28*:133, 1988. Copyright CRC Press, Inc., Boca Raton, FL.)

TECHNIQUE

The classic upper gastrointestinal examination begins at the level of the aortic arch. The act of swallowing, however, begins at the lips with the volitional carrying of a bolus to the mouth. Furthermore, pharyngeal contraction begins in the pharynx in the region of the superior constrictor. Thus the radiologist is faced with the question, "Where do I start?" Patients with dysphagia, odynophagia, and chest pain should have an examination of both pharynx and esophagus. Patients who have a feeling of "a lump in the throat" need careful examination of the pharynx. Disorders of the pharynx may be manifested by respiratory and speech problems as well as by swallowing dysfunction. Recurrent pneumonia, asthma, chronic bronchitis, coughing, or choking may indicate a pharyngeal disorder. Nasal regurgitation or nasal quality of voice may indicate soft palate insufficiency. Because symptoms poorly reflect the level of a lesion in the pharynx and esophagus, the pharynx should be evaluated even if an esophageal pathologic process is suspected or discovered.[16] Barium studies are also useful in assessing pharyngeal function and morphologic features in patients with a known history of neuromuscular disease, stroke,

pharyngeal tumor, or prior head and neck surgery or radiation. In general, if symptoms are referred to the mouth, neck, or suprasternal region, the radiologist should start with the pharynx. If symptoms are referred to the substernal or epigastric region, the radiologist should start with the esophagus.

Patient Preparation

Good barium coating requires dry pharyngeal mucosa. The patient is therefore instructed not to eat or drink after midnight. Activities that stimulate salivary secretion, such as smoking or chewing tobacco, gum, or throat lozenges, should be avoided. Diabetic patients should not take insulin the morning of the examination.

Plain Films

Contrast examination of the pharynx may be dangerous in patients with suspected airway obstruction, such as those with acute epiglottitis. A plain film of the neck should therefore constitute the initial examination if airway obstruction is suspected. Soft tissue scout-view films are also obtained when a neck mass is palpated or a foreign body, a fistula, an abscess, or perforation is suspected. The double contrast examination, however, obviates the need for plain films in most cases. Radiographic contrast between soft tissue and air is improved when barium coats the pharyngeal mucosa.

Routine Examination

Examination of the pharynx is tailored to the clinical problem and fluoroscopic results.[17,18] The patient should be studied initially in the lateral position because this position is the best for visualizing the entrance of barium into the laryngeal vestibule, either during swallowing (penetration) or during normal breathing (aspiration). A videotape and double contrast spot-film examination are integrated to assess both motility and morphologic characteristics. The general principles of double contrast interpretation are the same in the pharynx as elsewhere in the gastrointestinal tract (see Chapter 2).[9] The examination requires good mucosal coating, an adequate number of projections, and varying degrees of luminal distention.

Mucosal Coating

Adequate mucosal coating relies primarily on (1) dry pharyngeal mucosa and (2) properly prepared barium. A high-density barium (250% w/v) is used. If the barium is too "thin," the barium layer is of insufficient thickness and radiodensity to outline the pharyngeal mucosa. If the barium is too viscous, barium cannot wash mucus off the pharyngeal wall, resulting in artifactual strands of mucus.

Projection

In general, frontal and lateral films suffice for most diagnostic problems. Oblique films, however, help demonstrate the obliquely oriented aryepiglottic folds and the region of the cricopharyngeus.[19-21] The frontal film shows the en face surface features of the base of the tongue, the median and lateral glossoepiglottic folds, and the contours of the palatine fossae, valleculae, and hypopharynx (see Fig. 4–1).

The lateral film (see Fig. 4–1) better examines the palatine fossae en face and the contour of the soft palate, base of the tongue, posterior pharyngeal wall, epiglottis, aryepiglottic folds, and anterior hypopharyngeal wall.[22] The lateral view is crucial for evaluating laryngeal vestibule penetration (Fig. 4–9) and the region of the cricopharyngeus. Oblique views should be performed if the pharyngoesophageal segment is not well seen or if a structural abnormality is suspected or seen at fluoroscopy.[19-21]

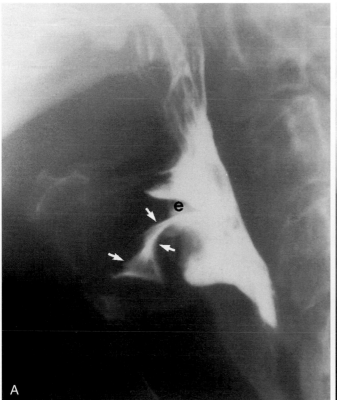
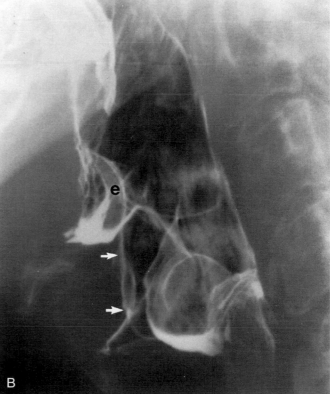

FIGURE 4–9. Laryngeal penetration is defined as barium entering the laryngeal vestibule while the patient is swallowing. Aspiration is defined as barium entering the laryngeal vestibule while the patient is breathing. *A,* Laryngeal penetration is best recorded in the lateral view during videofluoroscopy or cineradiography as barium enters the laryngeal vestibule *(arrows). e,* Epiglottis. *B,* During suspended respiration, barium coats the open laryngeal vestibule *(arrows). e,* Epiglottis.

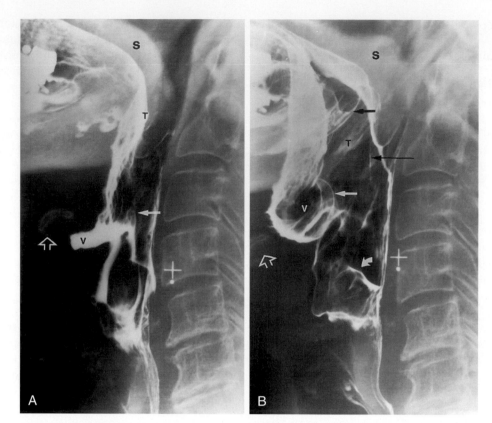

FIGURE 4–10. The effect of phonation. *A,* During suspended respiration the pharynx is partially collapsed. The soft palate (S) apposes the tongue, allowing communication of the nasopharynx and oropharynx. The pharyngoesophageal segment is closed to prevent swallowing of air or reflux of esophageal contents into the hypopharynx. T, Tonsillar fossa; V, valleculae; *open arrow,* hyoid; *solid white arrow,* epiglottic tip. *B,* With phonation (*Eeee . . .*), the hyoid bone *(open arrow)* moves anteriorly and inferiorly, and the tongue moves anteriorly. The soft palate *(S)* elevates, closing the velopharyngeal portal, which prevents the voice from having a nasal quality. These movements result in expansion of the valleculae (V), oropharynx, tonsillar fossa (T), and upper hypopharynx. The pharyngoesophageal segment remains closed. Phonation by *Eeee* results in better visualization of the epiglottic tip *(white arrow),* aryepiglottic folds *(curved white arrow),* tonsillar fossa (T), and base of the tongue. The palatoglossal *(short black arrow)* and palatopharyngeal *(long black arrow)* folds are shown. (From Rubesin, S.E., et al.: Contrast pharyngography: The importance of phonation. AJR Am. J. Roentgenol. *148:*269, 1987, with permission.)

Distention

Adequate distention is crucial for demonstration of mucosal surfaces and contours. Air cannot be generated by effervescent agents, however, or instilled through tube insufflation, as in other regions of the gastrointestinal tract. Instead, pharyngeal distention is achieved either with phonation (long vowel sounds Eee . . . or Ooo . . .)[22] or with some form of modified Valsalva maneuver (Fig. 4–10). Pharyngeal distention results in better visualization of many structures, including the soft palate, tonsillar fossa, epiglottic tip, valleculae, aryepiglottic folds, and asymmetry of the piriform sinus.[22]

POUCHES AND DIVERTICULA
Lateral Pharyngeal Pouches

Lateral pharyngeal pouches are *transient* protrusions of the lateral pharyngeal wall at sites of anatomic weak-ness, such as the posterior thyrohyoid membrane and the tonsillar fossa after tonsillectomy.[23] These pouches are common findings and usually occur as normal variants in asymptomatic patients. Rarely, some patients may complain of dysphagia, which is caused by the late spillage of pouch contents into the pharynx. The upper lateral pharyngeal wall is supported only by the superior constrictor muscle and tonsil. After palatine tonsillectomy or atrophy of the tonsil with age, a transient protrusion may occur at this site. Pouches usually protrude in the upper hypopharyngeal wall near the site of penetration of the thyrohyoid membrane by the superior laryngeal nerve (Fig. 4–11).

Lateral pharyngeal pouches (Fig. 4–12) appear on frontal views as transient, hemispherical protrusions in the upper hypopharynx above the calcified edge of the thyroid cartilage.[14] On lateral views, these pouches are recognized as ovoid barium collections or barium-coated rings in the anterior wall of the upper hypopharynx just below the hyoid bone at the level of the valleculae (see

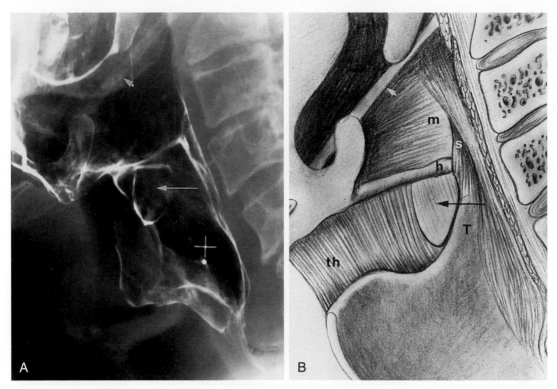

FIGURE 4–11. The lateral pharyngeal pouch *(long arrow)* is bounded superiorly by the hyoid bone (h) and the middle constrictor (m), posteriorly by the stylopharyngeus muscle (s) and the superior cornu of the thyroid cartilage (T), and anteriorly by the thyrohyoid muscle with its overlying thyrohyoid membrane (th). Calcified stylohyoid ligaments are also demonstrated *(short arrow).* (From Rubesin, S.E., Jessurun, J., Robertson, D., et al.: Lines of the pharynx. RadioGraphics *7*:217, 1987, with permission.)

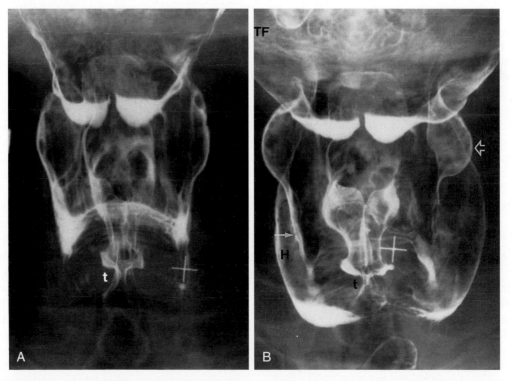

FIGURE 4–12. Lateral pharyngeal pouches. *A,* At the end of quiet inspiration the pharynx is relatively collapsed. The true vocal cords (t) are slightly open. *B,* During a modified Valsalva maneuver, the pharynx and oral cavity expand. The tonsillar fossae (TF) bulge laterally. Right and left lateral pouches are seen as smooth, hemispherical protrusions of the pharynx at the level of the thyrohyoid membrane *(open arrow).* The lateral hypopharyngeal wall (H) protrudes posteriorly around the lateral boundary of the thyroid cartilage *(white arrow).* The epiglottis is well coated. t, True vocal cords.

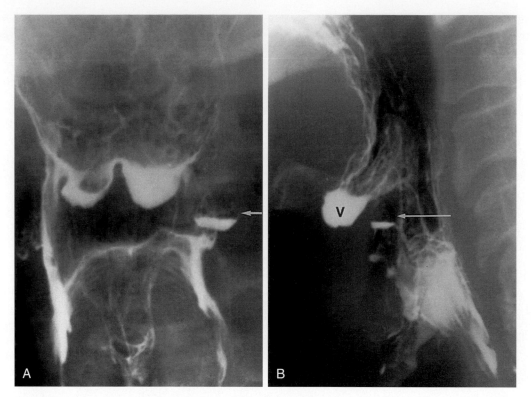

FIGURE 4–13. Lateral pharyngeal diverticulum. A round, barium-filled and air-filled structure *(arrow)* is lateral to the upper hypopharyngeal wall on the frontal view *(A)* and posterior to and at the level of the valleculae (V) on the lateral view *(B)*. (Reprinted with permission from Rubesin, S.E., and Glick, S.N.: The tailored double-contrast pharyngogram. Crit. Rev. Diagn. Imaging *28*:133, 1988. Copyright CRC Press, Inc., Boca Raton, FL.)

Fig. 4–11).[14] They are seen only during swallowing or during periods of increased intrapharyngeal pressure. Lateral pharyngeal pouches disappear at rest.

Lateral pharyngeal diverticula are *persistent* protrusions from the tonsillar fossa or region of the thyrohyoid membrane (Fig. 4–13). These diverticula are much less common than lateral pharyngeal pouches; they frequently occur in individuals who have markedly elevated pharyngeal pressure (glassblowers and wind instrument players).[23]

When stasis occurs in pharyngeal pouches or diverticula, delayed spillage of pouch contents into the hypopharynx after the bolus passes may result in dysphagia or aspiration.[24,25] Lateral pharyngeal diverticula may also appear as neck masses, or they may be sites of ulceration or neoplasia.

Radiographically, lateral pharyngeal diverticula appear as persistent pouches or saccular collections in the region of the posterior thyrohyoid membrane. Barium trapped in the lateral pharyngeal pouch or diverticulum spills into the piriform sinus after the swallow passes. If the volume of barium is large enough, the barium pooling in the piriform sinus will lie at a level above the interarytenoid notch. The barium will be aspirated into the laryngeal vestibule as the patient breathes or will penetrate the laryngeal vestibule during a subsequent swallow. Thus lateral pharyngeal pouches or diverticula that result in as-

piration are usually large, greater than 1 cm in craniocaudad dimension.[25] Overflow aspiration is seen in about 5% of patients with lateral pharyngeal pouches.[25]

Zenker's Diverticulum

Zenker's diverticulum (posterior hypopharyngeal diverticulum) is an acquired mucosal herniation through an area of anatomic weakness in the region of the cricopharyngeus (Killian's dehiscence).[26] This area of anatomic weakness has been variably described as being located between the thyropharyngeus and cricopharyngeus[27] or between the oblique and horizontal fibers of the cricopharyngeal muscle, occurring in approximately one third of people.[28,29] Patients with Zenker's diverticulum complain of dysphagia referred to the suprasternal notch, coughing after swallowing, food regurgitation, and halitosis. Many patients with Zenker's diverticulum have an associated hiatal hernia, gastroesophageal reflux, or both.[30,31] Rarely, these diverticula are complicated by ulceration,[32] fistula formation, bronchiectasis or lung abscess, massive gastrointestinal hemorrhage,[33] bezoar formation,[34] or malignancy.[35,36]

The pathogenesis of Zenker's diverticulum is controversial. Some radiographic and manometric studies suggest that either spasm (elevated pressure of the upper esophageal sphincter [UES]) or incoordination and abnormal relaxation ("achalasia") of the UES occur. Other manometric studies show normal coordination between pharyngeal contraction and relaxation of the UES and a normal resting UES pressure (i.e., there is no spasm).[37,38] The relationship between gastroesophageal reflux disease and Zenker's diverticulum is also controversial. Although most patients with a Zenker's diverticulum have a hiatal hernia and gastroesophageal reflux, whether gastroesophageal reflux predisposes the one third of patients with a large Killian's dehiscence to develop a Zenker's diverticulum is unknown.

During swallowing, in the lateral view, a Zenker's diverticulum appears as a posterior bulge of the distal pharyngeal wall above an anteriorly protruding cricopharyngeus (Fig. 4–14). At rest the barium-filled diverticulum extends below the level of the cricopharyngeus, posterior to the proximal cervical esophagus. In the frontal view the diverticulum lies midline, below the tips of the piriform sinuses. A large diverticulum may protrude to the left, compress the cervical esophagus, or do both.

Barium trapped between a prominent cricopharyngeus and the pharyngeal contraction wave may mimic Zenker's diverticulum. This small, trapped barium collection is termed a pseudo-Zenker's diverticulum (Fig. 4–15). The radiographic clues to differentiating true Zenker's diverticulum from pseudo-Zenker's diverticulum are (1) that the pseudo-Zenker's diverticulum is small and does not protrude from the expected contour of the posterior pharyngeal wall and (2) that the pseudo-Zenker's diverticulum disappears after the pharyngeal peristaltic wave passes the pharyngoesophageal segment.

Lateral Cervical Esophageal Pouches and Diverticula (Killian-Jamieson Pouches and Diverticula)

Another area of anatomic weakness lies just below the attachment of the cricopharyngeus on the cricoid cartilage, lateral to the insertion of the suspensory ligament of the esophagus on the cricoid cartilage. This area is known as the Killian-Jamieson space. Proximal cervical esophageal protrusions in this region are known as lateral cervical esophageal pouches or diverticula (also known as Killian-Jamieson pouches or diverticula for the space they protrude through). Radiographically, these pouches or diverticula are seen on the anterolateral wall of the proximal cervical esophagus just below the level of the cricopharyngeus (Fig. 4–16).[39] The pouches are more often bilateral than unilateral. During fluoroscopy, a unilateral diverticulum may be confused with Zenker's diverticulum.

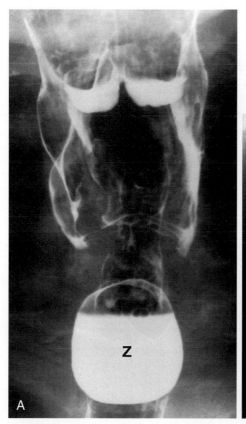
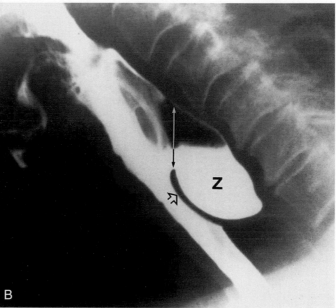

FIGURE 4–14. Zenker's diverticulum. *A,* The frontal view of the pharynx shows a barium-filled saccular structure (Z) in the midline, below the level of the hypopharynx. *B,* In the lateral view during midswallow, the Zenker's diverticulum (Z) appears as a barium-filled collection behind the posterior wall of the pharyngoesophageal segment *(open arrow)* and proximal cervical esophagus. Note the large opening *(double arrow)* into the Zenker's diverticulum seen during swallowing. (From Rubesin S.E.: Pharyngeal dysfunction. *In* Gore, R.M. (ed.): Categorical Course on Gastrointestinal Radiology. Reston, VA, American College of Radiology, 1991;1–9, with permission.)

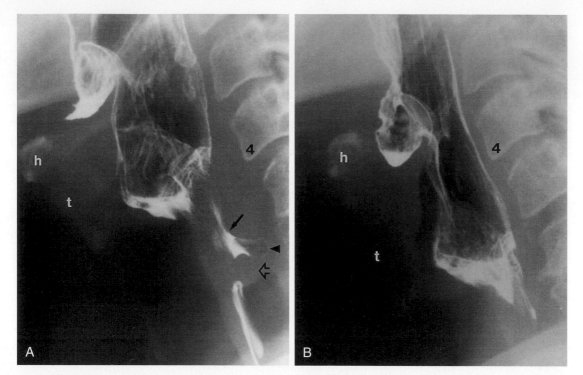

FIGURE **4–15. Pseudo-Zenker's diverticulum.** *A,* There is a small saclike collection of barium *(arrowhead)* above a prominent cricopharyngeus *(open arrow).* Note that this collection is not a true diverticulum, but rather air and barium trapped between the pharyngeal peristaltic wave in the inferior constrictor *(arrow)* and the prominent cricopharyngeus. The pseudo-Zenker's diverticulum does not protrude posteriorly in relation to the expected pharyngeal contour. Note that this film has been taken near the end of a swallow. The epiglottis has returned to the upright position, but laryngeal elevation and thyrohyoid apposition are still occurring. The laryngeal vestibule is just beginning to open. Peristalsis is just about to pass the cricopharyngeus. 4, Fourth cervical vertebra; h, hyoid bone; t, thyroid cartilage. *B,* After the swallow, the pseudo-Zenker's diverticulum has disappeared. The larynx and pharynx are no longer elevated. The thyroid cartilage (t) and hyoid bone (h) have returned to their resting locations.

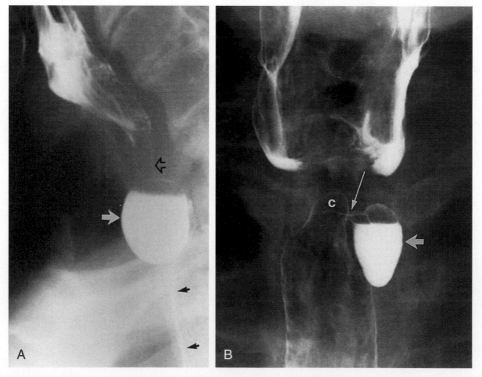

FIGURE **4–16. Lateral cervical esophageal diverticulum (Killian-Jamieson diverticulum).** *A,* On the lateral view, a round, barium-filled sac *(white arrow)* with an air-fluid level is seen just below the level of the pharyngoesophageal segment *(open arrow).* A radiographic clue that this diverticulum is not a Zenker's diverticulum is that the pouch protrudes anteriorly in relation to the cervical esophagus *(black arrows). B,* The frontal view shows that the origin *(long arrow)* of the Killian-Jamieson diverticulum *(short, thick arrow)* is in the proximal cervical esophagus (c) along the lateral wall.

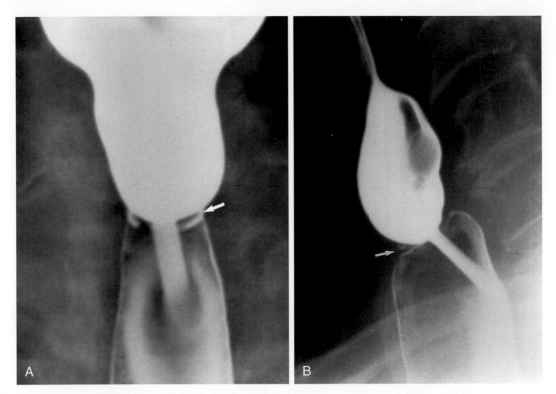

FIGURE 4–17. Cervical esophageal web. Frontal *(A)* and lateral *(B)* views during swallowing show a thin, 1-mm, radiolucent bar *(arrow)* encircling the cervical esophagus approximately 3 cm below the pharyngoesophageal junction. A jet of barium spurts through the center of the bar. Obstruction is implied by the jet phenomenon and proximal esophageal dilation.

WEBS

Hypopharyngeal and cervical esophageal webs are thin folds composed of mucosa and submucosa.[40] Radiographically, webs appear as shelflike filling defects that are 1 to 2 mm in width and that are seen along the anterior wall of the lower hypopharynx, pharyngoesophageal segment, or proximal cervical esophagus (Fig. 4–17).[40–43] Occasionally, webs are circumferential. Partial obstruction is suggested by a jet phenomenon[44,45] or by dilation of the esophagus or pharynx proximal to the web. Webs may be confused with redundant mucosa in the anterior wall of the hypopharynx at the level of the cricoid cartilage.[14] This "postcricoid defect" has been attributed to a venous plexus in the region,[46] but it more likely represents redundant mucosa (see Fig. 4–7).[14] Webs in the valleculae may be normal variants[47] or the sequelae of prior inflammation.

Most cervical esophageal webs are asymptomatic isolated findings seen in about 10% of patients. Some webs are associated with diseases of the esophagus that cause scarring, such as epidermolysis bullosa[48] or benign mucous membrane pemphigoid. Some cervical esophageal webs may be due to gastroesophageal reflux. The association between cervical esophageal webs and iron deficiency anemia, termed the Plummer-Vinson or Paterson-Kelly syndrome, is controversial.[42,43,46,49] In some countries this syndrome may be a premalignant condition associated with pharyngeal or esophageal carcinoma. In the United States, however, there is no association between webs and carcinoma.

INFLAMMATORY DISORDERS

Barium studies of the pharynx are usually of limited value in patients with acute sore throat due to viral, bacterial, or fungal infection.[50] Such patients have normal pharyngograms or nonspecific lymphoid hyperplasia of the palatine or lingual tonsils. A double contrast examination of the pharynx, however, may demonstrate the plaques of *Candida* pharyngitis (Fig. 4–18) or the ulcers of herpes pharyngitis, particularly in immunosuppressed patients or in patients with AIDS.[17] Barium studies may also be helpful in detecting underlying gastroesophageal reflux or reflux esophagitis in patients who have chronic sore throat.

Pharyngeal dysmotility is common in patients with marked gastroesophageal reflux or severe acute pharyngitis. Severe or long-standing inflammatory disorders of the pharynx can alter pharyngeal elevation, epiglottic tilt, or closure of the vocal cords and laryngeal vestibule. Thus pharyngeal dysmotility due to a local inflammatory process may result in laryngeal penetration.

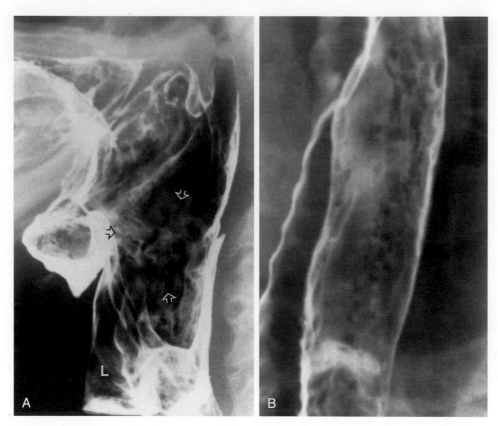

FIGURE 4–18. *Candida* **pharyngitis and esophagitis.** *A,* Lateral view of the pharynx during phonation shows multiple, irregular, 2- to 4-mm nodules *(arrows)* in the oropharynx and in the tonsillar fossa. Barium coating the laryngeal vestibule (L) and trachea reflects the motility disorder associated with severe pharyngeal inflammation. *B,* A coned-down view of the mid-esophagus shows multiple small, well-circumscribed plaques aligned longitudinally along the mucosal folds.

Lymphoid Hyperplasia

Lymphoid hyperplasia of the palatine tonsil or base of the tongue is associated with aging, chronic infections, or allergic states.[15] In addition, lymphoid hyperplasia may be a compensatory response after tonsillectomy.

In lymphoid hyperplasia of the lingual tonsil, multiple smooth, round or ovoid nodules are seen along the vertical surface of the tongue (Fig. 4–19).[15] With severe lymphoid hyperplasia, nodules may extend into the valleculae or piriform sinuses. The nodules of lymphoid hyperplasia are usually small, less than 5 mm in diameter, uniform, and symmetrically distributed. In contrast, the nodules of a pharyngeal carcinoma are large, irregular, and associated with a focal mass and obliteration of the normal mucosal contour. Lymphoid hyperplasia can occasionally appear as a polypoid mass of the base of the tongue and may be confused with a carcinoma of the base of the tongue.[15]

Other Inflammatory Disorders

A wide variety of disorders cause acute ulceration in the pharynx in patients who are not immunosuppressed. Barium studies, however, are not performed in these patients. Some of these disorders cause chronic inflammation or scarring, leading to distortion of pharyngeal contours, am-

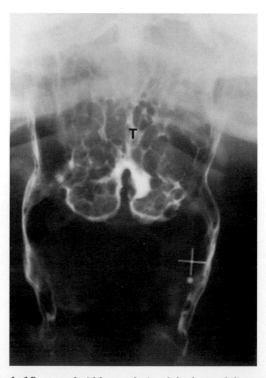

FIGURE 4–19. Lymphoid hyperplasia of the base of the tongue. A frontal view of the pharynx shows many 4- to 8-mm round/ovoid nodules uniformly distributed on the base of the tongue (T).

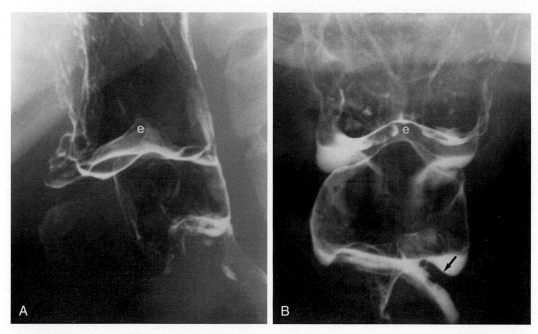

FIGURE **4–20.** **Corrosive ingestion.** *A,* Twenty years after the patient swallowed a corrosive agent (in this case, aqueous sodium hydroxide), the spot radiograph shows amputation of the epiglottic tip (e). *B,* The epiglottis is seen en face as a truncated, fixed structure. The median glossoepiglottic fold is broadened. The piriform sinuses are asymmetric because of scarring with a broad web *(arrow)* crossing the inferior left hypopharynx.

putation of the epiglottis, or pharyngeal dysmotility. Severe chronic inflammatory conditions include epidermolysis bullosa, benign mucous membrane pemphigoid,[18] and the sequelae of corrosive ingestion (Fig. 4–20).[51]

Infections related to branchial cleft cysts or branchial pouch fistulas often become symptomatic in adults 20 to

40 years of age (Fig. 4–21), as a fluctuant mass along the anterior border of the sternocleidomastoid muscle.[52,53] Branchial pouch sinuses arise from the tonsillar fossa (second pouch), upper anterolateral piriform fossa (third pouch), or lower anterolateral piriform fossa (fourth pouch).[54]

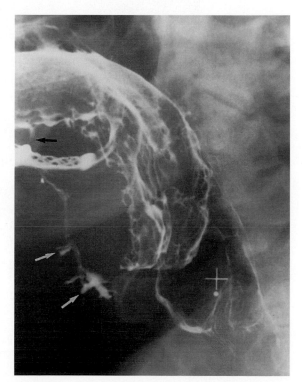

FIGURE **4–21.** **Second branchial pouch sinus.** A steep oblique view of the pharynx shows a sinus tract *(arrows)* arising in the retromolar trigone region just anterior to the tonsillar fossa. The tract extends inferiorly toward the hyoid bone. (Reprinted with permission from Rubesin, S.E., and Glick, S.N.: The tailored double-contrast pharyngogram. Crit. Rev. Diagn. Imaging *28*:133, 1988. Copyright CRC Press, Inc., Boca Raton, FL.)

DOUBLE CONTRAST MANIFESTATIONS OF PHARYNGEAL DYSMOTILITY

Review of double contrast spot films before review of the dynamic study aids in the interpretation of the videofluoroscopic images. Static radiographic signs of dysmotility are many. A coating of high-density barium on the laryngeal vestibule or vocal cords indicates penetration or aspiration. Barium coating of the posterior nasopharyngeal wall above the level of the soft palate indicates nasal regurgitation.[55] Excessive pooling of contrast agent in the valleculae or piriform sinuses may reflect unilateral or bilateral weakness. Smooth-surfaced, changeable asymmetry of the valleculae or lateral pharyngeal walls on the frontal view may indicate unilateral pharyngeal weakness. Excessive ballooning of the pharynx during the Valsalva maneuver may also indicate pharyngeal muscular weakness (Fig. 4–22). Distention of the normally tonically contracted pharyngoesophageal segment during the Valsalva maneuver also indicates muscular weakness (see Fig. 4–22). Rotation of the epiglottis may give it an asymmetric or a bulbous appearance on the lateral view.[56] A "ptotic" or posteriorly protruding epiglottis at rest may reflect epiglottic dysmotility.

BENIGN TUMORS

Whatever the underlying histologic characteristics, a benign pharyngeal tumor usually appears en face as a smooth, round, sharply circumscribed mass and in profile as a hemispheric line with acute angulation.[17] The most common benign lesions are retention cysts of the valleculae (Fig. 4–23) or aryepiglottic folds (Fig. 4–24).[57] Aryepiglottic fold cysts are usually filled with mucoid secretions, arising from the mucus-secreting glands of the saccule or appendix of the laryngeal ventricle.[57] Laryngoceles are expansions of the laryngeal ventricular apex or saccule into the submucosal portion of the anteroinferior aryepiglottic folds.[58–60] They are filled with air, fluid, or both. Laryngoceles do not communicate with the pharynx. True benign tumors include rare lipomas,[61] hamartomas,[62] and neural[63] and cartilaginous tumors.[64]

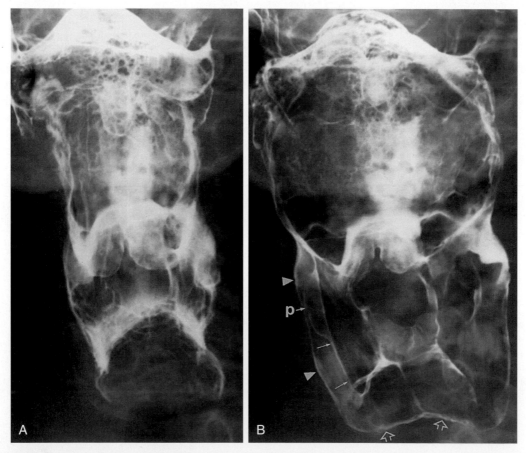

FIGURE 4–22. Ballooning of the pharynx due to muscle weakness. *A,* During suspended respiration in the supine position, the pharynx shows barium pooling along the posterior pharyngeal wall. *B,* During phonation, excessive distention of the pharynx occurs. The lateral pharyngeal walls *(arrowheads)* protrude laterally beyond the confines of the thyroid cartilage *(solid arrows)* and even beyond the anterolaterally located lateral pharyngeal pouch (P). The lower hypopharynx is usually collapsed, even during a Valsalva maneuver. In this patient, however, the lower hypopharynx is distended *(open arrows).* This distention is a sign of pharyngeal muscle weakness or hypotonicity.

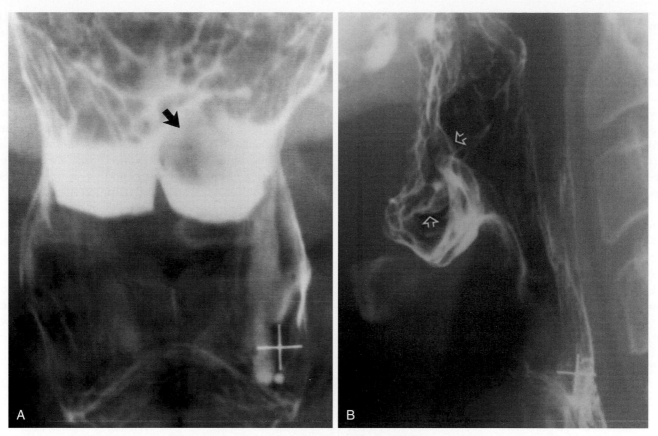

FIGURE **4–23. Retention cyst of the left vallecula.** The frontal view *(A)* shows a subtle filling defect *(arrow)* in the barium pool in the left vallecula. The lateral view *(B)* shows a smooth hemispheric line *(arrows)* protruding posteriorly in relation to the base of the tongue and partially obscured by the tip of the epiglottis.

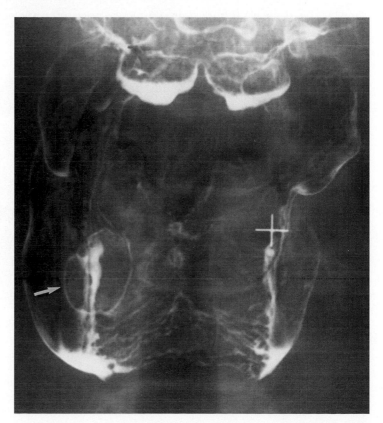

FIGURE **4–24. Squamous retention cyst in mucosa overlying muscular process right arytenoid cartilage.** A spot radiograph obtained during a modified Valsalva maneuver shows a well-circumscribed, smooth-surfaced mass *(arrow)* in the mucosa overlying the muscular process of the right arytenoid cartilage. This lesion was missed on the first endoscopic examination. (Reprinted with permission from Rubesin, S.E., and Glick, S.N.: The tailored double-contrast pharyngogram. Crit. Rev. Diagn. Imaging *28*:133, 1988. Copyright CRC Press, Inc., Boca Raton, FL.)

MALIGNANT TUMORS

Double contrast radiographs of the pharynx can accurately define the intraluminal size, level, and extent of a mucosal lesion. The radiologic examination demonstrates regions of the pharynx (the valleculae, lower hypopharynx, and cricopharyngeus) that are difficult to visualize by indirect examination or during endoscopy.[65,66] Although its accuracy is limited in the region of the palatine tonsil, the double contrast examination detects more than 95% of mucosal neoplasms in the pharynx below the level of the pharyngoepiglottic fold.[67]

In patients with known pharyngeal carcinoma, barium studies are also helpful for detecting separate, coexisting carcinomas of the pharynx or esophagus. About 10% of the patients with squamous cell carcinomas of the head and neck develop a second primary lesion,[68] and 1% develop synchronous or metachronous carcinomas of the esophagus.[69,70]

The most important radiographic signs of pharyngeal carcinoma are (1) intraluminal mass, (2) loss of distensi-

bility, and (3) mucosal irregularity (Fig. 4–25).[17,50] An intraluminal mass may be depicted by obliteration of the normal pharyngeal contour, barium-coated lines in an unusual location or shape, a filling defect in the barium pool, or a superimposed radiodensity. Loss of distensibility of a portion of the pharynx may indicate direct invasion by infiltrative tumor or neural damage. Tumors may have a lobulated, finely nodular, granular, or irregular mucosal surface texture. Pharyngeal carcinomas may also impair pharyngeal motility or cause stasis, resulting in laryngeal penetration or aspiration (see Fig. 4–25). Soft palate tumors may cause reflux of contents from the oropharynx into the nasopharynx (Fig. 4–26).[71]

Squamous cell carcinomas are by far the most common malignant tumor of the pharynx.[72] The overall 5-year survival rate is approximately 20%, a somewhat better prognosis than esophageal carcinoma.[60,73,74] Squamous cell carcinomas of the pharynx vary slightly in radiographic appearance and prognosis, depending on their location. Classification of tumors of the pharynx and larynx is confusing. Although the supraglottic laryngeal struc-

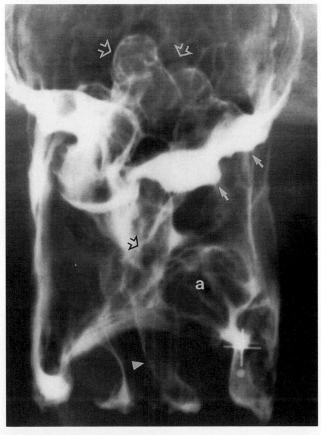

FIGURE 4–25. Radiographic findings in pharyngeal malignancy. A frontal view of the pharynx demonstrates the radiographic findings of malignancy: intraluminal mass, asymmetry and loss of distensibility, and mucosal irregularity. A large, lobulated mass replaces the normally smooth contour of the epiglottis *(open white arrows)*. Tumor extension into the left vallecula and pharyngoepiglottic fold is indicated by flattening and lobulation of the vallecular contour *(small arrows)*. Tumor extending down the laryngeal vestibule is seen as nodular mucosa en face *(open black arrow)*. Extension into the left false vocal cord is indicated by mass effect and an irregular mucosa of the left false cord *(arrowhead)*. Lobulation of the contour and mucosal irregularity of the mucosa overlying the muscular process of the arytenoid (a) can be seen. The left hypopharyngeal wall is less distensible than the right. Note the stasis of barium in the asymmetric left vallecula and the coating of the laryngeal vestibule due to laryngeal penetration. (Reprinted with permission from Rubesin, S.E., and Glick, S.N.: The tailored double-contrast pharyngogram. Crit. Rev. Diagn. Imaging *28*:133, 1988. Copyright CRC Press, Inc., Boca Raton, FL.)

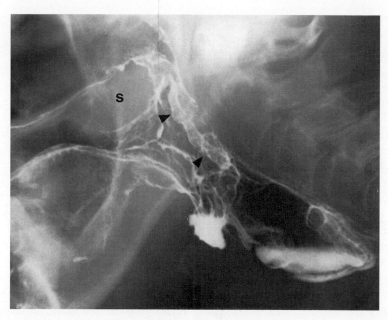

FIGURE 4–26. Soft palate and oropharyngeal carcinoma causing nasal regurgitation. A large tumor involves the soft palate and the posterolateral oropharyngeal wall. The soft palate (S) is enlarged with an irregular contour. The posterior pharyngeal wall has a lobulated contour *(arrowheads).* Irregular lines and nodules in the region of the tonsillar fossae also indicate tumor spread.

tures are part of the hypopharynx and are derived from pharyngobuccal anlage, supraglottic tumors confined by the aryepiglottic folds are classified as laryngeal carcinomas. Thus tumors of the false vocal cords, laryngeal surface of the epiglottis (Fig. 4–27), aryepiglottic fold, arytenoid cartilage, and ventricles are defined as laryngeal.

These supraglottic carcinomas are associated with approximately a 40% 5-year survival rate and often show early invasion of the preepiglottic space and lymph node metastasis.[50]

The palatine tonsil is the most common site of squamous cell carcinoma arising in the pharynx.[72] Bulky, exo-

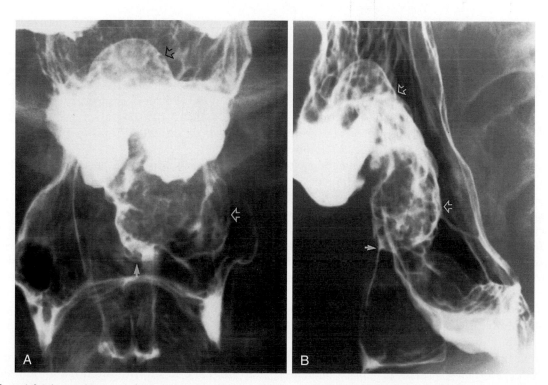

FIGURE 4–27. Epiglottic carcinoma. A frontal view *(A)* shows a nodular surface of the epiglottic tip *(black arrow)* and medial and lateral expansion of the left aryepiglottic fold *(open white arrow).* The lateral view *(B)* shows a mass *(open arrows)* involving the epiglottic tip and the superior portion of the anterior wall of the laryngeal vestibule *(arrow).* The anterior commissure is normal.

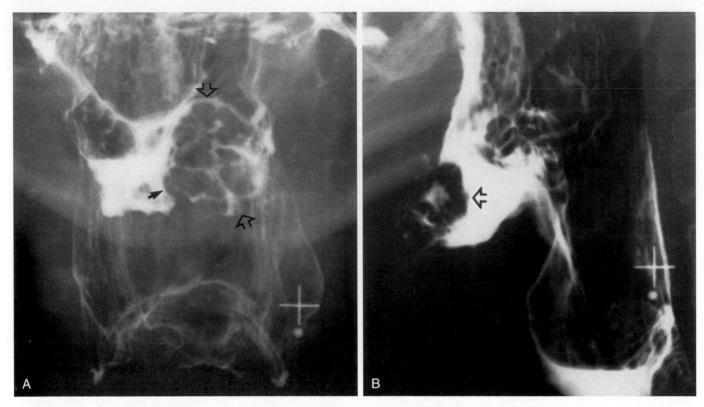

FIGURE 4–28. Carcinoma of the base of the tongue. *A,* The frontal view shows obliteration of the normal contour of the left vallecula and lateral glossoepiglottic fold. Irregular nodular mucosa is seen in the region of the left vallecula *(open arrows).* The median glossoepiglottic fold is deviated to the right *(solid arrow). B,* The lateral view shows a polypoid mass *(open arrow)* in the vallecula with barium tracks extending deep to the expected contour of the base of the tongue. (Reprinted with permission from Rubesin, S.E., and Glick, S.N.: The tailored double-contrast pharyngogram. Crit. Rev. Diagn. Imaging *28*:133, 1988. Copyright CRC Press, Inc., Boca Raton, FL.)

phytic tumors are easily detected radiographically. However, infiltrative tumors may be obscured by the nodular mucosa overlying the lymphoid tissue of the tonsillar fossa.

Carcinomas of the base of the tongue are usually clinically silent until they are advanced lesions with 70% lymph node metastasis. The 5-year survival rate approaches 15% to 40%.[75] Polypoid tumors project posteriorly from the base of the tongue (Fig. 4–28). Ulcerative tumors are seen as an irregular contrast collection extending anteriorly to disrupt the normal contour of the tongue.

Carcinomas of the piriform sinus metastasize early and are associated with 70% to 80% lymph node metastasis to the jugular chain at the time of diagnosis (Fig. 4–29).[73] Piriform sinus carcinomas are usually bulky and exophytic growths. Medial wall tumors infiltrate the aryepiglottic folds, arytenoid and cricoid cartilages, and the paraglottic space. Lateral wall tumors infiltrate the thyrohyoid membrane, thyroid cartilage, and soft tissue of the neck, including the carotid artery. Five-year survival of piriform sinus carcinomas is approximately 20% to 40%. Medial wall lesions have a better prognosis than lateral tumors because they present earlier with vocal cord and swallowing symptoms.

Posterior pharyngeal wall carcinomas are usually advanced when first seen, often presenting as a neck mass due to lymph node metastasis to the retropharyngeal or jugular chain. Posterior pharyngeal wall carcinomas have approximately a 20% 5-year survival rate.[50] These tumors are best seen on lateral films as large, fungating masses (Fig. 4–30).

Carcinomas arising in the region of the pharyngoesophageal segment (postcricoid carcinomas) are uncommon, except in Scandinavia. These tumors appear radiographically as annular, infiltrating lesions (Fig. 4–31). Postcricoid carcinomas may be difficult to detect while the pharyngoesophageal segment is constricted during suspended respiration or phonation. These lesions are best detected during swallowing, while a full column of barium distends the pharyngoesophageal segment.

Instillation of intranasal barium may be helpful in discovering or defining nasopharyngeal carcinomas (Fig. 4–32) or tumors of the soft palate.[76]

Lymphomas comprise 15% of oropharyngeal tumors and originate in the lymphoid tissue of Waldeyer's ring

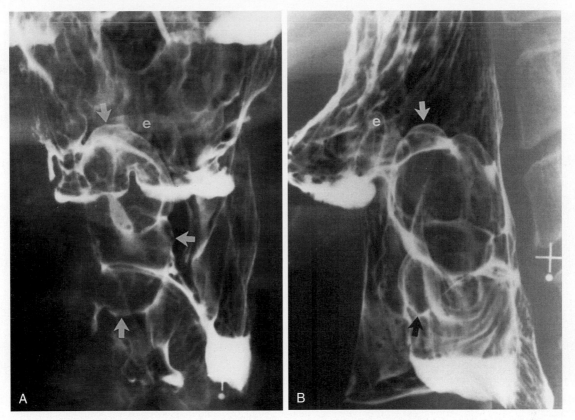

FIGURE 4–29. Carcinoma of the hypopharynx. A large polypoid tumor *(arrows)* obliterates the right hypopharyngeal wall and invades the right aryepiglottic fold and laryngeal vestibule. The contours of the epiglottic tip (e) and valleculae are preserved. (Reprinted with permission from Rubesin, S.E., and Glick, S.N.: The tailored double-contrast pharyngogram. Crit. Rev. Diagn. Imaging *28*:133, 1988. Copyright CRC Press, Inc., Boca Raton, FL.)

FIGURE 4–30. Carcinoma of the posterior pharyngeal wall. A large lobulated mass *(arrows)* involves the posterior oropharyngeal and hypopharyngeal walls. Note stasis in the valleculae and hypopharynx and barium coating of the laryngeal vestibule and trachea. a, Mucosa over muscular processes of arytenoid cartilages. (Reprinted with permission from Rubesin, S.E., and Glick, S.N.: The tailored double-contrast pharyngogram. Crit. Rev. Diagn. Imaging *28*:133, 1988. Copyright CRC Press, Inc., Boca Raton, FL.)

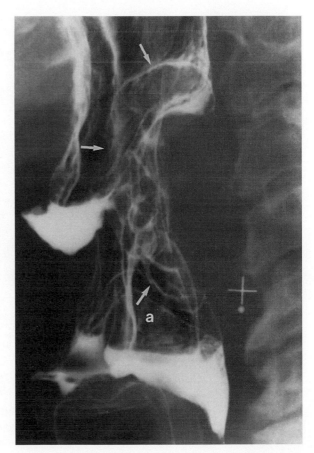

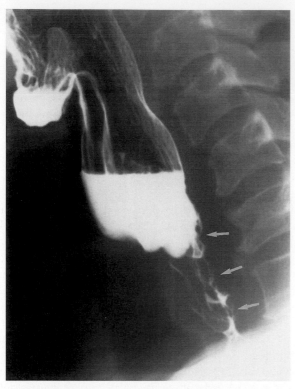

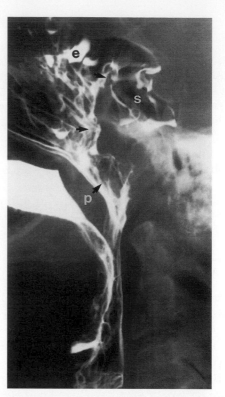

FIGURE 4–31. Postcricoid carcinoma. Lobulated mucosa and an irregular contour of the pharyngoesophageal segment are seen *(arrows).* (From Levine, M.S., et al.: Update on esophageal radiology. AJR Am. J. Roentgenol. *155*:993, 1990, with permission, © by American Roentgen Ray Society.)

FIGURE 4–32. Squamous cell carcinoma of the nasopharynx. A large lobulated mass involves the posterior nasopharyngeal wall *(arrows)* and extends into the sphenoid sinus and posterior ethmoidal sinus. Opacification of the posterior ethmoidal sinus (e) and sphenoid sinus (s) is present. The soft palate is identified (p).

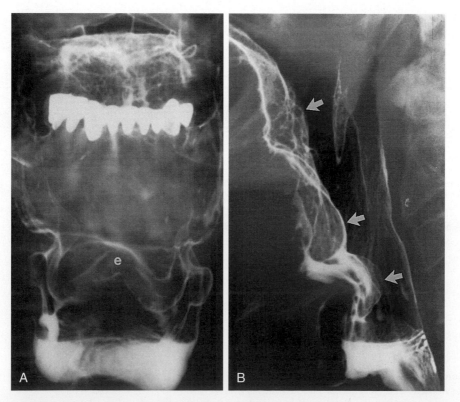

FIGURE 4–33. Lymphoma involving the tongue and epiglottis. The frontal *(A)* and lateral *(B)* views of the pharynx show a relatively smooth-surfaced mass *(arrows)* involving the base of the tongue and epiglottis. The frontal view shows obliteration of the normal surface features of the base of the tongue, resulting in a nearly smooth surface because of the submucosal location of the tumor.

distributed throughout the submucosa of the pharynx.[77,78] Almost all pharyngeal lymphomas are non-Hodgkins lymphoma, arising in the palatine tonsil (40% to 60%), nasopharynx (18% to 28%), and base of tongue (10%).[77,78] These tumors are manifested radiographically by masses with lobulated contours and a variably nodular or smooth mucosal surface (Fig. 4–33).[18]

Rare pharyngeal malignancies include adenoid cystic carcinoma,[79] Kaposi's sarcoma, synovial sarcoma,[80] melanoma,[81] and malignancies arising in minor salivary glands.[82]

TRAUMA AND RADIATION CHANGES

Contrast pharyngography may be helpful in evaluation of iatrogenic and other forms of trauma. Perforation of the pharynx usually occurs at the base of the piriform sinuses or in a Zenker's diverticulum. Thus the region of the pharyngoesophageal segment must be examined carefully. Blunt trauma to the neck may result in a hematoma of the larynx or pharynx (Fig. 4–34). If laryngeal penetration is suspected, barium or a nonionic water-soluble contrast agent should be used to demonstrate a leak into the soft tissue of the neck. If no laryngeal penetration is suspected, a water-soluble contrast is used, followed by barium if no leak is seen.

Squamous cell carcinoma of the head and neck may be treated and cured with radiotherapy. Acute mucositis and submucosal edema subside within 2 to 6 weeks after cessation of radiation therapy. Some postradiation therapy patients, however, have persistent symptoms because of submucosal edema or fibrosis. Pharyngography is used to evaluate patients with persistent or recurrent symptoms of dysphagia, odynophagia, hoarseness, and aspiration.[83–86] Late severe complications include chondronecrosis, osteomyelitis, or recurrent cancer.

Diffuse, symmetric swelling of the mucosa and submucosa of the pharynx occurs in the region of the radiation portal, manifested radiographically as smooth enlargement of the epiglottis.[50] Edema of the mucosa overlying the muscular processes of the arytenoid cartilages results in elevation of the mucosa over the cartilages. Arytenoid cartilage enlargement may be asymmetric with more enlargement occurring on the side of the tumor. The lumen of the laryngeal vestibule may be narrowed (Fig. 4–35). Dynamic examination may show diminished motility with one or more of the following signs: impairment of epiglottic tilt, paresis of the constrictor musculature, or diminished closure of the laryngeal vestibule.[83] Thus diminished motility may result in laryngeal penetration or aspiration. Mucosal irregularity, ulceration, nodularity, or a focal mass suggests tumor recurrence.

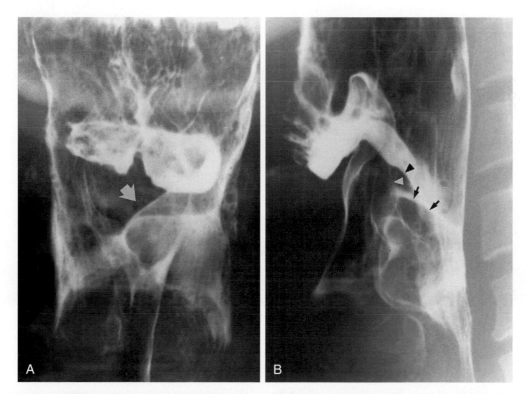

FIGURE 4–34. Hematoma following motor vehicle accident. Three days after a neck contusion, the patient complained of coughing. A frontal view *(A)* shows asymmetry and elevation of smooth mucosa overlying the muscular process of the left arytenoid cartilage *(arrow).* The lateral view *(B)* shows asymmetry of the aryepiglottic folds *(arrowheads),* elevation of mucosa overlying the muscular process of the left arytenoid cartilage *(arrows),* and barium coating the laryngeal vestibule. A hematoma overlying the muscular process of the arytenoid cartilage and the left aryepiglottic fold was seen during endoscopy.

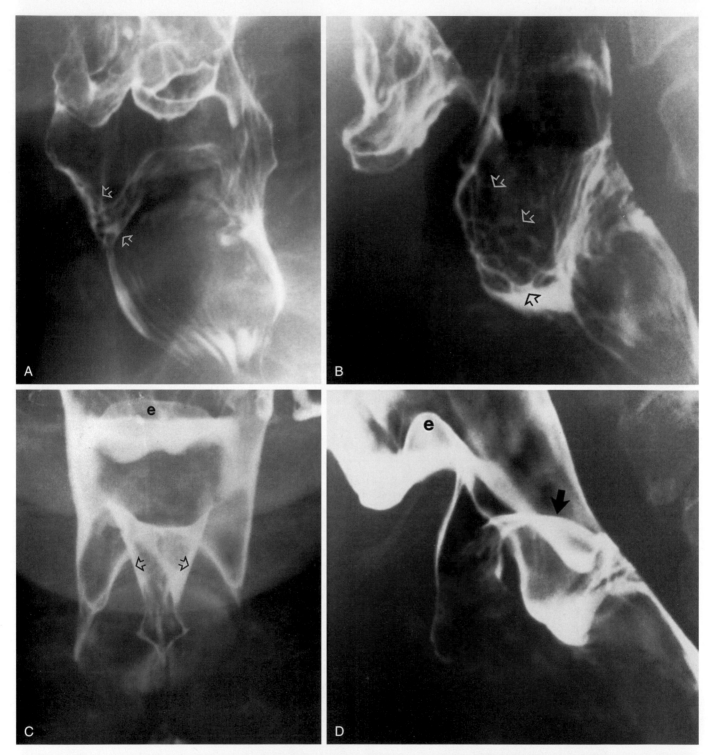

FIGURE 4–35. Early squamous cell carcinoma of the hypopharynx treated by radiotherapy. Slight oblique *(A)* and lateral *(B)* views show finely lobulated mucosa involving the anterolateral wall of the right piriform sinus *(arrows)*. The small nodules are nonuniform in size, are irregularly shaped, and cause mild lobulation of the contour. On biopsy, this squamous cell carcinoma invaded the submucosa. Nine months after radiotherapy, the nodularity in the right piriform sinus has disappeared, and the mucosa is now smooth (*C* and *D*). The epiglottis (e) is enlarged, with a bulbous shape and a smooth surface. Pooling of barium can be seen in the valleculae. The valleculae also have a flattened, smooth contour. The mucosa overlying the muscular processes of the arytenoid cartilages (*solid arrow* in *D*) is elevated, though smooth. Laryngeal penetration has occurred. The laryngeal vestibule appears smooth and narrowed (*open arrows* in *C*). Thus the squamous cell carcinoma has regressed, but changes from radiotherapy remain. (*A* and *B*, From Levine, M.S., et al.: Update on esophageal radiology. AJR Am. J. Roentgenol. *155*:993, 1990, with permission, © by American Roentgen Ray Society.)

POSTOPERATIVE CHANGES

Total Laryngectomy

Tumors of the larynx that extend into the laryngeal cartilages, extend more than 10 mm into the subepiglottic region, or cause vocal cord paralysis may be treated by total laryngectomy.[87,88] Total laryngectomy may also be performed when prior laryngeal conservation surgery has failed because of recurrent neoplasm or because of glottic insufficiency resulting in recurrent aspiration.

During total laryngectomy, the hyoid bone, thyroid and cricoid cartilages, and epiglottis are removed. The aryepiglottic folds and piriform fossae are removed, resulting in a defect of the anterior wall of the hypopharynx. The constrictor muscles are incised, resulting in retraction of the thyropharyngeus and cricopharyngeus. If there is insufficient mucosa to form a neopharyngeal tube, a graft (free flap, myocutaneous, or cutaneous) may be used. A radical neck dissection may be performed at the same time for enlarged cervical lymph nodes or for piriform sinus tumors that show early nodal spread.[87]

Radiographically, the resultant neopharyngeal tube resembles an inverted cone with smooth mucosa (Fig. 4–36). The hyoid bone, epiglottis, aryepiglottic folds, and piriform sinuses are absent. The neopharyngeal tube has a 1- to 2.5-cm luminal diameter and is 0.5 to 1 cm anterior to the anterior margin of the C3–C5 vertebral bodies. Oc-

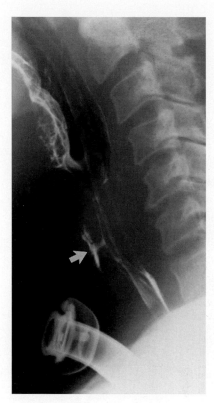

FIGURE 4–37. Pharyngocutaneous fistula following supraglottic laryngectomy. A lateral view shows a barium-filled tract along the junction line of the neopharyngeal tube *(arrow).*

casionally, there is sharp angulation or outpouching at the base of the tongue at the upper surgical line of closure. An abrupt transition to the cervical esophagus may be seen. A small cricopharyngeal impression may be noted. The pharynx should not be deviated from the midline more than approximately 0.5 cm.[87]

In the early postoperative period the complications of laryngectomy include formation of fistula, abscess, and edema with obstruction. Late complications following laryngectomy include stricture formation, dysphagia due to retracted constrictor muscles, and tumor recurrence.

Pharyngocutaneous Fistulae

Pharyngocutaneous fistulae occur in approximately 6% to 21% of patients following laryngectomy, usually in the immediate postoperative period.[87,89–91] If a pharyngocutaneous fistula occurs later, it may signify recurrent tumor. Fistulae usually develop along the anterior aspect of the neopharyngeal tube, at the base of the tongue, along the margin of a graft, or near the tracheostomy (Fig. 4–37). Fistulae may extend onto the skin or end blindly in the soft tissues of the neck. It is controversial whether preoperative irradiation of the neck may[91] or may not[90] increase the risk of postoperative fistula formation.

Benign Strictures

Luminal narrowing to a diameter of less than 5 mm is considered a postoperative stricture.[87] Benign strictures

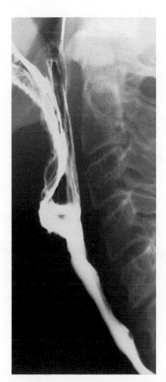

FIGURE 4–36. Radiographic changes following total laryngectomy. The normal features of the pharynx are not apparent. The epiglottis, piriform fossae, and aryepiglottic folds are not seen. The hyoid bone is missing. The neopharynx appears as a relatively featureless tube. Mild sacculation of the junction between the base of the tongue and neopharynx is seen, and there is mild nasal regurgitation.

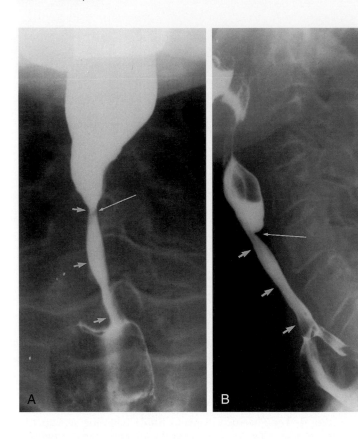

FIGURE **4–38. Stricture following total laryngectomy.** A diffuse, smooth narrowing *(short arrows)* of most of the neopharyngeal tube can be seen. The luminal diameter measures less than 5 mm. A short web *(long arrow)* is present at the proximal margin of the stricture.

following laryngectomy appear (1) as short, weblike narrowings less than 5 mm long at the upper or lower ends of the closure line or (2) as long, smooth, tapered symmetric narrowings greater than 3 cm long involving most of the neopharynx (Fig. 4–38). Pharyngeal luminal narrowings of intermediate length (1 to 3 cm) are often due to recurrent tumor. Deviation of pharyngeal strictures from the midline is uncommon and usually indicates tumor recurrence. Short strictures usually represent a postoperative change. Long strictures are usually the result of radiotherapy or insufficient pharyngeal mucosa at the time of the surgical closure.

Despite the presence of a radiologic stricture, patients may not complain of dysphagia. Patients may compensate for pharyngeal narrowing by altering diet or chewing their food carefully.

Retracted Cricopharyngeal Muscle

At the time of laryngectomy, the thyropharyngeus and cricopharyngeus are removed from their thyroid and cricoid cartilage attachments, respectively. These muscles retract toward the posterior pharyngeal wall. Innervation of the cricopharyngeus may be partially or completely destroyed. These retracted muscles, especially the retracted cricopharyngeus, may appear as an extrinsic mass impression on the posterior pharyngeal wall (Fig. 4–39) and may be confused with recurrent tumor. However, tumors remain fixed and have irregular contour, but the prominent cricopharyngeus causes a smooth impression that changes size, shape, and position with swallowing.[17,92]

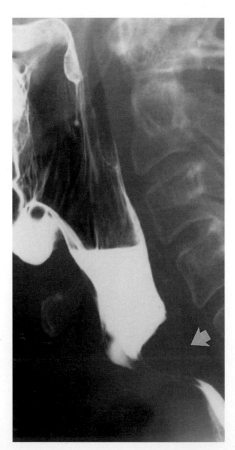

FIGURE **4–39. Retracted cricopharyngeal muscle following subtotal laryngectomy.** Lateral views of the pharynx show a smooth, broad-based mass impression *(arrow)* with tapered edges at the pharyngoesophageal segment. This "mass" changed over time.

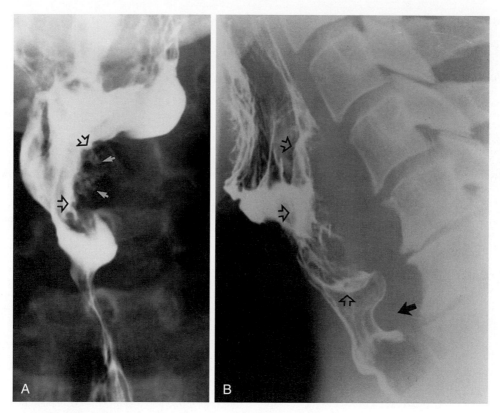

FIGURE 4-40. **Recurrent squamous cell carcinoma following laryngectomy.** A frontal view *(A)* shows a focal mass *(open arrows)* that is 4 cm long, has irregular mucosa *(white arrows),* and involves the left side of the neopharyngeal tube. The pharynx is mildly deviated to the right. The lateral view *(B)* shows lobulation of the posterior pharyngeal wall with increased thickness of the retropharyngeal space. This mass is superior to the smooth, 1-cm indentation of the cricopharyngeus *(black arrow).*

Recurrent Tumor

Tumor recurrence usually develops within the first 2 years following laryngectomy. The tumor is radiographically manifested as a focal mass that is larger than 1.5 to 2 cm and that does not change size or shape with swallowing (Fig. 4-40).[41] The mass deviates the pharynx more than 1 cm from the midline. The mass narrows the pharynx at the site of maximal deviation of the neopharyngeal tube. The mucosal surface is usually coarse or irregular. The posterior pharyngeal space may be widened, but this sign is not specific for tumor. Occasionally, fistulae into the soft tissues of the neck are seen. Thus any mass measuring 1.5 to 2 cm that deviates the pharynx more than 1 cm from the midline should arouse suspicion of recurrent tumor. Mucosal irregularity or ulceration seen in the remote postoperative pharynx suggests tumor recurrence.[14,93]

Other Procedures

If a pharyngeal or laryngeal tumor is relatively localized, the surgeon may choose a procedure designed to preserve voice or improve postoperative swallowing function. In a *supraglottic laryngectomy* the false vocal cords, epiglottis, superior half of the thyroid cartilage, and anterior portion of the hyoid bone are removed. In a *vertical hemilaryngectomy,* the ipsilateral true vocal cord, false vocal cord, and one half of the epiglottis and one half of the thyroid cartilage are removed. A detailed explanation of these procedures is available in references 1 and 94.[1,94]

REFERENCES

1. Jones, B., Kramer, S.S., and Donner, M.W.: Dynamic imaging of the pharynx. Gastrointest. Radiol. *10:*213, 1985.
2. Logemann, J.A.: Manual for the Videofluorographic Study of Swallowing, ed. 2. Austin, TX, Pro-Ed, 1993.
3. Logemann, J.A.: Evaluation and Treatment of Swallowing Disorders. Austin, TX, Pro-Ed, 1983.
4. Jones, B., and Donner, M.W.: Normal and Abnormal Swallowing. New York, Springer-Verlag, Inc., 1990.
5. Rubesin, S.E.: Pharyngeal dysfunction. *In* Gore, R.M. (ed.): Categorical Course on Gastrointestinal Radiology. Reston, VA, American College of Radiology, 1991, pp. 1–9.
6. Buchholz, D.W.: Dysphagia associated with neurological disorders. Acta Otorhinolaryngol. Belg. *48:*193, 1994.
7. Logemann, J.A.: Rehabilitation of oropharyngeal swallowing disorders. Acta Otorhinolaryngol. Belg. *48:*207, 1994.
8. Dodds, W.J., Stewart, E.T., and Logemann, J.A.: Physiology and radiology of the normal oral and pharyngeal phases of swallowing. AJR Am. J. Roentgenol. *154:*953, 1990.
9. Rubesin, S.E., and Laufer, I.: Pictorial review: Principles of double contrast pharyngography. Dysphagia *6:*170, 1991.
10. Rubesin, S.E.: Principles of performing a "modified barium swallow" examination. *In* Balfe, D.M., and Levine, M.S. (eds.): Categorical Course in Diagnostic Radiology: Gastrointestinal. Oak Brook, IL, Radiological Society of North America, 1997, pp. 7–19.

11. DuBrul, E.L.: Sicher's Oral Anatomy, ed. 7. St. Louis, C.V. Mosby, 1980, p. 319.
12. Donner, M.W., Bosma, J.F., and Robertson, D.L.: Anatomy and physiology of the pharynx. Gastrointest. Radiol. *10*:196, 1985.
13. Ekberg, O., and Nylander, G.: Double contrast examination of the pharynx. Gastrointest. Radiol. *10*:263, 1985.
14. Rubesin, S.E., Jessurun, J., Robertson, D., et al.: Lines of the pharynx. RadioGraphics *7*:217, 1987.
15. Gromet, M., Homer, M.J., and Carter, B.L.: Lymphoid hyperplasia at the base of the tongue. Radiology *144*:825, 1982.
16. Jones, B., Ravich, W.J., Donner, M.W., et al.: Pharyngoesophageal interrelationships: Observations and working concepts. Gastrointest. Radiol. *10*:225, 1985.
17. Rubesin, S.E., and Glick, S.N.: The tailored double-contrast pharyngogram. Crit. Rev. Diagn. Imaging *28*:133, 1988.
18. Levine, M.S., and Rubesin, S.E.: Radiologic investigation of dysphagia. AJR Am. J. Roentgenol. *154*:1157, 1990.
19. Jing, B.S.: Roentgen examination of the larynx and hypopharynx. Radiol. Clin. North Am. *8*:361, 1970.
20. Jing, B.S.: The pharynx and larynx: Roentgenographic technique. Semin. Roentgenol. *9*:259, 1974.
21. Taylor, A.J., Dodds, W.J., and Stewart, E.T.: Pharynx: Value of oblique projections for radiographic examination. Radiology *178*: 59, 1991.
22. Rubesin, S.E., Jones, B., and Donner, M.W.: Contrast pharyngography: The importance of phonation. AJR Am. J. Roentgenol. *148*: 269, 1987.
23. Bachman, A.L., Seaman, W.B., and Macken, K.L.: Lateral pharyngeal diverticula. Radiology *91*:774, 1968.
24. Curtis, D.J., Cruess, D.F., Crain, M., et al.: Lateral pharyngeal outpouchings: A comparison of dysphagic and asymptomatic patients. Dysphagia *2*:156, 1988.
25. Lindbichler, F., Raith, J., Uggowitzer, M., and Hausegger, K.: Aspiration resulting from lateral hypopharyngeal pouches. AJR Am. J. Roentgenol. *170*:129, 1998.
26. Ardran, G.M., Kemp, F.H., and Lund, W.S.: The aetiology of the posterior pharyngeal diverticulum: A cineradiographic study. J. Laryngol. Otol. *78*:333, 1964.
27. Perrott, J.W.: Anatomical aspects of hypopharyngeal diverticula. Aust. N. Z. J. Surg. *31*:307, 1962.
28. Zaino, C., Jacobson, H.G., Lepow, H., and Ozturk, C.: The pharyngoesophageal sphincter. Radiology *89*:639, 1967.
29. Zaino, C., Jacobson, H.G., Lepow, H., et al.: The pharyngoesophageal sphincter. Springfield, IL, Charles C Thomas, 1907.
30. Smiley, T.B., Caves, P.K., and Porter, D.C.: Relationship between posterior pharyngeal pouch and hiatus hernia. Thorax *25*:725, 1970.
31. Delahunty, J.E., Margulies, S.E., Alonso, U.A., et al.: The relationship of reflux esophagitis to pharyngeal pouch (Zenker's diverticulum). Laryngoscope *81*:570, 1971.
32. Shirazi, K.K., Daffner, R.H., and Gaede, J.T.: Ulcer occurring in Zenker's diverticulum. Gastrointest. Radiol. *2*:117, 1977.
33. Kensing, K.P., White, J.G., Korompai, F., and Dyck, W.P.: Massive bleeding from a Zenker's diverticulum: A case report and review of the literature. South. Med. J. *87*:1003, 1994.
34. Tolliver, B.A., and DiPalma, J.A.: Zenker's bezoar. South. Med. J. *88*:751, 1995.
35. Nanson, E.M.: Carcinoma in a long-standing pharyngeal diverticulum. Br. J. Surg. *63*:417, 1976.
36. Wychulis, A.R., Gunnulaugsson, G.H., and Claget, O.T.: Carcinoma arising in pharyngoesophageal diverticulum. Br. J. Surg. *63*:9786, 1969.
37. Knuff, T.E., Benjamin, S.B., and Castell, D.O.: Pharyngoesophageal (Zenker's) diverticulum: A reappraisal. Gastroenterology *82*:734, 1982.
38. Frieling, T., Berges, W., Lubke, H.J., et al.: Upper esophageal sphincter function in patients with Zenker's diverticulum. Dysphagia *3*:90, 1988.
39. Ekberg, O., and Nylander, G.: Lateral diverticula from the pharyngo-esophageal junction area. Radiology *146*:117, 1983.
40. Clements, J.L., Cox, G.W., Torres, W.E., and Weens, H.S.: Cervical esophageal webs—a roentgen-anatomic correlation. AJR Am. J. Roentgenol. *121*:221, 1974.
41. Seaman, W.B.: The significance of webs in the hypopharynx and upper esophagus. Radiology *89*:32, 1967.
42. Nosher, J.L., Campbell, W.L., and Seaman, W.B.: The clinical significance of cervical esophageal and hypopharyngeal webs. Radiology *117*:45, 1975.
43. Ekberg, O., and Nylander, G.: Webs and web-like formations in the pharynx and cervical esophagus. Diagn. Imaging *53*:10, 1983.
44. Shauffer, I.A., Phillips, H.E., and Sequeira, J.: The jet phenomenon: A manifestation of esophageal web. AJR Am. J. Roentgenol. *129*: 747, 1977.
45. Taylor, A.J., Stewart, E.T., and Dodds, W.J.: The esophageal jet phenomenon revisited. AJR Am. J. Roentgenol. *155*:289, 1990.
46. Pitman, R.G., and Fraser, G.M.: The post-cricoid impression on the oesophagus. Clin. Radiol. *16*:34, 1965.
47. Ekberg, O., Birch-Lensen, M., and Lindstrom, C.: Mucosal folds in the valleculae. Dysphagia *1*:68, 1986.
48. Kabakian, H.A., and Dahmash, M.S.: Pharyngoesophageal manifestations of epidermolysis bullosa. Clin. Radiol. *29*:91, 1978.
49. Chisholm, M., Ardran, G.M., Callender, S.T., and Wright, R.: Iron deficiency and autoimmunity in post-cricoid webs. Q. J. Med. *40*: 421, 1971.
50. Balfe, D.M., and Heiken, J.P.: Contrast evaluation of structural lesions of the pharynx. Curr. Probl. Diagn. Radiol. *15*:73, 1986.
51. Bosma, J.F., Gravkowski, E.A., and Tryostad, C.W.: Chronic ulcerative pharyngitis. Arch. Otolaryngol. *87*:85, 1968.
52. Maran, A.G.D., and Buchanan, D.R.: Branchial cysts, sinuses and fistulae. Clin. Otolaryngol. *3*:77, 1978.
53. Som, P.M., Sacher, M., Lanzieri, C.F., et al.: Parenchymal cysts of the lower neck. Radiology *157*:399, 1985.
54. Bhaskar, S.N., and Bernier, J.L.: Histogenesis of branchial cysts. Am. J. Pathol. *35*:407, 1959.
55. Dodds, W.J., Logemann, J.A., and Stewart, E.T.: Radiologic assessment of abnormal oral and pharyngeal phases of swallowing. AJR Am. J. Roentgenol. *154*:965, 1990.
56. Curtis, D.J., and Sepulveda, G.U.: Epiglottic motion: Video recording of muscular dysfunction. Radiology *148*:473, 1983.
57. Bachman, A.L.: Benign, non-neoplastic conditions of the larynx and pharynx. Radiol. Clin. North Am. *16*:273, 1978.
58. Lindell, M.M., Jing, B.S., Fischer, E.P., et al.: Laryngocele. AJR Am. J. Roentgenol. *131*:273, 1978.
59. Canalis, R.F., Maxwell, D.S., and Hemenway, W.G.: Laryngocele—an updated review. J. Otolaryngol. *6*:91, 1977.
60. Hyams, V.J., Batsakis, J.G., and Michaels, L.: Tumors of the upper respiratory tract and ear. *In* Atlas of Tumor Pathology. Second series. Fascicle 25, Bethesda, MD, Armed Forces Institute of Pathology, 1988.
61. Manson, T., Wilske, J., and Kindblom, L-G.: Lipoma of the hypopharynx: A case report and a review of the literature. J. Laryngol. Otol. *92*:1037, 1978.
62. Patterson, H.C., Dickerson, G.R., Pilch, B.Z., et al.: Harmartoma of the hypopharynx. Arch. Otolaryngol. *107*:767, 1981.
63. Haraguchi, J., Ohgaki, T., Hentona, J., and Komatsuzaki, A.: Schwannoma of the posterior pharyngeal wall: A case report. J. Laryngol. Otol. *110*:170, 1996.
64. Hyams, V.J., and Rabuzzi, D.D.: Cartilaginous tumors of the larynx. Laryngoscope *80*:755, 1970.
65. Levine, M.S., Rubesin, S.E., and Ott, D.J.: Update on esophageal radiology. AJR Am. J. Roentgenol. *155*:993, 1990.
66. Seaman, W.B.: Contrast radiography in neoplastic disease of the larynx and pharynx. Semin. Roentgenol. *9*:301, 1974.
67. Semenkovich, J.W., Balfe, D.M., Weyman, P.J., et al.: Barium pharyngography: Comparison of single and double contrast. AJR Am. J. Roentgenol. *144*:715, 1985.
68. Wagonfeld, D.J.H., Harwood, A.R., Bryce, D.P., et al.: Secondary primary respiratory tract malignant neoplasms in supraglottic carcinoma. Arch. Otolaryngol. *107*:135, 1981.
69. Goldstein, H.M., and Zornoza, J.: Association of squamous cell carcinoma of the head and neck with cancer of the esophagus. AJR Am. J. Roentgenol. *131*:791, 1978.
70. Thompson, W.M., Oddson, T.A., Kelvin, F., et al.: Synchronous and metachronous squamous cell carcinoma of the head, neck, and esophagus. Gastrointest. Radiol. *3*:123, 1978.
71. Rubesin, S.E., Jones, B., and Donner, M.W.: Radiology of the adult soft palate. Dysphagia *2*:8, 1978.
72. Dockerty, M.D., Parkhill, E.M., Dahlin, D.C., et al.: Tumors of the Oral Cavity and Pharynx. Washington, DC, Armed Forces Institute of Pathology, 1968.

73. Silver, C.E.: Surgical management of neoplasms of the larynx, hypopharynx and cervical esophagus. Curr. Probl. Surg. *14:*2, 1977.

74. Barrs, D.M., DeSanto, L.W., and O'Fallon, W.M.: Squamous cell carcinoma of the tonsil and tongue-base region. Arch. Otolaryngol. *105:*479, 1979.

75. Apter, A.J., Levine, M.S., and Glick, S.N.: Carcinomas of the base of the tongue: Diagnosis using double-contrast radiography of the pharynx. Radiology *151:*123, 1984.

76. Rubesin, S.E., Rabischong, P., Bilaniuk, L.T., et al.: Contrast examination of the soft palate with cross-sectional correlation. RadioGraphics *8:*641, 1988.

77. Banfi, A., Bonadonna, G., Carnevali, G., et al.: Lymphoreticular sarcomas with primary involvement of Waldeyer's ring. Cancer *26:*341, 1970.

78. Al-Saleem, R., Harwick, R., Robbins, R., et al.: Malignant lymphomas of the pharynx. Cancer *26:*1383, 1970.

79. Conley, J., and Dingman, D.L.: Adenoid cystic carcinoma in the head and neck (cylindroma). Arch. Otolaryngol. *101:*81, 1974.

80. Gatti, W.M., Strom, C.G., Orffei, E.: Synovial sarcoma of the laryngopharynx. Arch. Otolaryngol. *101:*633, 1975.

81. Johnson, I.J., Warfield, A.T., Smallman, L.A., and Watkinson, J.C.: Primary malignant melanoma of the pharynx. J. Laryngol. Otol. *108:*275, 1994.

82. Spiro, R.H., Koss, L.G., Hajdu, S.I., et al.: Tumors of minor salivary origin. Cancer *31:*117, 1973.

83. Ekberg, O., and Nylander, G.: Pharyngeal dysfunction after treatment for pharyngeal cancer with surgery and radiotherapy. Gastrointest. Radiol. *8:*97, 1983.

84. Larson, D.L., Lindberg, R.D., Lane, E., et al.: Major complications of radiotherapy in cancer of the oral cavity and oropharynx. A 10 year retrospective study. Am. J. Surg. *146:*431, 1983.

85. Goffinet, D.R., Eltringham, F.R., Glatstein, E., et al.: Carcinoma of the larynx: Results of radiation therapy in 213 patients. AJR Am. J. Roentgenol. *117:*553, 1973.

86. Keene, M., Harwood, A.R., Bryce, D.P., et al.: Histopathological study of radionecrosis in laryngeal carcinoma. Laryngoscope *92:* 173, 1982.

87. Balfe, D.M., Koehler, R.E., Setzen, M., et al.: Barium examination of the esophagus after total laryngectomy. Radiology *143:*501, 1982.

88. DiSantis, D.J., Balfe, D.M., Koehler, R.E., et al.: Barium examination of the pharynx after vertical hemilaryngectomy. AJR Am. J. Roentgenol. *141:*35, 1983.

89. Moses, B.L., Eisele, D.W., and Jones, B.: Radiologic assessment of the early postoperative total laryngectomy patient. Laryngoscope *103:*1157, 1993.

90. Fradis, M., Podoshin, L., and Ben David, J.: Post-laryngectomy pharyngocutaneous fistula—a still unresolved problem. J. Laryngol. Otol. *109:*321, 1995

91. Hier, M., Black, M.J., and Lafond, G.: Pharyngo-cutaneous fistulas after total laryngectomy: Incidence, etiology and outcome analysis. J. Otolaryngol. *22:*164, 1993.

92. Muller-Miny, H., Eisele, D.W., and Jones, B.: Dynamic radiographic imaging following total laryngectomy. Head Neck *154:*342,1993.

93. Quillen, S.P., Balfe, D.M., and Glick, S.N.: Pharyngography after head and neck irradiation: Differentiation of postirradiation edema from recurrent cancer. AJR Am. J. Roentgenol. *161:*205, 1993.

94. Wippold, F.J., and Balfe, D.M.: Imaging of the postoperative neck. *In* Gore, R.M., Levine, M.S., and Laufer, I. (eds): Textbook of Gastrointestinal Radiology. Philadelphia, W.B. Saunders Co., 1994, pp. 277–290.

Esophagus

MARC S. LEVINE
IGOR LAUFER

TECHNIQUE

Double contrast views of the esophagus are obtained at the beginning of the routine upper gastrointestinal examination. In patients with esophageal symptoms, double contrast views of the esophagus are also obtained as part of the routine esophagram. After ingesting an effervescent agent, the patient gulps a high-density barium suspension in the upright, left posterior oblique position so that the esophagus is projected free of the spine. One 3-on-1 or two 2-on-1 spot radiographs of the upper and lower esophagus taken in rapid succession usually provide excellent double contrast views of the distended esophagus (Fig. 5–1). If the study is being performed with digital fluoroscopic equipment, the ability to obtain almost instantaneous exposures (without need for changing cassettes) affords the radiologist an even larger window of opportunity for imaging the esophagus. Occasionally, when there is a high suspicion of esophageal disease, the cup of barium can be split in half; this maneuver allows the radiologist to obtain images of the esophagus in both the left posterior oblique and right posterior oblique positions to evaluate protruded or depressed lesions both en face and in profile.[1]

If the initial double contrast views of the esophagus are inconclusive, the examination of the stomach and duodenum should be completed before additional views of the esophagus are obtained at the end of the study. At that time, other maneuvers may be attempted to improve the quality of the esophageal examination. The patient may be asked to pinch the nose with one hand while gulping barium to increase the amount of air swallowing. Another dose of effervescent agent can also be given to improve gaseous distention of the esophagus. Better double contrast views of the distal esophagus can sometimes be obtained with the patient in the prone oblique position, particularly if the lower esophageal sphincter is incompetent (Fig. 5–2).[2]

Paralysis of the esophagus by relaxant drugs may also facilitate the double contrast examination. Anticholinergic agents such as Buscopan (hyoscine *N*-butyl bromide) and propantheline bromide (Pro-Banthine) are effective in abolishing esophageal peristalsis. However, it is important to be aware of the side effects associated with the use of these anticholinergic agents. Also, Buscopan has not been approved by the Federal Drug Administration for use in the United States. In contrast, glucagon relaxes the lower esophageal sphincter but does not affect esophageal peristalsis.[3] This drug therefore cannot be used to induce esophageal relaxation.

The greatest diagnostic difficulties usually occur in the distal esophagus, where poor distention or pooling of barium may obscure mucosal detail on routine double contrast radiographs. When an equivocal abnormality is identified, a tube esophagram occasionally may be performed for a more detailed examination by passing a small red rubber catheter into the proximal esophagus

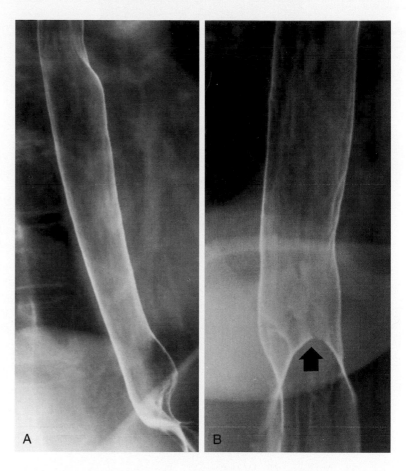

FIGURE **5–1. Normal esophagus, upright.** *A,* Normal appearance of thoracic esophagus. Note how esophageal mucosa is smooth and featureless and how mucosal folds have been completely effaced. *B,* The distal esophagus with typical arch-shaped configuration *(arrow)* at gastroesophageal junction.

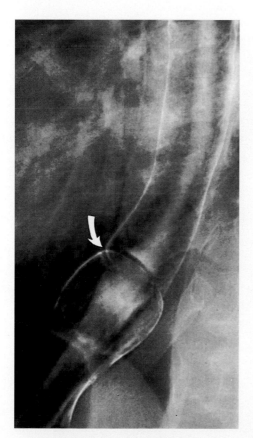

FIGURE **5–2. Prone oblique position.** Double contrast view of hiatal hernia, lower esophageal ring *(arrow),* and distal esophagus.

and having the patient swallow high-density barium as air is gently insufflated through the catheter.[4]

NORMAL APPEARANCES

The fully distended esophagus normally has a smooth, featureless appearance on double contrast radiographs (see Fig. 5–1A). During swallowing, the relaxed cardia produces a typical arch-shaped shadow at the gastroesophageal junction (see Fig. 5–1B). A small indentation is frequently seen on the anterior wall of the cervical esophagus (Fig. 5–3). This indentation probably is caused by a redundant mucosal fold and should not be mistaken for a cervical esophageal tumor or web (Fig. 5–4).[5] Typical indentations due to the aortic arch and left main bronchus may also be seen in the middle third of the esophagus (Fig. 5–5). In patients with a sliding hiatal hernia, a thin, zigzagging radiolucent line or "Z-line" demarcating the squamocolumnar junction is occasionally seen (Fig. 5–6).

As the esophagus collapses, the normal longitudinal folds become visible as thin, straight, parallel structures no more than several millimeters in width (Fig. 5–7). In some patients, fine transverse folds may also be seen intermittently in the esophagus (Fig. 5–8). These transverse folds were originally described as a normal feature of the feline esophagus.[6] However, they can also occur as a transient phenomenon in humans because of contraction of

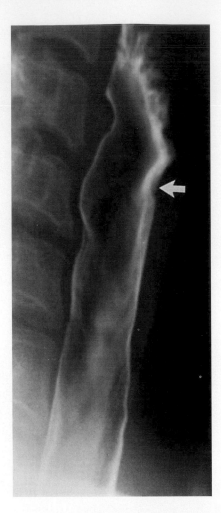

FIGURE 5–3. Normal cervical esophagus with anterior indentation by redundant mucosal fold *(arrow)*. Note slight posterior impression from cervical osteophyte.

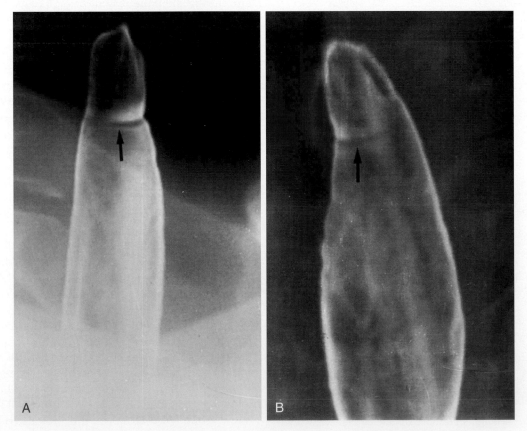

FIGURE 5–4. Cervical esophageal web *(arrows)* seen in lateral *(A)* and frontal *(B)* projections.

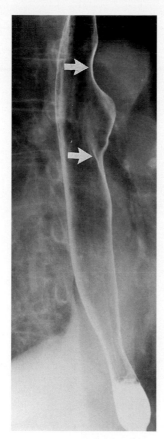

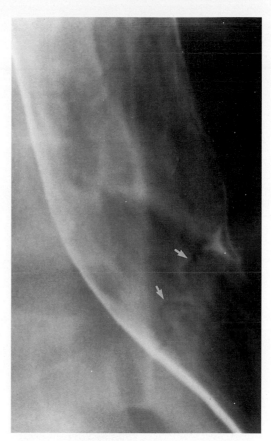

FIGURE 5–5. Normal impressions *(arrows)* due to aortic arch and left main bronchus.

FIGURE 5–6. Zigzagging radiolucent line or "Z-line" *(arrows),* probably representing the squamocolumnar junction.

FIGURE 5–7. Normal longitudinal folds in partially collapsed esophagus.

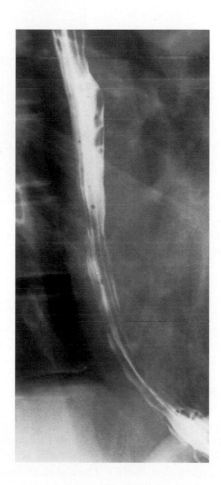

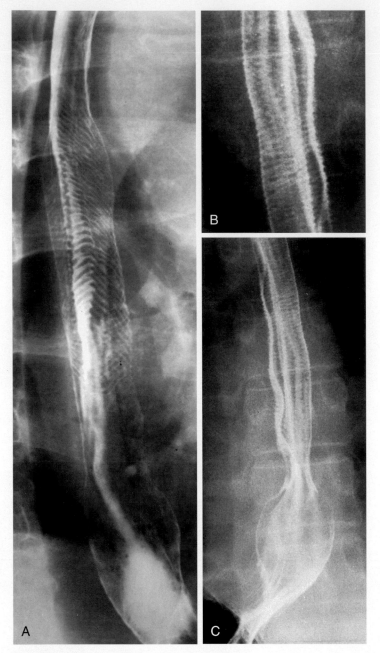

FIGURE 5–8. Three examples (*A* through *C*) of transverse folds in the esophagus. These folds are thought to result from contraction of the longitudinally oriented muscularis mucosae. (From Gohel, V.K., et al.: Transverse folds in the human esophagus. Radiology *128*:303, 1978, with permission.)

the longitudinal fibers of the muscularis mucosae.[7] These delicate transverse folds are only 1 to 2 mm wide and extend completely across the esophagus without interruption.[8] Because the folds are transient, they may be seen on one spot film and disappear moments later (Fig. 5–9). Although their clinical significance is uncertain, the folds have been observed with increased frequency in patients with gastroesophageal reflux.[8] These fine transverse folds should be distinguished from the broad transverse bands seen in patients with nonpropulsive tertiary esophageal contractions (Fig. 5–10). They should also be differenti-

ated from fixed transverse folds in the esophagus due to scarring from reflux esophagitis (see Fig. 5–35 and the later section, "Gastroesophageal Reflux Disease").

Focal spiculation of the upper thoracic esophagus may also be seen on double contrast radiographs as a normal variant.[9] This spiculation usually occurs as a transient finding above the level of the aortic arch at the leading edge of a lumen-obliterating peristaltic wave (Fig. 5–11*A*); the spiculation disappears when the esophagus is distended (Fig. 5–11*B*). This phenomenon is probably related to weakening of peristalsis or localized contraction

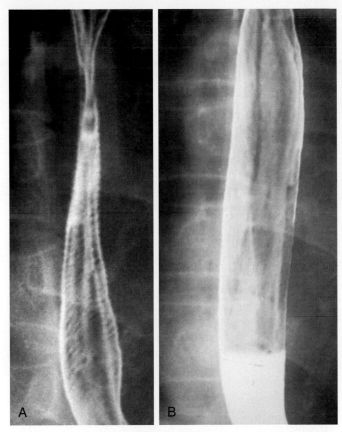

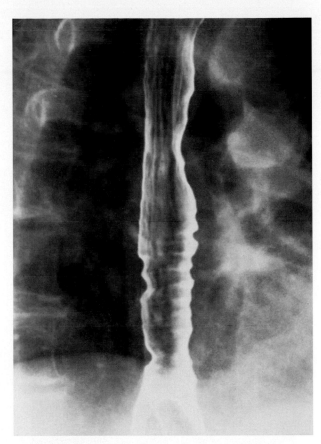

FIGURE 5–9. Transient nature of transverse folds. *A,* Transverse folds are present in middle and distal esophagus. *B,* Moments later, the folds are no longer visible.

FIGURE 5–10. Transverse bands due to contraction of muscularis propria. These bands are thicker than the transverse folds in Figures 5–8 and 5–9.

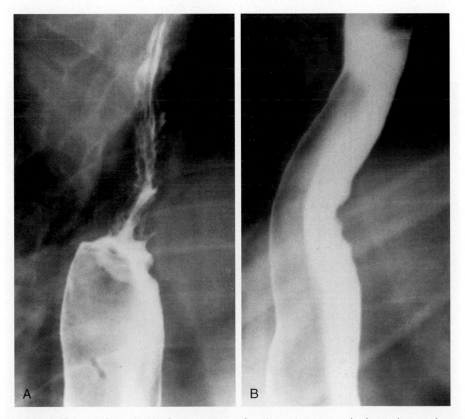

FIGURE 5–11. Focal spiculation of upper thoracic esophagus as normal variant. *A,* Note marked spiculation of upper esophagus just above level of lumen-obliterating peristaltic wave. *B,* Repeat view moments later with maximal distention shows normal-appearing esophagus at this level.

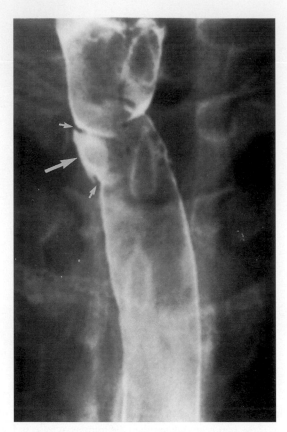

FIGURE 5–12. Ectopic gastric mucosa in upper esophagus. A flat depression *(large arrow)* is seen on right lateral border of upper thoracic esophagus with small indentations *(small arrows)* at superior and inferior borders of lesion. The appearance and location of this depression are characteristic of ectopic gastric mucosa.

of the longitudinally oriented muscularis mucosae at the junction of the striated-muscle and smooth-muscle portions of the esophagus. In one study transient spiculation of the upper esophagus was seen in about 10% of all patients who underwent double contrast examinations of the esophagus.[9] It therefore is important for radiologists to be familiar with this finding so that it is not mistaken for a focal area of esophagitis.

Congenital rests of ectopic gastric mucosa occasionally may be found in the upper esophagus at or near the level of the thoracic inlet (hence the term "inlet patch").[10,11] Affected individuals usually are asymptomatic. This ectopic gastric mucosa may be manifested on double contrast studies by the presence of a broad, relatively flat depression, most commonly on the right lateral wall of the upper esophagus, with small indentations superiorly and inferiorly (Fig. 5–12).[10,11] Because of its characteristic appearance and location, ectopic gastric mucosa can usually be differentiated radiographically from ulceration in the esophagus.

ARTIFACTS

Double contrast examinations of the esophagus may produce a variety of artifacts that simulate or obscure mucosal disease[12]:

1. *Localized noncoating* of a segment of the esophagus may suggest the presence of a tumor (Fig. 5–13*A*). With additional barium, however, the apparent abnormality disappears (Fig. 5–13*B*).

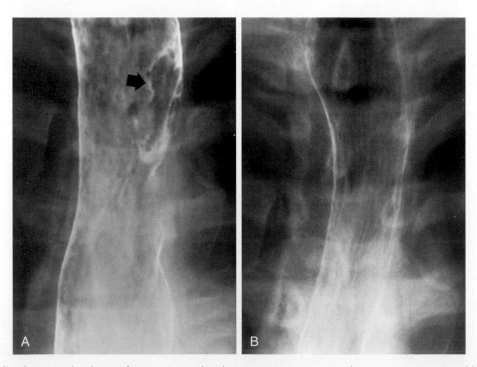

FIGURE 5–13. Localized noncoating in esophagus. *A,* Localized noncoating *(arrow)* simulating carcinoma. *B,* Additional view with improved coating shows that this area is normal.

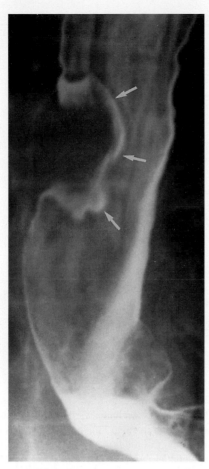

FIGURE 5–14. "Kissing" artifact in esophagus. Apparent polypoid lesion *(arrows)* is caused by adherence of anterior and posterior walls of esophagus ("kissing" artifact).

2. *"Kissing" artifact* in the esophagus due to incomplete distention with adherence of the anterior and posterior walls can also mimic the appearance of a mucosal or submucosal tumor on one or more films (Fig. 5–14).

3. *Undissolved effervescent agent* may be seen as a transient finding in the normal esophagus (Fig. 5–15) or as a persistent finding in the presence of esophageal obstruction. Undissolved effervescent granules should not be mistaken for the nodular mucosa of *Candida* esophagitis.

4. *Gas bubbles* can usually be recognized as artifacts by their smooth, round appearance on double contrast radiographs. Occasionally, however, small air bubbles in the esophagus may simulate mucosal nodularity due to *Candida* esophagitis or superficial spreading carcinoma (Fig. 5–16).

5. *Barium precipitates* may be seen as small, white dots on the esophageal mucosa (Fig. 5–17A). These precipitates can be distinguished from superficial ulcers or erosions by the absence of edema, marginal irregularity, or associated motor abnormalities. These problems can be avoided by choosing a suit-

able high-density barium suspension for the double contrast examination and by ensuring that the suspension is properly prepared.

6. A *pseudointraluminal diverticulum* may be seen in the esophagus when the barium column disintegrates, leaving a glob of barium surrounded by a thin, radiolucent halo (Fig. 5–17B).[13] This artifact is caused by the interaction of barium with retained fluid and debris due to esophageal stasis in patients with strictures or motility disorders.

7. *Flow artifact* occurs when mucosal detail is compromised by a thick coating or "sheen" of high-density barium in the esophagus.[14] Flow artifact is important because the nodular or granular mucosa of esophagitis can be obscured by residual high-density barium (Fig. 5–18A). However, this problem is minimized by delaying exposure of the films until the barium coating has thinned out enough to demonstrate the nodular mucosa of esophagitis (Fig. 5–18B) or other abnormalities. With digital fluoroscopic equipment, flow artifact can frequently be avoided by careful timing of the exposures because of the greater window of opportunity for visualizing the esophagus in double contrast.

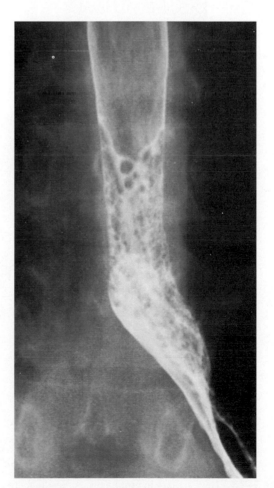

FIGURE 5–15. Undissolved effervescent granules in the distal esophagus.

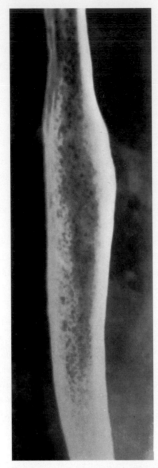

FIGURE 5–16. Gas bubbles throughout the esophagus, simulating diffuse mucosal nodularity.

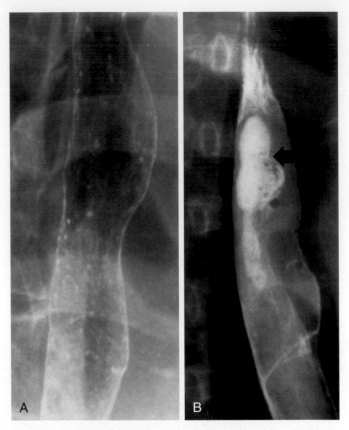

FIGURE 5–17. Barium-related artifacts. *A,* Barium precipitates in esophagus. *B,* Pseudointraluminal diverticulum *(arrow)* due to interaction of barium with retained fluid and debris in esophagus of a patient with a motility disorder. (*B,* From Levine, M.S.: Radiology of the Esophagus. Philadelphia, W.B. Saunders, 1989, p. 13.)

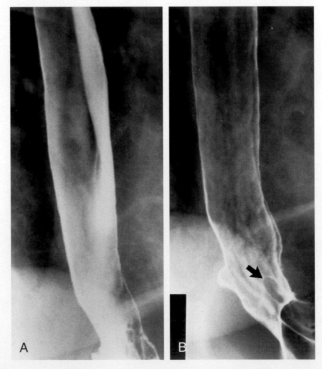

FIGURE 5–18. Flow artifact in esophagus. *A,* Residual layer of high-density barium obscures mucosal detail in distal esophagus. *B,* Repeat double contrast view moments later shows reflux esophagitis with mucosal nodularity and inflammatory esophagogastric polyp *(arrow)* not seen on earlier view. (From Levine, M.S., et al.: Double-contrast upper gastrointestinal examination: Technique and interpretation. Radiology *168:*593, 1988, with permission.)

INFLAMMATORY CONDITIONS

Gastroesophageal Reflux Disease

Reflux Esophagitis

Reflux esophagitis is by far the most common inflammatory condition in the esophagus. Traditional signs of esophagitis revealed by single contrast barium studies include thickened folds, decreased distensibility, marginal irregularity or ulceration, and abnormal motility. However, these findings are difficult to evaluate and are frequently found only in patients with severe reflux disease. Double contrast examinations permit a more detailed assessment of the esophageal mucosa to detect superficial ulceration or other changes of mild or moderate esophagitis that cannot be detected by conventional barium studies. As a result, double contrast esophagography has a sensitivity approaching 90% in diagnosing reflux esophagitis.[15,16]

Double contrast studies sometimes may reveal hiatal hernias and lower esophageal rings (see Fig. 5–2). However, the major purpose of upright double contrast views of the esophagus in patients with reflux symptoms is to demonstrate subtle findings of esophagitis that cannot be seen on single contrast views. In contrast, single contrast esophagrams obtained with the patient in the prone position permit optimal distention of the distal esophagus and gastroesophageal junction, allowing demonstration of hernias, strictures, or rings that are not visible on the double contrast phase of the examination (Fig. 5–19).[17] Thus the routine esophagram should be performed as a biphasic study that includes upright double contrast and prone single contrast views of the esophagus.

In the early stages of reflux esophagitis, edema and inflammation may be manifested by a finely nodular or granular appearance of the mucosa in the distal third or two thirds of the thoracic esophagus (Fig. 5–20).[18,19] This granularity results from trapping of barium between areas of edematous mucosa, producing innumerable tiny radiolucencies that merge with one another. Other patients may have more coarse nodularity of the mucosa with poorly defined nodules that lack discrete borders. In virtually all cases, the granular or nodular mucosa of reflux esophagitis extends proximally from the gastroesophageal junction as a continuous area of disease. Thus, the presence of a nodular mucosa that is confined to the upper or middle thirds of the esophagus should suggest another cause for the patient's disease.

Occasionally, severe reflux esophagitis may produce inflammatory exudates or pseudomembranes that are indistinguishable from the plaques of *Candida* esophagitis (Fig. 5–21*A*).[20] A single large pseudomembrane may also resemble a plaquelike carcinoma, particularly an adenocarcinoma arising in Barrett's esophagus (Fig. 5–21*B*).[20] However, pseudomembrane formation may be suggested by the presence of other discrete satellite lesions or by a change in the size or appearance of the lesion during the radiologic examination. When the radiographic findings are equivocal, endoscopy and biopsy may be required to rule out malignant tumor.

Reflux esophagitis may also be manifested by thick-

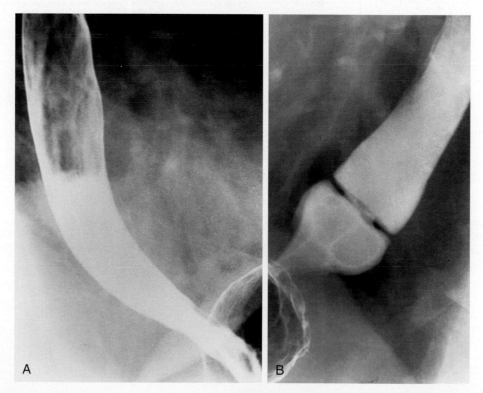

FIGURE 5–19. Schatzki ring only seen on prone single contrast esophagram. *A,* Upright double contrast view of distal esophagus shows no evidence of lower esophageal ring. *B,* However, prone single contrast view from same examination shows hiatal hernia with unequivocal Schatzki ring above hernia.

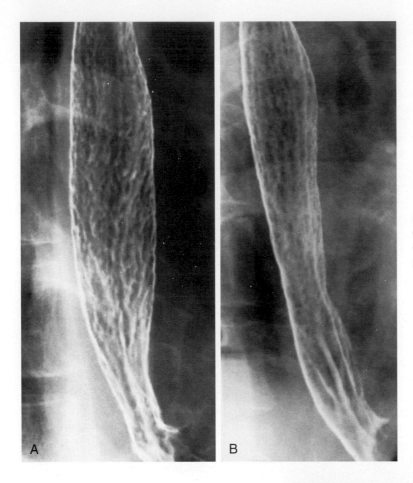

A

B

FIGURE 5–20. Two examples (*A* and *B*) of finely nodular or granular mucosa in distal half of esophagus due to reflux esophagitis. (From Levine, M.S.: Radiology of the Esophagus. Philadelphia, W.B. Saunders, 1989, p. 19.)

FIGURE 5–21. Reflux esophagitis with pseudomembranes. *A,* Multiple pseudomembranes in distal half of esophagus, mimicking the appearance of *Candida* esophagitis. (Courtesy of Howard Kessler, M.D., Philadelphia, Pennsylvania.) *B,* Hiatal hernia and peptic stricture with large pseudomembrane *(arrows)* on one wall of stricture. A plaquelike carcinoma arising in Barrett's esophagus could produce a similar appearance. (From Levine, M.S., et al.: Pseudomembranes in reflux esophagitis. Radiology *159:*43, 1986, with permission.)

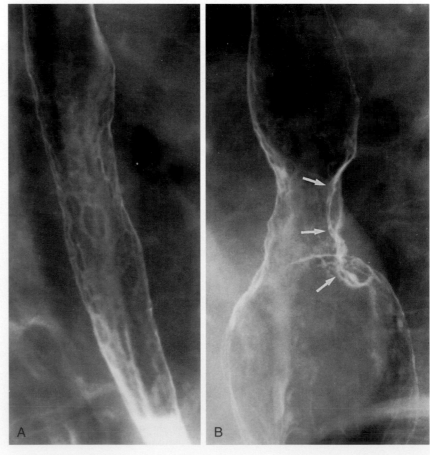

A

B

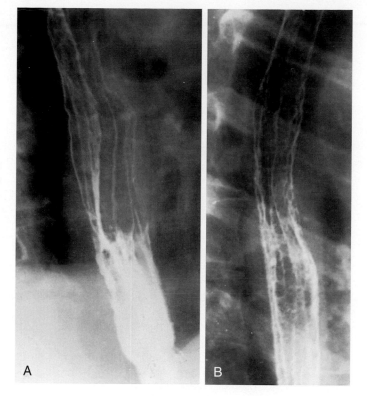

A   B

FIGURE 5–22. Two examples (*A* and *B*) of reflux esophagitis with thickened longitudinal folds. The folds in *B* are more serpiginous than those in *A* and could be mistaken for varices. (From Levine, M.S.: Radiology of the Esophagus. Philadelphia, W.B. Saunders, 1989, p. 25.)

ened longitudinal folds due to edema and inflammation that extend into the submucosa. However, thickened folds should be recognized as a nonspecific finding of esophagitis. These thickened folds may have a smooth, lobulated, or scalloped configuration, occasionally mimicking the appearance of esophageal varices (Fig. 5–22). Other patients with reflux esophagitis may have a single prominent fold that arises in the gastric fundus and ex-

tends above the gastroesophageal junction as a polypoid protuberance in the distal esophagus (Fig. 5–23*A;* see Fig. 5–18*B*).[21,22] Occasionally, this protuberance may be seen in a hiatal hernia or in the stomach when the hernia is reduced (Fig. 5–23*B*). These lesions are called "inflammatory" esophagogastric polyps and are thought to be a manifestation of chronic reflux esophagitis. Because these lesions have no malignant potential, endoscopy is

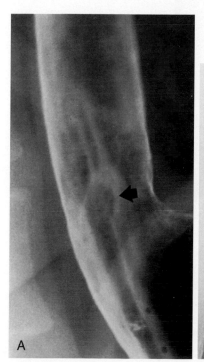

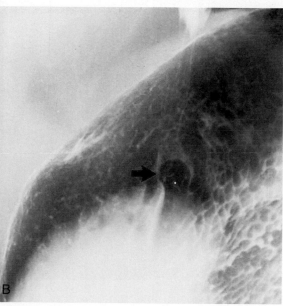

A   B

FIGURE 5–23. Inflammatory esophagogastric polyp. *A,* A prominent mucosal fold extends from the gastric fundus into the distal esophagus as a polypoid protuberance *(arrow).* *B,* With the esophagus collapsed, the polypoid fold is visible within the stomach *(arrow).*

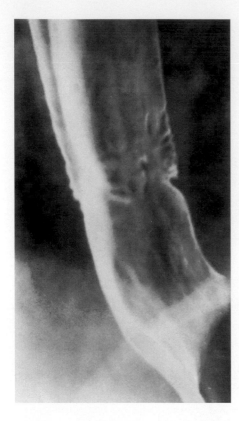

FIGURE 5–24. Reflux esophagitis with discrete, superficial ulcers in distal esophagus near the gastroesophageal junction. Note radiating folds and puckering of esophageal wall.

unwarranted when typical inflammatory polyps are found on double contrast studies.

Shallow ulcers and erosions caused by reflux esophagitis may appear as one or more streaks or dots of barium at or near the gastroesophageal junction (Fig. 5–24).[23,24]

Some ulcers may be irregular, whereas others may have a linear configuration with their long axis perpendicular to the gastroesophageal junction (Figs. 5–25 and 5–26). The ulcers may be surrounded by a radiolucent halo of edematous mucosa, and there may be fine radiating folds

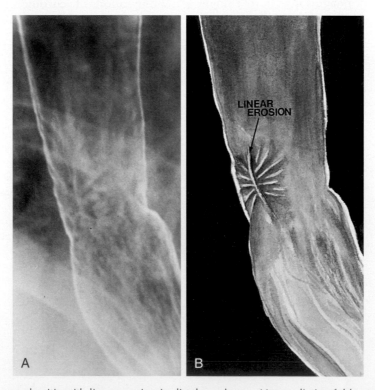

FIGURE 5–25. *A* and *B,* Reflux esophagitis with linear erosion in distal esophagus. Note radiating folds and retraction of adjacent esophageal wall. (Courtesy of Marc P. Banner, M.D., Philadelphia, Pennsylvania.)

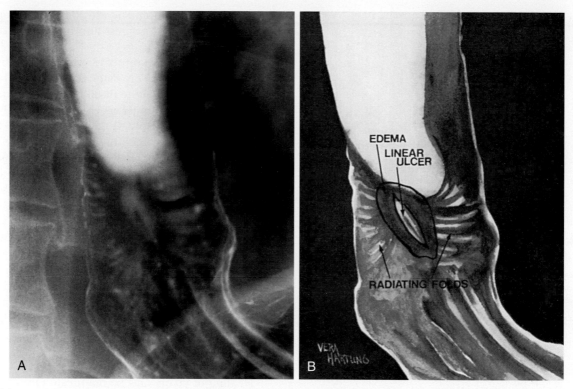

FIGURE 5—26. *A* and *B,* Reflux esophagitis with linear ulcer in distal esophagus. Note ulcer crater, surrounding edema, and radiating folds.

with slight retraction of the adjacent esophageal wall (Figs. 5–25 and 5–26). Occasionally, longitudinal ulcers may have a serpiginous or flowing appearance, with multiple transverse folds straddling the area of ulceration (Fig. 5 27).[25] Some patients may have more widespread

ulceration involving the distal third or even two thirds of the thoracic esophagus (Fig. 5–28). However, ulceration in reflux esophagitis tends to occur as a continuous area of disease that extends proximally from the gastroesophageal junction; the presence of superficial ulcers in

FIGURE 5–27. Two examples (*A* and *B*) of reflux esophagitis with serpiginous, longitudinally oriented ulcers *(small arrows).* In both cases, note multiple transverse folds straddling ulcers and associated peptic strictures *(large arrows).* (*A,* From Levine, M.S., and Goldstein, H.M.: Fixed transverse folds in the esophagus: A sign of reflux esophagitis. AJR Am. J. Roentgenol. *143:*275, 1984, with permission, © by American Roentgen Ray Society. *B,* Courtesy of Harvey M. Goldstein, M.D., San Antonio, Texas.)

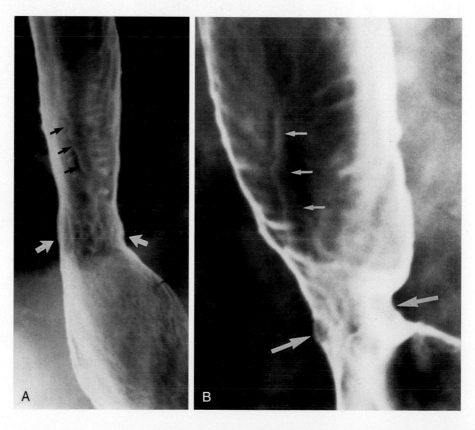

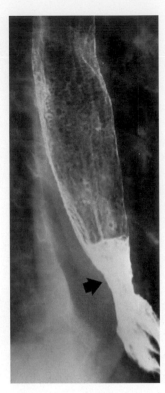

FIGURE 5–28. Reflux esophagitis with diffuse superficial ulceration of distal esophagus and associated peptic stricture *(arrow)* near gastroesophageal junction. (Courtesy of Henry I. Goldberg, M.D., San Francisco, California.)

the upper or midesophagus with distal esophageal sparing therefore should suggest another cause for the patient's esophagitis.

Other patients with reflux esophagitis may have a solitary, relatively large ulcer crater that tends to be located on the posterior wall of the distal esophagus near the gastroesophageal junction (Figs. 5–29 and 5–30). In one study, about 70% of these ulcers were found to be on the posterior wall.[26] It is uncertain why the ulcers have this characteristic location. However, gastroesophageal reflux often occurs during sleep, when secretion of peptic acid is at its peak and clearance of acid is delayed because of decreased esophageal peristalsis. It therefore has been postulated that patients who sleep primarily in the supine position are more likely to develop posterior wall ulcers due to prolonged exposure to refluxed acid that pools by gravity on the dependent or posterior esophageal wall.[26] These ulcers can be recognized en face (Fig. 5–30*B*) but are best visualized when they are projected tangentially beyond the normal contour of the esophagus (Figs. 5–29 and 5–30*A*).

Peptic Scarring and Strictures

Healing of ulcers may be manifested by localized flattening or puckering of the distal esophagus at the site of the previous ulcer (Fig. 5–31). Further scarring from reflux esophagitis may lead to the development of circumferential peptic strictures, which classically appear as

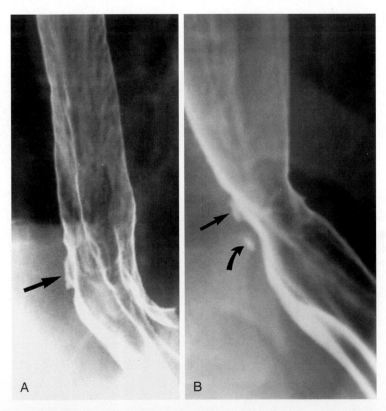

FIGURE 5–29. Two examples (*A* and *B*) of reflux esophagitis with relatively large, flat ulcers *(straight arrows)* on posterior wall of distal esophagus. In *B*, also note peptic scarring and esophageal intramural pseudodiverticulum *(curved arrow)* that appears to be floating outside wall of esophagus. (*A,* From Levine, M.S.: Radiology of the Esophagus. Philadelphia, W.B. Saunders, 1989, p. 24. *B,* From Hu, C., Levine, M.S., and Laufer, I.: Solitary ulcers in reflux esophagitis: Radiographic findings. Abdom. Imaging *22*:5, 1997, with permission.)

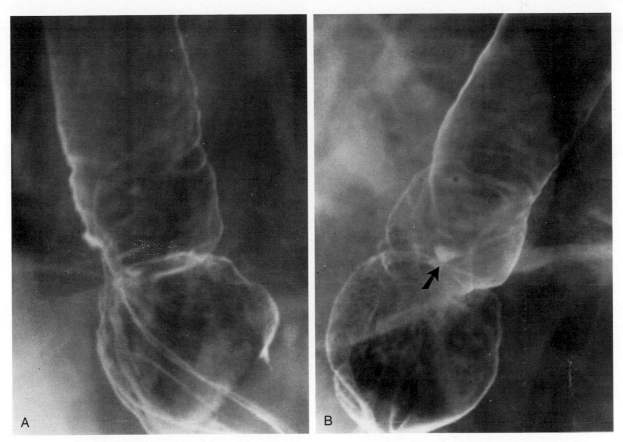

FIGURE 5–30. Reflux esophagitis with discrete ulcer *(arrow)* in distal esophagus. *A,* Profile view. *B,* En face view.

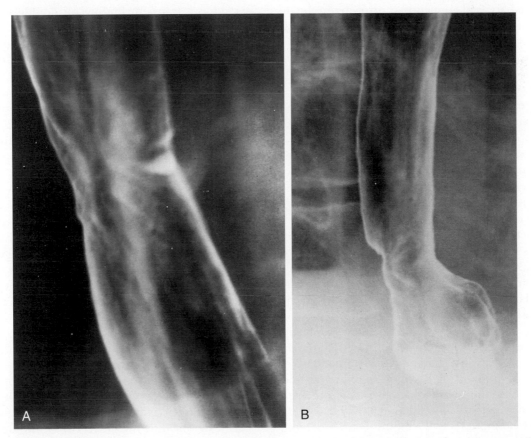

FIGURE 5–31. Two examples (*A* and *B*) of asymmetric puckering and retraction of posterior wall of distal esophagus, with radiating folds in this region due to scarring from reflux esophagitis.

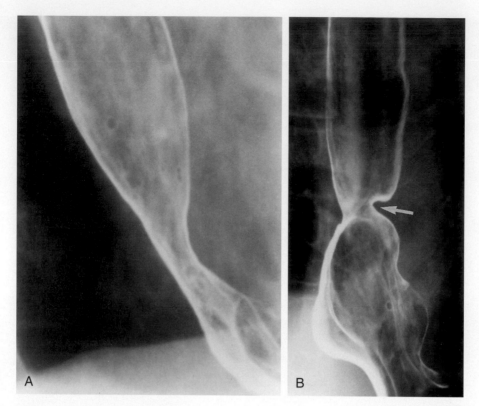

FIGURE 5–32. Peptic strictures. *A,* Typical peptic stricture with concentric narrowing and smooth, tapered margins. *B,* Eccentric stricture *(arrow)* in distal esophagus.

smooth, tapered areas of concentric narrowing in the distal esophagus above a sliding hiatal hernia (Fig. 5–32*A*). However, many strictures have an asymmetric appearance with puckering or deformity of one wall of the stricture due to asymmetric scarring from reflux esophagitis (Fig. 5–32*B*). As a result, a benign peptic stricture cannot always be differentiated radiographically from an infiltrating carcinoma, particularly an adenocarcinoma arising in Barrett's esophagus (see Chapter 6). Because almost all peptic strictures are associated with hiatal hernias, the absence of a hernia should also raise concern about the possibility of an underlying tumor. Whenever the radiographic findings are equivocal, endoscopy should be performed to rule out a malignant lesion.

Peptic strictures occasionally may be associated with the development of focal outpouching or sacculation of the distal esophagus due to ballooning of the esophageal wall between areas of fibrosis (Fig. 5–33). The latter finding is particularly common in patients with scleroderma because of the severe esophagitis that occurs in these individuals (Fig. 5–34). Scarring from reflux esophagitis may also be manifested by fixed transverse folds in the distal esophagus, producing a characteristic "stepladder" appearance due to pooling of barium between the folds (Fig. 5–35).[25] These transverse folds are usually 2 to 5 mm wide and do not extend more than halfway across the esophagus. They should be distinguished radiographically from the delicate transverse folds that are often ob-

served as a transient finding on double contrast studies (see Figs. 5–8 and 5–9).

Esophageal intramural pseudodiverticulosis occasionally may be found in patients with peptic strictures (Fig. 5–36).[27] The pseudodiverticula represent dilated excretory ducts of deep mucous glands in the esophagus. They usually appear as 1- to 3-mm collections of barium projecting outside the esophageal lumen. Although the pseudodiverticula can be mistaken for ulcers, these structures often seem to be "floating" outside the esophagus without apparent communication with the lumen (see Figs. 5–29*B* and 5–36), whereas true ulcers almost always communicate directly with the lumen. The majority of patients with esophageal intramural pseudodiverticulosis have associated reflux disease with localized pseudodiverticula in the region of a peptic stricture.[27] Thus, esophageal intramural pseudodiverticulosis probably represents a sequela of chronic reflux esophagitis, although the reason that so few patients with esophagitis develop this condition is unclear.

Barrett's Esophagus

Barrett's esophagus is a well-recognized entity in which there is progressive columnar metaplasia of the distal esophagus due to long-standing gastroesophageal reflux and reflux esophagitis. Barrett's esophagus is important because it is a premalignant condition associated with a significantly increased risk of the development of esophageal adenocarcinoma.

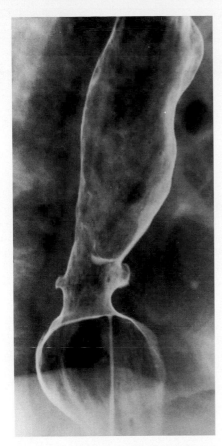

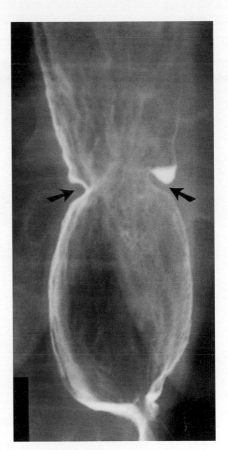

FIGURE 5–33. Peptic stricture with associated sacculations in distal esophagus. Note hiatal hernia below stricture.

FIGURE 5–34. Sacculated peptic stricture *(arrows)* in a patient with scleroderma.

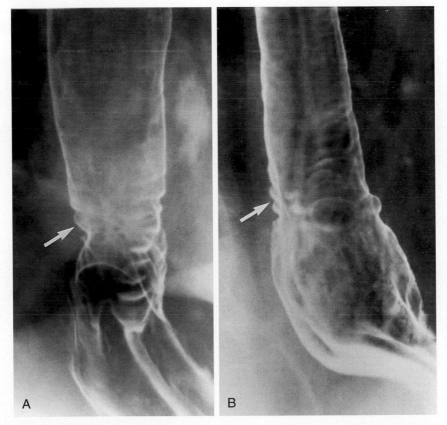

FIGURE 5–35. Two examples (*A* and *B*) of "stepladder" appearance with multiple transverse folds in distal esophagus due to scarring from reflux esophagitis. Note puckering of esophageal wall *(arrows).* (From Levine, M.S., and Goldstein, H.M.: Fixed transverse folds in the esophagus: A sign of reflux esophagitis. AJR Am. J. Roentgenol. *143:*275, 1984, with permission, © by American Roentgen Ray Society.)

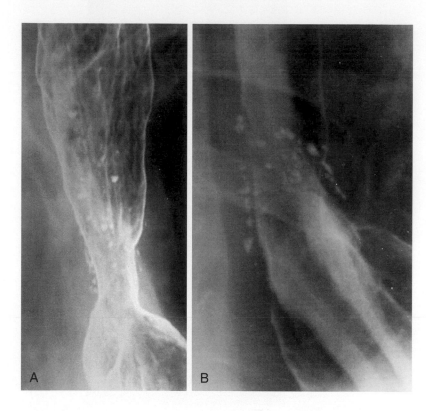

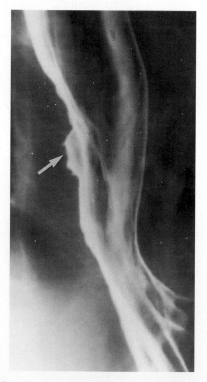

FIGURE 5–36. Two examples (*A* and *B*) of peptic strictures with localized esophageal intramural pseudodiverticulosis in region of stricture. Note how most pseudodiverticula, unlike ulcers, do not appear to communicate with esophageal lumen.

The classic radiologic features of Barrett's esophagus consist of a high stricture or ulcer associated with a sliding hiatal hernia, gastroesophageal reflux, or both (Figs. 5–37 and 5–38).[28] However, recent studies have found that strictures are actually more common in the distal esophagus and that most cases do not fit the classic description of a high stricture or ulcer.[29–31] A reticular mucosal pattern has also been described as a relatively specific sign of Barrett's esophagus on double contrast studies.[30] This reticular pattern is characterized by innu-

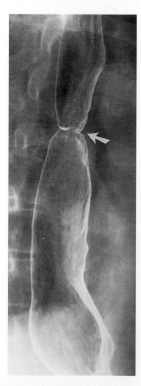

FIGURE 5–37. Barrett's esophagus with high stricture *(arrow)*. (From Levine, M.S.: Radiology of the Esophagus. Philadelphia, W.B. Saunders, 1989, p. 40.)

FIGURE 5–38. Barrett's esophagus with high ulcer *(arrow)*. Note the relatively large ulcer crater at a greater distance from the gastroesophageal junction than would be expected for uncomplicated reflux esophagitis. (From Levine, M.S.: Radiology of the Esophagus. Philadelphia, W.B. Saunders, 1989, p. 41.)

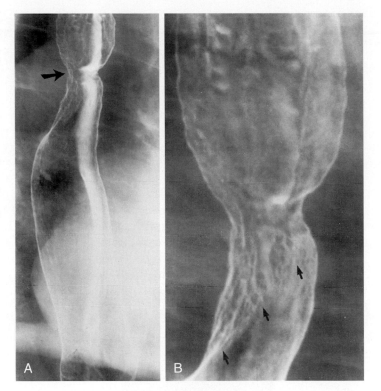

FIGURE 5–39. Barrett's esophagus with high stricture and reticular mucosal pattern. *A,* Midesophageal stricture *(arrow)* with reticular pattern adjacent to distal aspect of stricture. *B,* Close-up view better delineates this delicate reticular pattern *(arrows).* (From Levine, M.S., et al.: Barrett esophagus: Reticular pattern of the mucosa. Radiology *147*:663, 1983, with permission.)

merable, tiny, barium-filled grooves or crevices on the esophageal mucosa, often resembling the areae gastricae pattern found on double contrast studies of the stomach. In most cases, there is an associated stricture in the middle or, less frequently, distal esophagus, with the reticular pattern extending distally a short but variable distance from the stricture (Figs. 5–39 and 5–40). Occasionally, the reticular pattern may be detected as an isolated abnormality without an associated stricture.[32] However, this finding has been observed in only a minority of patients

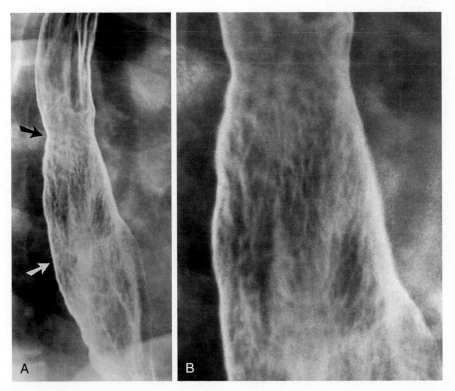

FIGURE 5–40. Barrett's esophagus with high stricture and reticular mucosal pattern. *A, Black arrow* indicates early stricture in midesophagus with reticular pattern extending distally to level of *white arrow. B,* Close-up view better delineates this reticular pattern. (From Levine, M.S., et al.: Barrett esophagus: Reticular pattern of the mucosa. Radiology *147*:663, 1983, with permission.)

with Barrett's esophagus.[30,33] Other more common findings in Barrett's esophagus, such as hiatal hernias, gastroesophageal reflux, reflux esophagitis, and peptic strictures, frequently occur in patients with uncomplicated reflux disease (Fig. 5–41). Thus, radiographic findings that are relatively specific for Barrett's esophagus are not sensitive, and findings that are sensitive are not specific. Many investigators therefore believe that esophagography has limited value as a screening examination for Barrett's esophagus and that endoscopy and biopsy are required to diagnose this condition.

In one study, however, Gilchrist and colleagues performed a blinded, retrospective review of 200 patients who underwent both double contrast esophagrams and endoscopy because of severe reflux symptoms.[34] Patients were classified at high risk for Barrett's esophagus if the radiographs revealed a high stricture, high ulcer, or reticular mucosal pattern; at moderate risk if the radiographs

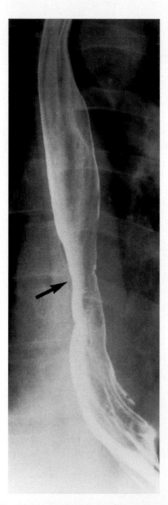

FIGURE 5–41. Barrett's esophagus with stricture *(arrow)* in distal esophagus above sliding hiatal hernia. An ordinary peptic stricture without Barrett's esophagus could produce identical findings. (From Gilchrist, A.M., et al.: Barrett's esophagus: Diagnosis by double-contrast esophagography. AJR Am. J. Roentgenol. *150:*97, 1988, with permission, © by American Roentgen Ray Society.)

revealed a distal stricture or reflux esophagitis; and at low risk if the esophagus appeared normal (i.e., if no esophagitis or strictures were noted). Using these radiologic criteria, the investigators found endoscopic proof of Barrett's esophagus in 9 of 10 patients (90%) at high risk, in 12 of 73 patients (16%) at moderate risk, and in only one of 117 patients (less than 1%) at low risk for Barrett's esophagus. Although mild esophagitis can be missed radiographically, the data suggest that esophagitis severe enough to cause Barrett's esophagus can almost always be detected on technically adequate double contrast examinations. Thus, the major value of double contrast esophagography is its ability to classify patients with reflux symptoms into these various risk groups for Barrett's esophagus to determine the relative need for endoscopy and biopsy.

Infections
Candida *Esophagitis*

Candida esophagitis is the most common infectious condition in the esophagus. It usually occurs as an opportunistic infection in patients who are immunocompromised as a result of underlying malignancy; other debilitating illnesses; treatment with radiation, steroids, or cytotoxic agents; or, most recently, acquired immunodeficiency syndrome (AIDS).[35–38] However, *Candida* esophagitis may also be caused by local esophageal stasis due to strictures, achalasia, or scleroderma.[39] Only about 50% of patients with *Candida* esophagitis are found to have oropharyngeal candidiasis (i.e., thrush), so that the absence of oropharyngeal disease in no way excludes this diagnosis. Occasionally, *Candida* esophagitis may occur in otherwise healthy, "immunocompetent" individuals who have no underlying esophageal diseases.[40] The possibility of fungal infection therefore should not be excluded simply because the classic predisposing factors are not present in a particular patient.

Despite its frequency, the radiologic diagnosis of *Candida* esophagitis has been limited because it is a superficial disease with mucosal abnormalities that are difficult to detect with conventional single contrast barium studies. However, double contrast esophagography has a sensitivity of about 90% in diagnosing *Candida* esophagitis.[41,42] The major advantage of this technique is its ability to demonstrate mucosal plaques that cannot easily be recognized by single contrast studies. As a result, only mild cases of *Candida* esophagitis are likely to be missed by the double contrast examination.

Candida esophagitis is first manifested radiographically by discrete plaquelike lesions corresponding to the characteristic white plaques seen during endoscopy. The plaques tend to be longitudinally oriented, appearing en face as linear or irregular filling defects with normal intervening mucosa (Fig. 5–42).[24,41] Because these lesions have discrete borders, they may be etched in white

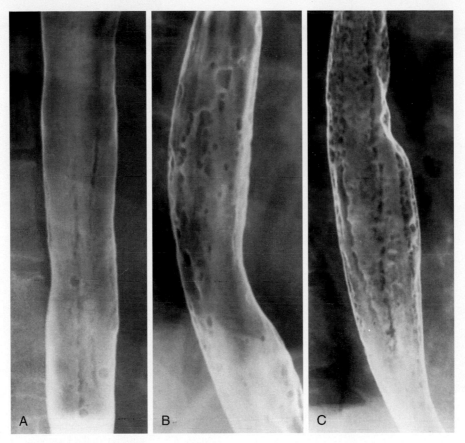

FIGURE 5–42. *Candida* **esophagitis with plaques.** *A,* Several linear plaques seen in middle and distal esophagus are due to relatively early *Candida* esophagitis. (Note round filling defects due to air bubbles.) *B,* More extensive plaque formation in another patient. Note irregular configuration of plaques. *C,* More advanced case with numerous discrete, longitudinal plaques in esophagus. (From Levine, M.S., et al.: *Candida* esophagitis: Accuracy of radiographic diagnosis. Radiology *154:*581, 1985, with permission.)

by a thin layer of barium trapped between the edge of the plaque and the adjacent mucosa. Whether these mucosal plaques are localized or diffuse, their typical en face appearance should strongly suggest the diagnosis of *Candida* esophagitis. In other patients the esophagus may have a finely nodular or granular appearance due to mucosal inflammation and edema or actual tiny plaques on the mucosa (Fig. 5–43).[18,43] When larger plaques are present, the lesions may coalesce, producing a distinctive "cobblestone" or "snakeskin" appearance (Fig. 5–44).[44]

During the past decade, a much more fulminant form of candidiasis has been encountered in patients with AIDS who may present with a grossly irregular or "shaggy" esophagus due to innumerable coalescent plaques and pseudomembranes with trapping of barium between these lesions (Fig. 5–45).[41,43] In one study, a shaggy esophagus was found in nearly 25% of AIDS patients with radiographically diagnosed *Candida* esophagitis.[43] Because this degree of esophagitis rarely occurs in other immunocompromised patients, the possibility of AIDS should be suspected when a shaggy esophagus is demonstrated by barium studies, particularly in high-risk patients. Some of

the plaques and pseudomembranes of severe *Candida* esophagitis may eventually slough, producing one or more deep ulcers superimposed on a background of diffuse plaque formation (Fig. 5–45*B*). Thus, ulceration in candidiasis is almost always associated with extensive plaque formation and rarely occurs on an otherwise normal background mucosa.

Candida esophagitis occasionally may be associated with polypoid lesions in the esophagus because of coalescent masses of heaped-up necrotic debris and fungal mycelia (i.e., fungus balls).[45] In patients with chronic esophageal stasis due to achalasia or scleroderma, *Candida* esophagitis may also be manifested by fine nodularity, polypoid folds, or a distinctive lacy appearance in the esophagus (Fig. 5–46).[39]

Candida esophagitis usually responds quickly to treatment with ketoconazole or other antifungal agents, so that the findings may regress dramatically on repeat esophagrams within several days of treatment. Occasionally, severe *Candida* esophagitis may lead to the development of strictures that typically appear as long, tapered areas of narrowing in the middle or distal esophagus (Fig. 5–47).[46] Strictures are more likely to develop in patients

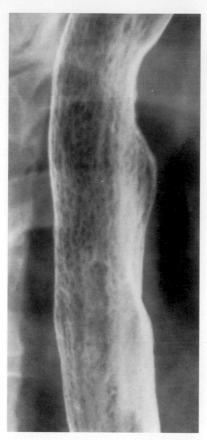

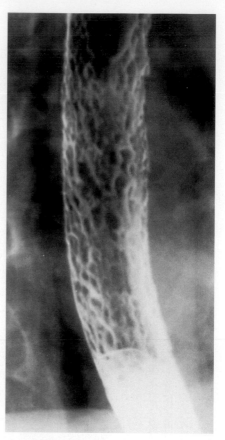

FIGURE 5–43. *Candida* esophagitis with finely nodular or granular mucosa due to tiny plaques in midesophagus.

FIGURE 5–44. *Candida* esophagitis with "cobblestone" or "snakeskin" appearance due to numerous coalescent plaques. (From Levine, M.S.: Radiology of the Esophagus. Philadelphia, W.B. Saunders, 1989, p. 54, with permission.)

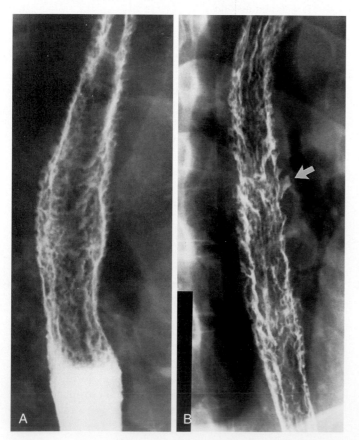

FIGURE 5–45. *Candida* esophagitis with "shaggy" esophagus. *A,* Note grossly irregular esophageal contour due to numerous plaques and pseudomembranes. (From Levine, M.S., et al.: *Candida* esophagitis: Accuracy of radiographic diagnosis. Radiology *154*:581, 1985, with permission.) *B,* Shaggy esophagus in a patient with AIDS. Although this finding results primarily from trapping of barium between plaques, an area of relatively deep ulceration *(arrow)* can be seen. (From Levine, M.S., et al.: Opportunistic esophagitis in AIDS: Radiographic diagnosis. Radiology *165*:815, 1987, with permission.)

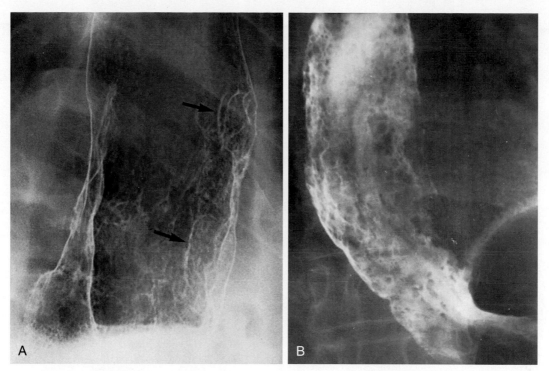

FIGURE 5–46. Chronic candidiasis in patients with esophageal stasis. *A,* Note lacy appearance of mucosa with large plaques *(arrows)* in a patient with achalasia. *B,* Note fine nodularity of the mucosa due to *Candida* esophagitis in another patient with scleroderma. Also note the dilated esophagus and patulous lower esophageal sphincter.

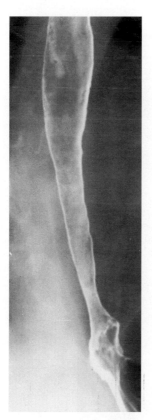

FIGURE 5–47. Long, tapered stricture involving middle and distal esophagus due to scarring from severe *Candida* esophagitis. (From Levine, M.S.: Radiology of the Esophagus. Philadelphia, W.B. Saunders, 1989, p. 56, with permission.)

who have chronic mucocutaneous candidiasis involving the nails, skin, mucous membranes, and esophagus.[47]

Herpes Esophagitis

Herpes simplex virus type 1 has been recognized as the second most frequent cause of opportunistic esophagitis in immunocompromised patients. Occasionally, however, an acute, transient form of herpes esophagitis may occur in otherwise healthy individuals who have no underlying immunologic problems.[48,49] Patients with herpes esophagitis usually present with acute odynophagia or dysphagia, so that the clinical presentation is indistinguishable from that of *Candida* esophagitis. Although herpes esophagitis tends to be a self-limited disease, acyclovir, a potent antiviral agent, has been used successfully to treat these patients.

Vesicle formation, the earliest endoscopic finding in herpes esophagitis, has not been demonstrated by radiologic studies. However, the vesicles subsequently rupture to form discrete, superficial ulcers on the esophageal mucosa that can readily be visualized on double contrast radiographs. In one study, double contrast esophagrams revealed discrete ulcers without plaques in more than 50% of patients with endoscopically proved herpes esophagitis.[50] These ulcers may have a punctate, linear, or stellate configuration and are often surrounded by a radiolucent halo of edematous mucosa (Figs. 5–48 and 5–49).[50,51] They may be clustered together or widely separated by intervening segments of normal mucosa. In the appropri-

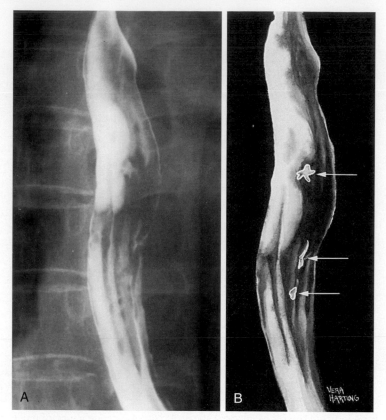

FIGURE 5–48. *A* and *B,* Herpes esophagitis with several shallow, widely separated ulcers *(arrows)* in midesophagus. Note stellate configuration of most proximal ulcer.

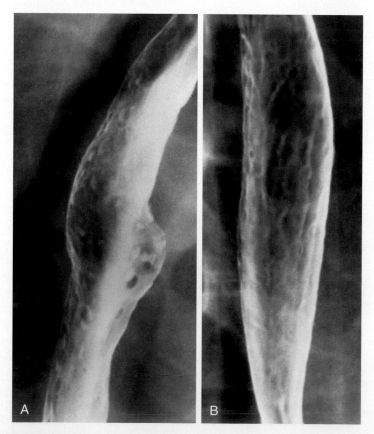

FIGURE 5–49. Herpes esophagitis with discrete ulcers. *A,* Multiple superficial ulcers in midesophagus. Note halos of edematous mucosa surrounding ulcers. *B,* Different patient with linear and serpiginous ulcers in midesophagus. (From Levine, M.S.: Radiology of the Esophagus. Philadelphia, W.B. Saunders, 1989, p. 62.)

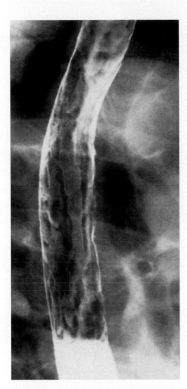

FIGURE 5–50. Advanced herpes esophagitis with multiple linear plaques indistinguishable from those of *Candida* esophagitis. (From Skucas, J., et al.: Herpes esophagitis: A case studied by air-contrast esophagography. AJR Am. J. Roentgenol. *128:*497, 1977, with permission, © by American Roentgen Ray Society.)

ate clinical setting, discrete ulcers on an otherwise normal background mucosa should strongly suggest herpes esophagitis because ulceration almost invariably occurs on a background of diffuse plaque formation in patients with candidiasis.[41,43] However, more advanced herpes esophagitis may be manifested by extensive ulceration, plaque formation, or a combination of ulcers and plaques in the esophagus (Fig. 5–50).[50–52] Advanced herpes esophagitis therefore may be indistinguishable radiographically from *Candida* esophagitis.

The ability to distinguish fungal and viral esophagitis on double contrast radiographs is important in the treatment of all immunocompromised patients, but particularly in the treatment of patients with AIDS, as many gastroenterologists are reluctant to perform endoscopy on these individuals for fear of contaminating their endoscopic instruments or exposing themselves to the AIDS virus. Recent data suggest that *Candida* esophagitis and herpes esophagitis can be accurately diagnosed in AIDS patients by their characteristic features on double contrast esophagrams, eliminating the need for endoscopic intervention in many cases (Fig. 5–51).[43] Nevertheless, endoscopy may be required for a definitive diagnosis if the radiographic findings are equivocal or if appropriate treatment with antifungal or antiviral agents fails to produce an adequate clinical response in these patients.

In contrast, herpes esophagitis in otherwise healthy patients is characterized by innumerable tiny ulcers that

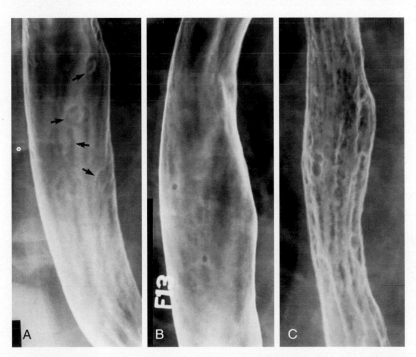

FIGURE 5–51. Herpes and *Candida* esophagitis in a patient with AIDS. *A,* Initial esophagram shows discrete, superficial ulcers *(arrows)* in midesophagus without evidence of plaques. Note halos of edematous mucosa surrounding ulcers. These findings should strongly suggest herpes esophagitis. *B,* Repeat esophagram obtained 2 weeks after treatment with intravenous acyclovir shows healing of ulcers with normal-appearing mucosa in this region. (Note air bubbles in esophagus.) *C,* Third esophagram obtained 3 months later shows linear plaquelike lesions in esophagus that are compatible with *Candida* esophagitis. The patient had a dramatic clinical response to treatment with ketoconazole. *(A, B,* and *C,* From Levine, M.S., et al.: Opportunistic esophagitis in AIDS: Radiographic diagnosis. Radiology *165:*815, 1987, with permission.)

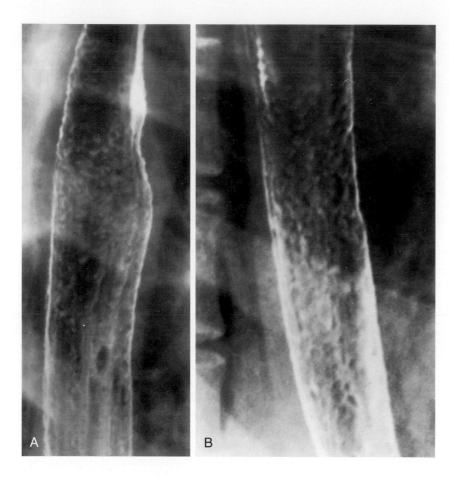

FIGURE 5–52. Two examples *(A and B)* of herpes esophagitis in otherwise healthy patients. In both cases, multiple tiny, superficial ulcers are clustered together in the midesophagus. *(A* From DeGaeta, L., et al.: Herpes esophagitis in an otherwise healthy patient. AJR Am. J. Roentgenol. *144:*1205, 1985, with permission, © by American Roentgen Ray Society.)

tend to be clustered together in the midesophagus below the level of the left main bronchus (Fig. 5–52).[49,53] It has been postulated that the ulcers are smaller than those in immunocompromised patients because these individuals have an intact immune system that prevents the ulcers from enlarging.[53] Affected individuals typically are young men with a recent history of exposure to sexual partners with oropharyngeal herpes. These patients often present with a characteristic flulike prodrome consisting of fever, headaches, myalgias, and upper respiratory infection for a period of 7 to 10 days before the sudden onset of severe odynophagia.[53] Thus, the diagnosis of herpes esophagitis in healthy patients can usually be suggested on the basis of the clinical and radiographic findings.

Cytomegalovirus Esophagitis

Cytomegalovirus (CMV) is another member of the herpesvirus group that has recently been recognized as a cause of opportunistic esophagitis in patients with AIDS. CMV esophagitis may be manifested radiographically by discrete, superficial ulcers that are indistinguishable from those of herpes esophagitis (Fig. 5–53).[54] More commonly, however, these patients have one or more large, relatively flat ulcers that are several centimeters or more in length (Fig. 5–54).[43,54] These giant ulcers may have an ovoid or diamond-shaped configuration and are often surrounded by a radiolucent rim of edematous mucosa. Because herpetic ulcers rarely become this large, the presence of one or more giant esophageal ulcers should

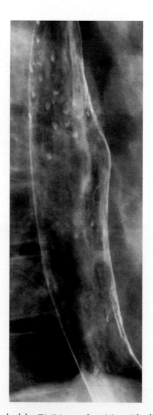

FIGURE 5–53. Probable CMV esophagitis with discrete, superficial ulcers separated by normal mucosa. Although endoscopic biopsy specimens were negative for CMV, this patient had elevated CMV titers at the time of the barium study. (From Levine, M.S.: Radiology of the Esophagus. Philadelphia, W.B. Saunders, 1989, p. 66.)

strongly suggest the possibility of CMV esophagitis in patients with AIDS. However, the treatment for CMV esophagitis includes relatively toxic antiviral agents (e.g., ganciclovir) that are associated with bone marrow suppression. Endoscopic brushings, biopsy specimens, and cultures are therefore required for a definitive diagnosis before treating these patients

Human Immunodeficiency Virus Esophagitis

In recent years, giant human immunodeficiency virus (HIV)–related esophageal ulcers have been encountered with increased frequency in HIV-positive patients with odynophagia.[55–57] Occasionally, affected individuals have associated palatal ulcers or a characteristic maculopapular rash on the upper half of the body.[56,57] Some of these patients have undergone recent seroconversion, so that they may have just become HIV positive at or near the time of clinical presentation. Endoscopic brushings, biopsy specimens, and cultures are all negative for CMV; HIV esophagitis is therefore a diagnosis of exclusion.[56,57] Finally, these patients may respond dramatically to treatment with oral steroids.[56,57] Thus, endoscopy should be performed on HIV-positive patients with giant esophageal

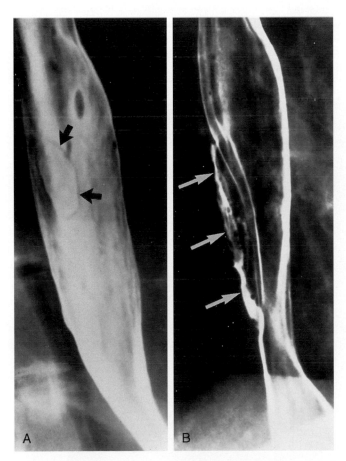

FIGURE 5–54. Two examples (*A* and *B*) of giant, relatively flat ulcers *(arrows)* in AIDS patients with CMV esophagitis. Note how ulcer is seen en face in *A* and in profile in *B*. (*A*, Courtesy of Kyunghee C. Cho, M.D., Bronx, New York. *B*, Courtesy of Patrick C. Freeny, M.D., Seattle, Washington.)

ulcers to differentiate HIV from CMV infection in the esophagus.

HIV esophagitis may be manifested on double contrast radiographs by one or more giant, flat ulcers that appear as ovoid or diamond-shaped collections of barium surrounded by a radiolucent rim of edematous mucosa (Fig. 5–55).[56,57] These giant ulcers are indistinguishable on barium studies from CMV ulcers in the esophagus. In fact, recent data suggest that most giant esophageal ulcers in HIV-positive patients are caused by HIV rather than CMV and that it is not possible to differentiate these infections by clinical or radiographic criteria.[57] Endoscopy is therefore required for a definitive diagnosis, so that appropriate therapy can be initiated in these patients.

Drug-Induced Esophagitis

Drug-induced esophagitis tends to involve the middle or upper esophagus with distal esophageal sparing.[58,59] About half of the cases are caused by antibiotics, particularly tetracycline and its derivative, doxycycline. Other oral medications implicated less frequently include potassium chloride, quinidine, aspirin, and other nonsteroidal anti-inflammatory drugs (NSAIDs). These patients typically have a history of ingesting the medication with little or no water immediately before going to bed. Prolonged exposure to the tablets or capsules is thought to cause a focal contact esophagitis, most frequently in the region of the aortic arch or left main bronchus. These patients often present with severe odynophagia, but rapid clinical improvement usually occurs after withdrawal of the offending agent.

Drug-induced esophagitis caused by tetracycline or doxycycline is usually manifested by a small solitary ulcer, several discrete ulcers, or a localized cluster of tiny ulcers distributed circumferentially on a normal background mucosa (Fig. 5–56).[58,59] The ulcers tend to be located in the upper or middle thirds of the esophagus near the level of the aortic arch or left main bronchus. When the ulcers are shallow, they may appear as ring shadows because of barium coating the rim of the unfilled ulcer crater (see Fig. 5–56*A*). Although herpes esophagitis may produce identical radiographic findings, a history of recent drug ingestion should suggest the correct diagnosis.

In contrast, drug-induced esophagitis caused by potassium chloride or quinidine can result in the development of large ulcers with considerable surrounding edema, occasionally mimicking the appearance of an ulcerated carcinoma.[58,60] Because of the degree of esophageal injury, these drugs can sometimes lead to the development of esophageal strictures, which typically are located above the level of an enlarged left atrium.[61] Aspirin and other NSAIDs have also been recognized as a cause of giant esophageal ulcers and strictures.[62,63] When esophageal ulcers are drug-induced, a repeat esophagram 7 to 10 days after withdrawal of the offending agent should show marked healing of the lesions.[58]

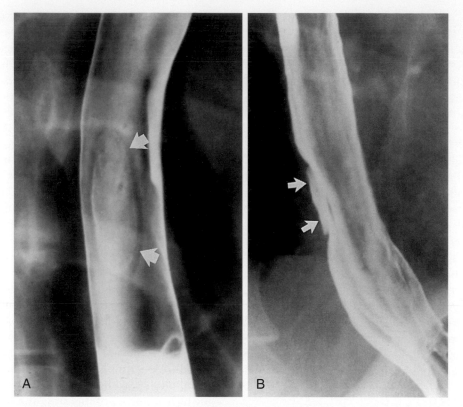

FIGURE 5–55. Two examples (*A* and *B*) of giant, relatively flat ulcers *(arrows)* in HIV-positive patients with HIV esophagitis. Note how ulcer is seen en face in *A* and in profile in *B*. These giant ulcers are impossible to differentiate from the ulcers of CMV esophagitis illustrated in Fig. 5–54. (*A,* From Levine, M.S., Loercher, G., Katzka, D.A., et al.: Giant, human immunodeficiency virus–related ulcers in the esophagus. Radiology *180:*323, 1991, with permission. *B,* From Sor, S., Levine, M.S., Kowalski, T.E., et al.: Giant ulcers of the esophagus in patients with human immunodeficiency virus: Clinical, radiographic, and pathologic findings. Radiology *194:*447, 1995, with permission.)

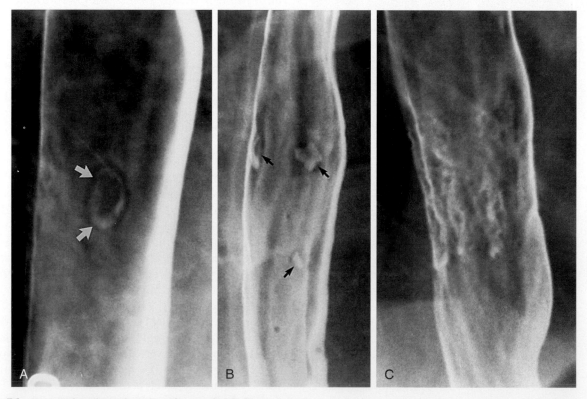

FIGURE 5–56. Drug-induced esophagitis with superficial ulcers. *A,* Solitary doxycycline-induced ulcer *(arrows)* in midesophagus. Note thin radiolucent halo surrounding ulcer. *B,* Several discrete ulcers *(arrows)* in midesophagus due to tetracycline ingestion. Note stellate configuration of largest ulcer. *C,* Doxycycline-induced esophagitis with multiple small, serpiginous ulcers clustered together in lower esophagus.

Other Types of Esophagitis
Nasogastric-Intubation Esophagitis

Nasogastric intubation occasionally may lead to the development of long strictures in the distal esophagus (Fig. 5–57). These patients probably have a severe form of reflux esophagitis induced by the tube.[64] The strictures are characterized by their tendency to progress rapidly in length and severity within a relatively short period.

Caustic Esophagitis

Long, ulcerated strictures may also be observed in patients who have ingested lye or other caustic agents. In severe cases, diffuse esophageal narrowing may reduce the thoracic esophagus to a thin, filiform structure (Fig. 5–58). Long-standing lye strictures apparently predispose patients to the development of esophageal carcinoma.[65] Thus, any mucosal irregularity in a chronic lye stricture should raise the possibility of carcinoma (Fig. 5–59).

Radiation Esophagitis

Radiation therapy to the chest or mediastinum may cause severe esophagitis and strictures when the dose to the esophagus exceeds 5000 rad.[66] Acute radiation esophagitis usually occurs 1 to 4 weeks after the onset of radiation therapy. This form of esophagitis may be manifested on double contrast studies by ulceration or, even more commonly, by a distinctive granular appearance of the mucosa and decreased distensibility due to edema and inflammation of the irradiated esophagus (Fig. 5–60A).[67] The involved segment typically has abrupt margins that conform to the borders of the radiation portal. In contrast, chronic radiation strictures typically appear as smooth, tapered areas of concentric narrowing within a preexisting radiation portal (Fig. 5–60B).

Miscellaneous

Other inflammatory diseases, such as Crohn's disease,[68,69] benign mucous membrane pemphigoid,[70] and epidermolysis bullosa dystrophica,[71] may also involve the esophagus. Rarely, esophageal Crohn's disease may be manifested by discrete "aphthous" ulcers similar to those found in granulomatous colitis (Fig. 5–61).[68,69] However, these patients almost always have advanced Crohn's disease in the small bowel or colon.

Some patients with esophageal intramural pseudodiverticulosis may have a small cluster of pseudodiverticula associated with a peptic stricture in the distal esophagus (see Fig. 5–36). However, others may have innumerable pseudodiverticula seen en face and in profile as tiny flask-shaped outpouchings in longitudinal rows parallel to the long axis of the esophagus (Fig. 5–62).[27] For reasons that are unclear, the diffuse form of esophageal intramural pseudodiverticulosis is often associated with strictures in the upper or middle thoracic esophagus (see Fig. 5–62A).

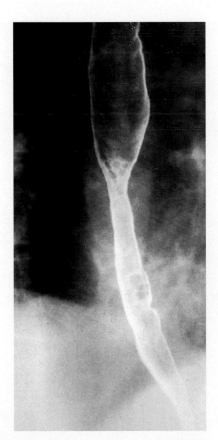

FIGURE 5–57. Long stricture in distal esophagus due to prolonged nasogastric intubation.

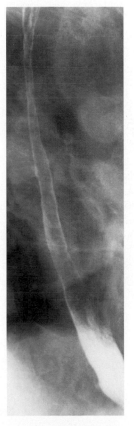

FIGURE 5–58. Lye stricture with diffuse narrowing of thoracic esophagus. This appearance should suggest caustic injury, as other conditions rarely cause such extensive esophageal narrowing.

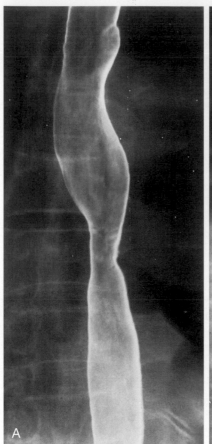

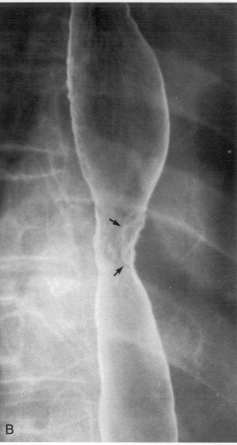

FIGURE 5–59. *A* and *B,* Carcinoma developing at the site of a lye stricture in a 70-year-old man who had ingested lye at the age of 4 years. Note focal stricture in midesophagus with superficial ulceration and nodularity of mucosa *(arrows)* in region of stricture. Endoscopic brushings and biopsy specimens revealed squamous cell carcinoma, but the patient refused surgery.

FIGURE 5–60. Radiation injury to the esophagus. *A,* Acute radiation esophagitis manifested by a granular mucosa and mild narrowing of upper thoracic esophagus. (From Collazzo, L.A., Levine, M.S., Rubesin, S.E., et al.: Acute radiation esophagitis: Radiographic findings. AJR Am. J. Roentgenol. *169:*1067, 1997, with permission, © by American Roentgen Ray Society.) *B,* Smooth, tapered stricture in midesophagus due to chronic radiation injury.

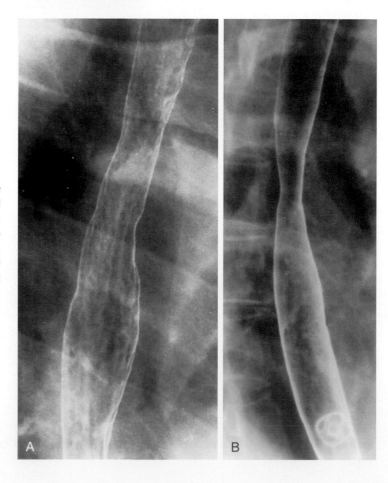

FIGURE **5–61. Esophageal Crohn's disease with "aphthous" ulcers.** *A,* Note tiny ulcers *(arrows)* in midesophagus with surrounding mounds of edema. *B,* Double contrast barium enema shows innumerable aphthous ulcers in colon due to associated granulomatous colitis. (*A* and *B,* Courtesy of Harvey M. Goldstein, M.D., San Antonio, Texas.)

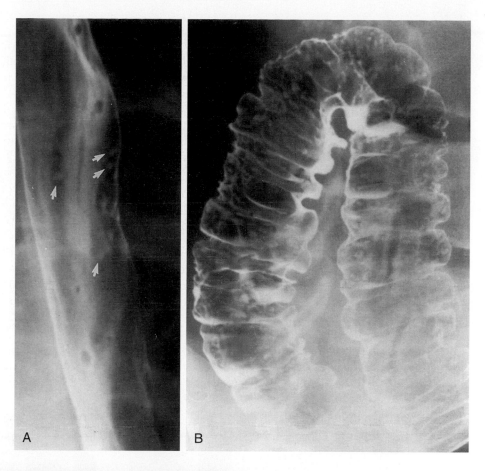

A

B

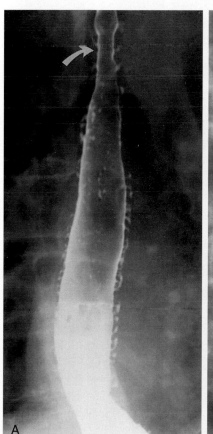

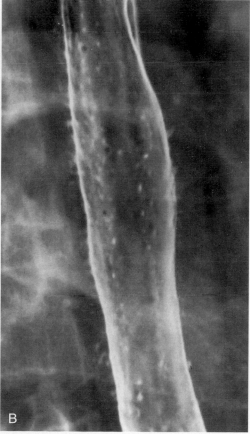

A

B

FIGURE **5–62. Esophageal intramural pseudodiverticulosis.** Two examples (*A* and *B*) of innumerable pseudodiverticula seen en face and in profile as tiny flask-shaped outpouchings in longitudinal rows parallel to the long axis of the esophagus. In *A,* there is an associated stricture *(arrow)* in the upper thoracic esophagus.

Differential Diagnosis of Esophagitis
Nodularity

Mucosal nodularity may be a feature of reflux esophagitis or infectious esophagitis. However, the nodules of reflux esophagitis tend to have poorly defined borders that fade peripherally into the adjacent mucosa, whereas the plaquelike lesions of *Candida* esophagitis usually have discrete borders separated by normal mucosa. Mucosal nodularity may also be caused by glycogenic acanthosis, a benign, degenerative condition in which cellular glycogen accumulates in the squamous epithelial lining of the esophagus. Double contrast esophagrams may reveal multiple small, rounded nodules or plaques indistinguishable from those of *Candida* esophagitis (Fig. 5–63; see Chapter 6).[72] However, patients with glycogenic acanthosis are almost always asymptomatic, whereas *Candida* esophagitis usually occurs in immunocompromised patients with odynophagia. Thus, the clinical history is extremely helpful for differentiating these conditions. Occasionally, a superficial spreading carcinoma, or even an advanced carcinoma, may cause localized or diffuse nodularity of the mucosa (Fig. 5–64; see Chapter 6).[73]

Ulceration

Mucosal ulceration may be simulated by transverse folds seen in profile (see Figs. 5–8 and 5–9) or by focal spiculation of the upper esophagus occurring as a normal variant (see Fig. 5–11A). Scarring from reflux esophagitis may produce one or more sacculations or outpouchings near the gastroesophageal junction that can also be mistaken for ulcers (see Figs. 5–33 and 5–34). However, these sacculations tend to have a more rounded configuration and are not associated with radiating folds or surrounding mounds of edema. Unlike ulcers, sacculations also tend to change in size and shape during the fluoroscopic examination. Esophageal intramural pseudodiverticulosis is another cause of barium projections that must be differentiated from ulcers. As indicated earlier, the pseudodiverticula often seem to be "floating" outside the esophagus on tangential views, a radiologic clue to the presence of these structures (see Figs. 5–29B and 5–36).[27]

Abnormal Mucosal Folds

Esophageal varices may resemble the enlarged folds of chronic esophagitis (Fig. 5–65). However, varices tend

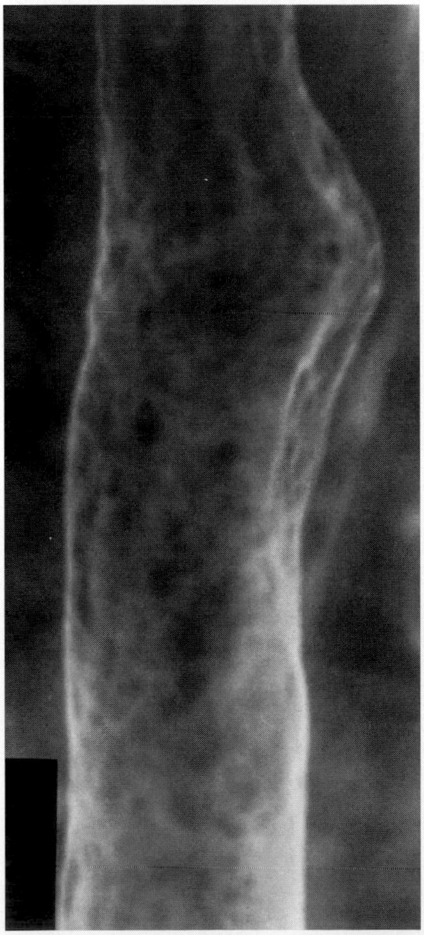

FIGURE 5–63. Glycogenic acanthosis with mucosal nodularity. Reflux esophagitis or *Candida* esophagitis could produce similar findings, but this patient was asymptomatic.

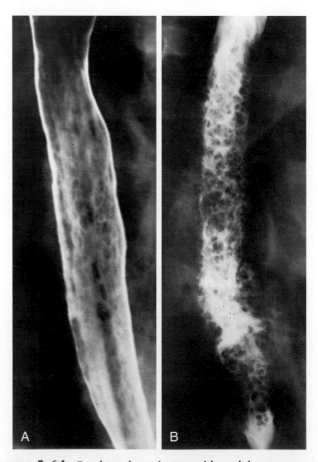

FIGURE 5–64. Esophageal carcinoma with nodular mucosa. *A,* Diffuse mucosal nodularity due to superficial spreading carcinoma. (Courtesy of Akiyoshi Yamada, M.D., Tokyo, Japan.) *B,* Diffuse mucosal nodularity due to advanced esophageal carcinoma. (Courtesy of Hans Herlinger, M.D., Philadelphia, Pennsylvania.)

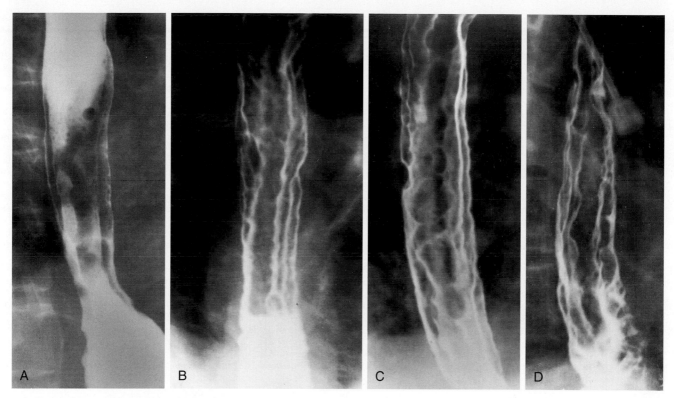

FIGURE 5–65. Four examples (*A* through *D*) of esophageal varices, with thickened longitudinal folds resembling those in patients with esophagitis. However, varices tend to have a more scalloped appearance.

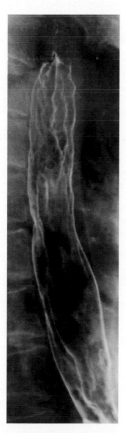

FIGURE 5–66. "Varicoid" carcinoma with thickened, tortuous folds, mimicking the appearance of esophageal varices. (Courtesy of Akiyoshi Yamada, M.D., Tokyo, Japan.)

to be more tortuous or serpiginous and can be effaced to a greater degree or even obliterated by esophageal distention, peristalsis, or Valsalva maneuvers. Occasionally, "varicoid" carcinomas may also be manifested by thickened, tortuous longitudinal folds due to submucosal spread of tumor (Fig. 5–66; see Chapter 6).[74,75]

REFERENCES

1. Levine, M.S., Rubesin, S.E., Herlinger, H.H., et al.: Double-contrast upper gastrointestinal examination: Technique and interpretation. Radiology *168*:593, 1988.
2. Cassel, D.M., Anderson, M.F., and Zboralske, F.F.: Double-contrast esophagrams: The prone technique. Radiology *139*:737, 1981.
3. Hogan, W.J., Dodds, W.J., Hoke, S.E., et al.: Effect of glucagon on esophageal motor function. Gastroenterology *69*:160, 1975.
4. Levine, M.S., Kressel, H.Y., Laufer, I., et al.: The tube esophagram: A technique for obtaining a detailed double-contrast examination of the esophagus. AJR Am. J. Roentgenol. *142*:293, 1984.
5. Friedland, G.W., and Filly, R.: The post-cricoid impression masquerading as an esophageal tumor. Am. J. Dig. Dis. *20*:287, 1985.
6. Goldberg, H.I., Dodds, W.J., and Jenis, E.H.: Experimental esophagitis: Roentgenographic findings after insufflation of tantalum powder. AJR Am. J. Roentgenol. *110*:288, 1970.
7. Gohel, V.K., Edell, S.L., Laufer, I., et al.: Transverse folds in the human esophagus. Radiology *128*:303, 1978.
8. Williams, S.M., Harned, R.K., Kaplan, P., et al.: Transverse striations of the esophagus: Association with gastroesophageal reflux. Radiology *146*:25, 1983.
9. Levine, M.S., Low, V., Laufer, I., et al.: Focal spiculation of the upper thoracic esophagus: Normal variant at double-contrast esophagography. Radiology *183*:807, 1992.
10. Ueno, J., Davis, S.W., Tanakami, A., et al.: Ectopic gastric mucosa in the upper esophagus: Detection and radiographic findings. Radiology *191*:751, 1994.

11. Takeji, H., Ueno, J., and Nishitani, H.: Ectopic gastric mucosa in the upper esophagus: Prevalence and radiographic findings. AJR Am. J. Roentgenol. *164*:901, 1995.

12. Gohel, V.K., Kressel, H.Y., and Laufer, I.: Double-contrast artifacts. Gastrointest. Radiol. *3*:139, 1978.

13. Cho, S.R., Henry, D.A., Shaw, C.I., et al.: Vanishing intraluminal diverticulum of the esophagus. Gastrointest. Radiol. 7:315, 1982.

14. Maglinte, D.D.T., Lappas, J.C., Chernish, S.M., et al.: Flow artifacts in double-contrast esophagography. Radiology *157*:535, 1985.

15. Creteur, V., Thoeni, R.F., Federle, M.P., et al.: The role of single and double-contrast radiography in the diagnosis of reflux esophagitis. Radiology *147*:71, 1983.

16. Graziani, L., De Nigris, E., Pesaresi, A., et al.: Reflux esophagitis: Radiologic-endoscopic correlation in 39 symptomatic cases. Gastrointest. Radiol. *8*:1, 1983.

17. Chen, Y.M., Ott, D.J., Gelfand, D.W., et al.: Multiphasic examination of the esophagogastric region for strictures, rings, and hiatal hernia: Evaluation of the individual techniques. Gastrointest. Radiol. *10*:311, 1985.

18. Kressel, H.Y., Glick, S.N., Laufer, I., et al.: Radiologic features of esophagitis. Gastrointest. Radiol. *6*:103, 1981.

19. Graziani, L., Bearzi, I., Romagnoli, A., et al.: Significance of diffuse granularity and nodularity of the esophageal mucosa at double-contrast radiography. Gastrointest. Radiol. *10*:1, 1985.

20. Levine, M.S., Cajade, A.G., Herlinger, H., et al.: Pseudomembranes in reflux esophagitis. Radiology *159*:43, 1986.

21. Bleshman, M.H., Banner, M.P., Johnson, R.C., et al.: The inflammatory esophagogastric polyp and fold. Radiology *128*:589, 1978.

22. Styles, R.A., Gibb, S.P., Tarshis, A., et al.: Esophagogastric polyps: Radiographic and endoscopic findings. Radiology *154*:307, 1985.

23. Laufer, I.: Radiology of esophagitis. Radiol. Clin. North Am. *20*:687, 1982.

24. Levine, M.S.: Radiology of the Esophagus. Philadelphia, W.B. Saunders, 1989.

25. Levine, M.S., and Goldstein, H.M.: Fixed transverse folds in the esophagus: A sign of reflux esophagitis. AJR Am. J. Roentgenol. *143*:275, 1984.

26. Hu, C., Levine, M.S., and Laufer, I.: Solitary ulcers in reflux esophagitis: Radiographic findings. Abdom. Imaging *22*:5, 1997.

27. Levine, M.S., Moolten, D.N., Herlinger, H., et al.: Esophageal intramural pseudodiverticulosis: A reevaluation. AJR Am. J. Roentgenol. *147*:1165, 1986.

28. Robbins, A.H., Hermos, J.A., Schimmel, E.M., et al.: The columnar-lined esophagus: Analysis of 26 cases. Radiology *123*:1, 1977.

29. Robbins, A.H., Vincent, M.E., Saini, M., et al.: Revised radiologic concepts of Barrett's esophagus. Gastrointest. Radiol. *3*:377, 1978.

30. Levine, M.S., Kressel, H.Y., Caroline, D.F., et al.: Barrett esophagus: Reticular pattern of the mucosa. Radiology *147*:663, 1983.

31. Agha, F.P.: Radiologic diagnosis of Barrett's esophagus: Critical analysis of 65 cases. Gastrointest. Radiol. *11*:123, 1986.

32. Glick, S.N., Teplick S.K., Amenta, P.S., et al.: The radiologic diagnosis of Barrett's esophagus: Importance of mucosal surface abnormalities on air-contrast barium studies. AJR Am. J. Roentgenol. *157*:951, 1991.

33. Chernin, M.M., Amberg, J.R., Kogan, F.J., et al.: Efficacy of radiologic studies in the detection of Barrett's esophagus. AJR Am. J. Roentgenol. *147*:257, 1986.

34. Gilchrist, A.M., Levine, M.S., Carr, R.F., et al.: Barrett's esophagus: Diagnosis by double-contrast esophagography. AJR Am. J. Roentgenol. *150*:97, 1988.

35. Sheft, D.J., and Shrago, G.: Esophageal moniliasis: The spectrum of the disease. JAMA *213*:1859, 1970.

36. Eras, P., Goldstein, M.J., and Sherlock, P.: *Candida* infection of the gastrointestinal tract. Medicine (Baltimore) *51*:367, 1972.

37. Wall, S.D., Ominsky, S., Altman, D.F., et al.: Multifocal abnormalities of the gastrointestinal tract in AIDS. AJR Am. J. Roentgenol. *146*:1, 1986.

38. Frager, D.H., Frager, J.D., Brandt, L.J., et al.: Gastrointestinal complications of AIDS: Radiological features. Radiology *158*:597, 1986.

39. Gefter, W.B., Laufer, I., Edell, S., et al.: Candidiasis in the obstructed esophagus. Radiology *138*:25, 1981.

40. Kodsi, B.E., Wickremesinghe, P.C., Kozinn, P.J., et al.: *Candida* esophagitis. Gastroenterology *71*:715, 1976.

41. Levine, M.S., Macones, A.J., Jr., and Laufer, I.: *Candida* esophagitis: Accuracy of radiographic diagnosis. Radiology *154*:581, 1985.

42. Vahey, T.N., Maglinte, D.D.T., and Chernish, S.M.: State-of-the-art barium examination in opportunistic esophagitis. Dig. Dis. Sci. *31*:1192, 1986.

43. Levine, M.S., Woldenberg, R., Herlinger, H., and Laufer, I.: Opportunistic esophagitis in AIDS: Radiographic diagnosis. Radiology *165*:815, 1987.

44. Goldberg, H.I., and Dodds, W.J.: Cobblestone esophagus due to monilial infection. AJR Am. J. Roentgenol. *104*:608, 1968.

45. Ho, C.S., Cullen, J.B., and Gray, R.R.: An unusual manifestation of esophageal moniliasis. Radiology *123*:287, 1977.

46. Agha, F.P.: Candidiasis-induced esophageal strictures. Gastrointest. Radiol. *9*:283, 1984.

47. Rohrmann, C.A., and Kidd, R.: Chronic mucocutaneous candidiasis: Radiologic abnormalities in the esophagus. AJR Am. J. Roentgenol. *130*:473, 1978.

48. Deschmukh, M., Shah, R., and McCallum, R.W.: Experience with herpes esophagitis in otherwise healthy patients. Am. J. Gastroenterol. *79*:173, 1984.

49. DeGaeta, L., Levine, M.S., Guglielmi, G.E., et al.: Herpes esophagitis in an otherwise healthy patient. AJR Am. J. Roentgenol. *144*:1205, 1985.

50. Levine, M.S., Loevner, L.A., Saul, S.H., et al.: Herpes esophagitis: Sensitivity of double-contrast esophagography. AJR Am. J. Roentgenol. *151*:57, 1988.

51. Levine, M.S., Laufer, I., Kressel, H.Y., et al.: Herpes esophagitis. AJR Am. J. Roentgenol. *136*:863, 1981.

52. Skucas, J., Schrank, W.W., Meyer, P.C., et al.: Herpes esophagitis: A case studied by air-contrast esophagography. AJR Am. J. Roentgenol. *128*:497, 1977.

53. Shortsleeve, M.J., and Levine, M.S.: Herpes esophagitis in otherwise healthy patients: Clinical and radiographic findings. Radiology *182*:859, 1992.

54. Balthazar, E.J., Megibow, A.J., Hulnick, D., et al.: Cytomegalovirus esophagitis in AIDS: Radiographic features in 16 patients. AJR Am. J. Roentgenol. *149*:919, 1987.

55. Rabeneck, L., Popovic, M., Gartner, S., et al.: Acute HIV infection presenting with painful swallowing and esophageal ulcers. JAMA *263*:2318, 1990.

56. Levine, M.S., Loercher, G., Katzka, D.A., et al.: Giant, human immunodeficiency virus–related ulcers in the esophagus. Radiology *180*:323, 1991.

57. Sor, S., Levine, M.S., Kowalski, T.E., et al.: Giant ulcers of the esophagus in patients with human immunodeficiency virus: Clinical, radiographic, and pathologic findings. Radiology *194*:447, 1995.

58. Creteur, V., Laufer, I., Kressel, H.Y., et al.: Drug-induced esophagitis detected by double contrast radiography. Radiology *147*:365, 1983.

59. Bova, J.G., Dutton, N.E., Goldstein, H.M., et al.: Medication-induced esophagitis: Diagnosis by double-contrast esophagography. AJR Am. J. Roentgenol. *148*:731, 1987.

60. Ravich, W.J., Kashima, H., Donner, M.W.: Drug-induced esophagitis simulating esophageal carcinoma. Dysphagia *1*:13, 1986.

61. Bonavina, L., DeMeester, T.R., McChesney, L, et al.: Drug-induced esophageal strictures. Ann. Surg. *206*:173, 1987.

62. Levine, M.S., Rothstein R.D., and Laufer, I.: Giant esophageal ulcer due to Clinoril. AJR Am. J. Roentgenol. *156*:955, 1991.

63. Levine, M.S., Borislow S.M., Rubesin, S.E., et al.: Esophageal stricture caused by a Motrin tablet (Ibuprofen). Abdom. Imaging *19*:6, 1994.

64. Graham, J., Barnes, M., and Rubenstein, A.S.: The nasogastric tube as a cause of esophagitis and stricture. Am. J. Surg. *98*:116, 1959.

65. Appleqvist, P., and Salmo, M.: Lye corrosion carcinoma of the esophagus: A review of 63 cases. Cancer *45*:2655, 1980.

66. Lepke, R.A., and Libshitz, H.I.: Radiation-induced injury of the esophagus. Radiology *148*:375, 1983.

67. Collazzo, L.A., Levine M.S., Rubesin S.E., et al.: Acute radiation esophagitis: Radiographic findings. AJR Am. J. Roentgenol. *169*:1067, 1997.

68. Gohel, V., Long, B.W., and Richter, G.: Aphthous ulcers in the esophagus with Crohn colitis. AJR Am. J. Roentgenol. *137*:872, 1981.

69. Degryse, H.R.M., and De Schepper, A.M.: Aphthoid esophageal ulcers in Crohn's disease of ileum and colon. Gastrointest. Radiol. *9*:197, 1984.

70. Agha, F.P., and Raji, M.R.: Esophageal involvement in pemphigoid:

Clinical and roentgen manifestations. Gastrointest. Radiol. *7:*109, 1982.

71. Agha, F.P., Francis, I.R., and Ellis, C.N.: Esophageal involvement in epidermolysis bullosa dystrophica: Clinical and roentgenographic manifestations. Gastrointest. Radiology *8:*111, 1983.

72. Glick, S.N., Teplick, S.K., Goldstein, J., et al.: Glycogenic acanthosis of the esophagus. AJR Am. J. Roentgenol. *139:*683, 1982.

73. Itai, Y., Kogure, T., Okuyama, Y., et al.: Diffuse finely nodular lesions of the esophagus. AJR Am. J. Roentgenol. *128:*563, 1977.

74. Lawson, T.L., Dodds, W.J., and Sheft, D.J.: Carcinoma of the esophagus simulating varices. AJR Am. J. Roentgenol. *107:*83, 1969.

75. Yates, C.W., LeVine, M.A., and Jensen, K.M.: Varicoid carcinoma of the esophagus. Radiology *122:*605, 1977.

6

Tumors of the Esophagus

MARC S. LEVINE
IGOR LAUFER
AKIYOSHI YAMADA

BENIGN TUMORS
Mucosal Lesions
Submucosal Lesions

ESOPHAGEAL CARCINOMA
Early Esophageal Cancer
Advanced Carcinoma

Associated Conditions
Posttreatment Studies

METASTATIC DISEASE

LYMPHOMA

OTHER MALIGNANT TUMORS

BENIGN TUMORS

Benign tumors of the esophagus are relatively uncommon. Most are small, asymptomatic lesions that are discovered as incidental findings on radiologic or endoscopic examinations. Occasionally, however, these tumors may cause dysphagia or gastrointestinal bleeding. Depending on their site of origin, benign tumors may be classified as mucosal or submucosal lesions that have typical radiologic features.

Mucosal Lesions

Squamous papillomas are the most frequent benign mucosal tumors in the esophagus. These lesions appear as coral-like excrescences containing a central fibrovascular core with multiple fingerlike projections covered by hyperplastic squamous epithelium.[1] Papillomas are difficult to detect on conventional single contrast barium studies because of the small size of the lesions. However, they are often recognized on double contrast studies as sessile, smooth, or slightly lobulated polyps less than 1 cm in size (Fig. 6–1).[2] Some papillomas may produce a ring shadow similar to that of colonic polyps on double contrast barium enemas as a result of barium trapped between the edge of the lesion and the adjacent mucosa (Fig. 6–1A). Because early esophageal cancers may also appear as small polypoid lesions, endoscopy and biopsy should be performed to differentiate a squamous papilloma from an early carcinoma. Occasionally, papillomas may be larger and more lobulated, or they

may have a bubbly appearance because of trapping of barium between the frondlike projections of the tumor (Fig. 6–2). Rarely, innumerable papillomas may be present in the esophagus in patients with esophageal papillomatosis.[3] The diagnosis of esophageal papillomatosis may be suggested on double contrast studies by the presence of multiple discrete, wartlike excrescences on the esophageal mucosa (Fig. 6–3). Even when multiple papillomas are present, however, these lesions rarely cause obstruction.

Multiple benign mucosal elevations are frequently found in the esophagus in patients with glycogenic acanthosis, a benign condition of unknown etiology in which cytoplasmic glycogen accumulates in the squamous epithelial cells that line the esophagus, causing focal plaquelike thickening of the mucosa.[4] Glycogenic acanthosis is a degenerative condition, predominantly occurring in middle-aged or elderly individuals. It usually is manifested on double contrast studies by multiple small, rounded nodules or plaques in the middle or distal esophagus (Fig. 6–4).[5–7] These lesions can sometimes be mistaken for the plaques of candidiasis. However, *Candida* esophagitis usually occurs in immunocompromised patients with odynophagia, whereas glycogenic acanthosis occurs in older people who have no esophageal symptoms. Also, the plaques in candidiasis tend to have a linear configuration (see Fig. 5–42), whereas the nodules in glycogenic acanthosis tend to have a more rounded appearance. Thus, it usually is possible to differentiate these conditions on the basis of the clinical and radiographic findings.

126

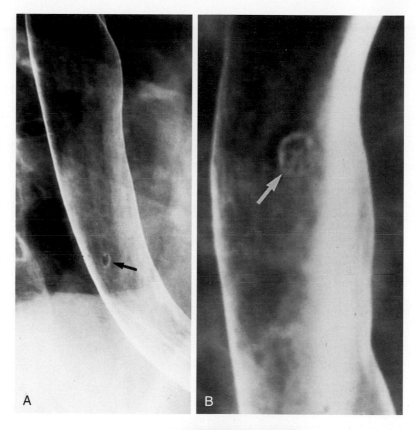

FIGURE 6–1. Squamous papillomas. *A,* Small papilloma in distal esophagus appears as ring shadow *(arrow)* because of barium trapped between edge of polyp and adjacent esophageal wall. (From Montesi, A., et al.: Small benign tumors of the esophagus: Radiological diagnosis with double-contrast examination. Gastrointest. Radiol. *8*:207, 1983, with permission.) *B,* Larger, more lobulated papilloma *(arrow)* in another patient. Early esophageal cancer could produce a similar appearance. (Courtesy of Harry Allen III, M.D., Norfolk, Virginia.)

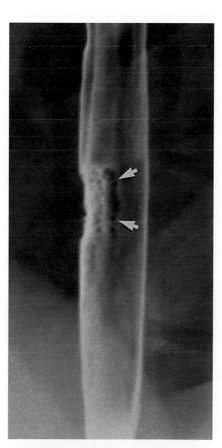

FIGURE 6–2. Squamous papilloma. This lesion in midesophagus has a bubbly appearance *(arrows)* due to trapping of barium in the frondlike projections of the tumor.

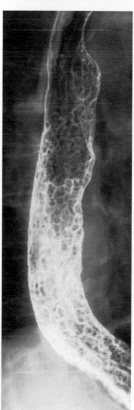

FIGURE 6–3. Esophageal papillomatosis with innumerable papillomas, appearing as wartlike excrescences on esophageal mucosa. Despite the dramatic radiographic findings, this patient had no esophageal symptoms. (Courtesy of Harvey M. Goldstein, M.D., San Antonio, Texas.)

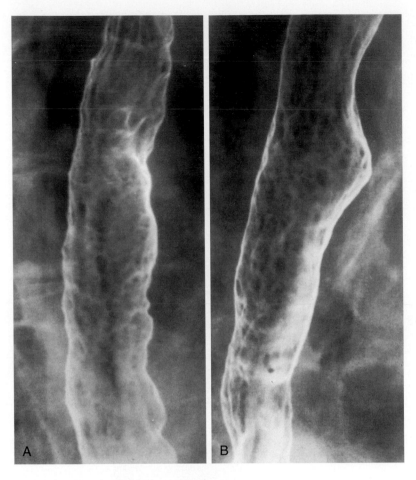

FIGURE 6–4. Two examples (*A* and *B*) of glycogenic acanthosis manifested by multiple small plaques and nodules in midesophagus. Although *Candida* esophagitis could produce similar findings, patients with glycogenic acanthosis are almost always asymptomatic. (From Levine, M.S.: Radiology of the Esophagus. Philadelphia, W.B. Saunders, 1989, p. 118.)

Submucosal Lesions

Most benign submucosal tumors in the esophagus are leiomyomas.[8] Histologically, these lesions consist of intersecting bands of smooth muscle and fibrous tissue surrounded by a well-defined capsule. Leiomyomas are frequently found in the middle or distal third of the esophagus, but they are much less common in the proximal third because of the presence of striated rather than smooth muscle in the esophagus above the level of the aortic arch. Most patients with esophageal leiomyomas are asymptomatic. However, lesions that are unusually large may cause dysphagia. Unlike smooth muscle tumors elsewhere in the gastrointestinal tract, esophageal leiomyomas almost never undergo sarcomatous degeneration.[9]

Leiomyomas usually appear radiographically as discrete submucosal masses in the esophagus (Figs. 6–5 through 6–7). When viewed in profile, the lesions have a smooth surface that is etched in white, and their upper and lower borders form either abrupt right angles or slightly obtuse angles with the adjacent esophageal wall (Figs. 6–6*A* and 6–7*A*). When viewed en face, the lesions may cause apparent widening of the esophageal lumen as barium flows around the lateral borders of the tumor (Fig. 6–7*B*). Unlike leiomyomas in the stomach, esophageal leiomyomas are almost never ulcerated. Although most leiomyomas range from 2 to 5 cm in size, they occasionally may be giant lesions (Fig. 6–8). Rarely, these tumors may contain areas of calcification (Fig. 6–9).[10]

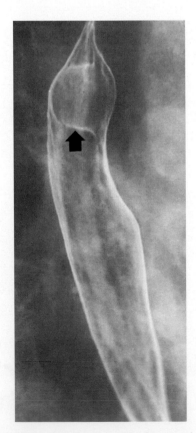

FIGURE 6–5. **Leiomyoma.** Note typical submucosal appearance of tumor (*arrow*) with smooth, stretched mucosa over lesion.

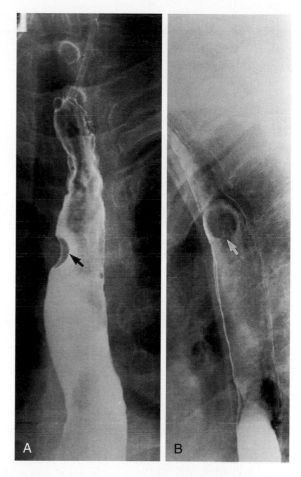

FIGURE 6–6. Leiomyoma. *A,* Tangential view shows characteristic features of submucosal mass *(arrow)* with smooth surface and slightly obtuse angle between edge of lesion and adjacent esophageal wall. *B,* En face view shows well-defined, ovoid filling defect *(arrow)* in esophagus.

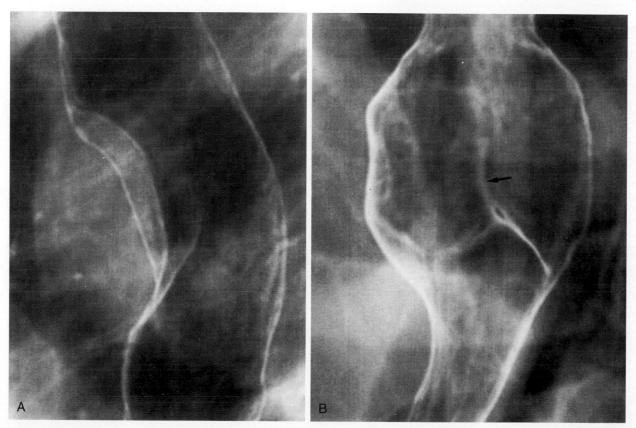

FIGURE 6–7. Leiomyoma. *A,* Tangential view shows large submucosal mass in esophagus. *B,* En face view shows widening of esophageal lumen with smooth mucosal surface and central furrow *(arrow).* (Courtesy of Marc P. Banner, M.D., Philadelphia, Pennsylvania.)

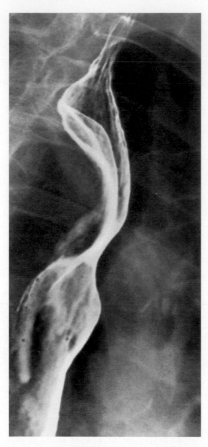

FIGURE 6–8. Giant leiomyoma. A large submucosal mass is seen in profile in upper esophagus.

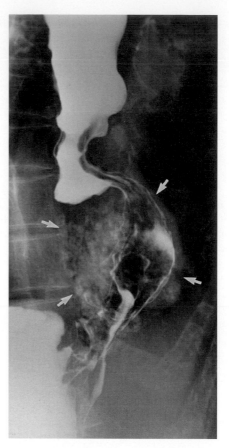

FIGURE 6–9. Calcified leiomyoma. Note large mass *(arrows)* in distal esophagus, with amorphous calcification in lesion.

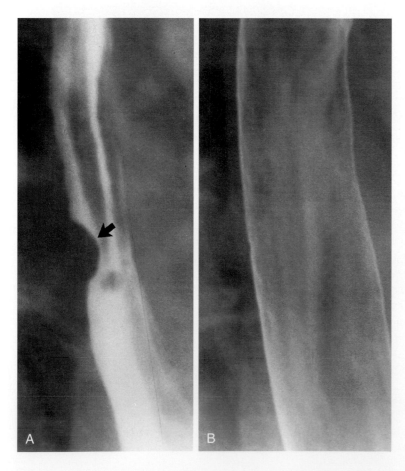

FIGURE 6–10. Idiopathic esophageal varix. *A,* View of partially collapsed esophagus shows solitary submucosal mass *(arrow)* indistinguishable from leiomyoma or other intramural lesion. *B,* Repeat double contrast view, however, shows obliteration of varix with greater esophageal distention. (From Trenkner, S.W., et al.: Idiopathic esophageal varix. AJR Am. J. Roentgenol. *141:*43–44, 1983, with permission, © by American Roentgen Ray Society.)

Although most submucosal masses in the esophagus are leiomyomas, other intramural lesions such as fibromas, neurofibromas, lipomas, hemangiomas, granular cell tumors, and duplication or retention cysts may produce identical radiographic findings.[11–14] Rarely, an isolated esophageal varix may also resemble a submucosal mass (Fig. 6–10*A*), but effacement or obliteration of the lesion by esophageal distention should suggest its vascular origin (Fig. 6–10*B*).[15] When multiple submucosal masses are present in the esophagus, the differential diagnosis should include not only multiple leiomyomas but also multiple neurofibromas, esophageal retention cysts (i.e., esophagitis cystica), hematogenous metastases from malignant melanoma, and leukemic or lymphomatous deposits in the esophagus (see Fig. 6–39*A*).[16]

Fibrovascular polyps are uncommon benign submucosal tumors in the esophagus that consist of varying amounts of fibrovascular and adipose tissue covered by normal squamous epithelium.[17] They almost always arise in the cervical esophagus, gradually forming a pedicle as they elongate distally into the thoracic esophagus because of the constant traction of esophageal peristalsis. These pedunculated masses are potentially life threatening because they may be regurgitated into the oropharynx, causing laryngeal obstruction with asphyxia and sudden death.[18] Fibrovascular polyps are classically manifested on double contrast studies by a smooth, expansile, sausage-shaped mass in the upper or midesophagus with a discrete pedicle extending proximally from the region of the cricopharyngeus (Fig. 6–11).[19,20] However, some polyps may be quite lobulated, so they cannot always be differentiated radiographically from malignant tumors in the esophagus.

ESOPHAGEAL CARCINOMA

Esophageal carcinoma is a deadly disease with 5-year survival rates of less than 10%. Unfortunately, dysphagia develops in most patients with esophageal cancer only after the tumor has invaded periesophageal lymphatic vessels or other mediastinal structures. As a result, affected individuals usually have advanced, unresectable lesions at the time of clinical presentation. Between 50% and 70% of these tumors are squamous cell carcinomas.[21] Although the major risk factors for squamous cell carcinoma are tobacco and alcohol,[22] other conditions associated with an increased risk of the development of esophageal cancer include achalasia,[23] lye strictures,[24] head and neck tumors,[25] celiac disease,[26] Plummer-Vinson syndrome,[27] and tylosis.[28] Some investigators advocate routine screening of patients with these conditions in the hope of detecting a superimposed carcinoma at the earliest possible stage (see the next section, "Early Esophageal Cancer").

The remaining 30% to 50% of esophageal cancers are adenocarcinomas,[29–31] so these tumors are more common than has previously been recognized. Unlike squamous cell carcinoma, esophageal adenocarcinoma virtually always arises on a background of Barrett's mucosa in the esophagus. The reported prevalence of adenocarcinoma in patients with Barrett's esophagus is about 10%.[32] Unfortunately, prevalence data tend to exaggerate the risk of cancer, as many patients with Barrett's esophagus remain asymptomatic until the development of a superimposed carcinoma. However, other studies (using incidence rather than prevalence data) indicate that the risk of adenocarcinoma developing in patients with Barrett's esophagus may be 30 to 40 times greater than that in the general population.[33,34] Esophageal adenocarcinoma apparently evolves through a sequence of progressively severe epithelial dysplasia in areas of preexisting columnar metaplasia. These dysplastic or early carcinomatous changes can be recognized by endoscopic biopsy or cytologic findings. As a result, many investigators advocate routine endoscopic surveillance of patients with Barrett's esophagus for early detection of cancer.

Squamous cell carcinoma and adenocarcinoma of the esophagus are common causes of dysphagia in older people. Although barium studies are often used to evaluate these individuals, some gastroenterologists believe that endoscopy is required for all patients with dysphagia who

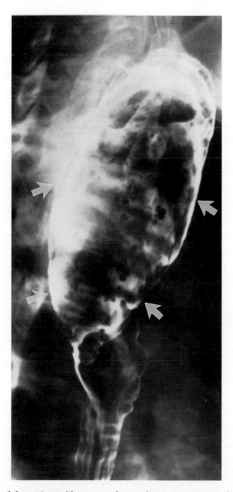

FIGURE 6–11. Giant fibrovascular polyp. Note smooth, sausage-shaped mass *(arrows)* that expands lumen of upper esophagus. (Courtesy of Duane Mezwa, M.D., Royal Oak, Michigan.)

have normal esophagrams to find tumors that are missed on the barium study. Recent data suggest that such views are not justified. In a large series of patients with esophageal cancer, the lesion was found on double contrast examinations in 98% of cases and malignant tumor was diagnosed or suspected in 96%.[35] This figure is comparable to the reported endoscopic sensitivity of 95% to 100% when multiple brushings and biopsy specimens are obtained.[36,37] An argument could be made that a high sensitivity is achieved in the radiographic diagnosis of esophageal cancer only by exposing an inordinate number of patients to unnecessary endoscopy. In the previous study, however, endoscopy was recommended to rule out malignant esophageal tumors in only about 1% of all patients who underwent double contrast examinations.[35] In other investigations, endoscopy also has failed to reveal any cases of esophageal carcinoma that were missed on double contrast studies.[38,39] We therefore believe that double contrast esophagography is a sensitive technique for the diagnosis of esophageal carcinoma and that endoscopy is not routinely warranted in patients who have normal findings on barium studies.

Early Esophageal Cancer

Various terms have been used to describe the earliest diagnosable form of esophageal cancer. *Early esophageal cancer* is defined histologically as cancer limited to the mucosa or submucosa without lymph node metastases.[40] Unlike advanced carcinoma, early esophageal cancer is a readily curable lesion with 5-year survival rates of approximately 95%.[41] Many of these cases have been found in parts of Northern China, where the high incidence of esophageal cancer has led to mass screening of the adult population to detect these lesions at the earliest possible stage. *Superficial esophageal cancer* is also confined to the mucosa or submucosa, but unlike early esophageal cancer, lymph node metastases may be present in this disease.[40] *Small esophageal cancer* is another term used to describe tumors less than 3.5 cm, regardless of the depth of invasion or the presence or absence of lymph node metastases.[42] Thus, some small or superficial esophageal cancers may be "early" lesions histologically, but others may have invaded regional lymph nodes with a prognosis comparable to that of advanced esophageal carcinoma. Although these distinctions are made on pathologic criteria, lesions that are small or superficial are more likely to be early cancers with the greatest possibility for cure.

The diagnosis of esophageal cancer is usually limited by the late onset of symptoms in patients with this disease. However, some patients do experience dysphagia or upper gastrointestinal bleeding while the tumor is still at an early stage. Patients with early adenocarcinoma arising in Barrett's mucosa may also seek medical attention because of their underlying reflux disease, so that early esophageal cancer may be detected fortuitously in patients with reflux symptoms.[43] Finally, early esophageal cancer may be diagnosed on radiologic or endoscopic examinations

performed as screening studies in asymptomatic patients with Barrett's esophagus, achalasia, lye strictures, or other conditions that predispose patients to the development of esophageal carcinoma.

Double contrast esophagography has been widely advocated as the best radiologic technique for diagnosing early esophageal cancer. Unfortunately, the higher sensitivity of this technique has resulted in a lower specificity, as more subtle lesions are identified and are suspected of representing cancer.[44] Nevertheless, it is probably best to accept a certain percentage of false-positive findings to avoid missing early cancers. The possibility of esophageal carcinoma should therefore be considered for any lesion that does not have a classically benign appearance. Although some benign lesions erroneously may be suspected of harboring malignancy, scrupulous endoscopic follow-up should clarify the diagnosis and lead to earlier detection of esophageal cancer.

In their early stages, esophageal cancers classically appear on double contrast radiographs as small, protruded lesions less than 3.5 cm in diameter (Figs. 6–12 through 6–14).[43–45] Some early cancers may be plaque-like lesions (often containing central ulceration) (Fig.

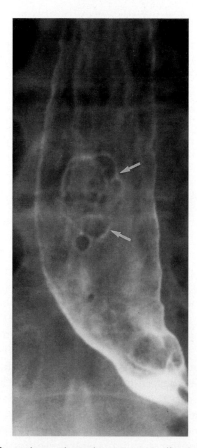

FIGURE 6–12. Early esophageal cancer. A small polypoid mass *(arrows)* is seen en face in distal esophagus. (From Levine, M.S., Chu, P., Furth, E.E., et al.: Carcinoma of the esophagus and esophagogastric junction: Sensitivity of radiographic diagnosis. AJR Am. J. Roentgenol. *168*:1423, 1997, with permission, © by American Roentgen Ray Society.)

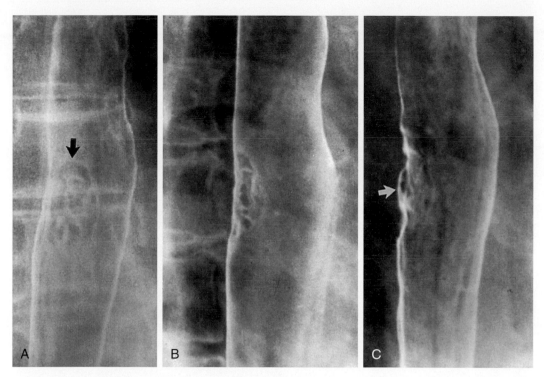

FIGURE 6–13. Ulcerated, plaquelike carcinoma seen in multiple projections. *A,* En face view shows poorly defined filling defect *(arrow)* in midesophagus. *B,* Oblique view better delineates irregular surface of lesion. *C,* Profile view shows plaquelike nature of lesion with central area of ulceration *(arrow).*

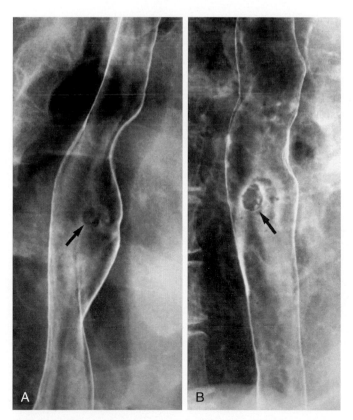

FIGURE 6–14. Two examples (*A* and *B*) of small esophageal cancers appearing as sessile, slightly lobulated polyps *(arrows)* in midesophagus. Note resemblance to squamous papilloma in Figure 6–1*B.*

6–13) or flat, sessile polyps with a smooth or slightly lobulated contour (Fig. 6–14). Other superficial cancers may cause focal irregularity, nodularity, puckering, or ulceration of the mucosa without a discrete mass (Fig. 6–15).[46,47] In patients with Barrett's esophagus the earliest manifestation of a developing adenocarcinoma may be a localized area of wall flattening or stiffening in a preexisting peptic stricture (Fig. 6–16).[43] Because small or superficial tumors may produce relatively subtle radiographic findings, double contrast views should be obtained in multiple projections to evaluate a possible lesion both en face and in profile. Tangential views are particularly helpful for assessing the degree of intraluminal protrusion and the presence of associated ulceration (see Fig. 6–13).

Superficial spreading carcinoma is another potentially curable form of esophageal cancer that extends longitudinally in the esophageal wall without invading beyond the mucosa or submucosa. These lesions are manifested radiographically by tiny, coalescent nodules or plaques, causing nodularity or granularity of the mucosa (Fig. 6–17).[43,46–48] Less frequently, an erosive form of superficial spreading cancer may be associated with shallow areas of ulceration (Fig. 6–18). The findings are often quite subtle, so that optimal radiographic technique is needed to demonstrate these lesions (Fig. 6–19).

Superficial spreading carcinoma occasionally can be mistaken for a localized area of *Candida* esophagitis. However, the plaquelike defects of candidiasis tend to be dis-

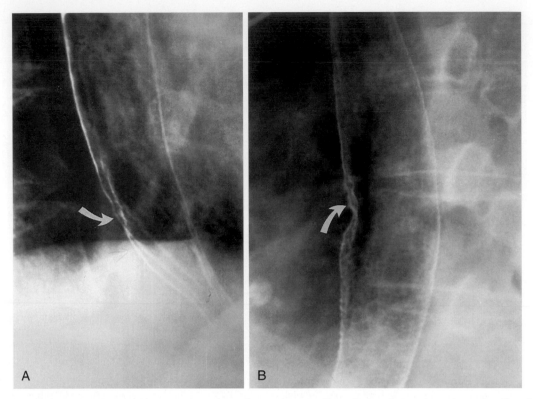

FIGURE 6–15. Two examples (*A* and *B*) of superficial esophageal carcinoma with focal irregularity of esophageal wall. In both cases, note puckering *(arrows)* of posterior esophageal wall by tumor.

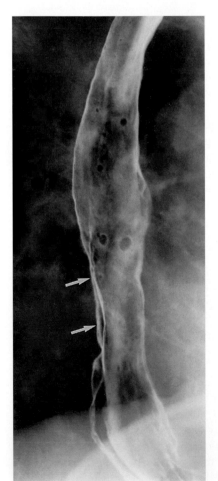

FIGURE 6–16. Early adenocarcinoma in Barrett's esophagus. Relatively long peptic stricture is present in distal esophagus with slight flattening of one wall of stricture *(arrows)*. (Note air bubbles in esophagus.) At surgery, this patient had carcinoma in situ within Barrett's mucosa.

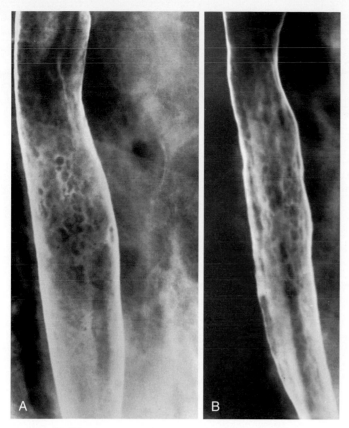

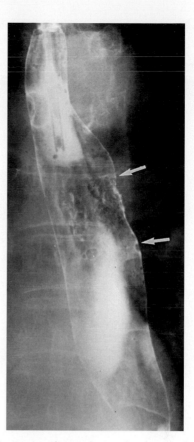

FIGURE 6–17. Two examples (*A* and *B*) of superficial spreading carcinoma. In both cases, note coarse, granular appearance of mucosa due to tiny mucosal elevations.

FIGURE 6–18. Erosive form of superficial spreading carcinoma with shallow, irregular areas of ulceration demarcated superiorly and inferiorly by arrows.

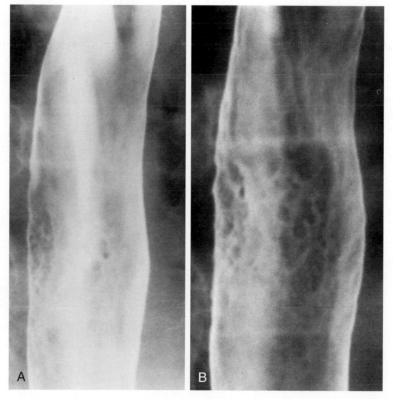

FIGURE 6–19. Superficial spreading carcinoma—importance of technique. *A,* Initial view shows barely discernible abnormality in mid-esophagus. Unfortunately, details of lesion are obscured by thick coating of high-density barium in esophagus—a phenomenon known as "flow artifact." *B,* Repeat view moments later reveals coalescent plaques and nodules due to superficial spreading carcinoma. This case shows how demonstration of these lesions requires optimal radiographic technique.

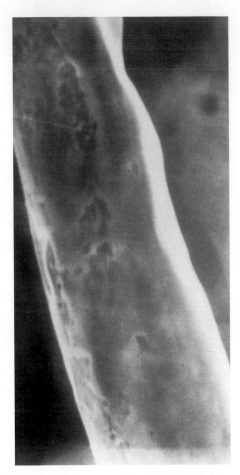

FIGURE 6–20. *Candida* **esophagitis with multiple plaques in mid-esophagus.** Although this appearance could be mistaken for that of a superficial spreading carcinoma, note how the plaquelike defects of candidiasis are discrete lesions with normal intervening mucosa.

crete lesions with sharp borders and normal intervening mucosa (Fig. 6–20),[49] whereas the nodules or plaques of superficial spreading carcinoma tend to coalesce, producing a continuous area of disease. Other considerations in the differential diagnosis include glycogenic acanthosis and esophageal papillomatosis.[3,5–7] However, these other conditions also tend to be manifested by discrete lesions rather than by a continuous area of mucosal disease. Finally, superficial spreading carcinoma may produce a reticulonodular appearance that closely resembles the reticular pattern of Barrett's mucosa (see Chapter 5). However, patients with Barrett's esophagus usually have a midesophageal stricture, with the reticular pattern extending distally a short but variable distance from the stricture (Fig. 6–21).[50]

Although early esophageal cancers are generally thought to be small lesions, some early cancers may appear as relatively large intraluminal masses greater than 3.5 cm in diameter (Fig. 6–22). Such polypoid lesions may be indistinguishable radiographically from advanced carcinomas.[43] Thus, early esophageal cancers are not necessarily small cancers, as they may undergo considerable intraluminal or intramural growth and still be classified histologically as early lesions.

Advanced Carcinoma

Advanced esophageal carcinomas (whether squamous cell carcinomas or adenocarcinomas) usually appear radiographically as infiltrating, polypoid, ulcerative, or varicoid lesions.[21,32,51] *Infiltrating* carcinomas are classically manifested by irregular narrowing and constriction of the lumen with nodular or ulcerated mucosa and abrupt, well-defined proximal and distal borders (Fig. 6–23). *Polypoid* carcinomas appear as lobulated or fungating intraluminal masses, usually greater than 3.5 cm in size (Fig. 6–24). *Ulcerative* carcinomas are relatively flat lesions in which the bulk of the tumor is replaced by ulceration. When viewed in profile, these lesions appear as irregular, meniscoid ulcers surrounded by a radiolucent rim of tumor (Fig. 6–25).[52] Finally, *varicoid* carcinomas are those in which submucosal spread of tumor produces thickened, tortuous longitudinal folds, mimicking the appearance of esophageal varices (Fig. 6–26).[53,54] However, these lesions have a rigid, fixed configuration at fluoroscopy, whereas true varices tend to change in size and shape with peristalsis, respiration, and Valsalva maneuvers. Varicoid carcinomas are also manifested by a relatively abrupt demarcation between the involved segment and the adjacent

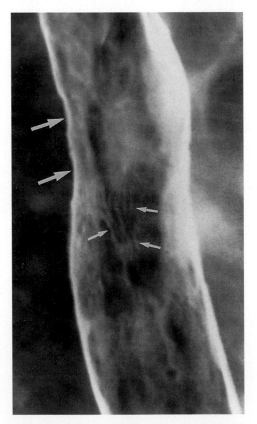

FIGURE 6–21. Barrett's esophagus with early stricture in midesophagus, manifested by slight flattening of esophageal wall *(large arrows)*. A delicate reticular pattern adjacent to distal aspect of stricture *(small arrows)* could be mistaken for superficial spreading carcinoma. However, the typical appearance and location of reticular pattern adjacent to stricture should suggest Barrett's mucosa. (From Levine, M.S., et al.: Barrett esophagus: Reticular pattern of the mucosa. Radiology *147*:663–667, 1983, with permission.)

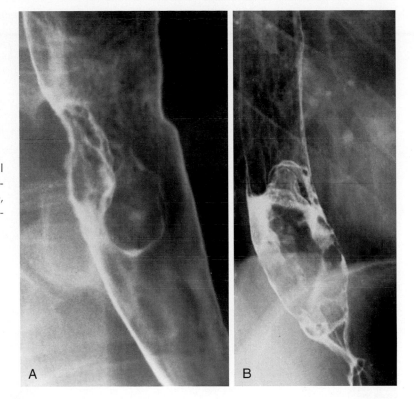

FIGURE 6–22. Two examples (*A* and *B*) of early esophageal cancers appearing as relatively large polypoid masses indistinguishable from advanced carcinomas. (*A*, From Levine, M.S.: Radiology of the Esophagus. Philadelphia, W.B. Saunders, 1989, p. 139.)

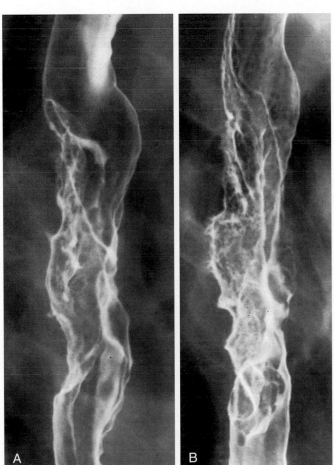

FIGURE 6–23. Infiltrating esophageal carcinomas (*A* and *B*) with irregular narrowing of lumen, ulceration, and relatively abrupt proximal and distal borders. (From Levine, M.S.: Radiology of the Esophagus. Philadelphia, W.B. Saunders, 1989, p. 141.)

normal mucosa and often spare the distal esophagus. Finally, varicoid carcinomas may cause dysphagia, a rare finding in patients with varices, since these are soft, compressible lesions. Thus, it usually is possible to differentiate varicoid carcinomas from varices on clinical and radiologic criteria.

Advanced esophageal carcinomas may be classified by their predominant morphologic features, but infiltrating lesions often have polypoid or ulcerated components (Fig. 6–27A and B), and polypoid lesions often have large areas of ulceration (see Fig. 6–27C). Thus many lesions have mixed radiographic patterns, so there is considerable overlap in the classification of these tumors.

Esophageal adenocarcinomas arising in Barrett's mucosa often cannot be distinguished radiographically from squamous cell carcinomas. However, squamous cell carcinomas tend to involve the upper or middle third of the esophagus, whereas adenocarcinomas are predominantly located in the distal third (Fig. 6–28). Unlike squamous cell carcinomas, esophageal adenocarcinomas also have a marked tendency to invade the gastric cardia or fundus.[55–57] In the past, these tumors at the gastroesophageal junction have almost always been classified as primary gastric carcinomas secondarily invading the lower end of the esophagus (see Chapter 8). However, data indicate that as many as 50% of adenocarcinomas at the gastroesophageal junction are Barrett's carcinomas invading the stomach.[55] Gastric involvement may be manifested radiographically by a polypoid or ulcerated mass in the fundus. In other patients, these tumors may cause obliteration of the normal anatomic landmarks at the cardia and irregular areas of ulceration without a discrete mass (Fig. 6–29).[55] The findings may be quite sub-

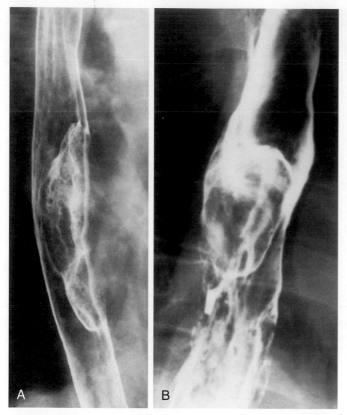

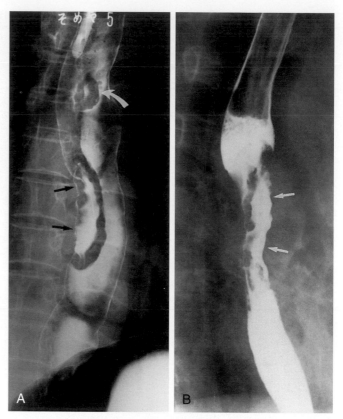

FIGURE 6–24. Polypoid carcinomas (*A* and *B*) appearing as lobulated intraluminal masses in esophagus. (*B*, From Levine, M.S.: Radiology of the Esophagus. Philadelphia, W.B. Saunders, 1989, p. 143.)

FIGURE 6–25. Ulcerative carcinomas (*A* and *B*) with large, meniscoid ulcers *(straight arrows)* and radiolucent rim of tumor adjacent to ulcers. Note discrete lymphatic metastasis with central ulceration *(curved arrow)* seen proximally in esophagus in *A*.

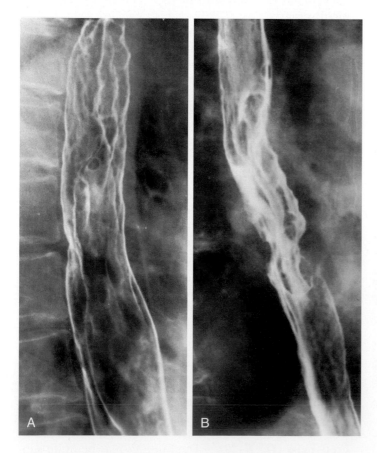

FIGURE 6–26. Varicoid carcinomas (*A* and *B*) in midesophagus with thickened, tortuous folds due to submucosal spread of tumor. These lesions could be mistaken for esophageal varices.

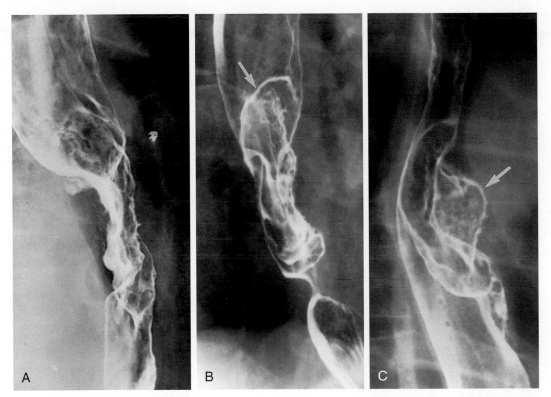

FIGURE 6–27. Mixed radiographic patterns in advanced esophageal carcinoma. *A,* Polypoid, infiltrating, and ulcerated carcinoma. *B,* Infiltrating carcinoma with polypoid superior component *(arrow). C,* Polypoid carcinoma with large area of ulceration *(arrow).*

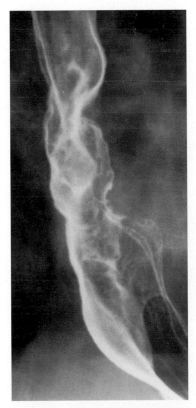

FIGURE 6–28. Infiltrating esophageal carcinoma arising in Barrett's mucosa. Note how lesion is located in distal esophagus above hiatal hernia. (From Levine, M.S.: Radiology of the Esophagus. Philadelphia, W.B. Saunders, 1989, p. 155.)

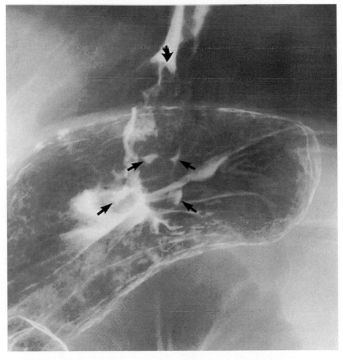

FIGURE 6–29. Barrett's esophagus with adenocarcinoma invading the stomach. Double contrast view of fundus shows obliteration of normal anatomic landmarks at cardia with irregular areas of ulceration *(straight arrows).* Note polypoid tumor in distal esophagus *(curved arrow).* (From Levine, M.S., et al.: Adenocarcinoma of the esophagus: Relationship to Barrett mucosa. Radiology *150:*305–309, 1984, with permission.)

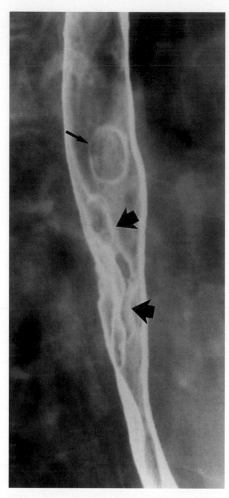

FIGURE 6–30. Advanced esophageal carcinoma with lymphatic metastasis. Note polypoid appearance of primary tumor *(large arrows)* in midesophagus with discrete metastatic implant seen as a small submucosal mass *(small arrow)* that is separated from main lesion by normal intervening mucosa.

tle, so that optimal double contrast views of the gastric cardia and fundus are required to determine the full extent of tumor in this region.

Dissemination of esophageal carcinoma by means of the rich submucosal lymphatic channels in the esophagus may also result in discrete implants adjacent to or remote from the primary tumor. These lymphatic metastases may appear radiographically as polypoid, plaquelike, or ulcerated lesions that are separated from the main tumor by normal intervening mucosa (Fig. 6–30; see Fig. 6–25A).[58] In other patients, tumor emboli from squamous cell carcinoma may spread subdiaphragmatically to the gastric fundus via submucosal esophageal lymphatic vessels. These squamous cell metastases to the stomach usually appear as large submucosal masses, often containing central areas of ulceration (Fig. 6–31).[59] Because the appropriate treatment for esophageal cancer depends on accurate staging of the tumor, the gastric cardia and fundus should be carefully examined in all patients with esophageal cancer to rule out unsuspected metastases to the stomach.

Once a lesion has been detected on double contrast studies, the presence of tumor can almost always be confirmed at endoscopy. Nevertheless, negative endoscopic brushings and biopsy specimens should not exclude the possibility of esophageal cancer if the radiographic findings are highly suggestive of tumor. In some cases, repeat radiologic or endoscopic examinations, or even surgery, may be necessary to establish the diagnosis.

Computed tomography, magnetic resonance imaging, and, most recently, endoscopic sonography have been used for preoperative staging of esophageal carcinoma.[60–62] Important prognostic features that can be assessed with these imaging techniques include the depth of esophageal wall invasion and the presence or absence

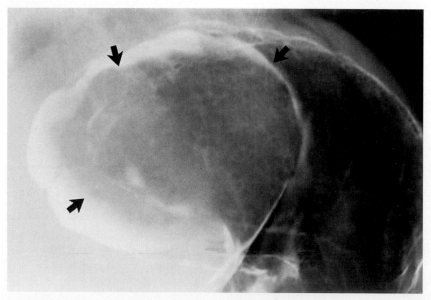

FIGURE 6–31. Squamous cell metastasis to stomach from esophageal carcinoma. Note giant submucosal mass *(arrows)* in gastric fundus. (From Glick, S.N., et al.: Squamous cell metastases to the gastric cardia. Gastrointest. Radiol. *10*:339, 1985, with permission.)

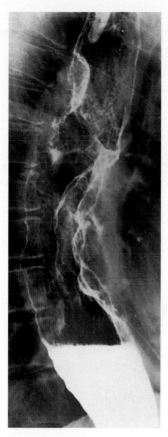

FIGURE 6–32. Advanced esophageal carcinoma in a patient with long-standing achalasia. Note barium level in distal esophagus below tumor.

of lymph node metastases or other metastatic lesions in the mediastinum. Even with these cross-sectional studies, however, it is difficult to detect lymph node metastases that are less than 1 cm.

Associated Conditions

Achalasia is a premalignant condition in the esophagus associated with a significantly increased risk of the development of esophageal carcinoma.[23] Because the esophagus is already dilated, these tumors often reach an enormous size before causing dysphagia. As a result, the lesions are usually discovered as bulky intraluminal masses, most frequently in the middle or upper esophagus (Fig. 6–32).[63] Because these tumors can be obscured by retained fluid and debris, esophageal lavage with a soft rubber catheter may be necessary to cleanse the esophagus before performing the double contrast examination. With adequate preparation a superimposed carcinoma can be demonstrated even in patients who have a massively dilated esophagus due to long-standing achalasia.

Patients with chronic lye strictures are also at increased risk for developing esophageal cancer.[24] It has been postulated that chronic inflammation and scarring from caustic ingestion are predisposing factors in the development of esophageal carcinoma. These lesions have a much better prognosis than other esophageal cancers,

probably because of dense scar tissue surrounding the tumor, which prevents early invasion of adjacent mediastinal structures.[24] Any change in swallowing function in patients with chronic lye strictures should therefore lead to further investigation to detect this complication. The development of cancer may be manifested radiographically by increasing stenosis, mass effect, nodularity, or ulceration within a preexisting lye stricture (Fig. 6–33). These lesions may be relatively subtle, so that any change in the appearance of a chronic lye stricture should be evaluated endoscopically to rule out a superimposed carcinoma.

Posttreatment Studies

Double contrast studies can be performed after palliative or, less frequently, curative radiotherapy for esophageal carcinoma. In general, squamous cell carcinomas of the esophagus are more radiosensitive than adenocarcinomas. Regression of tumor after radiotherapy is manifested by a decrease in the size or bulk of the lesion as compared with pretreatment studies. If the tumor regresses completely, follow-up barium studies may reveal a normal esophagus or a smooth, tapered stricture with a benign appearance at the site of the previous lesion

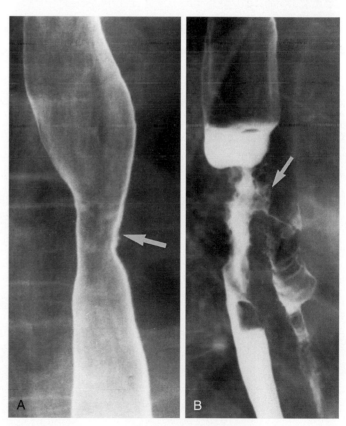

FIGURE 6–33. Esophageal carcinoma in lye stricture. *A,* Initial double contrast study shows focal stricture *(arrow)* in midesophagus due to previous lye ingestion. Note superficial ulceration and nodularity of mucosa in region of stricture. The patient refused surgery at this time. *B,* Repeat study 2 years later shows advanced esophageal carcinoma at site of previous stricture with esophagobronchial fistula *(arrow).* (From Levine, M.S.: Radiology of the Esophagus. Philadelphia, W.B. Saunders, 1989, p. 150.)

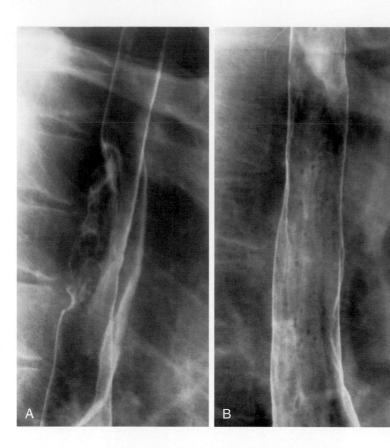

FIGURE 6–34. Total regression of esophageal carcinoma after radiation therapy. *A,* Polypoid carcinoma in upper esophagus. *B,* Normal appearance of esophagus without evidence of residual tumor 2 years after radiation therapy. (From Levine, M.S., et al.: Radiation therapy of esophageal carcinoma: Correlation of clinical and radiographic findings. Gastrointest. Radiol. *12*:99, 1987, with permission.)

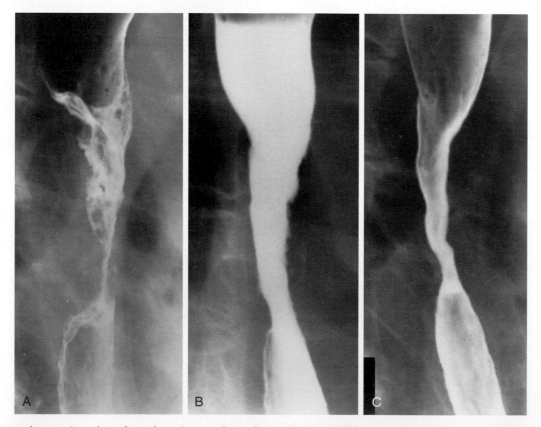

FIGURE 6–35. Total regression of esophageal carcinoma after radiation therapy with benign residual stricture. *A,* Infiltrating carcinoma in midesophagus. *B,* Partial regression of tumor with residual areas of ulceration 4 months after radiation therapy. *C,* Total regression of tumor with smooth, tapered stricture in this region 6 months after radiation therapy. (From Levine, M.S.: Radiology of the Esophagus. Philadelphia, W.B. Saunders, 1989, p. 164.)

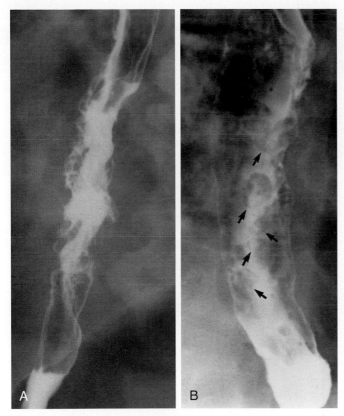

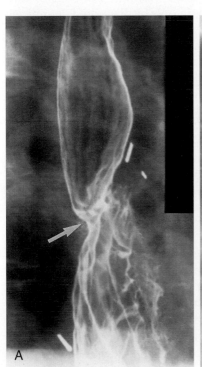

FIGURE 6–36. Herpes esophagitis after radiation therapy for esophageal carcinoma. *A,* Infiltrating carcinoma in distal esophagus. *B,* Repeat esophagram, obtained to evaluate recurrent dysphagia 18 months after radiation therapy, shows regression of tumor. However, note discrete ulcers with surrounding halos of edematous mucosa *(arrows)* due to herpes esophagitis. (From Levine, M.S., et al.: Radiation therapy of esophageal carcinoma: Correlation of clinical and radiographic findings. Gastrointest. Radiol. *12:*99, 1987, with permission.)

(Figs. 6–34 and 6–35).[64] However, the latter patients often die from distant metastases, so that disappearance of the cancer on radiologic or endoscopic examinations does not necessarily indicate a cure. Recurrent dysphagia after radiotherapy may result not only from recurrent tumor but also from benign radiation strictures, fistulas, or opportunistic esophageal infection (e.g., *Candida* or herpes esophagitis) (Fig. 6–36). Thus, double contrast studies are particularly helpful for differentiating recurrent carcinoma from other esophageal complications in these patients.[64]

Double contrast studies can also be used to evaluate patients who have undergone surgical resection of esophageal carcinoma. The most frequently performed operation is an esophagogastrectomy and gastric pull-through. With double contrast technique, it usually is possible to demonstrate the normal anatomy of the esophagogastric anastomosis and intrathoracic stomach (Fig. 6–37*A*), so that anastomotic strictures or recurrent tumor can be detected (Fig. 6–37*B*).[65]

METASTATIC DISEASE

Metastases to the esophagus can result from direct invasion by primary malignant tumors of the stomach, pharynx, or lung; from contiguous involvement by tumor-containing lymph nodes in the mediastinum; or from hematogenous metastases.[66] Direct extension of tumor from the adjacent lung or mediastinum may cause extensive mass effect, tethered folds, nodularity, ulceration, or in advanced cases, circumferential narrowing of the esophagus (Fig. 6–38). True bloodborne or hematogenous metastases are most frequently caused by carcinoma of the breast. They usually appear as short, eccentric stric-

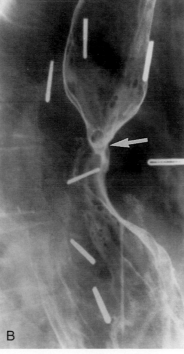

FIGURE 6–37. Appearances after esophagogastrectomy. *A,* Normal postoperative appearance of esophagogastric anastomosis *(arrow). B,* Benign anastomotic stricture *(arrow)* in another patient.

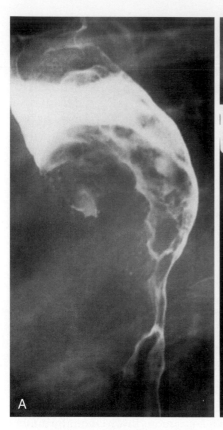
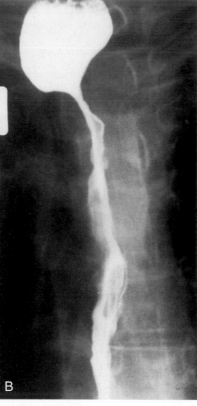

FIGURE 6–38. **Carcinoma of lung invading esophagus.** *A,* Eccentric mass effect and narrowing of esophagus with irregular areas of ulceration due to direct invasion by mediastinal tumor. (From Levine, M.S.: Radiology of the Esophagus. Philadelphia, W.B. Saunders, 1989, p. 171.) *B,* Another patient with a long segment of irregular narrowing in the upper thoracic esophagus due to circumferential involvement by metastatic tumor in the mediastinum. (Courtesy of Robert Goren, M.D., Philadelphia, Pennsylvania.)

tures in the midesophagus.[66] Occasionally, carcinoma of the breast can metastasize to the esophagus many years after treatment of the original lesion.

LYMPHOMA

Both non-Hodgkin's and, less frequently, Hodgkin's lymphoma may involve the esophagus. These patients almost always have generalized lymphoma with direct invasion of the esophagus by lymphomatous nodes in the mediastinum, contiguous spread of lymphoma from the gastric fundus, or synchronous development of lymphoma in the wall of the esophagus. Esophageal lymphoma may be manifested by a spectrum of findings, including submucosal masses, enlarged folds, polypoid lesions, and strictures.[67] Occasionally, the esophagus may have a diffusely nodular appearance as a result of innumerable tiny, submucosal nodules extending from the thoracic inlet to the gastroesophageal junction (Fig. 6–39).[16] Other rare causes of submucosal nodules include leukemic infiltrates, hematogenous metastases, esophageal retention cysts, and multiple leiomyomas, but the lesions tend to be larger and less numerous in these conditions.

OTHER MALIGNANT TUMORS

Polypoid malignant tumors of the esophagus containing both carcinomatous and sarcomatous elements are rare. In the past these lesions have been called carcinosarcomas or pseudosarcomas. However, they are now classified as spindle cell carcinomas, as they are thought to represent carcinomas that have undergone varying degrees of spindle cell metaplasia.[68] Spindle cell carcinomas typically appear radiographically as polypoid intraluminal masses that expand the esophageal lumen without causing obstruction (Fig. 6–40).[68,69] Other esophageal neoplasms may produce similar findings, however, so that spindle cell carcinomas can only be diagnosed definitively on histologic grounds.

Primary malignant melanoma of the esophagus is a rare tumor that may be manifested radiographically by a polypoid, expansile esophageal mass indistinguishable from spindle cell carcinoma (Fig. 6–41).[70] Small cell carcinoma of the esophagus is another rare but aggressive malignant tumor that may appear on double contrast studies as a smoothly marginated, sessile, centrally ulcerated mass in the midesophagus near the level of the carina (Fig. 6–42).[71] Leiomyosarcoma is a rare smooth muscle tumor characterized by a large intramural mass with a frequent exophytic component, ulceration, or tracking (Fig. 6–43).[72] Recently, esophageal involvement by Kaposi's sarcoma has also been recognized with increased frequency in patients with AIDS. These tumors are characterized by multiple submucosal masses or by a single polypoid or infiltrating lesion in the esophagus (Fig. 6–44).[73,74] Double contrast studies are particularly helpful for differentiating opportunistic esophagitis from Kaposi's sarcoma involving the esophagus in patients with AIDS.

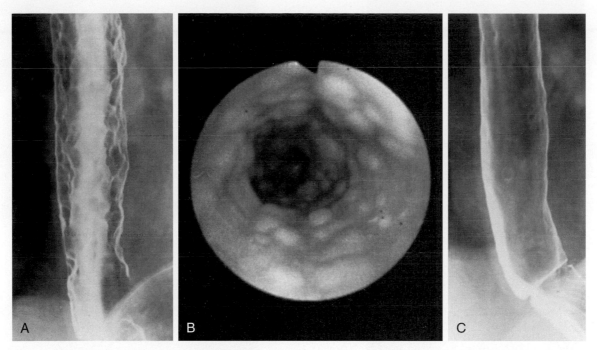

FIGURE 6–39. Non-Hodgkin's lymphoma involving esophagus. *A,* Initial esophagram shows innumerable small submucosal-appearing defects in thoracic esophagus. Note resemblance to varices. *B,* Endoscopic photograph reveals multiple, discrete submucosal nodules. *C,* Repeat esophagram 2 months after chemotherapy shows virtually complete regression of lesions seen on earlier study. (Note air bubbles in esophagus.) (From Levine, M.S., et al.: Diffuse nodularity in esophageal lymphoma. AJR Am. J. Roentgenol. *145*:1218–1220, 1985, with permission, © by American Roentgen Ray Society.)

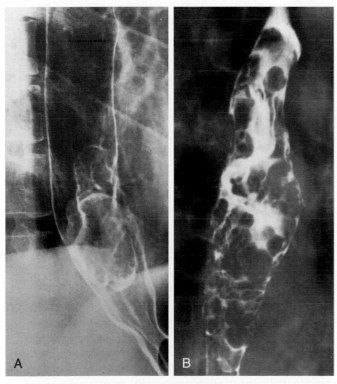

FIGURE 6–40. Two examples of spindle cell carcinoma. *A,* Polypoid intraluminal mass in distal esophagus. *B,* More extensive intraluminal mass that locally expands esophagus without causing obstruction. Note scalloped borders of lesion.

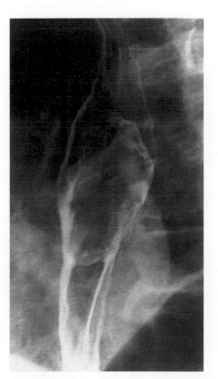

FIGURE 6–41. Primary malignant melanoma. A large polypoid mass is seen in midesophagus. Note how tumor expands the esophagus. Spindle cell carcinoma may produce identical findings (see Fig. 6–40). (From Yoo, C.C., Levine, M.S., McLarney, J.K., et al.: Primary malignant melanoma of the esophagus: Radiographic findings in seven patients. Radiology *209*:455, 1998, with permission.)

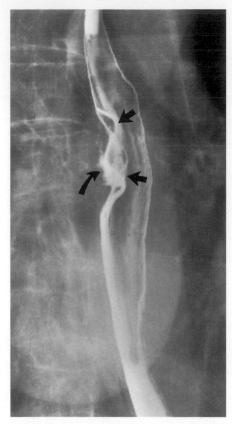

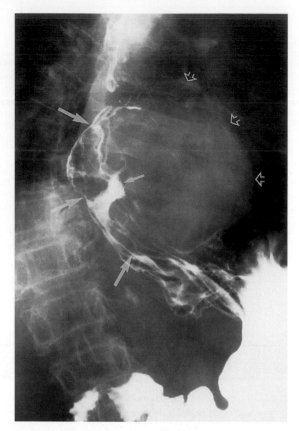

FIGURE 6–42. Small cell carcinoma. Smoothly marginated, polypoid mass *(straight arrows)* contains a relatively flat central ulcer *(curved arrow)* on right posterolateral wall of midesophagus just below level of carina. This appearance is typical of small cell carcinoma. (From Levine, M.S., Pantongrag-Brown, L., Buck, J.L., et al.: Small-cell carcinoma of the esophagus: Radiographic findings. Radiology *199:*703, 1996, with permission.)

FIGURE 6–43. Leiomyosarcoma. A giant intramural mass *(large arrows)* in the distal esophagus with a bulky exophytic component *(open arrows)* is seen extending into the mediastinum. Also note small central ulcer filling with barium *(small arrow)*. (From Levine, M.S., Buck, J.L., Pantongrag-Brown, L., et al.: Leiomyosarcoma of the esophagus: Radiographic findings in 10 patients. AJR Am. J. Roentgenol. *167:*27, 1996, with permission, © by American Roentgen Ray Society.)

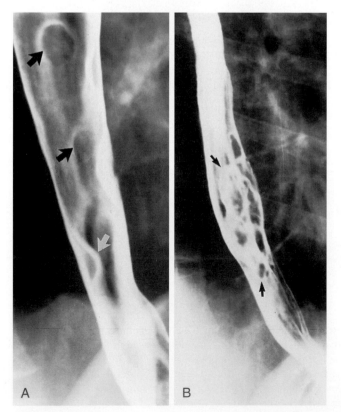

FIGURE 6–44. Kaposi's sarcoma involving esophagus. *A,* Several discrete submucosal masses *(arrows)* are present in esophagus in AIDS patient with Kaposi's sarcoma. (Courtesy of Robert Goren, M.D., Philadelphia, Pennsylvania.) *B,* Another patient with Kaposi's sarcoma manifested by large polypoid mass *(arrows)* in distal esophagus. (From Rose, H.S., et al.: Alimentary tract involvement in Kaposi sarcoma: Radiographic and endoscopic findings in 25 homosexual men. AJR Am. J. Roentgenol. *139:*661–666, 1982, with permission, © by American Roentgen Ray Society.)

REFERENCES

1. Miller, B.J., Murphy, F., and Lukie, B.E.: Squamous cell papilloma of esophagus. Can. J. Surg. *21*:538, 1978.
2. Montesi, A., Alessandro, P., Graziani, L., et al.: Small benign tumors of the esophagus: Radiological diagnosis with double-contrast examination. Gastrointest. Radiol. *8*:207, 1983.
3. Nuwayhid, N.S., Ballard, E.T., and Cotton, R.: Esophageal papillomatosis. Ann. Otol. Rhinol. Laryngol. *86*:623, 1977.
4. Rywlin, A.M., and Ortega, R.: Glycogenic acanthosis of the esophagus. Arch. Pathol. *90*:439, 1970.
5. Berliner, L., Redmond, P., Horowitz, L., et al.: Glycogen plaques (glycogenic acanthosis) of the esophagus. Radiology *141*:607, 1981.
6. Glick, S.N., Teplick, S.K., Goldstein, J., et al.: Glycogenic acanthosis of the esophagus. AJR Am. J. Roentgenol. *139*:683, 1982.
7. Ghahremani, G.G., and Rushovich, A.M.: Glycogenic acanthosis of the esophagus: Radiographic and pathologic features. Gastrointest. Radiol. *9*:93, 1984.
8. Plachta, A.: Benign tumors of the esophagus: Review of literature and report of 99 cases. Am. J. Gastroenterol. *38*:639, 1962.
9. Glanz, I., and Grunebaum, M.: The radiological approach to leiomyoma of the oesophagus with a long-term follow-up. Clin. Radiol. *28*:197, 1977.
10. Gutman, E.: Posterior mediastinal calcification due to esophageal leiomyoma. Gastroenterology *63*:665, 1972.
11. Nora, P.F.: Lipoma of the esophagus. Am. J. Surg. *108*:353, 1964.
12. Govoni, A.F.: Hemangiomas of the esophagus. Gastrointest. Radiol. *7*:113, 1982.
13. Rubesin, S.E., Herlinger, H., and Sigal, H.: Granular cell tumors of the esophagus. Gastrointest. Radiol. *10*:11, 1985.
14. Farman, J., Rosen, Y., Dallemand, S., et al.: Esophagitis cystica: Lower esophageal retention cysts. AJR Am. J. Roentgenol. *128*:495, 1977.
15. Trenkner, S.W., Levine, M.S., Laufer, I., et al.: Idiopathic esophageal varix. AJR Am. J. Roentgenol. *141*:43, 1983.
16. Levine, M.S., Sunshine, A.G., Reynolds, J.C., et al.: Diffuse nodularity in esophageal lymphoma. AJR Am. J. Roentgenol. *145*:1218, 1985.
17. Avezzano, E.A., Fleischer, D.E., Merida, M.A., et al.: Giant fibrovascular polyp of the esophagus. Am. J. Gastroenterol. *85*:299, 1990.
18. Cochet, B., Hohl, P., Sans, M., et al.: Asphyxia caused by laryngeal impaction of an esophageal polyp. Arch. Otolaryngol. *106*:176, 1980.
19. Carter, M.M., and Kulkarni, M.V.: Giant fibrovascular polyp of the esophagus. Gastrointest. Radiol. *9*:301, 1984.
20. Levine, M.S., Buck, J.L., Pantongrag-Brown, L., et al.: Fibrovascular polyps of the esophagus: Clinical, radiographic, and pathologic findings in 16 patients. AJR Am. J. Roentgenol. *166*:781, 1996.
21. Levine, M.S.: Esophageal cancer: Radiologic diagnosis. Radiol. Clin. North Am. *35*:265, 1997.
22. Wynder, E.L., and Mabuchi, K.: Cancer of the esophagus: Etiological and environmental factors. JAMA *226*:1546, 1973.
23. Carter, R., and Brewer, L.A.: Achalasia and esophageal carcinoma. Am. J. Surg. *130*:114, 1975.
24. Appleqvist, P., and Salmo, M.: Lye corrosion carcinoma of the esophagus: A review of 63 cases. Cancer *45*:2655, 1980.
25. Goldstein, H.M., and Zornoza, J.: Association of squamous cell carcinoma of the head and neck with cancer of the esophagus. AJR Am. J. Roentgenol. *131*:791, 1978.
26. Collins, S.M., Hamilton, J.D., Lewis, T.D., and Laufer, I.: Small-bowel malabsorption and gastrointestinal malignancy. Radiology *126*:603, 1978.
27. Chisholm, M.: The association between webs, iron and postcricoid carcinoma. Postgrad. Med. J. *50*:215, 1974.
28. Harper, P.S., Harper, R.M.J., and Howel-Evans, A.W.: Carcinoma of the oesophagus with tylosis. QJM *39*:317, 1970.
29. Pera, M., Cameron, A.J., Trastek, V.F., et al.: Increasing incidence of adenocarcinoma of the esophagus and esophagogastric junction. Gastroenterology *104*:510, 1993.
30. Hesketh, P.J., Clapp, R.W., Doos, W.G., et al.: The incidence of adenocarcinoma of the esophagus. Cancer *64*:526, 1989.
31. Skinner, D.B., Ferguson, M.K., Soriano, A., et al.: Selection of operation for esophageal cancer based on staging. Ann. Surg. *204*:391, 1986.
32. Levine, M.S., Herman, J.B., and Furth, E.E.: Barrett's esophagus and esophageal adenocarcinoma: The scope of the problem. Abdom. Imaging *20*:291, 1995.
33. Spechler, S.J., Robbins, A.H., Rubins, H.B., et al.: Adenocarcinoma and Barrett's esophagus: An overrated risk? Gastroenterology *87*:927, 1984.
34. Cameron, A.J., Ott, B.J., and Payne, W.S.: The incidence of adenocarcinoma in columnar-lined (Barrett's) esophagus. N. Engl. J. Med. *313*:857, 1985.
35. Levine, M.S., Chu, P., Furth, E.E., et al.: Carcinoma of the esophagus and esophagogastric junction: Sensitivity of radiographic diagnosis. AJR Am. J. Roentgenol. *168*:1423, 1997.
36. Sherlock, P., Ehrlich, A.N., and Winawer, S.J.: Diagnosis of gastrointestinal cancer: Current status and recent progress. Gastroenterology *63*:672, 1972.
37. Bemvenuti, G.A., Hattori, K., Levin, B., et al.: Endoscopic sampling for tissue diagnosis in GI malignancy. Gastrointest. Endosc. *21*:159, 1975.
38. DiPalma, J.A., Prechter, G.C., and Brady, C.E.: X-ray-negative dysphagia: Is endoscopy necessary? J. Clin. Gastroenterol. *6*:409, 1984.
39. Halpert, R.D., Feczko, P.J., Spickler, E.M., et al.: Radiologic assessment of dysphagia with endoscopy. Radiology *157*:599, 1985.
40. Japanese Society for Esophageal Diseases: Guidelines for the clinical and pathologic studies on carcinoma of the esophagus. Jpn. J. Surg. *6*:69, 1976.
41. Guojun, H., Lingfang, S., Dawei, Z., et al.: Diagnosis and surgical treatment of early esophageal carcinoma. Chin. Med. J. *94*:229, 1981.
42. Zornoza, J., and Lindell, M.M.: Radiologic evaluation of small esophageal carcinoma. Gastrointest. Radiol. *5*:107, 1980.
43. Levine, M.S., Dillon, E.C., Saul, S.H., et al.: Early esophageal cancer. AJR Am. J. Roentgenol. *146*:507, 1986.
44. Moss, A.A., Koehler, R.E., and Margulis, A.R.: Initial accuracy of esophagograms in detection of small esophageal carcinoma. AJR Am. J. Roentgenol. *127*:909, 1976.
45. Koehler, R.E., Moss, A.A., and Margulis, A.R.: Early radiographic manifestations of carcinoma of the esophagus. Radiology *119*:1, 1976.
46. Itai, Y., Kogure, T., Okiyama, Y., et al.: Superficial esophageal carcinoma: Radiological findings in double-contrast studies. Radiology *126*:597, 1978.
47. Sato, T., Sakai, Y., Kajita, A., et al.: Radiographic microstructures of early esophageal carcinoma: Correlation of specimen radiography with pathologic findings and clinical radiography. Gastrointest. Radiol. *11*:12, 1986.
48. Itai, Y., Kogure, T., Okiyama, Y., et al.: Diffuse finely nodular lesions of the esophagus. AJR Am. J. Roentgenol. *128*:563, 1977.
49. Levine, M.S., Macones, A.J., and Laufer, I.: *Candida* esophagitis: Accuracy of radiographic diagnosis. Radiology *154*:581, 1985.
50. Levine, M.S., Kressel, H.Y., Caroline, D.F., et al.: Barrett esophagus: Reticular pattern of the mucosa. Radiology *147*:663, 1983.
51. Goldstein, H.M., Zornoza, J., and Hopens, T.: Intrinsic diseases of the adult esophagus: Benign and malignant tumors. Semin. Roentgenol. *16*:183, 1981.
52. Gloyna, R.E., Zornoza, J., and Goldstein, H.M.: Primary ulcerative carcinoma of the esophagus. AJR Am. J. Roentgenol. *129*:599, 1977.
53. Lawson, T.L., Dodds, W.J., and Sheft, D.J.: Carcinoma of the esophagus simulating varices. AJR Am. J. Roentgenol. *107*:83, 1969.
54. Yates, C.W., LeVine, M.A., and Jensen, K.M.: Varicoid carcinoma of the esophagus. Radiology *122*:605, 1977.
55. Levine, M.S., Caroline, D., Thompson, J.J., et al.: Adenocarcinoma of the esophagus: Relationship to Barrett mucosa. Radiology *150*:305, 1984.
56. Agha, F.P.: Barrett carcinoma of the esophagus: Clinical and radiographic analysis of 34 cases. AJR Am. J. Roentgenol. *145*:41, 1985.
57. Keen, S.J., Dodd, G.D., and Smith, J.L.: Adenocarcinoma arising in Barrett's esophagus: Pathologic and radiologic features. Mt. Sinai J. Med. *51*:442, 1984.
58. Steiner, H., Lammer, J., and Hackl, A.: Lymphatic metastases to the esophagus. Gastrointest. Radiol. *9*:1, 1984.
59. Glick, S.N., Teplick, S.K., Levine, M.S., et al.: Gastric cardia metastasis in esophageal carcinoma. Radiology *160*:627, 1986.
60. Halvorsen, R.A., and Thompson, W.M.: CT of esophageal neoplasms. Radiol. Clin. North Am. *27*:667, 1989.
61. Takashima, S., Takeuchi, N., Shiozaki, H., et al.: Carcinoma of the esophagus: CT vs. MR imaging in determining resectability. AJR Am. J. Roentgenol. *156*:297, 1991.
62. Vilgrain, V., Mompoint, D., Palazzo, L., et al.: Staging of esophageal carcinoma: Comparison of results with endoscopic sonography and CT. AJR Am. J. Roentgenol. *155*:277, 1990.

63. Hankins, J.R., and McLaughlin, J.S.: The association of carcinoma of the esophagus with achalasia. J. Thorac. Cardiovasc. Surg. *69:* 355, 1975.

64. Levine, M.S., Langer, J., Laufer, I., et al.: Radiation therapy of esophageal carcinoma: Correlation of clinical and radiographic findings. Gastrointest. Radiol. *12:*99, 1987.

65. Owen, J.W., Balfe, D.M., Koehler, R.E., et al.: Radiologic evaluation of complications after esophagogastrectomy. AJR Am. J. Roentgenol. *140:*1163, 1983.

66. Anderson, M.F., and Harell, G.S.: Secondary esophageal tumors. AJR Am. J. Roentgenol. *135:*1243, 1980.

67. Carnovale, R.L., Goldstein, H.M., Zornoza, J., et al.: Radiologic manifestations of esophageal lymphoma. AJR Am. J. Roentgenol. *128:*751, 1977.

68. Agha, F.P., and Keren, D.F.: Spindle-cell squamous carcinoma of the esophagus: A tumor with biphasic morphology. AJR Am. J. Roentgenol. *145:*541, 1985.

69. Olmsted, W.W., Lichtenstein, J.E., and Hyams, V.J.: Polypoid epithelial malignancies of the esophagus. AJR Am. J. Roentgenol. *140:* 921, 1983.

70. Yoo, C.C., Levine, M.S., McLarney, J.K., et al.: Primary malignant melanoma of the esophagus: Radiographic findings in seven patients. Radiology *209:*455, 1998.

71. Levine, M.S., Pantongrag-Brown, L., Buck, J.L., et al.: Small-cell carcinoma of the esophagus: Radiographic findings. Radiology *199:* 703, 1996.

72. Levine, M.S., Buck, J.L., Pantongrag-Brown, L., et al.: Leiomyosarcoma of the esophagus: Radiographic findings in 10 patients. AJR Am. J. Roentgenol. *167:*27, 1996.

73. Rose, H.S., Balthazar, E.J., Megibow, A.J., et al.: Alimentary tract involvement in Kaposi sarcoma: Radiographic and endoscopic findings in 25 homosexual men. AJR Am. J. Roentgenol. *139:*661, 1982.

74. Umerah, B.C.: Kaposi sarcoma of the oesophagus. Br. J. Radiol. *53:*807, 1980.

7

Stomach

MARC S. LEVINE
IGOR LAUFER

NORMAL APPEARANCES

The normal appearance of the stomach is familiar to all physicians. The double contrast examination provides additional detail, however, about the anatomic structure of the stomach, including (1) the surface pattern, (2) the cardia, and (3) compression by adjacent structures.

Surface Pattern

Although single contrast barium studies of the stomach rely heavily on analysis of the rugal fold pattern, gastric distention effaces the normal rugal folds on double contrast studies. Abnormal folds, such as those associated with a healing gastric ulcer or early gastric cancer, may be stiffer than normal and therefore tend to resist effacement. As a result, they may become particularly prominent when the surrounding normal folds are flattened.

When adequate mucosal coating and gaseous distention of the stomach have been achieved, the surface pattern or areae gastricae can be seen (Fig. 7–1).[1] The frequency of visualization of the normal areae gastricae depends not only on radiographic technique but also on the amount and viscosity of mucus in the stomach. With high-density barium suspensions, the areae gastricae can be detected on routine double contrast studies in about 70% of patients.[2] This surface pattern is observed most frequently in the antrum or body of the stomach (Fig. 7–1A), but it can also be seen in the fundus (Fig. 7–1B). Areae gastricae are easier to visualize on barium studies than on endoscopy, presumably because of the thin layer of mucus that obscures these tiny crevices in the mucosa on endoscopic examinations. However, the normal surface pattern of the stomach can be well demonstrated on scanning electron micrographs (Fig. 7–2).

Variations in the size and appearance of the areae gastricae are sometimes seen on double contrast studies. In the past it was postulated that the size of the areae gastricae depended on parietal cell mass.[1] As a result, hypersecretory states or duodenal ulcers have been associated with enlarged areae gastricae, particularly in the upper body and fundus of the stomach (Fig. 7–3).[3,4] More recently, however, enlarged areae gastricae have been demonstrated in patients with *Helicobacter pylori* gastritis (Fig. 7–4).[5] In fact, the high frequency of *H. pylori* gastritis in patients with duodenal ulcers may account for the apparent association between ulcers and enlarged areae gastricae. Focal enlargement or distortion of the areae gastricae may also be caused by nonspecific inflammation, intestinal metaplasia (Fig. 7–5), or even mucosal spread of cancer (Fig. 7–6).[6] Conversely, patients with at-

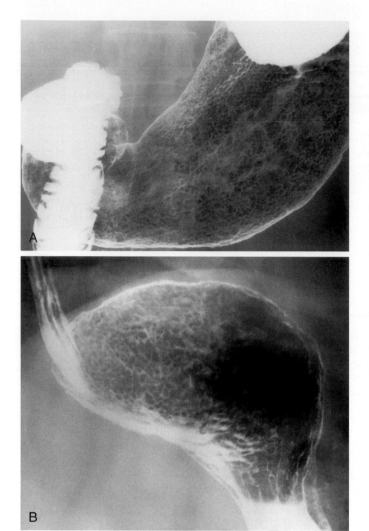

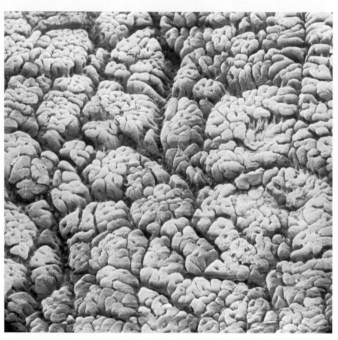

FIGURE 7–2. Scanning electron micrograph showing normal surface pattern of stomach. Innumerable gastric sulci account for reticular appearance seen on radiographs. The tiny black dots represent openings of gastric pits. (Magnification, × 20.) (Courtesy of Gerald D. Dodd, M.D., and J.D. Anderson, M.D., Houston, Texas, and Harvey M. Goldstein, M.D., San Antonio, Texas.)

FIGURE 7–1. Normal surface pattern of stomach. *A,* Areae gastricae in antrum and body. *B,* Areae gastricae in fundus.

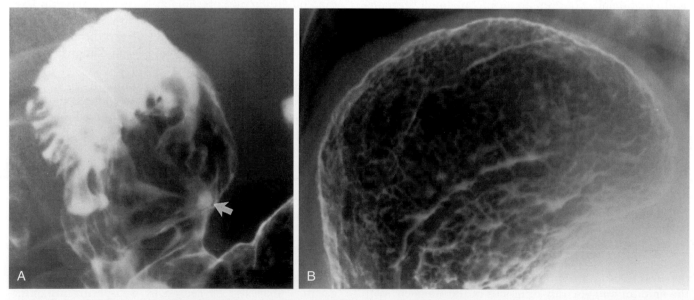

FIGURE 7–3. Duodenal ulcer with enlarged areae gastricae in fundus. *A,* Small ulcer *(arrow)* at base of duodenal bulb. *B,* Enlarged areae gastricae in fundus, probably a result of hypersecretion of acid associated with peptic ulcer.

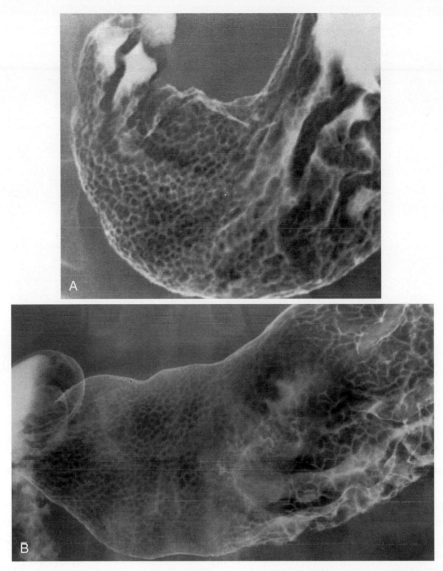

FIGURE 7–4. Two examples (*A* and *B*) of *H. pylori* gastritis with enlarged areae gastricae in antrum and body of stomach.

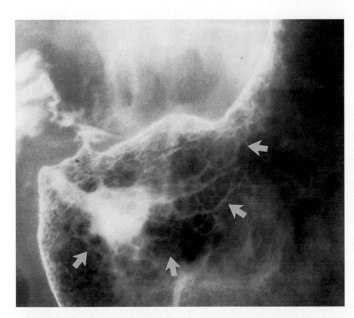

FIGURE 7–5. Intestinal metaplasia in antrum, causing focal irregularity and enlargement of areae gastricae *(arrows)*.

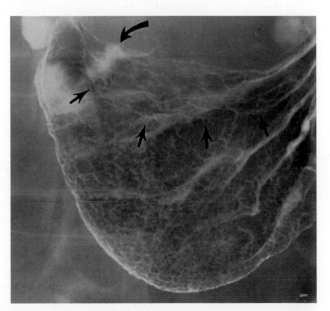

FIGURE 7–6. Ulcerated carcinoma *(curved arrow)* on lesser curvature of antrum. Note enlarged, distorted areae gastricae *(straight arrows)* in adjacent stomach due to mucosal spread of tumor.

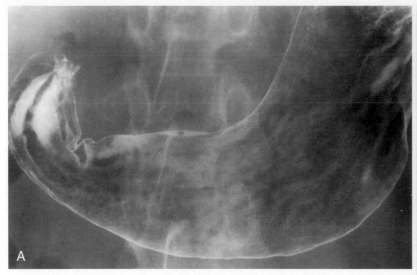

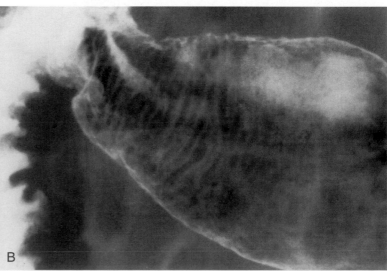

FIGURE 7–7. Atrophic gastritis with tiny, barely discernible areae gastricae in stomach. Note decreased distensibility and paucity of mucosal folds in antrum, body, and fundus. (From Levine, M.S., et al.: Atrophic gastritis in pernicious anemia: Diagnosis by double-contrast radiography. Gastrointest. Radiol. *14:*215, 1989, with permission.)

rophic gastritis tend to have small or absent areae gastricae (Fig. 7–7), presumably because of achlorhydria and the loss of parietal cells that occurs in these individuals.[7] However, other investigators have found no correlation between the size of the areae gastricae and the presence or absence of superficial or atrophic gastritis.[8] As a result, it is generally difficult to diagnose abnormalities on the basis of the areae gastricae. When there is a striking focal alteration, however, endoscopic biopsy specimens should be obtained to rule out an early gastric cancer.

Occasionally, fine transverse folds or striae may also be seen in the gastric antrum (Fig. 7–8).[9,10] Unlike transverse folds in the esophagus, which occur as a transient phenomenon, these gastric folds are more persistent. Some patients have associated antral gastritis.[10] The pathophysiologic basis and clinical significance of these folds are

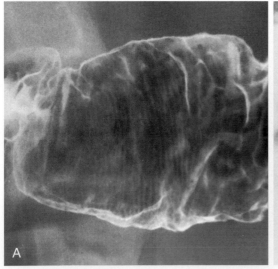

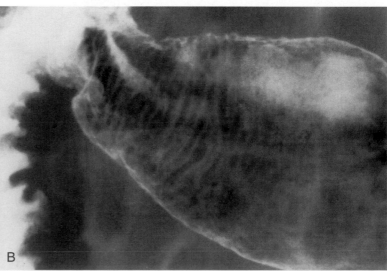

FIGURE 7–8. Two examples (*A* and *B*) of fine transverse folds or striae in antrum, probably occurring as a normal variant.

uncertain, however, and we tend to consider them a normal variant.

Cardia

The gastric cardia and fundus are particularly well demonstrated by double contrast technique.[11,12] The radiographic appearance of the cardia on double contrast studies depends on how firmly it is anchored by the surrounding phrenoesophageal membrane to the esophageal hiatus of the diaphragm. When the cardia is well anchored, protrusion of the distal esophagus into the fundus produces a circular elevation containing four or five stellate folds that radiate to a central point at the gastroesophageal junction (the cardiac "rosette") (Fig. 7–9A).[11,12] The circular elevation may be etched in white or may appear as a filling defect in the surrounding barium pool, depending on the amount of barium in the fundus. This elevation is demarcated from the adjacent fundus by a "hooding" fold that surrounds it laterally and

superiorly. In the past, this hooding fold has been called the "sign of the burnous" because of its resemblance to the cloaklike garment worn by Arabs and Moors.[13] Several longitudinal folds characteristically extend inferiorly from the cardiac rosette along the posterior wall and lesser curvature.

When the cardia is less firmly anchored, an esophageal rosette may be visible without an associated protrusion or circular elevation (see Fig. 7–9B).[12] With further ligamentous laxity, the rosette may also vanish, and the cardia may be recognized by only a single crescentic line that crosses the area of the esophageal orifice (see Fig. 7–9C).[12] Finally, severe ligamentous laxity may lead to the formation of a hiatal hernia, so that no cardiac structure is identified below the diaphragm (see Fig. 7–9D).

Radiologists should be familiar with the range of appearances of the cardia to avoid mistaking the normal anatomic landmarks in this region for ulcers or mass lesions. At the same time, abnormalities at the cardia may

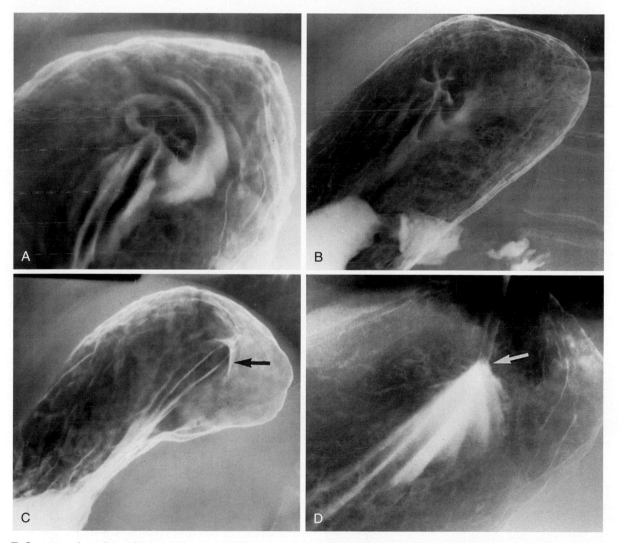

FIGURE 7–9. Normal cardia and its variations. *A,* Well-anchored cardia appearing as circular elevation with centrally radiating folds (the cardiac "rosette"). *B,* Stellate folds without surrounding elevation due to laxity of ligamentous attachments. *C,* Further weakening of ligaments with obliteration of cardiac rosette. Note crescentic line *(arrow)* that crosses area of esophageal orifice. *D,* Severe ligamentous laxity with gastric folds in small hiatal hernia converging superiorly *(arrow)* above esophageal hiatus of diaphragm.

be manifested by relatively subtle findings. For example, an ulcer adjacent to the cardia can be mistaken for the esophageal orifice (Fig. 7–10A). Carcinoma of the cardia may cause distortion or obliteration of the cardiac rosette without a discrete mass (Fig. 7–10B; see Chapter 8). Finally, gastric varices may be manifested by enlarged, scalloped folds adjacent to the cardia (see Fig. 7–9C). Thus, radiologic evaluation of the cardia requires meticulous attention to anatomic detail in this region.

Extrinsic Impressions

The double contrast examination results in considerable distention of the stomach, particularly when a hypotonic agent is used. As a result, neighboring structures may produce a variety of extrinsic impressions on the distended stomach. On lateral views, the posterior wall of the stomach may be compressed by normal retrogastric structures such as the pancreas and spleen (Fig. 7–11A). This finding may be particularly prominent in thin patients (Fig. 7–11B). Although impressions caused by the liver are usually quite subtle, enlargement of the left lobe of the liver or anomalous lobulation of the liver may produce an extrinsic impression on the lesser curvature of the gastric body, mimicking the appearance of an intramural gastric lesion (Fig. 7–12). A gas-filled or stool-filled splenic flexure of the colon may also cause an impression on the posterolateral wall of the upper stomach.

Retrogastric masses can be recognized en face by an ill-defined translucency in the stomach (Fig. 7–13A) or on oblique views by a double contour seen through the gas-filled stomach, with one line representing the edge of the mass. However, lateral views are best for showing

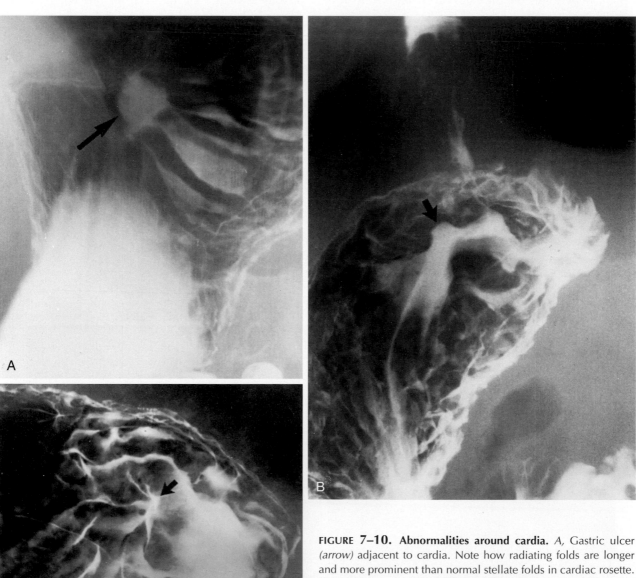

FIGURE 7–10. Abnormalities around cardia. *A,* Gastric ulcer *(arrow)* adjacent to cardia. Note how radiating folds are longer and more prominent than normal stellate folds in cardiac rosette. *B,* Carcinoma of cardia with obliteration of normal cardiac structures and associated ulceration *(arrow).* Note how tumor extends into distal esophagus. *C,* Gastric varices with enlarged, lobulated folds adjacent to cardia. The central button of cardiac rosette is indicated by *arrow.*

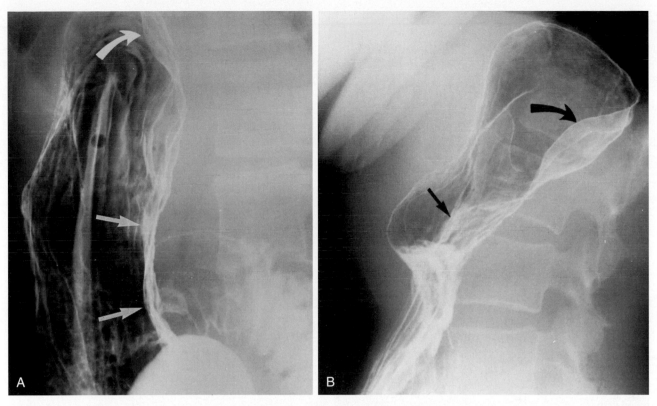

FIGURE 7–11. Normal retrogastric impressions. *A,* Subtle impressions on posterior wall of stomach from normal retrogastric structures such as pancreas *(straight arrows)* and spleen *(curved arrow)*. *B,* In thin patients, these impressions from pancreas *(straight arrow)* and spleen *(curved arrow)* may become more prominent but are still normal.

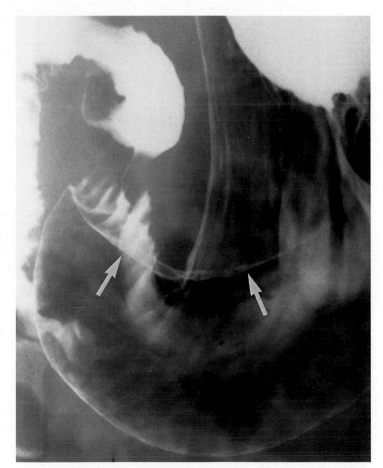

FIGURE 7–12. Enlarged left lobe of liver causing smooth extrinsic impression *(arrows)* on superior border of antrum. This appearance could be mistaken for an intramural mass.

these extrinsic impressions on the posterior gastric wall in profile (Fig. 7–13*B*). If an abnormal extrinsic mass lesion is suspected on double contrast studies, computed tomography (CT) may be helpful in determining the origin, extent, and nature of the lesion (Fig. 7–13*C*).

Mucosal Folds

The rugal folds in the antrum should be completely effaced on routine double contrast studies. Persistence of the folds despite adequate distention should suggest antral gastritis, particularly if the folds have a scalloped or irregular appearance (Fig. 7–14). Rarely, other causes of thickened, lobulated antral folds, such as arteriovenous malformations, may be encountered (Fig. 7–15).[14]

The rugal folds in the body and fundus of the stomach are more difficult to evaluate on double contrast studies. Even with optimal gaseous distention, the folds are often visible as persistent structures, particularly along the

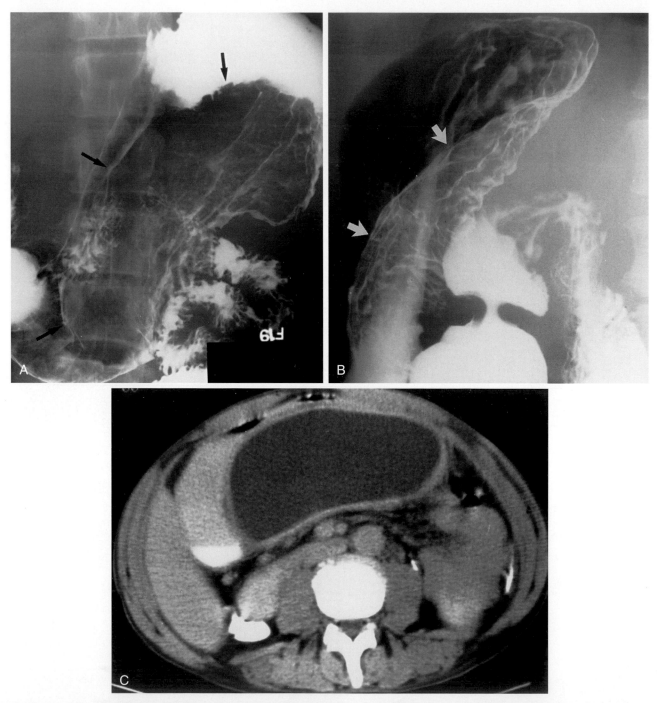

FIGURE 7–13. Abnormal retrogastric mass. *A,* Supine film shows ill-defined translucency *(arrows)* suggestive of extrinsic mass lesion compressing stomach. *B,* Lateral film confirms presence of large retrogastric mass causing extrinsic impression *(arrows)* on posterior gastric wall. *C,* CT scan shows giant pancreatic pseudocyst compressing and displacing stomach.

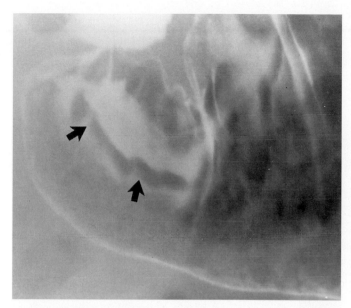

FIGURE 7–14. Antral gastritis with thickened, scalloped fold *(arrows)* in antrum.

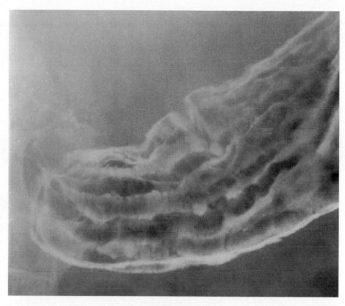

FIGURE 7–15. Arteriovenous malformation with thickened, tortuous folds in antrum. (From Lewis, T.D., et al.: Arteriovenous malformation of the stomach: Radiologic and endoscopic features. Am. J. Dig. Dis. *23*:467, 1978, with permission.)

greater curvature. However, the folds should have a relatively smooth, straight contour in the normal stomach. In contrast, folds that are unusually thickened and lobulated should be considered abnormal. In our experience, *H. pylori* gastritis is the most common cause of thickened, lobulated gastric folds (Fig. 7–16). Other less common causes include hypertrophic gastritis (Fig. 7–17*A*), Ménétrier's disease (Fig. 7–17*B*), lymphoma (Fig. 7–17*C*),

or even a submucosally infiltrating adenocarcinoma (Fig. 7–17*D*). Occasionally, folds in the upper body or fundus of the stomach may appear abnormal because of inadequate gaseous distention, erroneously suggesting an infiltrating process (Fig. 7–18*A*). In such cases, administration of additional effervescent agent to increase gastric distention should allow demonstration of these folds as normal (Fig. 7–18*B*).

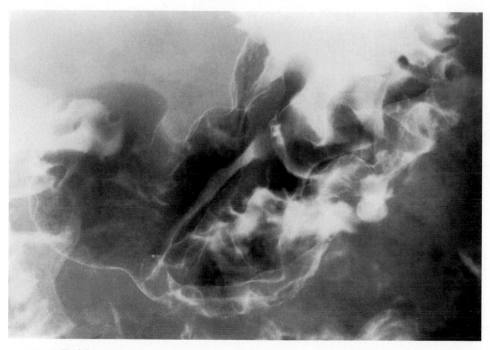

FIGURE 7–16. *H. pylori* gastritis with markedly thickened, lobulated folds in gastric body.

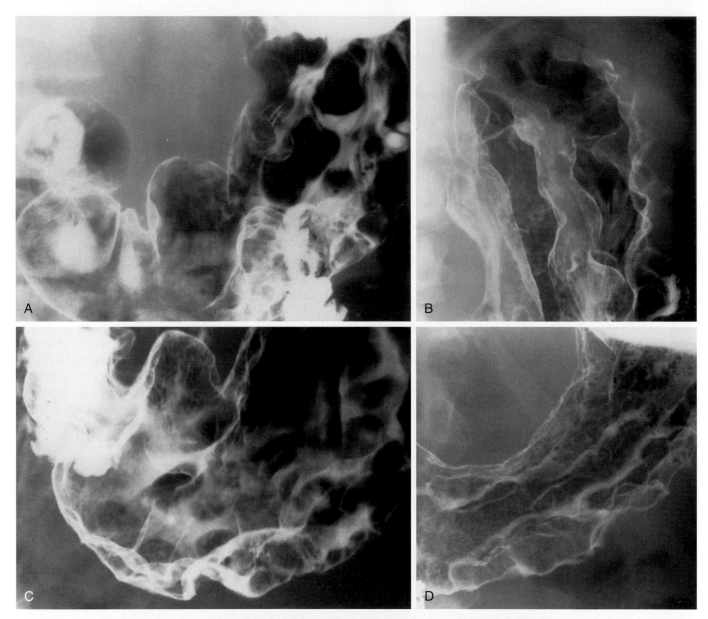

FIGURE 7–17. Other causes of thickened folds in stomach. *A,* Thickened, lobulated folds in body due to hypertrophic gastritis. *B,* Grossly thickened folds in fundus due to Ménétrier's disease. *C,* Thickened, polypoid folds in antrum and body due to lymphoma. Note how stomach retains its normal distensibility. *D,* Thickened, irregular folds in body due to gastric carcinoma. Unlike lymphoma, infiltrating carcinomas typically limit gastric distensibility, as in this case. (*D,* From Levine, M.S., et al.: Scirrhous carcinoma of the stomach: Radiologic and endoscopic diagnosis. Radiology *175:*151, 1990, with permission.)

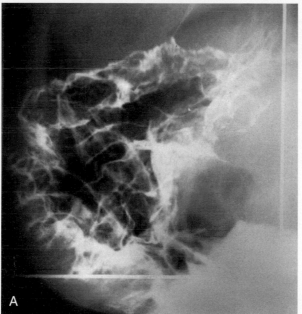

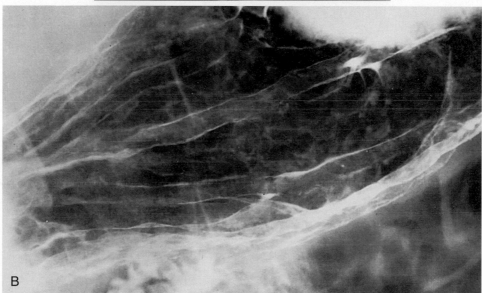

FIGURE 7–18. Importance of distention for evaluating gastric folds. *A,* Right lateral view of fundus shows apparently thickened, irregular folds in proximal portion of stomach, suggesting diffuse infiltration by tumor. *B,* With further distention, the folds are seen to straighten, and there is no evidence of tumor.

ARTIFACTS

The general nature of double contrast artifacts has been discussed in Chapter 2. Some of the major artifacts that can simulate disease in the stomach are listed in the following[15]:

1. *"Kissing" artifacts* due to underdistention of the stomach with adherence of the anterior and posterior walls can mimic the appearance of mucosal or submucosal masses (Figs. 7–19 and 7–20).
2. *Undissolved effervescent agent* or *gas bubbles* in the stomach can also be mistaken for polypoid lesions.
3. *Barium precipitates* may appear as tiny, white dots on the gastric mucosa that resemble gastric erosions (see the next section, "Erosive Gastritis") (Fig. 7–21).
4. *See-through artifacts* due to overlying structures such as calcified vessels or barium-filled duodenal or colonic diverticula can simulate polyps or ulcers in a particular projection (Fig. 7–22).
5. *Stalactites* or droplets of barium suspended from folds on the anterior wall of the stomach can also be mistaken for ulcers (Fig. 7–23).

The transient nature of these various artifacts usually can be recognized during fluoroscopy by turning the patient into different positions or, if necessary, by obtaining additional views of the stomach after reviewing the films.

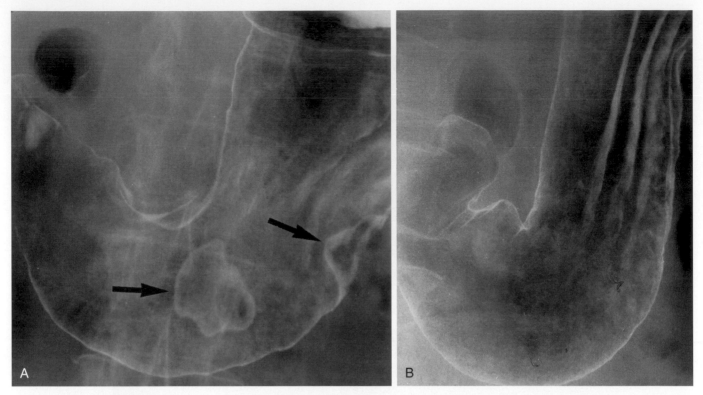

FIGURE 7–19. "Kissing" artifacts simulating gastric lesions. *A,* In supine position, anterior and posterior walls are adherent *(arrows)*. The resulting artifacts could be mistaken for polypoid lesions in stomach. *B,* With further distention the walls are separated, and these artifacts disappear. (From Laufer, I.: A simple method for routine double contrast study of the upper gastrointestinal tract. Radiology *117:*513, 1975, with permission.)

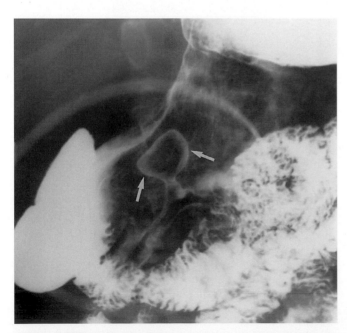

FIGURE 7–20. "Kissing artifact" mimicking pedunculated polyp *(arrows)* in gastric antrum.

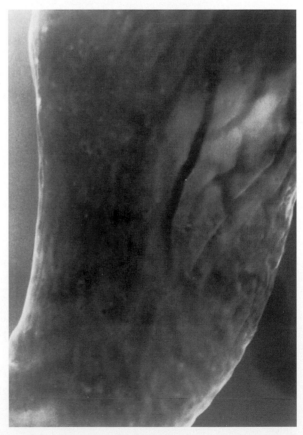

FIGURE 7–21. Barium precipitates simulating gastric erosions. Unlike gastric erosions, however, the precipitates are sharp and distinct and have no surrounding radiolucent halos.

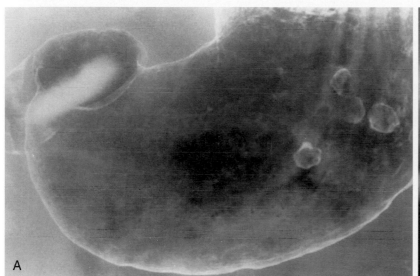

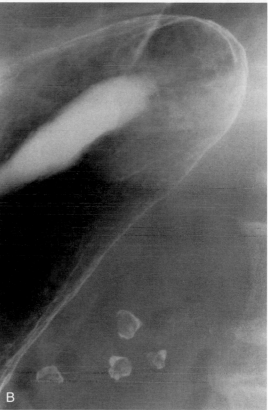

FIGURE 7–22. See-through artifacts simulating gastric polyps. *A,* Supine view shows multiple ring shadows in gastric body that could represent anterior wall polyps etched in white. *B,* Lateral view shows barium-filled colonic diverticula behind stomach.

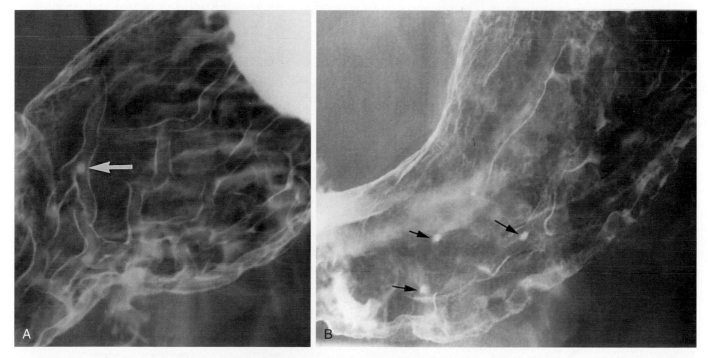

FIGURE 7–23. Stalactite phenomenon. *A,* Small, rounded density *(arrow)* overlying anterior wall fold. This hanging droplet of barium or stalactite could be mistaken for a tiny ulcer. *B,* Multiple stalactites *(arrows).*

GASTRITIS

Erosive Gastritis

Erosions are defined histologically as epithelial defects that do not penetrate beyond the muscularis mucosae. In approximately 50% of patients with erosive gastritis, there are no apparent predisposing factors.[16] However, known causes include alcohol, aspirin, other nonsteroidal antiinflammatory drugs (NSAIDs), steroids, stress, trauma, burns, Crohn's disease, and viral or fungal infection.[17-20] Patients with erosive gastritis may have vague dyspepsia, ulcerlike symptoms, or, less frequently, upper gastrointestinal bleeding.[21] However, some patients with this condition are asymptomatic. Thus, it may be difficult to establish the clinical significance of gastric erosions demonstrated on radiologic or endoscopic examination.

Although gastric erosions are frequently seen at endoscopy, they have been diagnosed only rarely on single contrast barium studies. By comparison, erosive gastritis has become a relatively frequent finding on double contrast studies, with an overall incidence of 0.5% to 20%.[22-27] Two types of erosions may be identified. The most common type is the complete or "varioliform" erosion, in which a punctate or slitlike collection of barium representing the epithelial defect is surrounded by a radiolucent halo of edematous, elevated mucosa.[16,24,26] Varioliform erosions typically occur in the gastric antrum and are often aligned on rugal folds (Fig. 7–24).[21,24,26] Because they are shallow lesions, erosions on the dependent or posterior wall may be better delineated by using flow technique to manipulate a thin layer of barium over the mucosal surface (Fig. 7–25).[28] Occasionally, barium may fail to enter the central defect of the erosions, so that they may be recognized as rounded filling defects due to the surrounding mounds of edema. In other patients, erosive

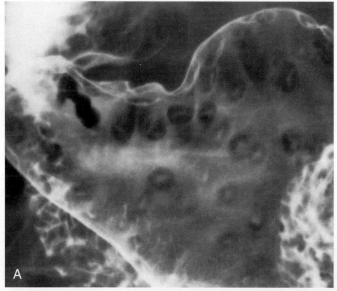

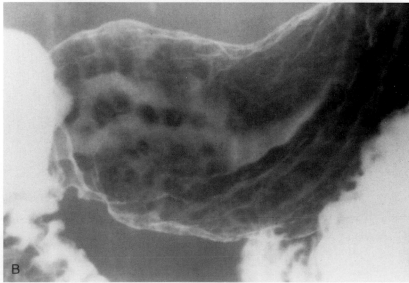

FIGURE 7–24. Two examples (*A* and *B*) of varioliform erosions in antrum with central barium collections surrounded by radiolucent halos of edematous mucosa. In *B*, note how erosions are aligned on rugal folds.

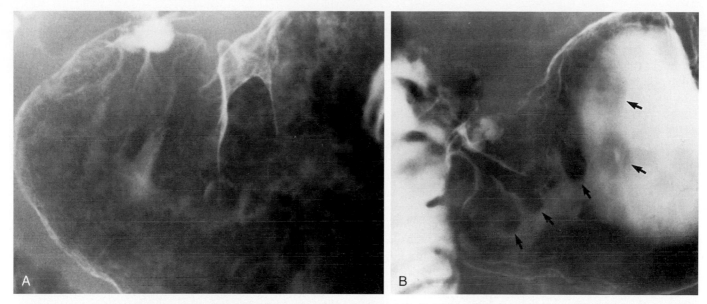

FIGURE 7–25. Value of flow technique for demonstrating gastric erosions. *A,* Initial view of antrum shows irregular, nodular mucosa without discrete lesions. *B,* Flow technique shows varioliform erosions as circular filling defects *(arrows)* in barium pool because of mounds of edema surrounding central part of erosions. Even in retrospect, these lesions are barely discernible on earlier view. (From Kikuchi, Y., et al.: Value of flow technique for double-contrast examination of the stomach. AJR Am. J. Roentgenol. *147:*1183, 1986, with permission, © by American Roentgen Ray Society.)

gastritis may be manifested only by scalloped or nodular antral folds. Depending on the quality of the mucosal coating, erosions may be faintly seen on the crests of the folds (Fig. 7–26*A*). In some cases, these scalloped antral folds may persist after the erosions have healed (Fig. 7–26*B*). Occasionally, residual epithelial nodules may also

be detected at the site of the healed erosions. These hyperplastic nodules or polyps are thought to represent the sequelae of chronic erosive gastritis.[21,29] In other patients, erosions may persist for years, even in the absence of clinical symptoms.[30]

Incomplete or "flat" erosions are epithelial defects

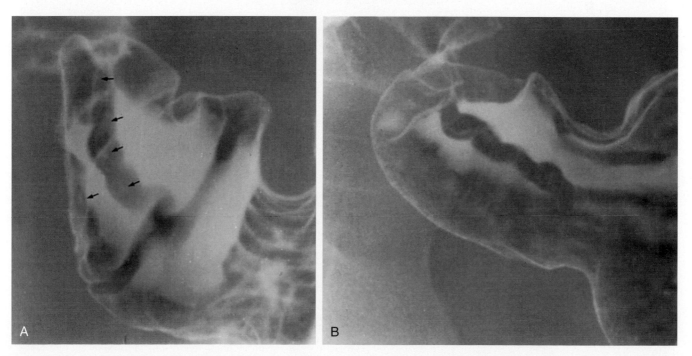

FIGURE 7–26. Erosive gastritis with scalloped folds. *A,* Scalloped antral folds with erosions *(arrows)* faintly seen on crests of folds. *B,* Persistent scalloped fold after erosions have healed.

without elevation of the surrounding mucosa. They appear radiographically as linear streaks or dots of barium (Fig. 7–27).[16,27] As a result, they are much more difficult to detect than are varioliform erosions, and they account for less than 5% of all erosions seen on double contrast studies.[27] Occasionally, incomplete erosions may be associated with slight flattening or deformity of the adjacent gastric wall (Fig. 7–27*B*).

Although no etiologic significance is usually attributed to the shape or location of gastric erosions seen on double contrast studies, aspirin and other NSAIDs may produce distinctive linear or serpiginous erosions that tend to be clustered in the body of the stomach, on or near the greater curvature (Fig. 7–28).[31] It has been postulated that these erosions result from localized mucosal injury that occurs as the dissolving tablets collect by gravity in the dependent portion of the stomach. Other patients taking NSAIDs may have linear erosions in the antrum or body away from the greater curvature (Fig. 7–29). Still other patients taking NSAIDs may have characteristic flattening, straightening, or retraction of the greater curvature of the distal antrum (Fig. 7–30), presumably due to scarring associated with multiple cycles of recurrent erosion formation and healing.[32] Detection of any of these findings therefore should lead to careful questioning of the patient about a possible history of NSAID use. If recent ingestion of these drugs is confirmed in symptomatic patients, with-

drawal of the offending agent often produces a rapid clinical response.[31]

Other conditions may also be manifested by erosive gastritis. In some patients, gastric erosions are seen as an early sign of Crohn's disease with multiple "aphthous ulcers" in the stomach (Fig. 7–31) (see Chapter 14).[18,19] Severe erosive gastritis or ulceration may also result from opportunistic infection by cytomegalovirus in patients with AIDS.[33] Rarely, one or more shallow ulcers may develop as a complication of endoscopic heater-probe therapy or of other iatrogenic trauma (Fig. 7–32).[34]

Gastric erosions must be differentiated on double contrast studies from barium precipitates in the stomach (see Fig. 7–21).[15] However, barium precipitates are sharp, crisp, and well defined. They do not have a radiolucent halo, and when viewed in profile, they appear as small clumps of barium on the mucosal surface rather than as projections of barium beyond the gastric contour. Varioliform gastric erosions must also be differentiated from centrally ulcerated submucosal masses, also known as "bull's-eye" or "target" lesions (see Figs. 8–43 and 8–47). However, bull's-eye lesions tend to be larger and more sporadic, occurring anywhere in the stomach. In contrast, varioliform erosions are smaller and more numerous and tend to be located in the antrum, often on the crests of the folds. Thus, it usually is possible to differentiate gastric erosions from true bull's-eye lesions on the basis of the radiographic findings.

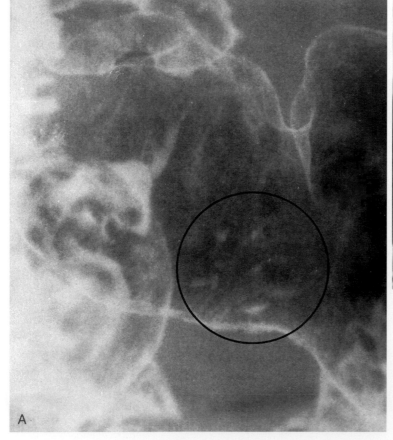

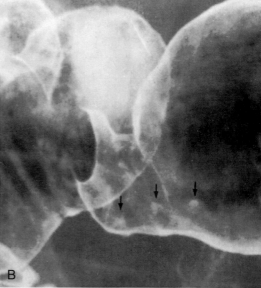

FIGURE 7–27. Incomplete erosions. *A,* Linear streaks and dots of barium in antrum *(inside circle)* are due to incomplete erosions. *B,* Another patient with incomplete erosions *(arrows)* in antrum. Note associated flattening of adjacent greater curvature.

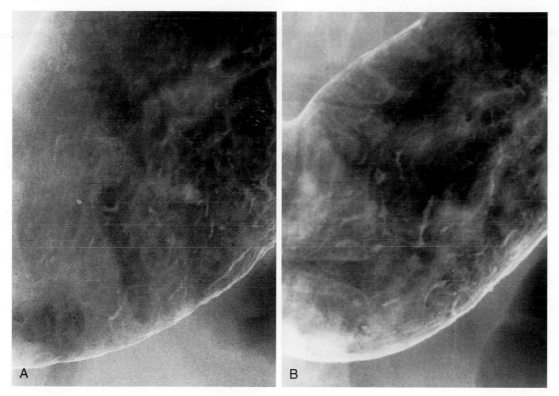

FIGURE 7–28. Two examples (*A* and *B*) of distinctive linear and serpiginous erosions in body of stomach near greater curvature due to aspirin in *A* and indomethacin in *B*. (From Levine, M.S., et al.: Serpiginous gastric erosions caused by aspirin and other nonsteroidal antiinflammatory drugs. AJR Am. J. Roentgenol. *146:*31, 1986, with permission, © by American Roentgen Ray Society.)

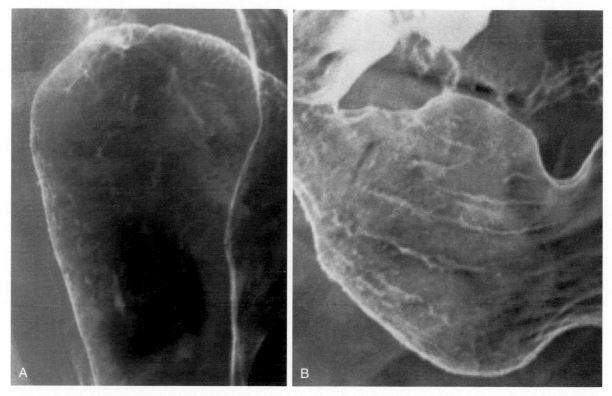

FIGURE 7–29. Linear erosions in antrum due to NSAIDs. *A,* Numerous linear erosions seen in antrum are due to naproxen. (From Levine, M.S., et al.: Serpiginous gastric erosions caused by aspirin and other nonsteroidal antiinflammatory drugs. AJR Am. J. Roentgenol. *146:*31, 1986, with permission, © by American Roentgen Ray Society.) *B,* Long, linear erosions are seen in antrum in another patient who was taking aspirin.

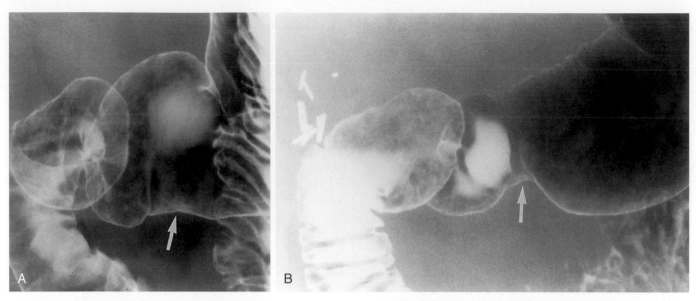

FIGURE 7–30. These two examples of flattening and retraction *(arrows)* of greater curvature of distal antrum are due to chronic aspirin therapy with associated scarring.

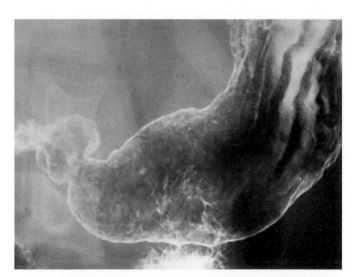

FIGURE 7–31. Erosive gastritis with multiple aphthous ulcers in antrum due to Crohn's disease involving stomach. Note duodenal ulcer. This patient had typical changes of Crohn's disease in terminal ileum. Subsequent endoscopy confirmed presence of superficial gastric erosions, and biopsy specimens revealed noncaseating granulomas. (From Laufer, I., et al.: Multiple superficial gastric erosions due to Crohn's disease of the stomach: Radiologic and endoscopic diagnosis. Br. J. Radiol. *49:*726, 1976, with permission.)

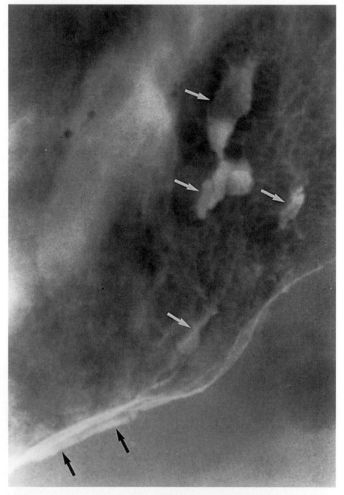

FIGURE 7–32. Heater probe ulcers in stomach. Note shallow, irregular ulcers *(white arrows)* on posterior wall and flat ulcer *(black arrows)* on greater curvature. (From Rumerman, J., et al.: Gastric ulceration caused by heater probe coagulation. Gastrointest. Radiol. *13:*200, 1988, with permission.)

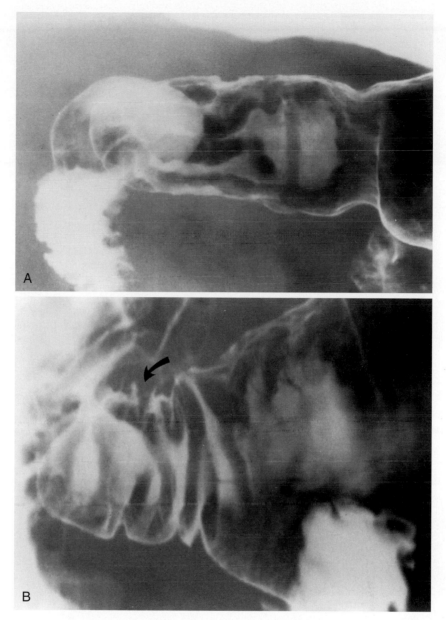

FIGURE 7–33. Antral gastritis. *A,* Thickened, scalloped longitudinal folds are present in gastric antrum. *B,* This patient has thickened transverse folds in antrum with nodularity and crenulation of adjacent lesser curvature *(arrow).*

Antral Gastritis

Antral gastritis is a form of gastritis that is confined to the gastric antrum. A number of factors have been implicated in the development of this condition, including alcohol, tobacco, coffee, and, more recently, *H. pylori.*[5,35] Some patients with antral gastritis have one or more thickened, scalloped folds oriented longitudinally in the antrum (Fig. 7–33A; see Fig. 7–14), whereas others have thickened transverse antral folds, often associated with fine nodularity and crenulation of the adjacent lesser curvature (Fig. 7–33B).[36] Still other patients have a single lobulated fold that arises on the lesser curvature of the distal antrum and extends across the pylorus into the base of the duodenal bulb (Fig. 7–34).[37] Because of its characteristic appearance and location, this hypertrophied antral-pyloric fold can almost always be differentiated from a polypoid or plaquelike antral carcinoma. If the radiographic findings are equivocal, however, endoscopy should be performed for a more definitive diagnosis.

Helicobacter pylori Gastritis

Since its original description by Warren and Marshall in 1983,[38] *H. pylori* has been recognized as a major cause of gastritis, gastric or duodenal ulcers, gastric carcinoma, and even gastric lymphoma (see Chapter 8). The gastric antrum is the most common site of infection, but the proximal stomach or even the entire stomach may be involved by this disease.[39] The prevalence of *H. pylori* gastritis increases with age; more than 50% of Americans over 60 years of age are infected by this organism.[40] However,

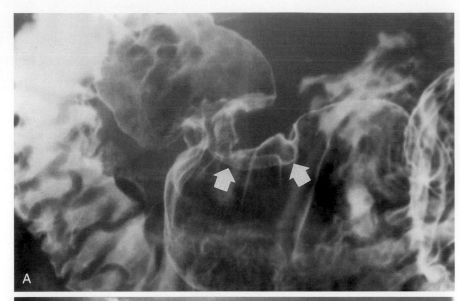

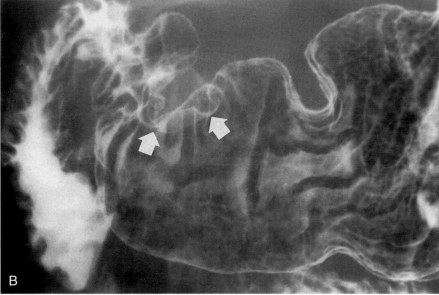

FIGURE 7–34. Two examples (*A* and *B*) of a hypertrophied antral-pyloric fold *(arrows)* in patients with antral gastritis. In both cases, the lesion is seen as a single lobulated fold on lesser curvature of distal antrum that extends across pylorus into base of duodenal bulb. These findings are characteristic of a hypertrophied fold.

only a small percentage of infected individuals have dyspepsia or epigastric pain; most are asymptomatic. Although *H. pylori* can be eradicated from the stomach by treatment with omeprazole and antibiotics, routine treatment of asymptomatic patients does not appear to be warranted because of the cost and side effects of drug therapy.

H. pylori gastritis may be manifested on double contrast studies by thickened folds, predominantly in the gastric antrum and body (Fig. 7–35).[5,35] Although fold thickening is a nonspecific radiographic finding, *H. pylori* should be a leading consideration in the differential diagnosis of thickened gastric folds in patients with dyspepsia or epigastric pain. Other patients with this infection may have enlarged areae gastricae in the stomach (see Fig. 7–4); the combination of thickened folds and enlarged areae gastricae therefore should be highly suggestive of *H. pylori* gastritis. Still other patients may have a polypoid form of gastritis with markedly thickened, lobulated folds in the stomach (Fig. 7–36; see Fig. 7–16), mimicking the appearance of hypertrophic gastritis, lym-

phoma, or even Ménétrier's disease.[5,35] Occasionally, these polypoid folds may have a focal distribution, so that the radiographic findings erroneously may suggest an infiltrating neoplasm (Fig. 7–37).[5] In such cases, endoscopy is required to rule out malignant tumor. In our experience, however, most patients with enlarged, polypoid folds on double contrast studies are found to have *H. pylori* gastritis.

Hypertrophic Gastritis

In the past, hypertrophic gastritis was thought to be a relatively common condition characterized pathologically by glandular hyperplasia with increased parietal cell mass and increased acid secretion in the stomach.[41] This condition is manifested on double contrast studies by moderately to markedly thickened gastric folds, predominantly in the gastric body and fundus (see Fig. 7–17A). In retrospect, however, many patients with a presumed diagnosis of hypertrophic gastritis may have had unrecognized infection by *H. pylori*.

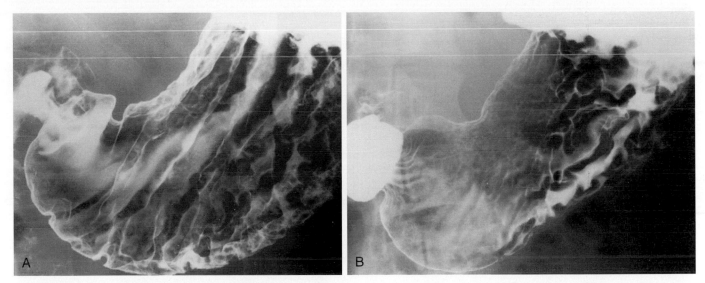

FIGURE 7–35. *H. pylori* gastritis. *A,* Thickened folds are seen in gastric antrum and body. *B,* In another patient, thickened folds are present only in gastric body. (*B,* From Levine, M.S., and Rubesin, S.E.: The *Helicobacter pylori* revolution: Radiologic perspective. Radiology *195:* 593, 1995, with permission.)

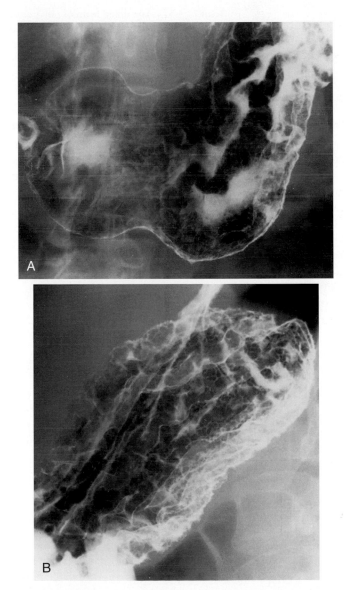

FIGURE 7–36. Polypoid *H. pylori* gastritis. Markedly thickened, lobulated folds are seen in gastric body *(A)* and fundus *(B)* in this patient with severe gastritis due to *H. pylori.* (From Sohn, J., Levine, M.S., Furth, E.E., et al.: *Helicobacter pylori* gastritis: Radiographic findings. Radiology *195:*763, 1995, with permission.)

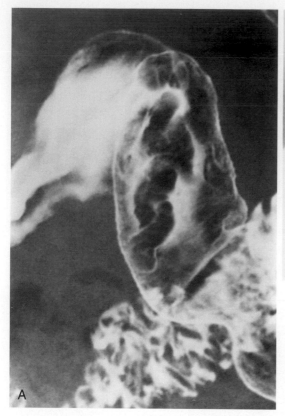

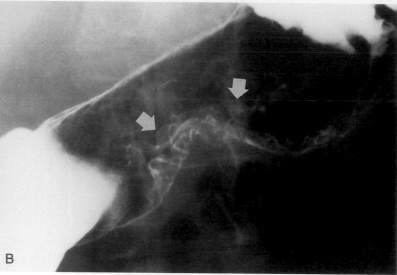

FIGURE 7–37. **Localized form of polypoid *H. pylori* gastritis mimicking tumor.** *A,* Focally thickened, polypoid folds are present in antrum. Lymphoma could produce similar findings. *B,* Another patient has focally thickened, polypoid folds *(arrows)* on greater curvature of gastric body that could be mistaken for a polypoid carcinoma. (*B,* From Sohn, J., Levine, M.S., Furth, E.E., et al.: *Helicobacter pylori* gastritis: Radiographic findings. Radiology *195:*763, 1995, with permission.)

Atrophic Gastritis

Pernicious anemia is a megaloblastic anemia associated with vitamin B_{12} malabsorption due to decreased synthesis of intrinsic factor. More than 90% of patients with pernicious anemia have atrophic gastritis. These patients are at increased risk for the development of gastric carcinoma,[42] but the risk of cancer probably is not high enough to warrant routine screening. Nevertheless, early diagnosis of pernicious anemia is important, so that vitamin B_{12} replacement therapy can be initiated before the development of irreversible neurologic sequelae. Because the average adult has a 3 to 6 year bodily store of vitamin B_{12}, gastric involvement by pernicious anemia may antedate the hematologic and neurologic abnormalities in this condition by several years. The radiologic diagnosis of atrophic gastritis therefore might permit these patients to be treated before the development of fully blown pernicious anemia. Atrophic gastritis may be manifested on double contrast studies by decreased distensibility of the stomach (which often has a smooth, tubular configuration), decreased or absent rugal folds, and small or absent areae gastricae (see Fig. 7–7).[7] Although false-positive radiologic diagnoses of atrophic gastritis can occur, it is easy and inexpensive to obtain blood tests for vitamin B_{12} to determine whether vitamin B_{12} replacement therapy is required.

GASTRIC ULCERS

The radiologic diagnosis of gastric ulcers is important not only because of the frequent occurrence of ulcer symptoms or complications but also because a small percentage of these lesions are found to be malignant. The double contrast examination permits not only detection of small ulcers but also assessment of the en face appearance of the surrounding gastric mucosa for more accurate differentiation between benign and malignant ulcers. As a result, gastric ulcers that have an unequivocally benign appearance on double contrast studies can be followed radiographically until healing without the need for endoscopic intervention.

Technical Points
Mucosal Coating

In the search for gastric ulcers, adequate mucosal coating is critical. In the absence of adequate coating, small or even large ulcers can easily be overlooked (Fig. 7–38). Mucosal coating is adequate when a uniform white line is visible along the contour of the stomach. The normal areae gastricae should also be visualized in most patients.

Distention

Gastric distention is important because overlying mucosal folds may obscure small ulcers, and small collections of barium trapped between folds may simulate ulcers. The stomach therefore must be distended sufficiently to efface the normal mucosal folds. This technique improves our ability to detect ulcers and also accentuates abnormal folds or areas of decreased distensibility in relation to ulcers (Fig. 7–39).

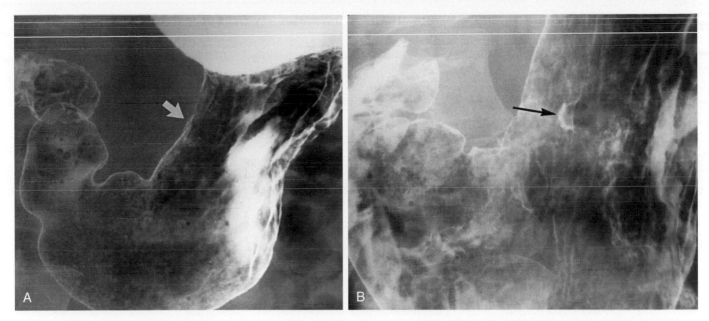

FIGURE 7–38. Danger of poor coating. *A,* Supine film shows no definite abnormality in stomach. However, note area of incomplete coating *(arrow)* near lesser curvature. *B,* With improved coating, semilunar shadow of ulcer crater *(arrow)* is clearly seen.

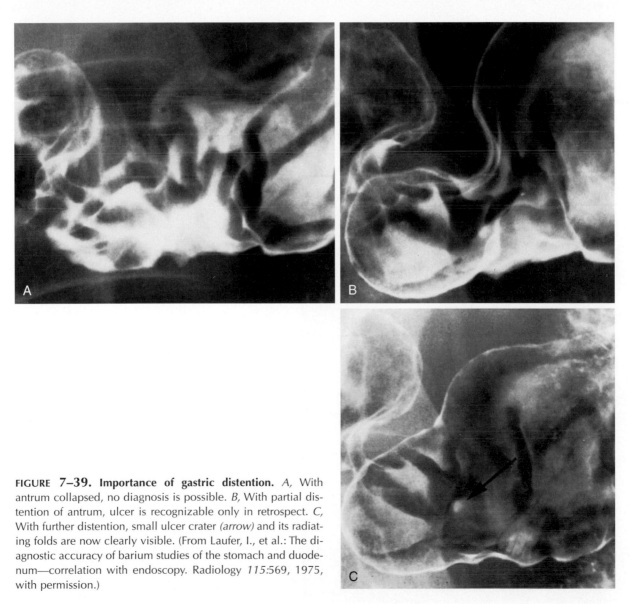

FIGURE 7–39. Importance of gastric distention. *A,* With antrum collapsed, no diagnosis is possible. *B,* With partial distention of antrum, ulcer is recognizable only in retrospect. *C,* With further distention, small ulcer crater *(arrow)* and its radiating folds are now clearly visible. (From Laufer, I., et al.: The diagnostic accuracy of barium studies of the stomach and duodenum—correlation with endoscopy. Radiology *115:*569, 1975, with permission.)

171

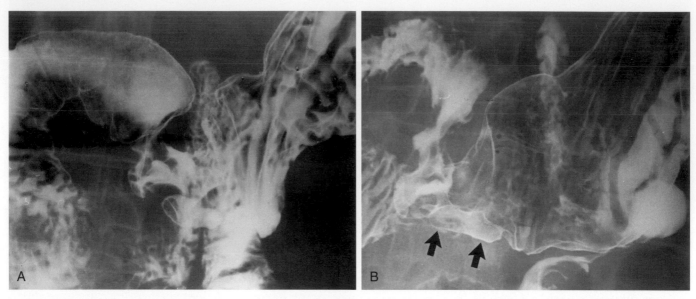

FIGURE 7–40. Importance of projection. *A,* Small bowel loops overlap greater curvature of antrum in left posterior oblique projection, obscuring this region. *B,* Overlapping loops are thrown clear of greater curvature in supine projection, and large greater curvature ulcer *(arrows)* is now seen.

Positioning

An adequate number of views must be obtained to show each area of the stomach clearly. It is particularly important to obtain multiple projections because a peristaltic wave may conceal a small ulcer, and overlapping loops of small bowel may obscure surface detail on a single radiograph (Fig. 7–40). In addition, the duodenal bulb may overlap the distal antrum and pyloric channel, so that small degrees of rotation may demonstrate lesions that are hidden in other projections. Ulcers high on the lesser curvature of the stomach may also be difficult to detect in profile because of prominent rugal folds that are normally found in this area. En face views of the proximal stomach with the patient turned to the right and barium drained out of the fundus are particularly important for evaluating this area (Fig. 7–41).

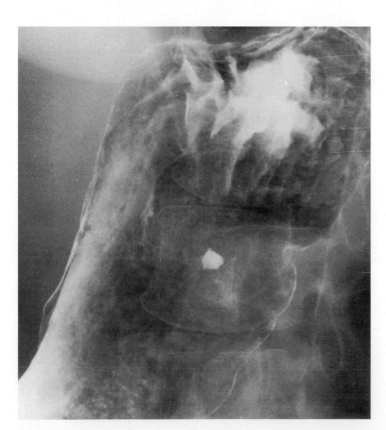

FIGURE 7–41. High lesser curvature ulcer seen en face in right posterior oblique projection.

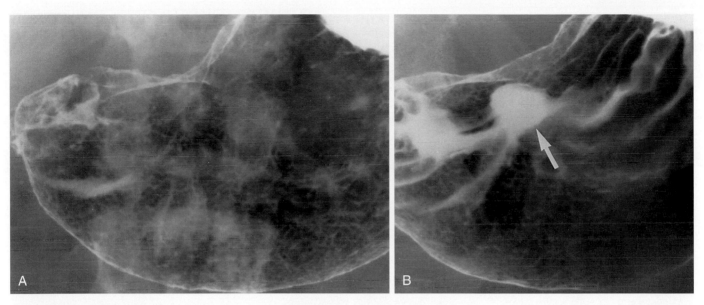

FIGURE 7–42. Importance of flow technique. *A,* Supine film shows no evidence of ulcer, even in retrospect. *B,* With flow technique, ulcer *(arrow)* is now seen on posterior wall of antrum. Note folds radiating to edge of crater.

Flow Technique

Flow technique can be used to better delineate ulcers on the posterior wall or lesser curvature (Fig. 7–42).[28] Slow rotation of the patient from side to side allows manipulation of the barium pool across the dependent surface of the stomach. This technique is particularly helpful for demonstrating shallow ulcers on the posterior wall and ulcers high on the lesser curvature near the gastric cardia.[28]

Compression Study

Because of the effects of gravity, ulcers on the nondependent or anterior wall of the stomach do not fill with barium on double contrast radiographs obtained in the usual supine or supine oblique projections (Fig. 7–43*A* and 7–44*A*). Prone compression views of the gastric antrum and body therefore should be obtained routinely to demonstrate ulcers on the anterior wall (Fig. 7–43*B* and 7–44*B*).

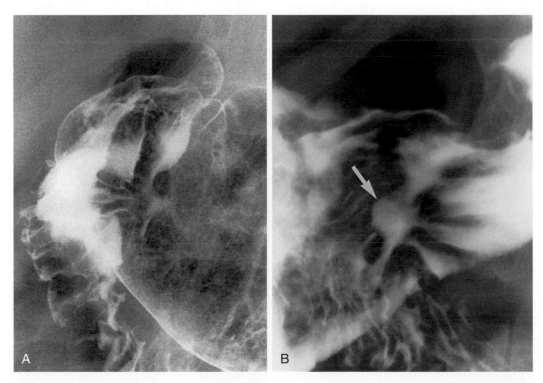

FIGURE 7–43. Importance of prone compression for anterior wall ulcers. *A,* Supine film shows abnormal folds in antrum without definite ulcer. *B,* Prone compression view results in filling of anterior wall ulcer *(arrow).* Note folds radiating to ulcer crater.

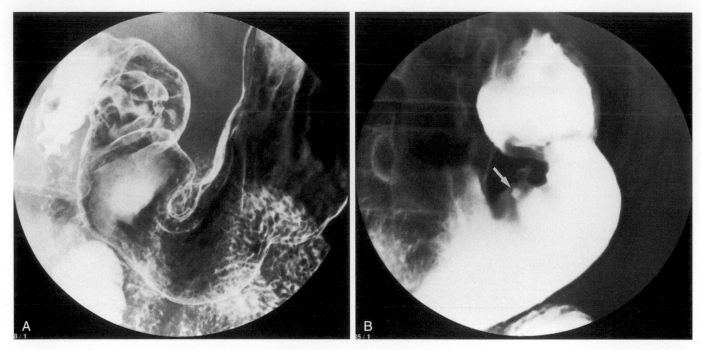

FIGURE 7–44. **Importance of prone compression for anterior wall ulcers.** *A,* Supine oblique film shows no definite abnormality in antrum. *B,* Prone compression view demonstrates filling of small anterior wall ulcer *(arrow)* that cannot be seen, even in retrospect, on double contrast image in *A.*

Recognition of Gastric Ulcers

The presence of a gastric ulcer may be suggested on conventional single contrast barium studies by secondary signs such as radiating folds, edema, or spasm. However, a definitive diagnosis of a gastric ulcer requires demonstration of a barium collection representing the ulcer crater. Ideally, the ulcer should be visualized both en face and in profile.

The appearance of a gastric ulcer on double contrast studies depends on whether it is located on the dependent or nondependent wall of the stomach. An ulcer on the dependent or posterior wall may fill with barium, producing the conventional appearance of an ulcer crater (Fig. 7–45). However, shallow ulcers on the dependent wall may be coated by only a thin layer of barium, producing a ring shadow (Fig. 7–46A). In such cases the use

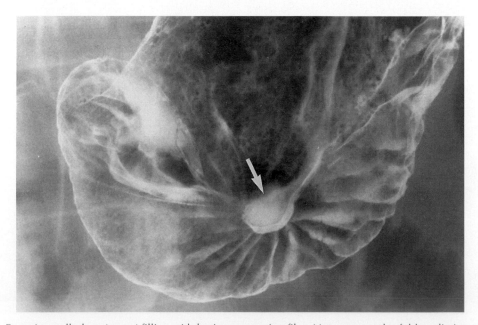

FIGURE 7–45. Posterior wall ulcer *(arrow)* filling with barium on supine film. Note spectacular folds radiating to edge of crater.

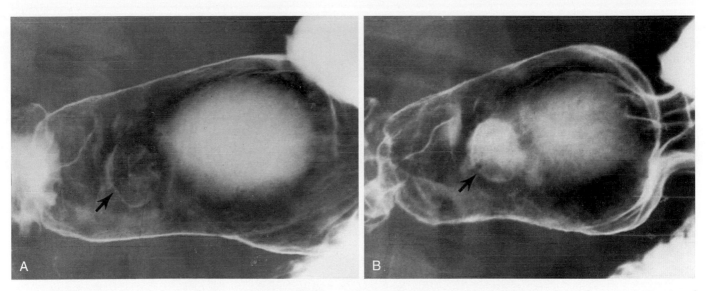

FIGURE 7–46. Ring shadow due to shallow posterior wall ulcer. *A,* Supine film shows ring shadow *(arrow)* due to barium coating rim of unfilled ulcer crater on posterior wall of antrum. *B,* Use of flow technique to manipulate barium pool over surface of ulcer shows filling of crater *(arrow).*

of flow technique to manipulate the barium pool over the surface of the ulcer should result in filling of the crater (Fig. 7–46B).[28]

An ulcer on the nondependent or anterior wall of the stomach may also appear as a ring shadow because of barium's coating the rim of the unfilled ulcer crater tangential to the central beam of the radiograph (Fig. 7–47A).[43] The ulcer may be manifested by a partial or incomplete ring shadow if one wall is sloping and the other is vertical in relation to the x-ray beam (Fig. 7–48A). In such patients, the ulcer may be demonstrated by visualizing the crater in profile or by turning the patient 180 degrees to

the prone position and obtaining prone compression views, so that the ulcer is located on the dependent wall and fills with barium (Figs. 7–47B and 7–48B). Occasionally, when the base of a nondependent ulcer is broader than the neck, a double ring shadow may be seen (Fig. 7–49).

A ring shadow therefore must be recognized as an important sign of an ulcer. This ring shadow may represent (1) a shallow, dependent wall ulcer coated with barium (see Fig. 7–46), (2) a nondependent wall ulcer coated with barium (see Figs. 7–47 through 7–49), or (3) a dependent wall ulcer containing a filling defect such as a

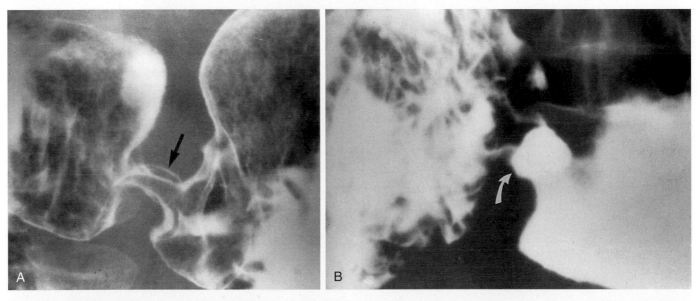

FIGURE 7–47. Ring shadow due to anterior wall ulcer. *A,* Supine film shows ring shadow *(arrow)* in pyloric channel. *B,* Prone film shows anterior wall ulcer *(arrow)* filling with barium.

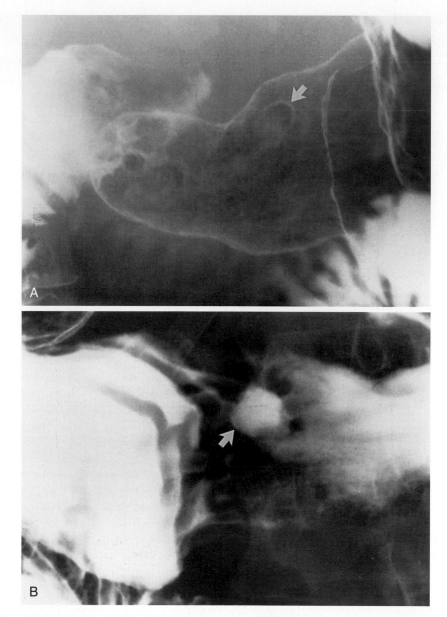

FIGURE 7–48. Partial ring shadow due to anterior wall ulcer. *A,* Supine film shows partial ring shadow *(arrow)* in antrum. *B,* Prone compression film shows anterior wall ulcer *(arrow)* filling with barium.

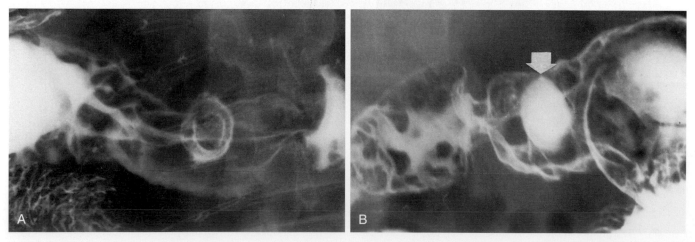

FIGURE 7–49. *A,* Double ring shadow due to empty ulcer crater on posterior wall with patient in prone position. This appearance occurs because base of nondependent ulcer is wider than neck. *B,* Posterior wall ulcer *(arrow)* fills with barium in supine position.

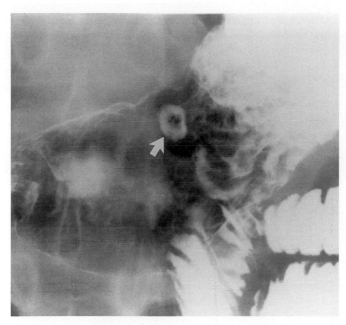

FIGURE 7–50. Ring shadow *(arrow)* due to blood clot at base of posterior wall ulcer in body of stomach.

blood clot at its base (Fig. 7–50). Use of flow technique and prone compression views to supplement the routine double contrast study should allow differentiation of these lesions in most patients.

An ulcer crater may have several other appearances on double contrast studies. When an ulcer is seen obliquely but not quite in profile, it may be manifested by only a crescentic or semilunar line (Fig. 7–51A). When the patient is rotated under fluoroscopic control, the le-

sion can usually be demonstrated to represent a projecting ulcer crater (Fig. 7–51B). In elderly or debilitated patients who are unable to turn 360 degrees, an uncoated ulcer crater may be manifested by a collection of gas outside the contour of the stomach before entry of barium (Fig. 7–52).

Radiologists must also be aware of the various artifacts of the double contrast examination that may simulate gastric ulcers (see Chapter 2).[15] These artifacts include the stalactite phenomenon (see Fig. 7–23); the see-through effect, in which an overlying colonic or small bowel diverticulum can mimic the appearance of a gastric ulcer (Fig. 7–53); and patchy coating due to mucus in the stomach, which can simulate a shallow, irregular ulcer. Normal anatomic structures can also mimic the appearance of ulcers. Radiating folds are usually seen at the gastric cardia (the cardiac rosette) (see Fig. 7–9).[11,12] If the cardia is slightly open, it may collect a drop of barium, erroneously suggesting an ulcer. Similarly, the normal pylorus may be seen en face, particularly in the right posterior oblique projection. The pyloric channel may appear as a ring shadow with radiating folds, or a drop of barium may be trapped in the pyloric channel, resembling a shallow ulcer (Fig. 7–54). However, familiarity with the normal double contrast appearance of the cardia and pylorus should prevent confusion in these areas.

Features of Gastric Ulcers
Shape

Radiologists are accustomed to looking for a circular collection of barium as a sign of a gastric ulcer. With double contrast techniques, however, linear ulcers can be demonstrated (Fig. 7–55).[44–46] Linear ulcers often occur

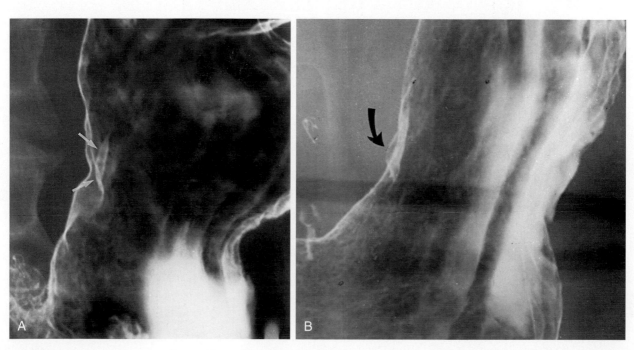

FIGURE 7–51. *A,* Ulcer crater, not quite seen in profile, is manifested by crescentic line *(arrows). B,* With slight rotation of patient, projecting ulcer *(arrow)* is clearly seen.

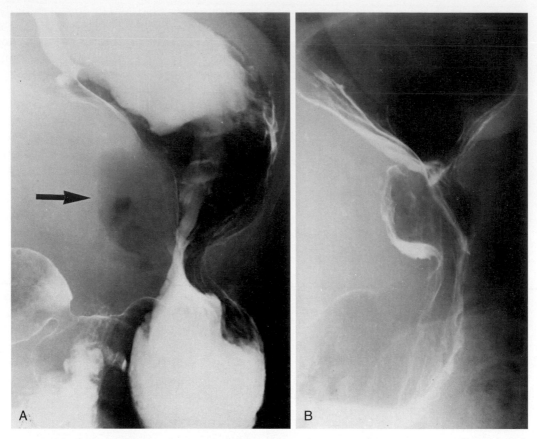

FIGURE 7–52. Uncoated ulcer filling with gas. *A,* Early film from double contrast study shows large gas collection *(arrow)* adjacent to lesser curvature. *B,* With additional turning of patient, barium-coated ulcer crater is seen on lesser curvature.

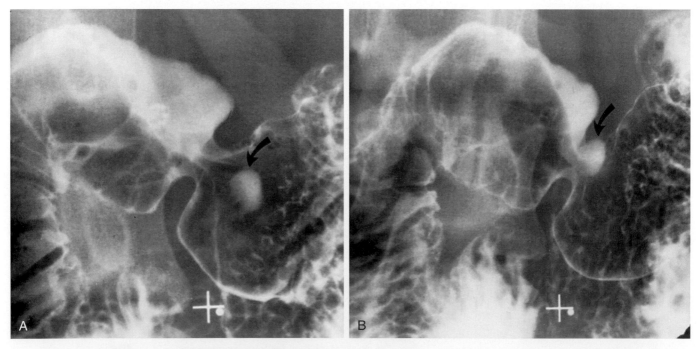

FIGURE 7–53. Duodenal diverticulum *(arrows)* simulating antral ulcer.

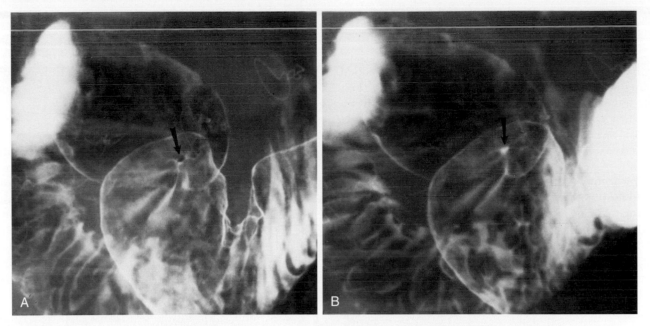

FIGURE 7–54. Normal pyloric channel *(arrows)* simulating tiny ulcer.

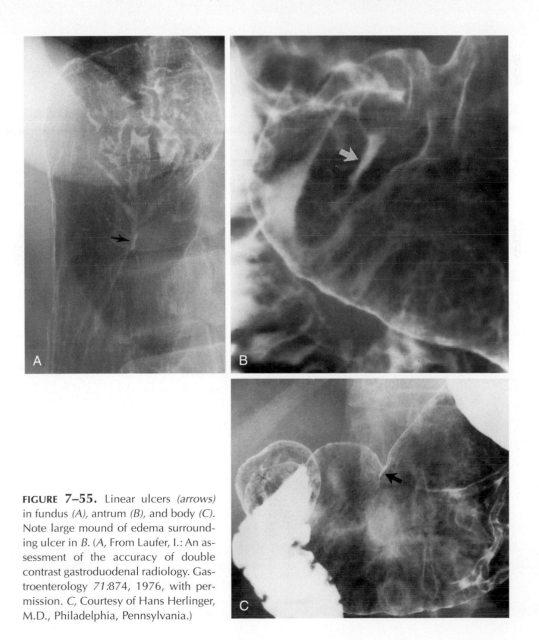

FIGURE 7–55. Linear ulcers *(arrows)* in fundus *(A)*, antrum *(B)*, and body *(C)*. Note large mound of edema surrounding ulcer in *B*. (*A*, From Laufer, I.: An assessment of the accuracy of double contrast gastroduodenal radiology. Gastroenterology *71*:874, 1976, with permission. *C*, Courtesy of Hans Herlinger, M.D., Philadelphia, Pennsylvania.)

during the healing phase of larger ulcers.[46] Ulcer craters may have other unusual forms, appearing as rod-shaped, rectangular, serpiginous, or flame-shaped lesions (Figs. 7–56 and 7–57). Radiologists therefore should be aware that ulcer craters may have a variety of shapes and configurations.

Size

Gastric ulcers may be of any size, and it is now accepted that the size of the ulcer has no relationship to the presence of carcinoma. However, a major advantage of the double contrast technique is its ability to distend the stomach and efface the normal mucosal folds to demonstrate small ulcers (Figs. 7–58 through 7–60). As a result, most gastric ulcers diagnosed on double contrast studies are less than 1 cm in size.[46] The increasing prevalence of small ulcers may also be related to the aggressive medical treatment these patients often receive before undergoing radiologic investigations.

Location

Most gastric ulcers are located on the lesser curvature or posterior wall of the antrum or body of the stomach.[46–49] Ulcers on the lesser curvature typically project beyond the adjacent gastric contour and may be associated with smooth, symmetric mucosal folds that radiate to the edge of the crater (Fig. 7–61). Fewer than 15% of gastric ulcers are located on the anterior wall or greater curvature.[46,47,49] In younger patients, ulcers tend to occur in the distal part of the stomach (Fig. 7–62), whereas in

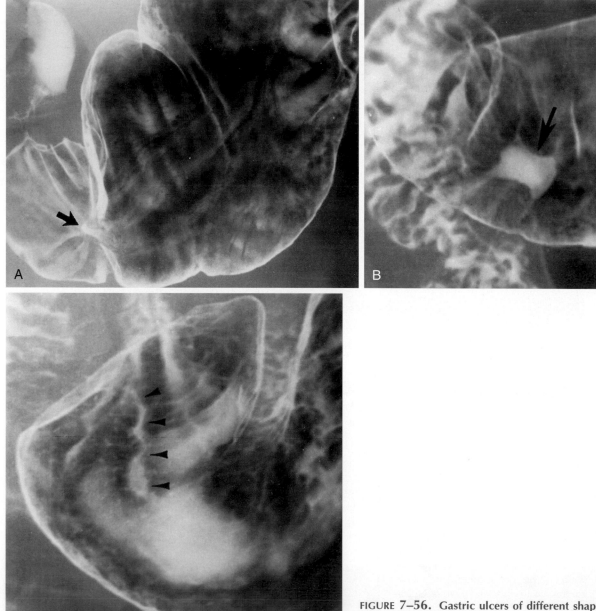

FIGURE 7–56. Gastric ulcers of different shapes. *A,* Rod-shaped ulcer *(arrow). B,* Rectangular ulcer *(arrow). C,* Serpiginous ulcer *(arrowheads).*

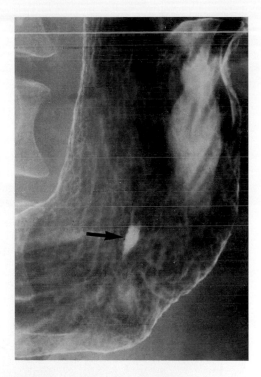

FIGURE 7–57. Flame-shaped ulcer *(arrow)* on posterior gastric wall. Note slight retraction of greater curvature due to scarring. Also note enlarged areae gastricae due to inflammation of mucosa adjacent to ulcer. (From Laufer, I.: An assessment of the accuracy of double contrast gastroduodenal radiology. Gastroenterology *71*:874, 1976, with permission.)

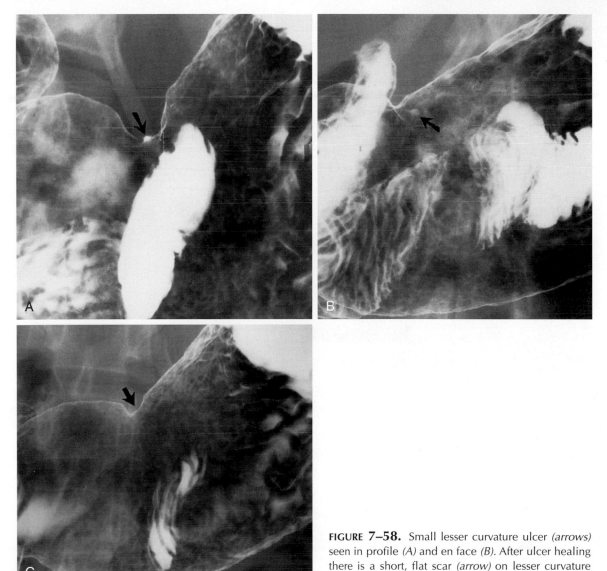

FIGURE 7–58. Small lesser curvature ulcer *(arrows)* seen in profile *(A)* and en face *(B)*. After ulcer healing there is a short, flat scar *(arrow)* on lesser curvature *(C)*.

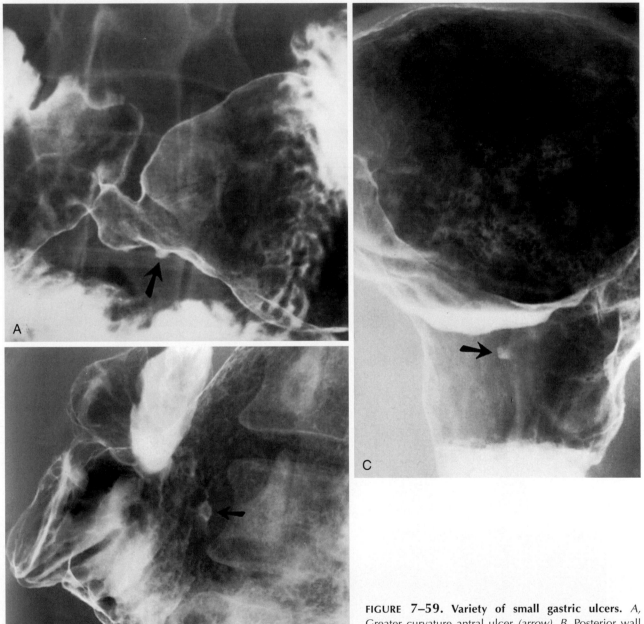

FIGURE 7–59. Variety of small gastric ulcers. *A,* Greater curvature antral ulcer *(arrow). B,* Posterior wall antral ulcer *(arrow). C,* Posterior wall ulcer *(arrow)* high in body of stomach.

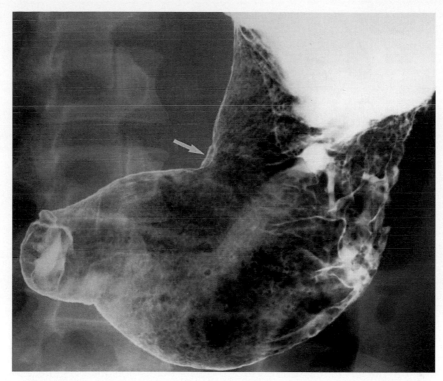

FIGURE 7–60. Broad, shallow ulcer *(arrow)* on lesser curvature at angle of stomach.

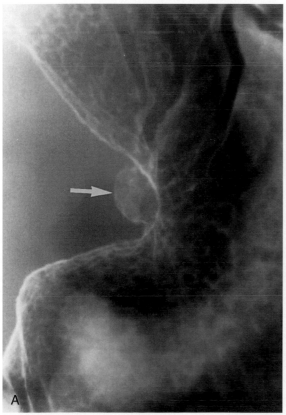

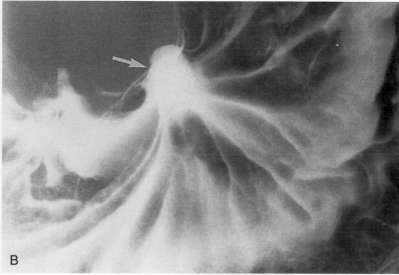

FIGURE 7–61. Lesser curvature ulcers. *A,* Smooth, round ulcer *(arrow)* projecting beyond lesser curvature. Note radiating folds and enlarged areae gastricae in adjacent mucosa due to associated inflammation and edema. (From Levine, M.S., et al.: Benign gastric ulcers: Diagnosis and follow-up with double contrast radiography. Radiology *164:*9, 1987, with permission.) *B,* Ulcer *(arrow)* straddling lesser curvature. Note smooth, symmetric folds radiating to edge of crater. Both these cases demonstrate classic features of benign gastric ulcers.

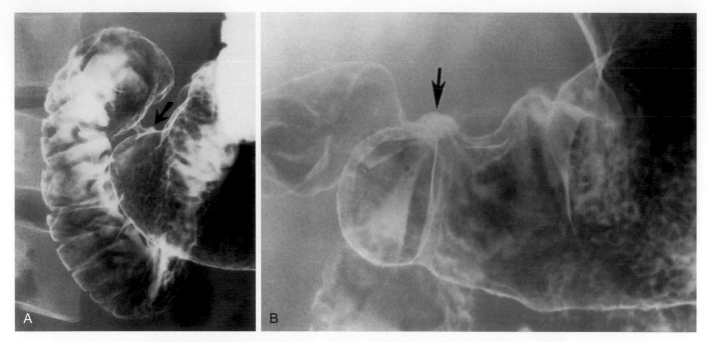

FIGURE 7–62. Antral ulcers *(arrows)* in two young patients.

older patients, they tend to be located more proximally in the stomach, particularly on the lesser curvature (Fig. 7–63).[50,51] The latter ulcers have been described as "geriatric ulcers."[50] Thus, the distribution of gastric ulcers is influenced by the age of the patients being studied.

Benign greater curvature ulcers are almost always located in the distal half of the stomach (Figs. 7–64 through 7–67).[46,52,53] Almost all of these ulcers are caused by in-

gestion of aspirin or other NSAIDs.[46,53] The dissolving aspirin tablets presumably collect by gravity on the greater curvature, causing localized ulceration. This phenomenon may also explain why aspirin-induced erosions are frequently located near the greater curvature (see Fig. 7–28 and the earlier discussion, Erosive Gastritis).[31]

Unlike benign ulcers on the lesser curvature, greater curvature ulcers often appear to have an intraluminal lo-

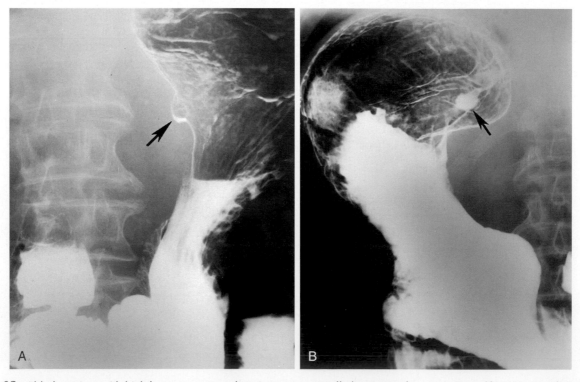

FIGURE 7–63. Elderly patient with high lesser curvature ulcer *(arrows),* a so-called geriatric ulcer, seen in profile *(A)* in upright position and en face *(B)* in prone position.

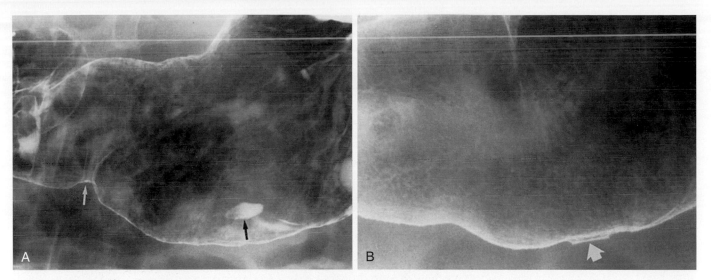

FIGURE 7–64. Greater curvature ulcers due to aspirin and indomethacin. *A,* Small ulcer *(black arrow)* in body of stomach adjacent to greater curvature. Note area of scarring more distally *(white arrow)* due to healed greater curvature ulcer in antrum. *B,* Extremely shallow ulcer *(arrow)* on greater curvature due to indomethacin. Note absence of radiating folds or of other signs of inflammatory disease. This ulcer could easily be missed without optimal radiographic technique.

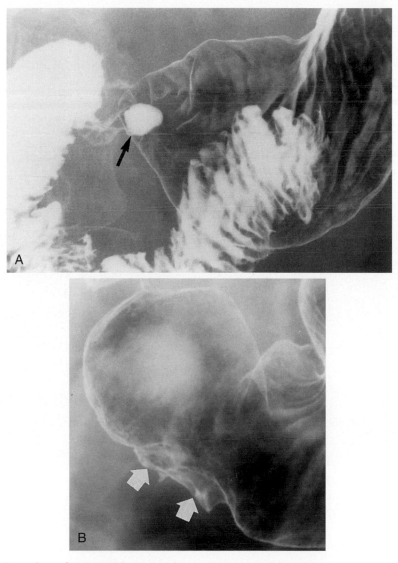

FIGURE 7–65. Greater curvature ulcers due to aspirin. *A,* An ulcer *(arrow)* is seen adjacent to greater curvature of distal antrum with folds radiating toward ulcer crater. *B,* This patient has a very flat ulcer *(arrows)* on greater curvature.

FIGURE 7–66. **Greater curvature ulcer due to aspirin.** *A,* Double contrast view of ulcer *(arrows)* on greater curvature of distal antrum. Note how ulcer crater appears to lie within contour of stomach. *B,* The ulcer crater *(arrows)* has filled with barium.

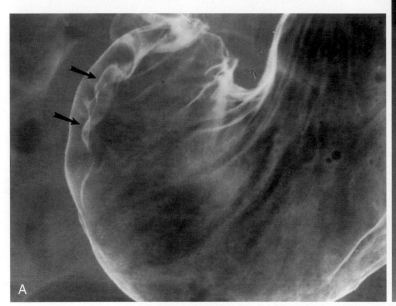

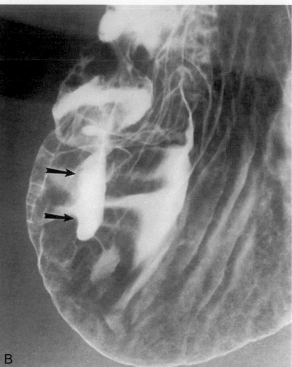

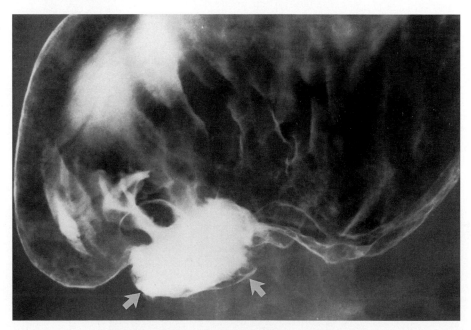

FIGURE 7–67. Giant greater curvature ulcer *(arrows)* due to aspirin. Note apparent intraluminal location of ulcer with thickened, irregular folds and considerable mass effect due to an adjacent mound of edema. These morphologic features should arouse suspicion of a malignant ulcer. However, endoscopic biopsy specimens revealed no evidence of tumor, and after medical therapy, repeat barium study showed complete healing of ulcer.

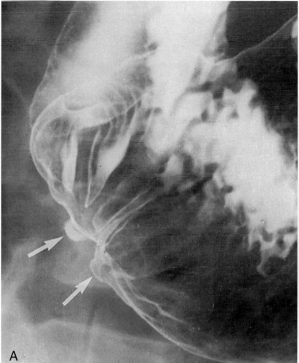

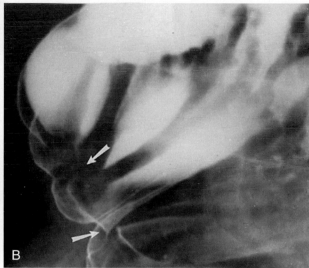

FIGURE 7–68. Multiple ulcer scars on greater curvature. *A,* Several outpouchings *(arrows)* are seen on greater curvature with radiating folds. These outpouchings could be mistaken for active ulcers. *B,* In steep oblique projection, however, it is apparent that these outpouchings are two separate ulcer scars *(arrows)* associated with radiating folds.

cation and may be associated with considerable mass effect and thickened, irregular folds as a result of marked edema and inflammation surrounding the ulcer (see Figs. 7–66 and 7–67).[46,54] Because of these morphologic features, endoscopy and biopsy may be required for some greater curvature ulcers despite a history of aspirin ingestion. When these greater curvature ulcers heal, they also tend to result in considerable deformity of the adjacent gastric wall, producing one or more outpouchings that can be mistaken for active ulcers (Fig. 7–68A). Careful

evaluation of the mucosa en face, however, may reveal that this appearance has resulted from radiating folds and scarring (Fig. 7–68B).

Greater curvature ulcers also have a tendency to penetrate inferiorly into the gastrocolic ligament, eventually leading to the development of a gastrocolic fistula (Fig. 7–69).[55,56] Affected individuals may have a dramatic clinical presentation with diarrhea, feculent vomiting, and foul-smelling eructations. In today's pill-oriented society, these NSAID-induced greater curvature ulcers have be-

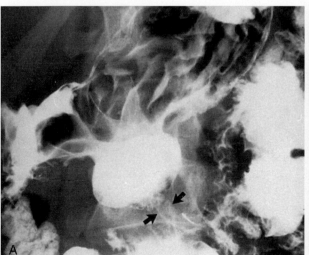

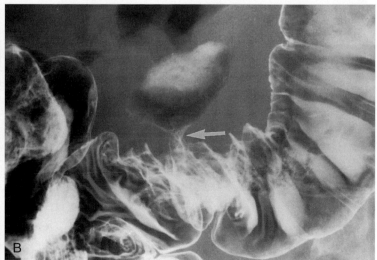

FIGURE 7–69. Gastrocolic fistula due to aspirin-induced greater curvature ulcer. *A,* Double contrast upper gastrointestinal study shows giant ulcer on greater curvature of stomach, with barium entering fistula *(arrows)* that communicates with transverse colon. *B,* Double contrast barium enema better delineates fistula *(arrow)* between transverse colon and greater curvature ulcer. Note inflammatory changes in transverse colon, with spiculated, tethered mucosal folds adjacent to fistula. (From Laufer, I., et al.: Gastrocolic fistula as a complication of benign gastric ulcer. Radiology *119:7,* 1976, with permission.)

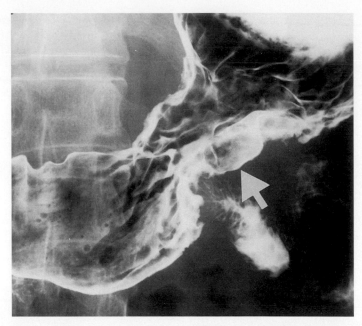

FIGURE 7–70. Malignant ulcer *(arrow)* on greater curvature of upper body of stomach. Note intraluminal location of ulcer with considerable mass effect and infiltration of adjacent gastric wall. Greater curvature ulcers in proximal half of stomach are almost always found to be malignant.

come a more common cause of gastrocolic fistulas than carcinoma of the stomach or transverse colon.

Benign gastric ulcers are much less common in the fundus than in the antrum or body of the stomach and are rarely found on the proximal half of the greater curvature.[46,47,49] Thus, any ulcer in this location should be considered malignant until proved otherwise (Fig. 7–70). Except for these ulcers high on the greater curvature, the location of the ulcer has no relationship to the presence of carcinoma.

Gastric ulcers occasionally may be found in hiatal hernias.[57] They tend to occur on the lesser curvature aspect of the hernia, where the hernial sac is compressed by the esophageal hiatus of the diaphragm.[57] Because the hernia is inaccessible to palpation, double contrast technique is particularly helpful for demonstrating these lesions (Fig. 7–71).

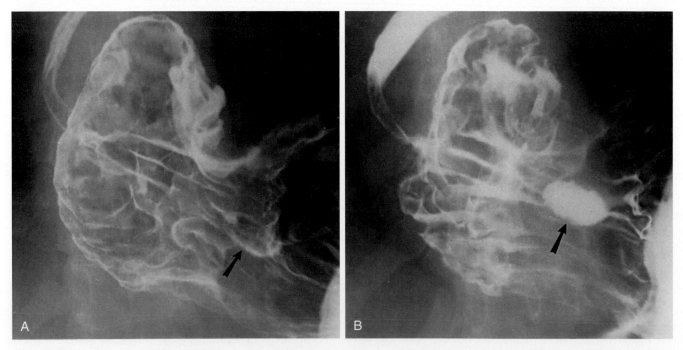

FIGURE 7–71. Gastric ulcer in hiatal hernia. *A,* Ring shadow *(arrow)* due to unfilled ulcer in hiatal hernia. *B,* Moments later, ulcer crater *(arrow)* has filled with barium.

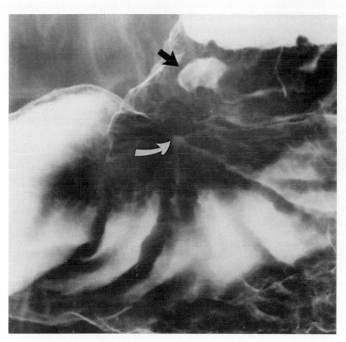

FIGURE 7–72. Multiple gastric ulcers. Note small satellite ulcer *(white arrow)* adjacent to large ulcer *(black arrow)* in antrum.

Multiplicity

The frequency of multiple ulcers on conventional single contrast barium studies has ranged from 2% to 8%.[58,59] However, data based on autopsy, surgical, or endoscopic findings indicate a much higher incidence of multiple ulcers, ranging from 20% to 30%.[60–62] Thus, it seems clear that the conventional barium study has led to underestimation of the frequency of multiple gastric ulcers. Furthermore, it has been shown that multiplicity of ulcers is not necessarily a sign of benignity. In one series

of 29 patients with multiple ulcers, 20% had malignant lesions.[63] Each ulcer must therefore be evaluated separately for signs of malignancy. With double contrast technique, multiple ulcers have been detected in nearly 25% of patients with ulcers or ulcer scars.[64] This finding more closely approximates the findings at autopsy, surgery, or endoscopy, indicating that double contrast studies are more sensitive than single contrast studies in detecting gastric ulcers.

When multiple gastric ulcers are present, they tend to be found in the antrum or body (Figs. 7–72 and 7–73). There is often a marked discrepancy between the size of the ulcers, so that one may see a small satellite ulcer adjacent to a large ulcer (Fig. 7–72). Multiple gastric ulcers or ulcer scars occur more frequently in patients who are taking aspirin or other NSAIDs (see Figs. 7–64A and 7–68). In one study, more than 80% of patients with multiple ulcers had a history of aspirin ingestion.[62]

Healing of Gastric Ulcers

The radiologic assessment of ulcer healing is important not only for evaluating the success or failure of medical therapy but also for confirming the presence of benign ulcer disease (see the next discussion, Benign Versus Malignant Ulcers). Ulcer healing may be manifested radiographically not only by a decrease in the size of the ulcer crater but also by a change in its shape. Previously round or oval ulcers often have a linear appearance on follow-up studies, so that linear ulcers presumably represent a stage of ulcer healing (Fig. 7–74).[46] Other ulcers may undergo splitting, so that the original crater is replaced by two separate ulcer niches at the periphery of the healing ulcer (Fig. 7–75).[46] This phenomenon probably occurs because the rate of healing and re-epithelial-

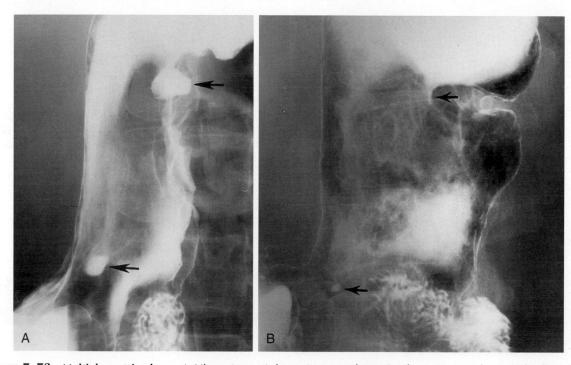

FIGURE 7–73. Multiple gastric ulcers. *A,* Ulcers *(arrows)* shown in acute phase. *B,* Ulcers *(arrows)* shown in healing phase.

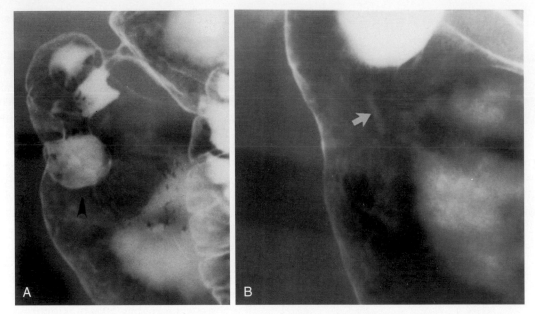

FIGURE 7–74. Development of linear ulcer during healing. *A,* Large, round ulcer *(arrowhead)* on posterior wall of antrum. *B,* Follow-up study 8 weeks later shows linear configuration of ulcer *(arrow)* with healing. (From Levine, M.S., et al.: Benign gastric ulcers: Diagnosis and follow-up with double-contrast radiography. Radiology *164:*9, 1987, with permission.)

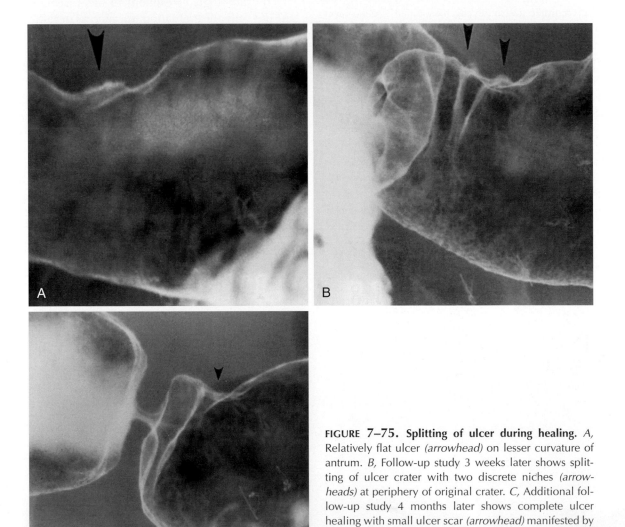

FIGURE 7–75. Splitting of ulcer during healing. *A,* Relatively flat ulcer *(arrowhead)* on lesser curvature of antrum. *B,* Follow-up study 3 weeks later shows splitting of ulcer crater with two discrete niches *(arrowheads)* at periphery of original crater. *C,* Additional follow-up study 4 months later shows complete ulcer healing with small ulcer scar *(arrowhead)* manifested by retraction of adjacent gastric wall. (From Levine, M.S., et al.: Benign gastric ulcers: Diagnosis and follow-up with double-contrast radiography. Radiology *164:*9, 1987, with permission.)

ization is more rapid in the central portion of the ulcer than in the periphery.

Benign gastric ulcers usually respond dramatically to conservative medical treatment with histamine-receptor antagonists (H_2 blockers) or proton pump inhibitors. The average interval between the initial barium study showing the ulcer and the follow-up study showing complete healing is approximately 8 weeks.[46] Follow-up barium studies to document ulcer healing therefore should be performed after 6 to 8 weeks of medical treatment because those studies performed sooner are unlikely to show complete healing.

In general, complete radiologic healing of a gastric ulcer has been considered a reliable sign that the ulcer is benign. Rarely, complete healing of malignant ulcers may occur with medical therapy.[65,66] However, nodularity of the ulcer scar or irregularity, clubbing, or amputation of radiating folds should suggest the possibility of an underlying malignancy. The surrounding gastric mucosa therefore must be evaluated carefully after ulcer healing has occurred. If suspicious findings are present, endoscopy and biopsy are still required to rule out a malignant lesion.

Ulcer healing may be associated with the development of an ulcer scar. Although ulcer scars are not often detected on single contrast barium studies, 90% of healed gastric ulcers produce a visible ulcer scar on double contrast studies.[46] Double contrast technique is particularly well suited for demonstrating ulcer scars, as gaseous distention of the stomach permits recognition of relatively subtle areas of wall flattening or deformity or of abnormal folds associated with scars. The discovery of an ulcer scar is important because it indicates that the patient has suffered from peptic ulcer disease in the past.

Ulcer scars may be manifested radiographically by a central pit or depression, radiating folds, or retraction of the adjacent gastric wall.[46,67,68] The location of the ulcer is a major determinant of the morphologic features of the scar. Healing of ulcers on the lesser curvature may lead to the development of relatively innocuous scars manifested by slight flattening or retraction of the adjacent gastric wall with or without radiating folds (Fig. 7–76; see Figs. 7–58 and 7–75).[46,67] In contrast, healing of ulcers on the greater curvature or posterior wall often leads to the development of a spectacular collection of radiating folds (Fig. 7–77; see Fig. 7–68).[46,67] Occasionally, healing of greater curvature ulcers may result in some unusual or picturesque scars (Fig. 7–78).

When radiating folds are present, they may converge to a central point or to a circular or linear pit or depression. This central depression can be mistaken radiographically for a shallow, residual ulcer crater (Fig. 7–79). In other cases, this depression may have a bald, featureless appearance, so that it is unclear whether complete ulcer healing has occurred (Fig. 7–80). However, the central depression of an ulcer scar tends to have more gradually sloping margins than an ulcer crater and should remain unchanged on sequential follow-up studies. A reepithelialized ulcer scar can also be differentiated radiographically from an active ulcer by the presence of normal areae gastricae within the central portion of the scar (Fig. 7–81).[46] The latter finding indicates complete ulcer healing, so that further radiologic or endoscopic evaluation is unnecessary.

In some patients, ulcer healing may lead to the development of severe scar formation, manifested by antral narrowing and deformity (Fig. 7–82A), or, less frequently, focal narrowing of the gastric body, producing an "hourglass" stomach (Fig. 7–82B). Although 90% of healed gastric ulcers produce a radiographically visible ulcer scar, the remaining 10% undergo healing without producing a

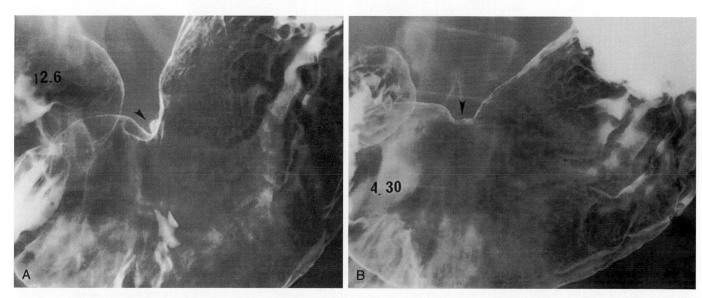

FIGURE 7–76. Healing of lesser curvature ulcer with scarring. *A,* Small, benign-appearing ulcer *(arrowhead)* on lesser curvature. *B,* Follow-up study 5 months later shows complete healing of ulcer with slight flattening and retraction of adjacent gastric wall *(arrowhead).*

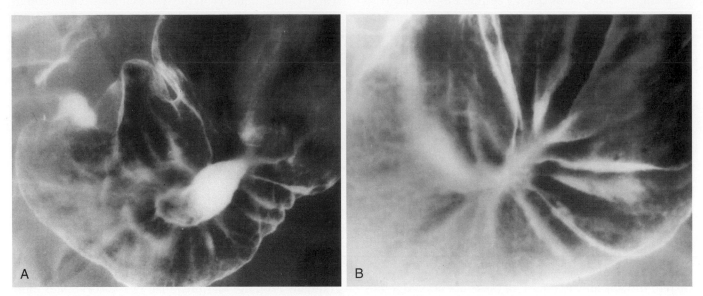

FIGURE 7–77. Healing of posterior wall ulcer with scarring. *A,* Large posterior wall ulcer with multiple folds seen radiating to edge of crater. *B,* Follow-up study 8 weeks later shows complete healing of ulcer with spectacular folds radiating to site of previous crater.

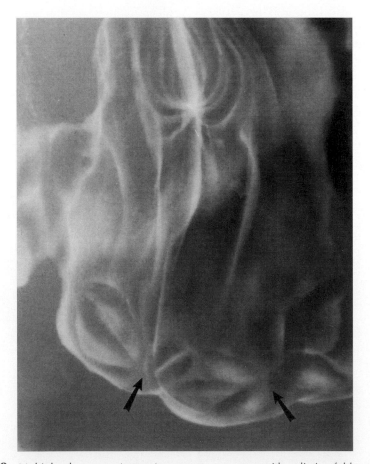

FIGURE 7–78. Multiple ulcer scars *(arrows)* on greater curvature with radiating folds and retraction.

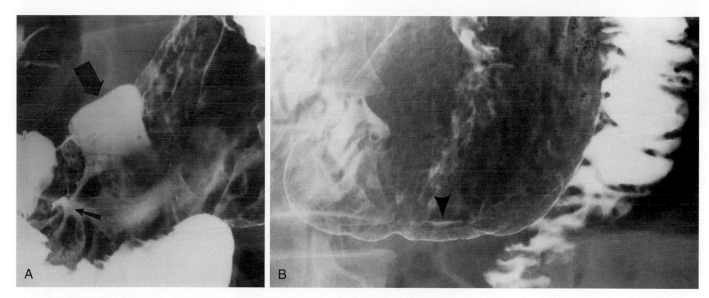

FIGURE 7–79. **Ulcer scars mimicking active ulcers.** *A,* Ulcer scar *(small arrow)* with radiating folds and central, epithelialized depression that resembles active ulcer crater. (*Large arrow* indicates site of cystogastrostomy for decompression of pancreatic pseudocyst.) *B,* Linear ulcer scar in another patient. Note linear barium collection *(arrowhead)* adjacent to greater curvature with slight retraction of gastric wall proximally and distally. Although a linear ulcer could produce identical findings, endoscopy revealed a reepithelialized ulcer scar.

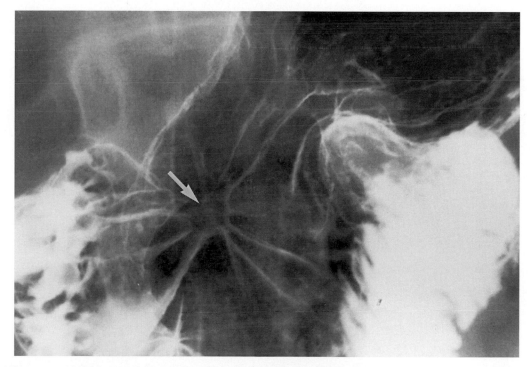

FIGURE 7–80. Ulcer scar with folds seen radiating toward a bald, featureless central area *(arrow)* that could be mistaken for a shallow, residual ulcer crater. (From Levine, M.S., et al.: Benign gastric ulcers: Diagnosis and follow-up with double-contrast radiography. Radiology *164:*9, 1987, with permission.)

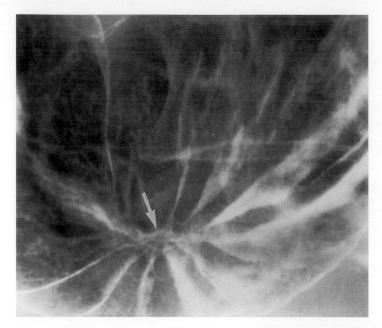

FIGURE 7–81. Reepithelialized ulcer scar with centrally radiating folds. This scar can be differentiated from an active ulcer by the presence of normal areae gastricae within central portion of scar *(arrow).* (From Levine, M.S., et al.: Benign gastric ulcers: Diagnosis and follow-up with double-contrast radiography. Radiology *164:*9, 1987, with permission.)

FIGURE 7–82. Severe gastric scarring due to ulcer disease. *A,* Marked antral narrowing and deformity *(arrow)* due to previous antral ulcer. When scarring is this severe, gastric outlet obstruction may ensue. *B,* Hourglass deformity of stomach due to scarring associated with healing ulcer *(arrowhead)* in body.

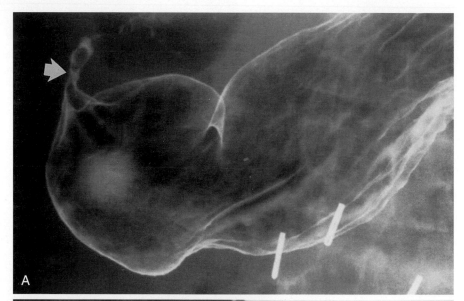

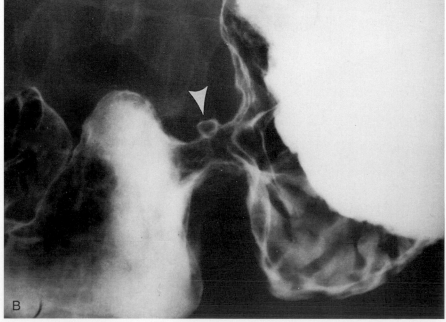

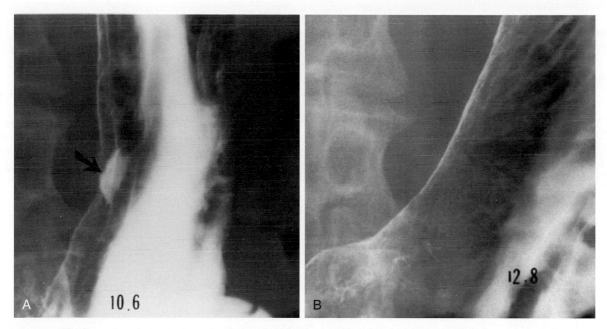

FIGURE 7–83. Healing of gastric ulcer without scarring. *A,* Relatively shallow lesser curvature ulcer *(arrow)* in body of stomach. *B,* Follow-up study 2 months later shows complete healing of ulcer without evidence of scar. (From Levine, M.S., et al.: Benign gastric ulcers: Diagnosis and follow-up with double-contrast radiography. Radiology *164:*9, 1987, with permission.)

scar (Fig. 7–83).[46] Thus, the absence of an ulcer scar in no way excludes the possibility that the patient has had ulcer disease in the past.

Benign Versus Malignant Ulcers

More than 95% of gastric ulcers diagnosed in the United States are benign.[69,70] The typical distinguishing features of a benign ulcer demonstrated by conventional single contrast barium studies include projection of the ulcer beyond the contour of the stomach, radiating folds to the edge of the ulcer crater, Hampton's line, and intact surrounding mucosa.[69,71] However, single contrast studies are thought to be unreliable in differentiating benign ulcers from ulcerated carcinomas. Previous reports indicate that 6% to 16% of gastric ulcers that appear benign on single contrast upper gastrointestinal examinations are malignant.[72–75] Although these studies were performed between 1955 and 1975, many gastroenterologists have used these data as justification for performing endoscopy and biopsy on all radiographically diagnosed gastric ulcers to rule out cancer in these patients.

With double contrast techniques, however, it is possible to obtain a much more detailed study of the mucosa surrounding the ulcer to detect signs of malignancy, such as irregular mass effect, nodularity, rigidity, or mucosal destruction. Several recent studies have shown that virtually all gastric ulcers with an unequivocally benign appearance on double contrast studies are in fact benign lesions.[46,76] In those studies, about two thirds of all benign ulcers had a benign radiographic appearance, so that unnecessary endoscopy could be avoided in most patients with gastric ulcers diagnosed on double contrast examinations. This finding has enormous implications for the evaluation of gastric ulcers in general because barium studies are safer and less expensive than endoscopy.

On double contrast studies, unequivocally benign gastric ulcers are characterized en face by a discrete ulcer crater surrounded by a smooth mound of edema or regular, symmetric mucosal folds that radiate to the edge of the crater (see Figs. 7–45, 7–74, and 7–77).[46,76,77] The areae gastricae adjacent to the ulcer may be enlarged as a result of inflammation and edema of the surrounding mucosa (see Figs. 7–57 and 7–61A). However, the areae gastricae can often be seen to extend to the edge of the ulcer crater without evidence of nodularity, mass effect, or tumor infiltration. When viewed in profile, benign gastric ulcers project outside the gastric lumen and are often associated with a smooth, symmetric ulcer mound or collar or with smooth, straight mucosal folds that radiate to the edge of the ulcer crater (see Figs. 7–61 and 7–76).

In contrast, malignant ulcers are characterized en face by an irregular ulcer crater eccentrically located in an irregular mass with distortion or obliteration of the normal areae gastricae surrounding the ulcer.[46,77] Although radiating folds may be present, they tend to be nodular and irregular and may stop well short of the ulcer crater (Fig. 7–84). In addition, the tips of the folds may be fused, clubbed, or amputated.[78] When viewed in profile, malignant ulcers do not project beyond the expected gastric contour (Fig. 7–85), and often a discrete tumor mass forms acute angles with the gastric wall rather than the obtuse, gently sloping angles expected for a benign mound of edema. Nodularity of the adjacent mucosa or thickened, lobulated folds radiating to the ulcer may also be present because of infiltration by tumor (Fig. 7–86).

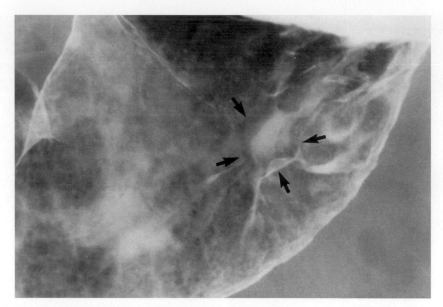

FIGURE 7–84. Malignant gastric ulcer *(arrows)* with tumor nodule in its wall. Note how radiating folds are nodular and irregular. (Courtesy of Frederick M. Kelvin, M.D., Indianapolis, Indiana. From Laufer, I: Double contrast radiology in the diagnosis of gastrointestinal cancer. *In* Glass, G.B.J. [ed.]: Progress in Gastroenterology, vol. 3., New York, Grune & Stratton, 1977, p. 643, with permission.)

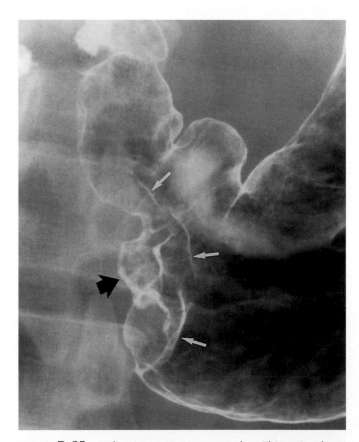

FIGURE 7–85. Malignant greater curvature ulcer. This patient has a mass etched in white *(white arrows)* on greater curvature of antrum, with a large central ulcer *(black arrow).* Note how ulcer projects within expected contour of gastric wall. These are features of a malignant ulcer. (From Levine, M.S.: Erosive gastritis and gastric ulcers. Radiol. Clin. North Am. *32*:1203, 1994, with permission.)

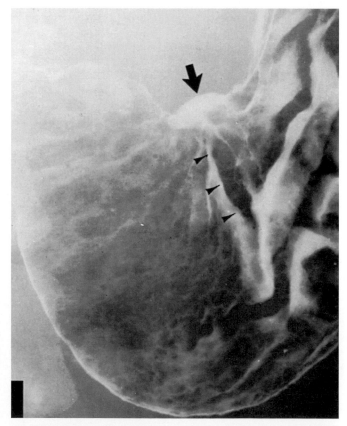

FIGURE 7–86. Early gastric cancer with lesser curvature ulcer *(large arrow).* Note how surrounding mucosal folds *(small arrowheads)* are disorganized and lobulated and taper as they approach ulcer. (From Laufer, I: Double contrast radiology in the diagnosis of gastrointestinal cancer. *In* Glass, G.B.J. [ed.]: Progress in Gastroenterology, vol. 3., New York, Grune & Stratton, 1977, p. 643, with permission.)

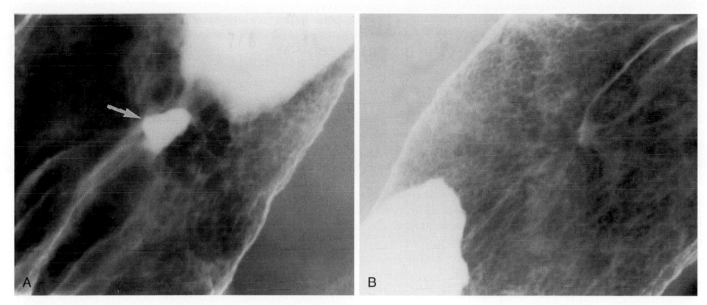

FIGURE 7–87. Benign ulcer with suspicious radiographic appearance. *A,* Posterior wall ulcer *(arrow)* in upper body of stomach. Enlarged, nodular areae gastricae adjacent to ulcer raise possibility of mucosal spread of tumor. However, endoscopic biopsy specimens revealed no evidence of malignancy. *B,* Follow-up study 3 months later shows return of normal areae gastricae in this region with ulcer healing. (From Levine, M.S., et al.: Benign gastric ulcers: Diagnosis and follow-up with double-contrast radiography. Radiology *164:*9, 1987, with permission.)

Equivocal ulcers are those that have mixed features of benign and malignant disease, so that a confident diagnosis cannot be made on radiologic criteria.[46,77] For example, edema and inflammation surrounding an acute ulcer may result in enlarged, distorted areae gastricae, mass effect, or thickened, irregular folds, producing an indeterminate radiographic appearance (Figs. 7–87 and 7–88). Similarly, greater curvature ulcers that have an ap-

parent intraluminal location or considerable associated mass effect and shouldered edges may result in equivocal radiographic findings (see Fig. 7–67). Most ulcers that have an equivocal appearance are ultimately found to be benign.[46,76] However, it seems prudent to err on the side of caution by suggesting the possibility of malignancy in some benign lesions to avoid missing an early carcinoma.

Gastric ulcers that have an unequivocally benign ap-

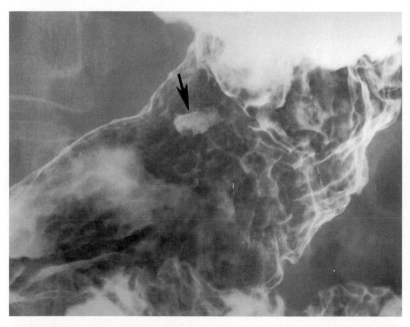

FIGURE 7–88. Benign ulcer with malignant appearance. A 1-cm ulcer *(arrow)* is located near lesser curvature with considerable mass effect surrounding ulcer. Note how adjacent mucosa has nodular appearance, suggestive of malignancy. However, endoscopic biopsy specimens revealed no evidence of tumor, and repeat endoscopy 1 month later showed complete healing of ulcer.

pearance on double contrast studies can be followed radiographically until complete healing without the need for endoscopic intervention.[46,77] However, ulcers that have an equivocal or suspicious appearance should undergo endoscopy and biopsy. Although endoscopy is an extremely accurate technique for diagnosing gastric carcinoma,[79] false-negative endoscopic brushings and biopsy specimens have been reported in some patients with malignant lesions.[80] If the radiographic findings are suggestive of malignancy, negative endoscopic or cytologic findings therefore should not be taken as definitive evidence of a benign ulcer. Instead, follow-up barium studies should be performed at regular intervals until complete healing is documented. If the ulcer fails to heal with adequate medical treatment or if it continues to have a suspicious appearance, repeat endoscopy may be necessary. Even if endoscopic brushings and biopsy specimens remain negative, surgical resection should be considered when the radiographic findings suggest malignancy.

Helicobacter pylori and Gastric Ulcers

H. pylori is currently thought to be a major factor in the development of gastric ulcers; the prevalence of _H. pylori_ ranges from 60% to 80% in these patients.[35] It has been shown that eradication of _H. pylori_ from the stomach with antibiotics and antisecretory agents leads to more rapid healing of gastric ulcers and a lower rate of recurrence.[81] As a result, an expert panel convened by the National Institutes of Health concluded that all patients with gastric ulcers who are infected by _H. pylori_ should be treated with antibiotics as well as conventional antiulcer agents.[82] An argument could therefore be made that all patients with gastric ulcers should undergo endoscopy and biopsy to look for this organism. However, noninvasive tests for _H. pylori_, such as a urea breath test and a serum antibody test, which are highly sensitive and specific for this infection, are now widely available.[83,84] Thus, in the future, clinical decisions about the use of antisecretory agents, antibiotics, or both could be made based on the combination of a double contrast study and a noninvasive test for _H. pylori_ without need for endoscopy.[35]

POSTOPERATIVE STOMACH

A high-quality double contrast examination can often be performed on patients who have undergone a partial gastrectomy.[85,86] These patients may have a "Billroth I" with an antrectomy and gastroduodenostomy or, more commonly, a "Billroth II" with an antrectomy and gastrojejunostomy. Unless a Roux-en-Y anastomosis is created, a Billroth II usually consists of an end-to-side gastrojejunostomy with an afferent loop that terminates in a blind-ending duodenal stump and an efferent loop of proximal jejunum. In both procedures, rapid spillage of barium from the gastric remnant through the anastomosis may compromise the radiologic study. As a result the examination technique must be modified to obtain adequate double contrast views of the gastric remnant and anastomotic region (i.e., the gastroenterostomy) before emptying of barium has occurred. It is important to be aware of the normal radiographic appearances of the postoperative stomach and the complications that occur in these patients.

Examination Technique

The patient is given 1 mg of intravenous glucagon at the outset of the examination. This higher dose of glucagon is needed to induce maximal gastric hypotonia and prevent rapid spillage of barium from the gastric remnant. After administration of effervescent agent, less barium may be given than usual to avoid flooding the gastric remnant. The table is gradually lowered to the horizontal or near horizontal position and the patient slowly rotated to obtain optimal coating of the stomach. Careful fluoroscopic control is needed to prevent rapid loss of barium or gas through the anastomosis into the small bowel. Double contrast views of the gastric remnant are routinely obtained with the patient in the supine, oblique, lateral, and upright positions. The gastrojejunal or gastroduodenal anastomoses usually are best visualized with the patient in supine oblique positions, but the optimal projection for demonstrating the anastomotic region depends on the precise anatomic configuration in each case. An overhead film may also be obtained to demonstrate the afferent and efferent loops of proximal jejunum.

If the gastric remnant contains too much barium or is overdistended with gas, the table may be moved to the upright or horizontal positions to facilitate emptying of barium or gas from the stomach. Conversely, if the gastric remnant contains insufficient barium or is inadequately distended, additional barium or effervescent agent may be administered to ensure that adequate double contrast views are obtained.

Normal Postoperative Findings

The normal gastric remnant, gastroduodenal or gastrojejunal anastomosis, and adjacent small bowel can be well visualized on double contrast examinations (Fig. 7–89).[85,86] After a Billroth II, the cut end of the stomach frequently is oversewn and inverted to restrict the size of the gastrojejunal stoma. This produces typical anastomotic deformities or plication defects that should not be mistaken for plaquelike or polypoid tumors in the gastric remnant (Fig. 7–90). Occasionally, trapping of barium between distorted mucosal folds or in postsurgical outpouchings at or near the anastomosis may produce discrete collections that are difficult to distinguish from recurrent ulcers.

Postoperative Complications

After a partial gastrectomy, reflux of bile through a gastroduodenal or gastrojejunal anastomosis may cause bile

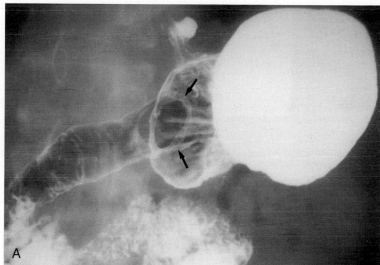

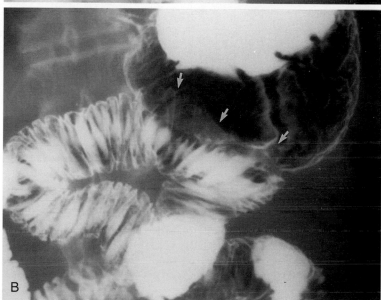

FIGURE 7–89. Normal postoperative appearances after partial gastrectomy. *A,* Billroth I with gastroduodenostomy *(arrows). B,* Billroth II with gastrojejunostomy *(arrows).*

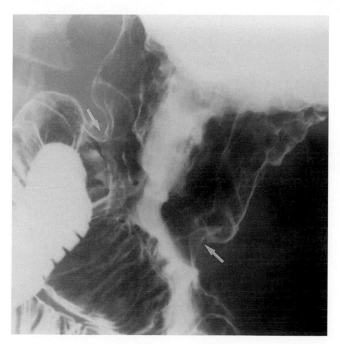

FIGURE 7–90. Billroth II with plication defects. Plication defects *(arrows)* are seen along both borders of gastrojejunal anastomosis. These defects could be mistaken for neoplastic lesions.

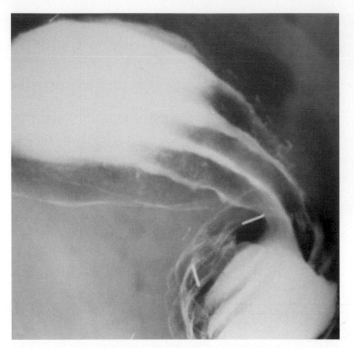

FIGURE 7–91. **Billroth II with bile reflux gastritis.** Thickened, edematous folds present in gastric remnant are due to reflux of bile.

reflux gastritis with thickened, nodular gastric folds due to edema and inflammation of the gastric remnant (Fig. 7–91). In patients who underwent surgery for benign ulcer disease, recurrent ulcers can often be demonstrated on double contrast studies. After a Billroth II, these recurrent ulcers tend to occur in the proximal jejunum, directly adjacent to the distal aspect of the gastrojejunal anastomosis (hence the term *marginal ulcers*) (Fig. 7–92).

A Billroth II may occasionally be complicated by gastrojejunal intussusception (Fig. 7–93) or, more commonly, retrograde jejunogastric intussusception, with a striated or coiled-spring defect in the gastric remnant representing the invaginated small bowel. Postsurgical scarring of the gastrojejunal or gastroduodenal anastomosis may lead to gastric outlet obstruction or even the development of a bezoar in the gastric remnant (Fig. 7–94). Finally, scarring at the gastrojejunal anastomosis may produce an afferent loop syndrome with marked dilatation of the afferent loop associated with obstruction or bacterial overgrowth.

The radiologic diagnosis of recurrent gastric carcinoma and primary gastric stump carcinoma after partial gastrectomy is considered in Chapter 8.

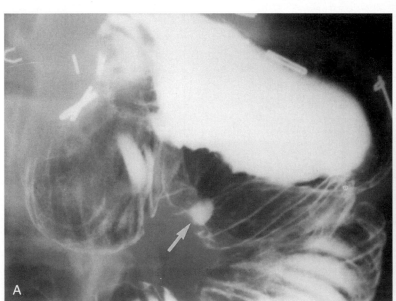

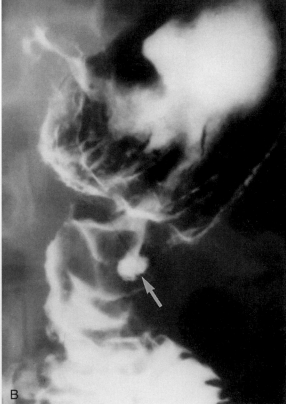

FIGURE 7–92. Two examples (*A* and *B*) of marginal ulcers *(arrows)* after Billroth II partial gastrectomy. In both cases, note how ulcers are located on jejunal side of anastomosis.

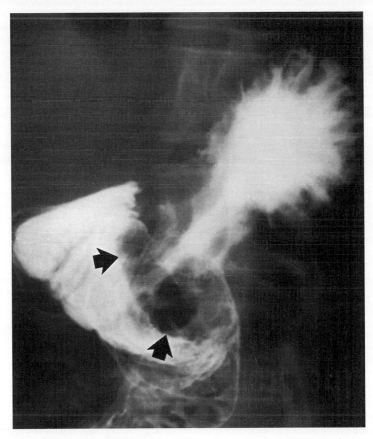

FIGURE 7–93. Billroth II with gastrojejunal intussusception. Note filling defect *(arrows)* in proximal jejunum due to invagination of gastric remnant through anastomosis.

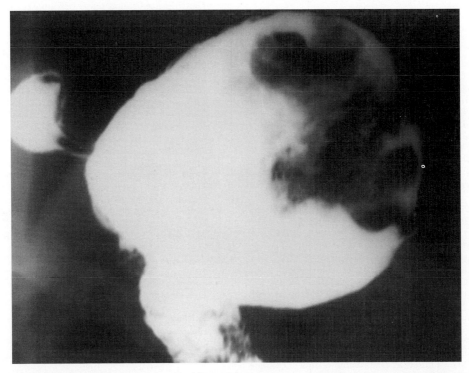

FIGURE 7–94. Billroth II with bezoar. The large, irregular filling defect in gastric remnant is due to a conglomerate of retained food and debris. Other views showed narrowing of the gastrojejunostomy as the cause of this finding.

REFERENCES

1. Mackintosh, C.E., and Kreel, L.: Anatomy and radiology of the areae gastricae. Gut *18*:855, 1977.
2. Rubesin, S.E., and Herlinger, H.: The effect of barium suspension viscosity on the delineation of areae gastricae. AJR Am. J. Roentgenol. *146*:35, 1986.
3. Rose, C., and Stevenson, G.W.: Correlation between visualization and size of the areae gastricae and duodenal ulcer. Radiology *139*:371, 1981.
4. Watanabe, H., Magota, S., Shiiba, S., et al.: Coarse areae gastricae in the proximal body and fundus: A sign of gastric hypersecretion. Radiology *146*:303, 1983.
5. Sohn, J., Levine, M.S., Furth, E.E., et al.: *Helicobacter pylori* gastritis: Radiographic findings. Radiology *195*:763, 1995.
6. Koga, M., Nakata, H., and Kuyonari, H.: Minute mucosal patterns in gastric carcinoma: Magnification radiography on resected gastric specimens. Radiology *120*:199, 1976.
7. Levine, M.S., Palman, C.L., Rubesin, S.E., et al.: Atrophic gastritis in pernicious anemia: Diagnosis by double-contrast radiography. Gastrointest. Radiol. *14*:215, 1989.
8. Keto, P., Suoranta, H., Myllarniemi, H., et al.: Areae gastricae in gastritis: Lack of correlation between size and histology. AJR Am. J. Roentgenol. *141*:693, 1983.
9. Seymour, E.Q., and Meredith, H.C.: Antral and esophageal rimple: A normal variation. Gastrointest. Radiol. *3*:147, 1978.
10. Cho, K.C., Gold, B.M., and Printz, D.A.: Multiple transverse folds in the gastric antrum. Radiology *164*:339, 1987.
11. Freeny, P.C.: Double-contrast gastrography of the fundus and cardia: Normal landmarks and their pathologic changes. AJR Am. J. Roentgenol. *133*:481, 1979.
12. Herlinger, H., Grossman, R., Laufer, I., et al.: The gastric cardia in double-contrast study: Its dynamic image. AJR Am. J. Roentgenol. *135*:21, 1980.
13. Cimmino, C.V.: Sign of the burnous in the stomach. Radiology *75*:722, 1960.
14. Lewis, T.D., Laufer, I., and Goodacre, R.L.: Arteriovenous malformation of the stomach: Radiologic and endoscopic features. Am. J. Dig. Dis. *23*:467, 1978.
15. Gohel, V.K., Kressel, H.Y., and Laufer, I.: Double-contrast artifacts. Gastrointest. Radiol. *3*:139, 1978.
16. Laufer, I., Hamilton, J., and Mullens, J.E.: Demonstration of superficial gastric erosions by double contrast radiography. Gastroenterology *68*:387, 1975.
17. Lanza, F., Royer, G., and Nelson, R.: An endoscopic evaluation of the effects of non-steroidal anti-inflammatory drugs on the gastric mucosa. Gastrointest. Endosc. *21*:103, 1975.
18. Laufer, I., Trueman, T., and de Sa, D.: Multiple superficial gastric erosions due to Crohn's disease of the stomach: Radiologic and endoscopic diagnosis. Br. J. Radiol. *49*:726, 1976.
19. Ariyama, J., Wehlin, L., Lindstrom, C.G., et al.: Gastroduodenal erosions in Crohn's disease. Gastrointest. Radiol. *5*:121, 1980.
20. Cronan, J., Burrell, M., and Trepeta, R.: Aphthoid ulcerations in gastric candidiasis. Radiology *134*:607, 1980.
21. McLean, A.M., Paul, R.E., Philipps, E., et al.: Chronic erosive gastritis—clinical and radiological features. J. Can. Assoc. Radiol. *33*:158, 1982.
22. Poplack, W., Paul, R.E., Goldsmith, M., et al.: Demonstration of erosive gastritis by the double-contrast technique. Radiology *117*:519, 1975.
23. Laufer, I.: An assessment of the accuracy of double contrast gastroduodenal radiology. Gastroenterology *71*:874, 1976.
24. Op den Orth, J.O., and Dekker, W.: Gastric erosions: Radiological and endoscopic aspects. Radiologica Clinica (Belg.) *45*:88, 1976.
25. Op den Orth, J.O., and Dekker, W.: Gastric polyps or erosions. AJR Am. J. Roentgenol. *129*:357, 1977.
26. Tragardh, B., Wehlin, L., and Ohashi, K.: Radiologic appearance of complete gastric erosions. Acta Radiol. (Stockh.) *19*:634, 1978.
27. Catalano, D., and Pagliaru, U.: Gastroduodenal erosions: Radiological findings. Gastrointest. Radiol. *7*:235, 1982.
28. Kikuchi, Y., Levine, M.S., Laufer, I., et al.: Value of flow technique for double-contrast examination of the stomach. AJR Am. J. Roentgenol. *147*:1183, 1986.
29. Elta, G.H., Fawaz, K.A., Dayal, Y., et al.: Chronic erosive gastritis: A recently recognized disorder. Dig. Dis. Sci. *28*:7, 1983.
30. McAdam, W.A.F., Morgan, A.G., Jackson, A., et al.: Multiple persisting idiopathic gastric erosions. Gut *16*:410, 1975.
31. Levine, M.S., Verstandig, A., and Laufer, I.: Serpiginous gastric erosions caused by aspirin and other nonsteroidal antiinflammatory drugs. AJR Am. J. Roentgenol. *146*:31, 1986.
32. Laveran-Stiebar, R.L., Laufer, I., and Levine, M.S.: Greater curvature antral flattening: A radiologic sign of NSAID-related gastropathy. Abdom. Imaging *19*:295, 1994.
33. Balthazar, E.J., Megibow, A.J., and Hulnick, D.H.: Cytomegalovirus esophagitis and gastritis in AIDS. AJR Am. J. Roentgenol. *144*:1201, 1985.
34. Rumerman, J., Rubesin, S.E., Levine, M.S., et al.: Gastric ulceration caused by heater probe coagulation. Gastrointest. Radiol. *13*:200, 1988.
35. Levine, M.S., and Rubesin, S.E.: The *Helicobacter pylori* revolution: Radiologic perspective. Radiology *195*:593, 1995.
36. Turner, C.J., Lipitz, L.R., and Pastore, R.A.: Antral gastritis. Radiology *113*:305, 1974.
37. Glick, S.N., Cavanaugh, B., and Teplick, S.K.: The hypertrophied antral-pyloric fold. AJR Am. J. Roentgenol. *145*:547, 1985.
38. Warren, J.R., and Marshall, B.J.: Unidentified curved bacilli on gastric epithelium in active chronic gastritis. Lancet *1*:1273, 1983.
39. Bayerdorffer, E., Lehn, N., Hatz, R., et al.: Difference in expression of *Helicobacter pylori* gastritis in antrum and body. Gastroenterology *102*:1575, 1992.
40. Dooley, C.P., Cohen, H., Fitzgibbons, P.L., et al.: Prevalence of *Helicobacter pylori* infection and histologic gastritis in asymptomatic persons. N. Engl. J. Med. *321*:1562, 1989.
41. Tan, D.T.D., Stempien, S.J., and Dagradi, A.E.: The clinical spectrum of hypertrophic hypersecretory gastropathy. Gastrointest. Endosc. *18*:69, 1971.
42. Elsborg, L., and Mosbech, J.: Pernicious anaemia as a risk factor in gastric cancer. Acta Med. Scand. *206*:315, 1979.
43. Lubert, M., and Krause, G.R.: The "ring" shadow in the diagnosis of ulcer. AJR Am. J. Roentgenol. *90*:767, 1963.
44. Poplack, W., Paul, R.E., Goldsmith, M., et al.: Linear and rod-shaped peptic ulcers. Radiology *122*:317, 1977.
45. Braver, J.M., Paul, R.E., Philipps, E., et al.: Roentgen diagnosis of linear ulcers. Radiology *132*:29, 1979.
46. Levine, M.S., Creteur, V., Kressel, H.Y., et al.: Benign gastric ulcers: Diagnosis and follow-up with double-contrast radiography. Radiology *164*:9, 1987.
47. Sun, D.C.H., and Stempien, S.J.: The Veterans' Administration Cooperative Study on Gastric Ulcer. Site and size of the ulcer as determinants of outcome. Gastroenterology *61*:576, 1971.
48. Thompson, G., Stevenson, G.W., and Somers, S.: Distribution of gastric ulcers by double-contrast barium meal with endoscopic correlation. J. Can. Assoc. Radiol. *34*:296, 1983.
49. Gelfand, D.W., Dale, W.J., and Ott, D.J.: The location and size of gastric ulcers: Radiologic and endoscopic evaluation. AJR Am. J. Roentgenol. *143*:755, 1984.
50. Amberg, J.R., and Zboralske, F.F.: Gastric ulcers after seventy. AJR Am. J. Roentgenol. *96*:393, 1966.
51. Sheppard, M.C., Holmes, G.K.T., and Cockel, R.: Clinical picture of peptic ulceration diagnosed endoscopically. Gut *18*:524, 1977.
52. Findley, J.W.: Ulcers on the greater curvature of the stomach. Gastroenterology *40*:183, 1961.
53. Kottler, R.E., and Tuft, R.J.: Benign greater curve gastric ulcer: The "sump-ulcer." Br. J. Radiol. *54*:651, 1981.
54. Zboralske, F.F., Stargardter, F.L., and Harell, G.S.: Profile roentgenographic features of benign greater curvature ulcers. Radiology *127*:63, 1978.
55. Laufer, I., Thornley, G.D., and Stolberg, H.: Gastrocolic fistula as a complication of benign gastric ulcer. Radiology *119*:7, 1976.
56. Levine, M.S., Kelly, M.R., Laufer, I., et al.: Gastrocolic fistulas: The increasing role of aspirin. Radiology *187*:359, 1993.
57. Hocking, B.V., and Alp, M.H.: Gastric ulceration within hiatus hernia. Med. J. Aust. *2*:207, 1976.
58. Welch, C.E., and Allen, A.W.: Gastric ulcer: Study of Massachusetts General Hospital cases during the 10-year period 1938–1947. N. Engl. J. Med. *240*:277, 1949.
59. Smith, F.H., Boles, R.S., and Jordon, S.M.: Problem of gastric ulcers reviewed. JAMA *153*:1505, 1953.
60. Portis, S.A., and Jaffee, R.H.: Study of peptic ulcer based on necropsy records. JAMA *106*:6, 1938.

61. Dolphin, J.A., Smith, L.A., and Waugh, J.M.: Multiple gastric ulcers: Their occurrence in benign and malignant lesions. Gastroenterology 25:202, 1953.

62. Dagradi, A.E., Falkner, R.E., and Lee, E.R.: Multiple benign gastric ulcers. Am. J. Gastroenterol. 62:36, 1974.

63. Taxin, R.N., Livingston, P.A., and Seaman, W.B.: Multiple gastric ulcers: A radiographic sign of benignity? Radiology 114:23, 1975.

64. Bloom, S.M., Paul, R.E., Matsue, H., et al.: Improved radiologic detection of multiple gastric ulcers. AJR Am. J. Roentgenol. 128:949, 1977.

65. Sakita, T., Ogura, Y., and Takasu, S.: Observations on the healing of ulcerations in early gastric cancer. Gastroenterology 60:835, 1971.

66. Kagan, A.R., and Steckel, R.J.: Gastric ulcer in a young man with apparent healing. AJR Am. J. Roentgenol. 128:831, 1977.

67. Keller, R.J., Wolf, B.S., and Khilnani, M.T.: Roentgen features of healing and healed benign gastric ulcers. Radiology 97:353, 1970.

68. Gelfand, D.W., and Ott, D.J.: Gastric ulcer scars. Radiology 140:37, 1981.

69. Nelson, S.W.: The discovery of gastric ulcers and the differential diagnosis between benignancy and malignancy. Radiol. Clin. North Am. 7:5, 1969.

70. Wenger, J., Brandborg, L.L., and Spellman, F.A.: Cancer: Part I. Clinical aspects. Gastroenterology 61:598, 1971.

71. Wolf, B.S.: Observations on roentgen features of benign and malignant ulcers. Semin. Roentgenol. 6:140, 1971.

72. Hayes, M.A.: The gastric ulcer problem. Gastroenterology 29:609, 1955.

73. Kirsh, I.E.: Benign and malignant gastric ulcers: Roentgen differentiation. Radiology 64:357, 1955.

74. Elliott, G.V., Wald, S.M., and Benz, R.I.: A roentgenologic study of ulcerating lesions of the stomach. AJR Am. J. Roentgenol. 77:612, 1957.

75. Schulman, A., and Simpkins, K.C.: The accuracy of radiological diagnosis of benign, primarily and secondarily malignant gastric ulcers and their correlation with three simplified radiological types. Clin. Radiol. 26:317, 1975.

76. Thompson, G., Somers, S., and Stevenson, G.W.: Benign gastric ulcer: A reliable radiologic diagnosis? AJR Am. J. Roentgenol. 141:331, 1983.

77. Levine, M.S.: Erosive gastritis and gastric ulcers. Radiol. Clin. North Am. 32:1203, 1994.

78. Ichikawa, H.: Differential diagnosis between benign and malignant ulcers of the stomach. Clin. Gastroenterol. 2:329, 1973.

79. Qizilbash, A.H., Castelli, M., Kowalski, M.A., and Churly, A.: Endoscopic brush cytology and biopsy in the diagnosis of cancer of the upper gastrointestinal tract. Acta Cytol. (Baltimore) 24:313, 1980.

80. Segal, A.W., Healy, M.J.R., Cox A.G., et al.: Diagnosis of gastric cancer. BMJ 2:669, 1975.

81. Graham, D.Y., Lew, G.M., Klein, P.D., et al.: Effect of treatment of *Helicobacter pylori* infection on the long-term recurrence of gastric or duodenal ulcer. Ann. Intern. Med. 116:705, 1992.

82. NIH consensus conference: *Helicobacter pylori* in peptic ulcer disease. JAMA 272:65, 1994.

83. Graham, D.Y.: Treatment of peptic ulcers caused by *Helicobacter pylori* (editorial). N. Engl. J. Med. 328:349, 1993.

84. Talley, N.J., Kost, L., Haddad, A., et al.: Comparison of commercial serological tests for detection of *Helicobacter pylori* antibodies. J. Clin. Microbiol. 30:3146, 1992.

85. Gold, R.P., and Seaman, W.B.: The primary double-contrast examination of the postoperative stomach. Radiology 124:297, 1977.

86. Gohel, V.K., and Laufer, I.: Double contrast examination of the postoperative stomach. Radiology 129:601, 1978.

8

Tumors of the Stomach

MARC S. LEVINE
IGOR LAUFER

BENIGN TUMORS

Mucosal Polyps

Gastric polyps are generally considered to be uncommon lesions. However, the routine use of double contrast technique has dramatically improved our ability to detect gastric polyps, which are found in 1% to 2% of double contrast studies.[1,2] Because gastric polyps are usually small lesions, it is likely that most are being missed on conventional single contrast examinations.

On double contrast studies, a gastric polyp on the dependent or posterior wall typically appears as a smooth, round filling defect in the thin barium pool (Fig. 8–1). Conversely, a polyp on the nondependent or anterior wall of the stomach is etched in white because of barium coating the edge of the polyp (Fig. 8–2). As a result, anterior wall polyps may be manifested by one or more ring shadows in the stomach (Fig. 8–3). If the polyp is pedunculated, its stalk may be seen en face overlying the head of the polyp, producing the "Mexican hat" sign (Fig. 8–2). Not infrequently, a droplet of barium or "stalactite" may be seen hanging down from an anterior wall polyp.[3] When this hanging droplet is viewed en face, it can be mistaken for a central area of ulceration (Figs. 8–3 and 8–4A). However, it occurs as a transient finding, since the droplet of barium invariably falls off the polyp during fluoroscopic observation. Occasionally, a stalactite may be the only clue to the presence of a protruded lesion on the anterior wall (see Chapter 2).[4] When ring shadows or stalactites are observed in the stomach (Fig. 8–4A), careful examination of the area with prone compression views should demonstrate the underlying polyps responsible for these findings (Fig. 8–4B).

Most polypoid lesions in the stomach are hyperplastic polyps.[5] They are almost always less than 1 cm and tend to occur as multiple lesions, most frequently in the fundus or body (Fig. 8–5).[1] Occasionally, the stomach may contain innumerable hyperplastic polyps (Fig. 8–6). Because these polyps are not premalignant, small (less than 1 cm), asymptomatic gastric polyps detected on double contrast studies should be considered innocuous lesions not requiring endoscopic biopsy or removal.

Although adenomatous polyps make up less than 10% of all gastric polyps,[1,2,5] they are dysplastic lesions that are capable of undergoing malignant degeneration by means of an adenoma-carcinoma sequence similar to that found in the colon. The risk of cancer is related to polyp size and becomes significant when the polyp reaches a diameter of 2 cm.[6] Nevertheless, adenocarcinoma is about 30 times more common than adenomatous polyps in the stomach, so that most gastric cancers are thought to originate de novo and not from preexisting polyps.[7] Adenomatous polyps are almost always greater than 1 cm.[7,8] The majority occur as solitary lesions, most frequently in the antrum (Fig. 8–7), but multiple lesions are occasionally found (Fig. 8–8).[8] Adenomatous polyps may be sessile or pedunculated and tend to be more lobulated than hyperplastic polyps (Figs. 8–7 and 8–8). Thus, polyps that are pedunculated or lobulated or those that are greater than 1 cm should be evaluated by endoscopy. If biopsy re-

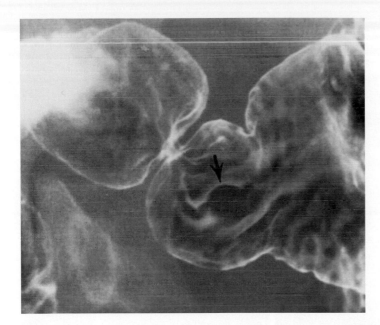

FIGURE 8–1. Polyp on posterior wall of antrum seen as radiolucent filling defect *(arrow)* in thin barium pool.

FIGURE 8–2. Anterior wall polyps are etched in white *(small arrows)* because of barium coating edge of polyp. Note that largest polyp exhibits Mexican hat sign *(large arrow),* with central lucency representing stalk of polyp.

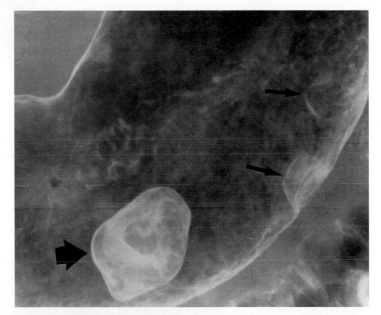

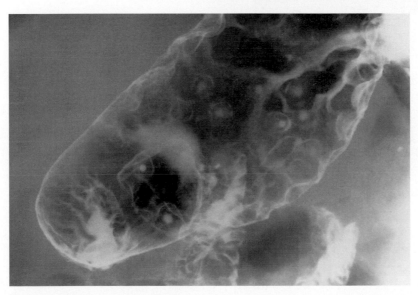

FIGURE 8–3. Multiple anterior wall polyps appearing as ring shadows in stomach. Note hanging droplets of barium or stalactites that could be mistaken for central areas of ulceration.

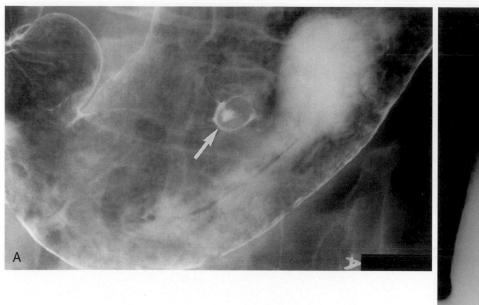

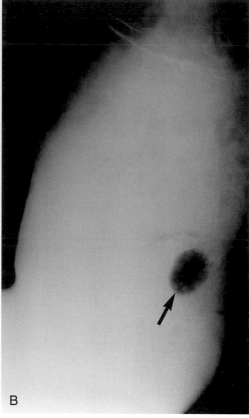

FIGURE 8–4. Anterior wall polyp with stalactite. *A,* Anterior wall polyp seen as ring shadow *(arrow)* in gastric body. Also note central barium collection representing a hanging droplet of barium or stalactite. *B,* Prone compression view shows this anterior wall polyp as a filling defect *(arrow)* in barium pool.

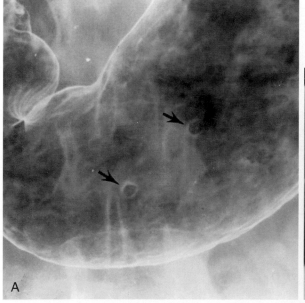

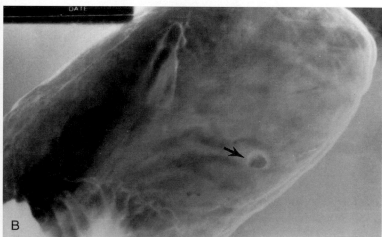

FIGURE 8–5. Multiple small hyperplastic polyps *(arrows)* in body *(A)* and fundus *(B)* of stomach.

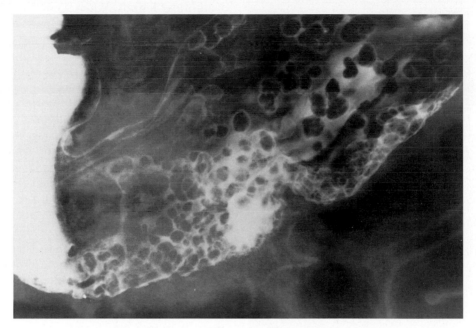

FIGURE 8–6. Innumerable hyperplastic polyps in stomach.

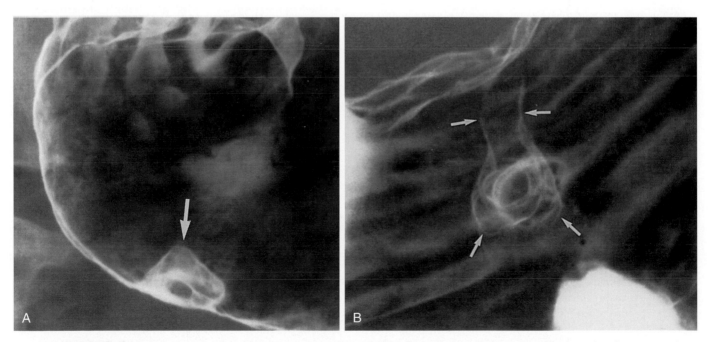

FIGURE 8–7. Solitary adenomatous polyps *(arrows)* in antrum. Note that polyp is sessile in *A* and pedunculated in *B*.

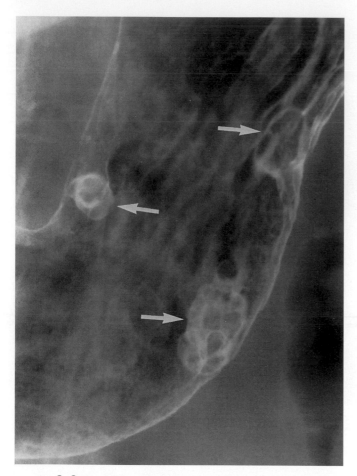

FIGURE 8–8. Multiple adenomatous polyps *(arrows)* in stomach. Note that lesions are larger and more lobulated than hyperplastic polyps.

sults confirm the presence of an adenomatous polyp, it should be resected because of the risk of malignant degeneration (Fig. 8–9). Adenomatous polyps are also important because they are associated with a high incidence of separate, coexisting gastric carcinomas.[5,7]

Submucosal Tumors

Leiomyomas are by far the most common submucosal tumors in the stomach.[9] Other less common submucosal lesions include leiomyoblastomas, lipomas, hemangiomas, neurofibromas, and granular cell tumors.[10] Although most of these lesions are discovered as incidental findings, ulcerated submucosal masses may cause abdominal pain or upper gastrointestinal bleeding. Submucosal tumors of smooth muscle origin are also important because of an associated risk of malignancy.

Submucosal tumors are often difficult to visualize at endoscopy because the overlying mucosa appears normal. However, these lesions are readily detected on double contrast studies. When viewed en face, submucosal tu-

mors have very abrupt, well-defined borders, with adjacent mucosal folds that fade out at the periphery of the lesion (Fig. 8–10A). Because the mucosa is usually intact, a normal areae gastricae pattern can often be seen overlying these lesions. When viewed in profile, submucosal tumors also have a very smooth surface, and their borders form right angles or slightly obtuse angles with the adjacent gastric wall (Fig. 8–10B). Although it is difficult to distinguish the various submucosal tumors on radiographic criteria, a lipoma may be suspected if the lesion changes in size or shape at fluoroscopy (Figs. 8–11A and B).[11] The fatty density of a lipoma can be confirmed by computed tomography (CT) (Fig. 8–11C).[12,13]

Submucosal tumors may vary in size from tiny lesions of several millimeters to enormous masses that encroach significantly on the gastric lumen (Fig. 8–12). Some exogastric lesions may grow outward from the stomach into the peritoneal cavity. Tumors greater than 2 cm frequently contain areas of ulceration, manifested by a central barium-filled crater within the mass (Fig. 8–13A). Ulceration is generally considered an indication for surgery because of the risk of upper gastrointestinal bleeding. However, complete healing of ulceration in a gastric leiomyoma has been reported (Fig. 8–13B)[14]; conservative medical treatment therefore may lead to cessation of bleeding when surgery is contraindicated. Occasionally, a hanging droplet of barium or stalactite on an anterior wall leiomyoma can mimic the appearance of ulceration (see Fig. 8–10A). However, the stalactite can be recognized as a transient finding at fluoroscopy. Although leiomyomas and leiomyosarcomas cannot be reliably differentiated on radiologic criteria, malignancy should be suspected when the lesion is larger than 2 to 3 cm, is lobulated, or contains extensive areas of ulceration (Fig. 8–14).[9]

Other types of lesions can mimic submucosal tumors. An ectopic pancreatic rest may be manifested radiographically by a submucosal mass, most frequently on the greater curvature of the distal antrum (Fig. 8–15).[15,16] Approximately 50% of these lesions have a central umbilication, representing the orifice of a primitive ductal system.[15] As a result, the radiographic appearance may suggest an ulcerated submucosal tumor. An acute antral ulcer with a large mound of edema may also simulate an intramural lesion. With ulcers, however, the transition between the edematous mound and the adjacent gastric mucosa tends to be more gradual. Finally, extrinsic compression of the stomach by a normal or enlarged liver, spleen, pancreas, or kidney may be indistinguishable from an exophytic submucosal tumor (Fig. 8–16). However, the presence of a central dimple or spicule at the apex of the mass should suggest an exogastric lesion such as a leiomyoma or leiomyosarcoma.[17] In such patients, CT is often helpful for establishing the correct diagnosis.

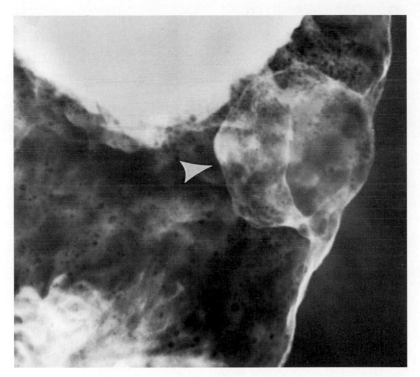

FIGURE 8–9. Giant adenomatous polyp *(arrowhead)* found to contain a central focus of adenocarcinoma.

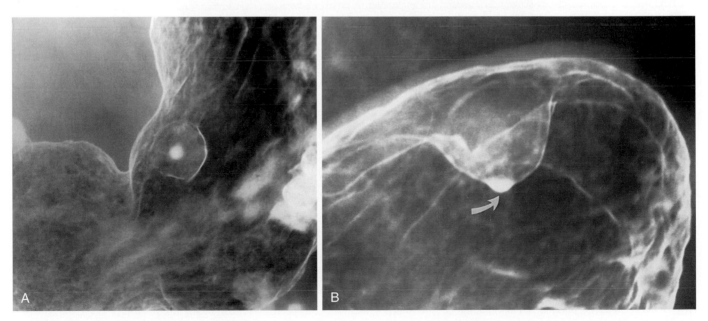

FIGURE 8–10. Gastric leiomyomas. *A,* Small leiomyoma seen en face in gastric body. This lesion has typical features of submucosal mass with smooth, well-defined borders. Also note hanging droplet of barium or stalactite on surface of this anterior wall lesion. *B,* Another leiomyoma seen in profile in gastric fundus. Note that borders of lesion form slightly obtuse angles with adjacent gastric wall. This view was taken with patient upright, and barium stalactite *(arrow)* is seen hanging down from inferior surface of lesion.

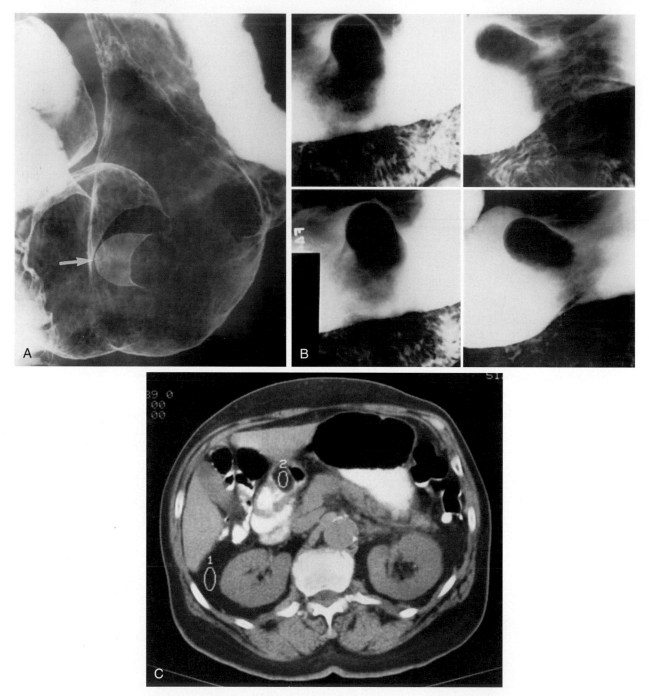

FIGURE 8–11. Gastric lipoma. *A,* Double contrast view shows smooth submucosal mass *(arrow)* in antrum. *B,* Prone single contrast views show how lesion changes in size and shape with varying degrees of compression. This changing appearance should be highly suggestive of a lipoma. *C,* CT scan shows how lesion in antrum *(cursor 2)* has same density as perirenal fat *(cursor 1),* confirming presence of lipoma.

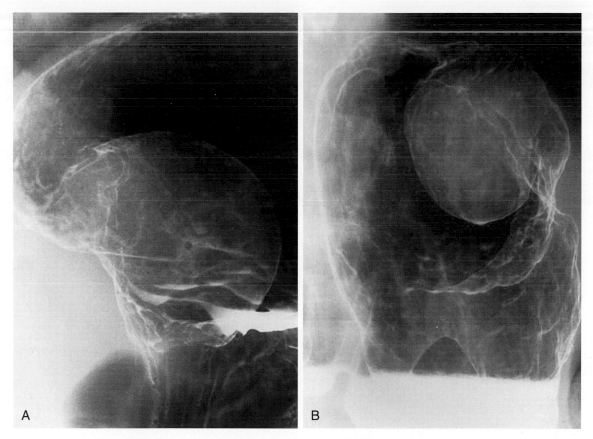

FIGURE 8–12. Two examples (*A* and *B*) of giant leiomyomas in gastric fundus.

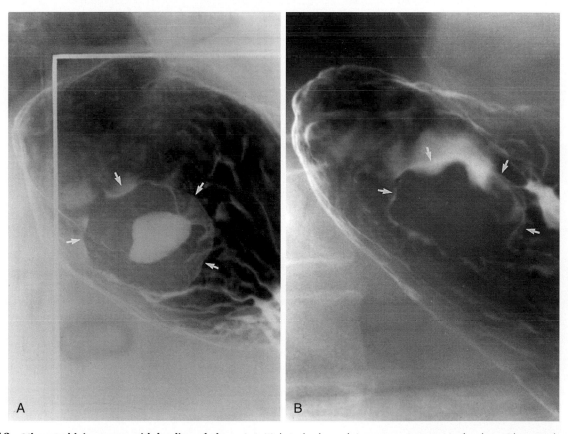

FIGURE 8–13. Ulcerated leiomyoma with healing of ulcer. *A,* Initial study shows leiomyoma *(arrows)* in fundus with central area of ulceration. *B,* Follow-up study 3½ years later shows complete healing of ulcer in leiomyoma *(arrows)*. (From O'Riordan, D., et al.: Complete healing of ulceration within a gastric leiomyoma. Gastrointest. Radiol. *10:*47, 1985, with permission.)

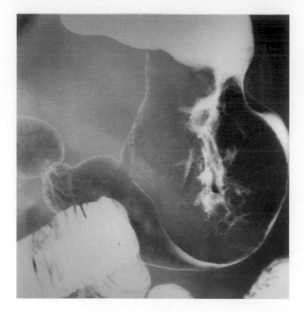

FIGURE 8–14. Large leiomyosarcoma on posterior wall of stomach with irregular areas of ulceration. (Courtesy of Hans Herlinger, M.D., Philadelphia, Pennsylvania.)

FIGURE 8–15. Ectopic pancreatic rest appearing as submucosal mass *(arrows)* on greater curvature of antrum.

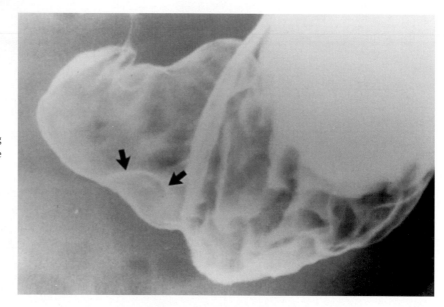

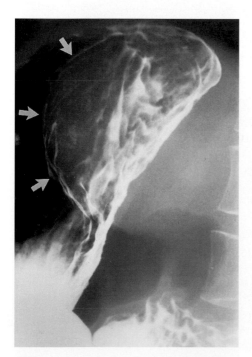

FIGURE 8–16. Pancreatic pseudocyst with extrinsic compression of posterior wall of fundus *(arrows),* simulating appearance of giant submucosal mass.

MALIGNANT TUMORS

Carcinoma

Accurate diagnosis of gastric carcinoma has always been an important aim of barium studies of the upper gastrointestinal tract. Unfortunately, the average sensitivity of single contrast barium studies for the diagnosis of gastric carcinoma has only been about 75%.[18] Concern about missing gastric cancer on barium studies therefore has been used as the rationale for performing endoscopy as the initial diagnostic procedure in patients with signs or symptoms of upper gastrointestinal disease. However, in a recent series of 80 patients with proven gastric carcinoma, double contrast studies showed the lesions in 99% of cases and malignant tumor was diagnosed or suspected in 96%.[18] This figure is comparable to the reported endoscopic sensitivity of 94% to 99% when multiple endoscopic biopsy specimens and brushings are obtained.[19–21] In the same radiologic series, only about 4% of all patients who underwent double contrast studies were referred for endoscopy because of equivocal radiographic findings.[18] Thus, a high sensitivity can be achieved in the radiographic diagnosis of gastric carcinoma without exposing an inordinate number of patients to unnecessary endoscopy.

Early Tumors

Early gastric cancer is defined histologically as carcinoma in which malignant invasion is limited to the mucosa or submucosa.[22] During the past several decades, detection of early gastric cancer has increased dramatically in Japan as the result of mass screening of asymptomatic patients who undergo periodic double contrast upper gastrointestinal studies and endoscopy. This aggressive approach to gastric cancer by the Japanese has also resulted in a dramatic increase in patient survival, with 5-year survival rates as high as 95% for patients with early gastric cancer.[23] The Japanese have devised an elaborate system for classifying these tumors on the basis of the predominant morphologic (elevated, flat, or depressed) features of the lesions.[22]

Type I early gastric cancers are usually small, protruded lesions in the stomach (Fig. 8–17A).[24,25] Because adenomatous polyps can degenerate into invasive adenocarcinoma, any polypoid lesions that are lobulated or greater than 1 cm in size should be evaluated by endoscopy and biopsy to rule out an early cancer. Other type I lesions may protrude considerably into the lumen and still be classified as early gastric cancers.[25] Type II early gastric cancers are superficial lesions with elevated, flat, or depressed components. These tumors may be manifested by plaquelike lesions, mucosal nodularity, or shallow areas of ulceration (Fig. 8–17B).[24,25] Rarely, type II lesions may be superficial spreading cancers that occupy a considerable surface area of the stomach. Finally, type III early gastric cancers are depressed lesions character-ized by shallow, irregular ulcer craters, often associated with nodularity of the adjacent mucosa and clubbing, fusion, or amputation of radiating folds (Fig. 8–17C and D).[24,25] Careful analysis of the radiographic findings enables differentiation of these lesions from benign ulcers in most patients (see Chapter 7). Although some lesions with a suspicious appearance are found to be benign, endoscopy and biopsy should be performed for all lesions with equivocal radiographic findings to avoid missing early cancers.

Radiologists in Western countries should be aware of the various appearances of early gastric cancer because occasional cases may be encountered (see Fig. 8–17). However, the widespread use of double contrast radiographic techniques and fiberoptic endoscopy has not led to an increased detection rate of early gastric cancer in the West.[26] This discrepancy from the Japanese experience can be attributed primarily to the fact that mass screening programs are not used in Western countries because of the lower incidence of gastric carcinoma. Thus, radiologists should recognize that they are unlikely to experience a significant increase in the detection of early gastric cancer as long as these examinations are performed predominantly on symptomatic patients.

Advanced Tumors

Most symptomatic patients with gastric carcinoma present with advanced tumors. These lesions may be polypoid (Fig. 8–18), plaquelike (Fig. 8–19), ulcerated (Fig. 8–20), or infiltrating (Fig 8–21); or, less frequently, they may be manifested by thickened, irregular folds (Fig. 8–22). Despite the advanced stage of these tumors, approximately 25% of gastric carcinomas are missed or misinterpreted on conventional single contrast barium studies.[18] Infiltrating tumors and tumors involving the proximal portion of the stomach are the ones most likely to be missed on single contrast studies.[27] Yet these are precisely the lesions that require accurate radiologic diagnosis because endoscopic biopsy specimens and brushings are often negative for tumor in these patients.[28] Fortunately, double contrast studies are particularly well suited for demonstrating infiltrating lesions or lesions involving the proximal portion of the stomach (Fig. 8–23).

Localized areas of rigidity or decreased distensibility due to infiltrating tumors are accentuated by gastric distention on the double contrast examination (see Fig. 8–23). In general, the greater the degree of distention, the easier it is to detect infiltrating lesions that limit distensibility. However, it should be recognized that overdistention may obscure some of the morphologic features of the lesion that are better seen when the stomach is less distended. Conversely, inadequate gaseous distention can accentuate the appearance of the rugal folds, erroneously suggesting an infiltrating tumor (Fig. 8–24A). With adequate distention, however, normal folds usually can be effaced, ruling out the possibility of malignancy (Fig. 8–24B).

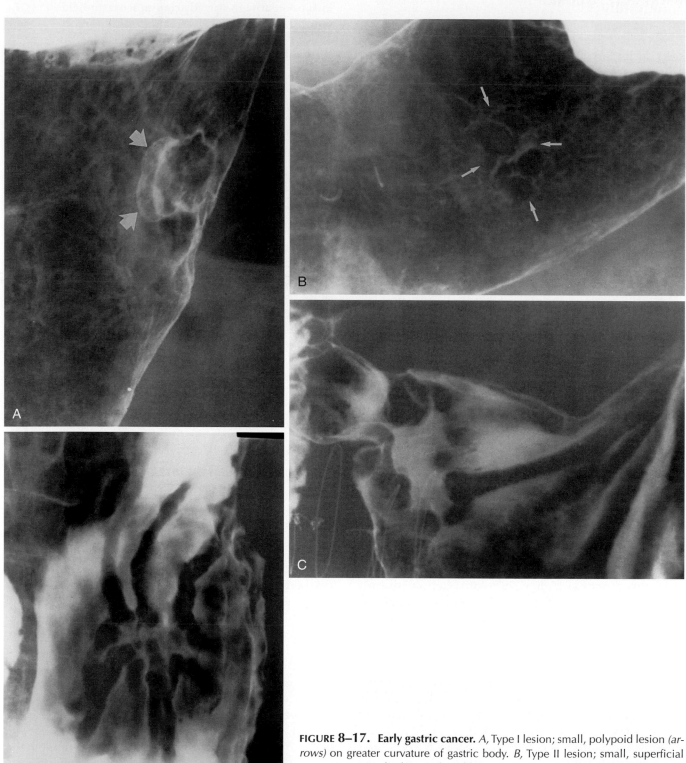

FIGURE 8–17. Early gastric cancer. *A,* Type I lesion; small, polypoid lesion *(arrows)* on greater curvature of gastric body. *B,* Type II lesion; small, superficial cancer in gastric body manifested by nodular, irregular elevations *(arrows)*. *C,* Type III lesion; malignant ulcer on posterior wall of antrum, with scalloped borders and nodular, clubbed folds surrounding ulcer. (*C,* From Levine, M.S., et al.: Benign gastric ulcers: Diagnosis and follow-up with double contrast radiography. Radiology *164:*9, 1987, with permission.) *D,* Type III lesion; malignant ulcer on posterior wall of body, with scalloped, nodular folds abutting ulcer. (*D,* Courtesy of Toyohiko Honda, M.D., Kyoto, Japan.)

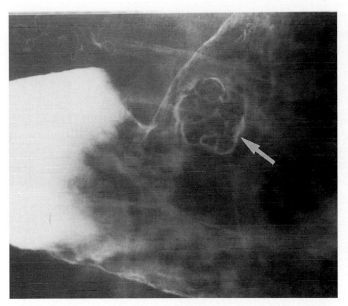

FIGURE 8–18. Small polypoid carcinoma *(arrow)* in gastric body.

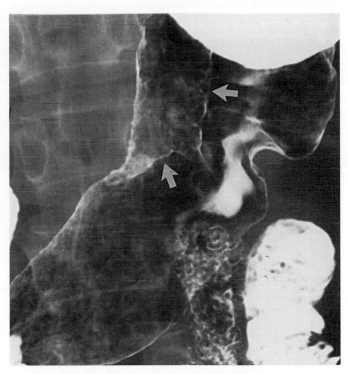

FIGURE 8–19. Plaquelike carcinoma *(arrows)* high on lesser curvature of stomach.

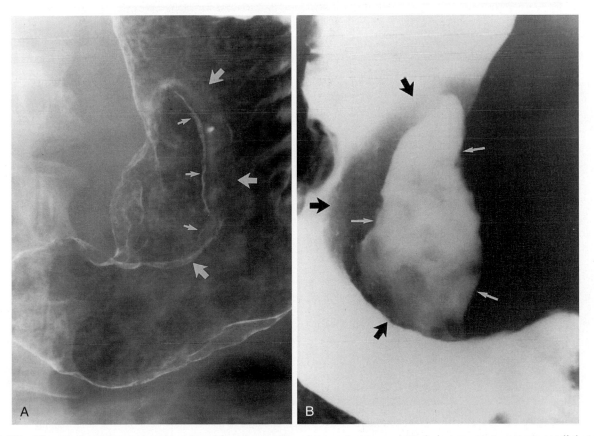

FIGURE 8–20. Ulcerated gastric carcinoma. *A,* Double contrast view of stomach shows relatively large mass on anterior wall that is etched in white *(large arrows)*. Also note second curvilinear density *(small arrows)* due to barium coating rim of unfilled central ulcer. *B,* Prone compression view shows mass as radiolucent filling defect *(black arrows)* on anterior wall of stomach. Note how central ulcer fills with barium *(white arrows)* when patient is in prone position.

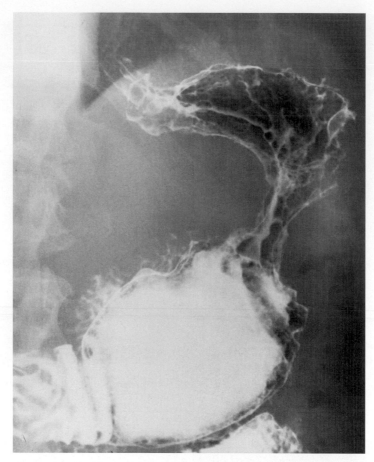

FIGURE 8–21. Advanced, infiltrating carcinoma with irregular narrowing of proximal portion of stomach.

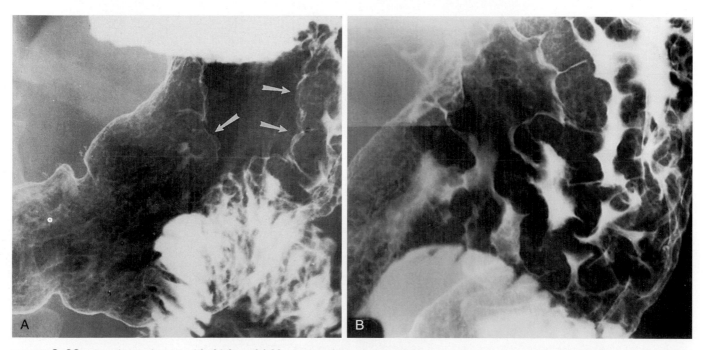

FIGURE 8–22. Gastric carcinoma with thickened folds. *A,* Note large, lobulated folds *(arrows)* in gastric body. *B,* Close-up view shows disorganization of folds due to infiltration by tumor.

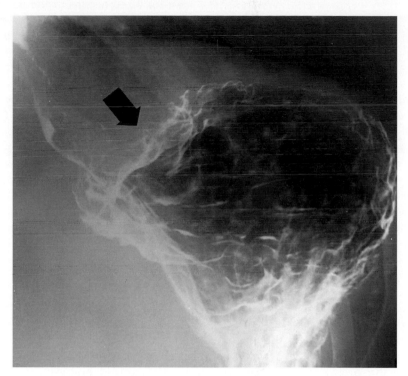

FIGURE 8–23. Gastric carcinoma with localized infiltration of medial aspect of fundus *(arrow)*. Optimal distention of fundus is needed to demonstrate this lesion.

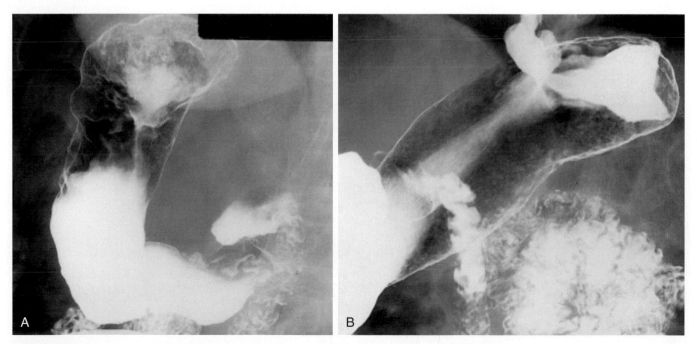

FIGURE 8–24. Danger of inadequate gaseous distention. *A,* Thickened folds are seen in proximal portion of stomach, raising the possibility of tumor. However, the fundus is inadequately distended on this view. *B,* With greater gaseous distention, the folds are effaced in the fundus, eliminating the possibility of tumor.

Scirrhous Tumors

Scirrhous carcinoma of the stomach is an infiltrating type of gastric cancer in which the tumor spreads predominantly in the submucosa, inciting a marked desmoplastic response in the gastric wall. Less frequently, the stomach can be infiltrated by metastatic breast cancer. Whether primary or metastatic, these scirrhous tumors are classically manifested radiographically by irregular narrowing and rigidity of the stomach, producing a "linitis plastica" or "leather bottle" appearance (Fig. 8–25). Not infrequently, however, scirrhous tumors of the stomach cause only mild loss of distensibility. As a result, these lesions may be recognized on double contrast studies primarily by distortion of the normal surface pattern of the stomach with mucosal nodularity, spiculation, ulceration, or thickened, irregular folds (Fig. 8–26).[29] Thus, some lesions are likely to be missed if the radiologist relies too heavily on gastric narrowing as the major criterion for diagnosing these tumors.

Scirrhous gastric carcinomas are classically thought to involve the distal half of the stomach, arising near the pylorus and gradually extending upward from the antrum into the body and fundus. Although some localized lesions may be confined to the prepyloric region of the antrum (Fig. 8–27),[30] it is difficult to find cases in the literature of lesions involving the proximal stomach that spare the antrum. With double contrast technique, however, nearly 40% of patients with these scirrhous tumors have localized lesions in the gastric fundus or body with antral sparing (Figs. 8–28 and 8–29).[29] Detection of these lesions is presumably related to gaseous distention of the proximal stomach on double contrast studies. In any case, radiologists should be aware that a significant percentage of patients with scirrhous tumors have localized lesions involving the gastric fundus or body rather than the classic form of linitis plastica involving the distal stomach.

The limitations of endoscopy in diagnosing scirrhous carcinoma of the stomach should also be recognized. False-negative endoscopic biopsy specimens and brushings are frequently obtained not only because these tumors are located predominantly in the submucosa but also because the tumor cells are often separated by extensive areas of fibrosis.[28-31] Excessive reliance on negative endoscopic findings therefore can lead to a significant delay in the diagnosis and treatment of these tumors.

Carcinoma of the Cardia

During the past 50 years, the distribution of gastric cancer has gradually shifted from the antrum proximally to the cardia and fundus.[32-34] In one study, nearly 50% of all gastric cancers diagnosed on double contrast examinations involved the cardia or fundus.[18] These patients often present with recent onset of dysphagia caused by tumor obstructing the cardia. Some may complain of food sticking behind the lower sternum, but others may have a sensation of blockage that is referred upward to the tho-

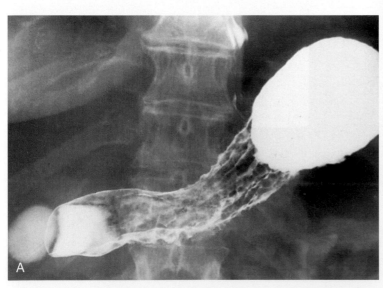
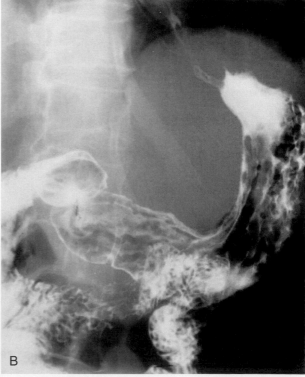

FIGURE 8–25. Scirrhous tumors of stomach. *A,* Linitis plastica with irregular narrowing of antrum and body due to metastatic breast cancer involving stomach. Note absent left breast shadow. *B,* Diffuse gastric narrowing due to primary scirrhous carcinoma of stomach. The distal esophagus was also involved, producing an achalasia-like picture. This patient presented with dysphagia.

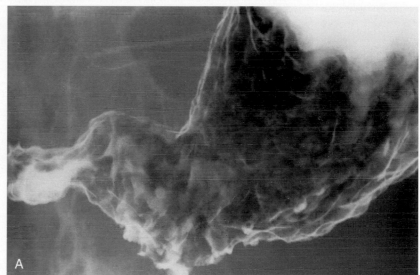

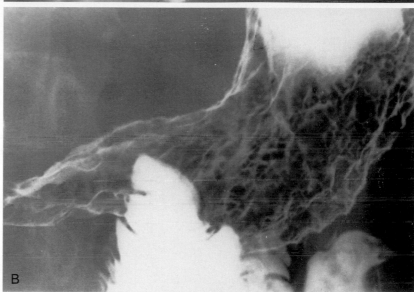

FIGURE 8–26. Two examples (*A* and *B*) of metastatic breast cancer involving stomach with only mild loss of distensibility. However, normal surface pattern is distorted, with nodular, irregular mucosa in both cases. (From Levine, M.S., et al.: Scirrhous carcinoma of the stomach: Radiologic and endoscopic diagnosis. Radiology *175*:151, 1990, with permission.)

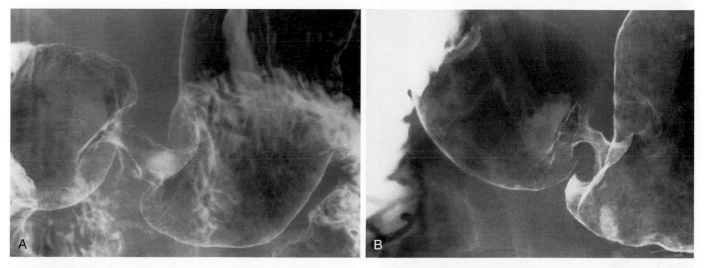

FIGURE 8–27. Localized scirrhous carcinomas of distal antrum. In both cases, there is a short, annular lesion in prepyloric region of antrum. Note abrupt, shelflike borders of lesions. (*A*, From Levine, M.S., et al.: Scirrhous carcinoma of the stomach: Radiologic and endoscopic diagnosis. Radiology *175*:151, 1990, with permission.)

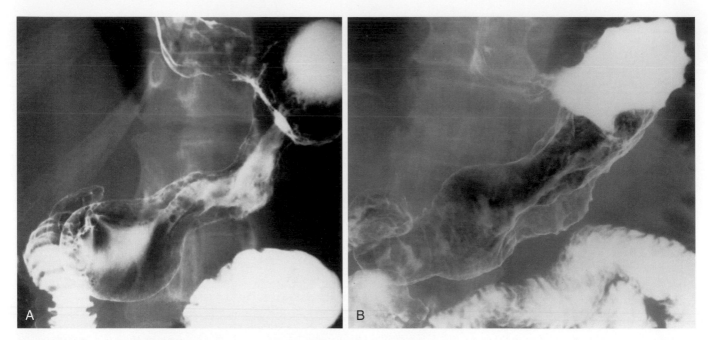

FIGURE 8–28. Localized scirrhous carcinomas of proximal stomach. *A,* Marked narrowing of gastric body with normal distensibility of antrum and fundus. *B,* Irregular narrowing of fundus and body with antral sparing. (*A,* From Levine, M.S., et al.: Scirrhous carcinoma of the stomach: Radiologic and endoscopic diagnosis. Radiology *175:*151, 1990, with permission.)

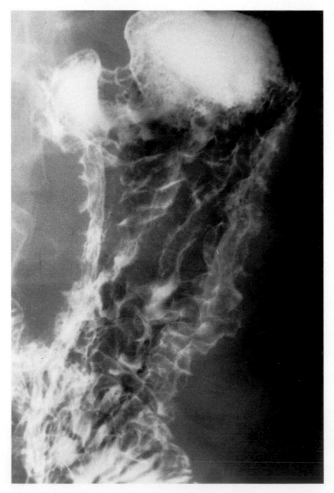

FIGURE 8–29. Metastatic breast cancer causing linitis plastica in proximal half of stomach with antral sparing. Note how gastric fundus and body have irregular contour with thickened, spiculated folds. Despite the dramatic radiographic findings, biopsy specimens and brushings from initial endoscopic examination failed to confirm presence of tumor. (From Levine, M.S., et al.: Scirrhous carcinoma of the stomach: Radiologic and endoscopic diagnosis. Radiology *175:*151, 1990, with permission.)

racic inlet or even the pharynx. The cardia and fundus therefore should be carefully evaluated in all patients with dysphagia to rule out a carcinoma of the cardia masquerading as a pharyngeal or esophageal disorder. Also, a small percentage of these patients are under the age of 40, so radiologists should not be lulled into a false sense of security about the possibility of malignant tumor because of the patient's age.[35]

Carcinoma of the cardia is notoriously difficult to detect on conventional single contrast barium studies. Because the overlying rib cage precludes manual palpation or compression of the fundus, even large lesions at the cardia may be obscured by crowded folds or relatively opaque barium that prevents adequate visualization of this region (Fig. 8–30A). With gaseous distention of the fundus, however, it is possible to evaluate the normal anatomic landmarks at the cardia and the surrounding gastric mucosa for evidence of malignancy (Fig. 8–30B).

When viewed en face, the normal cardia often appears on double contrast studies as a circular elevation containing four or five stellate folds that radiate to a central button at the gastroesophageal junction (the cardiac "rosette"; see Chapter 7).[36,37] Some lesions at the cardia may be recognized only by relatively subtle nodularity, mass effect, or ulceration in this region with distortion, effacement, or obliteration of these landmarks (Fig. 8–31).[35–39] Enlargement or lobulation of the surrounding elevation should also suggest a neoplastic lesion (Fig.

8–32). If the radiographic findings are equivocal, the patient should be instructed to swallow an additional bolus of barium. The protrusion surrounding a normal cardia should disappear when barium is swallowed because this landmark is obliterated by relaxation of the lower esophageal sphincter. A lesion therefore should be suspected if this protrusion or other abnormalities persist during passage of the barium bolus at fluoroscopy (Fig. 8–33). Conversely, an apparent abnormality at the cardia must be an artifact if it vanishes as the cardia opens.

Advanced carcinomas of the gastric cardia or fundus usually are exophytic or infiltrating lesions, often containing irregular areas of ulceration (Fig. 8–34B).[39,40] Secondary esophageal involvement by advanced lesions may be manifested radiographically by a polypoid or fungating mass that extends from the fundus into the distal esophagus (see Fig. 8–31) or by thickened folds or irregular narrowing of the distal esophagus without a discrete lesion.[39,40] Submucosal spread of tumor may also result in "secondary achalasia" with tapered, beaklike narrowing of the distal esophagus at or just above the gastroesophageal junction (Fig. 8–34A).[40,41] However, careful examination of the gastric cardia and fundus almost always demonstrates the underlying gastric lesion (Fig. 8–34B). The possibility of secondary achalasia should also be suspected when the narrowed segment is asymmetric or ulcerated or extends several centimeters proximally from the gastroesophageal junction.[42]

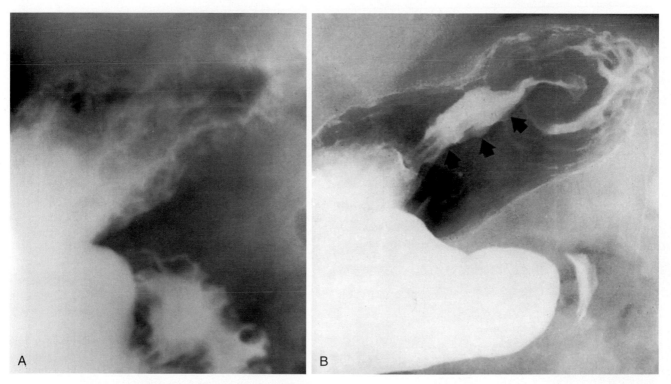

FIGURE 8–30. Limitation of single contrast barium study in diagnosis of carcinoma of the cardia. *A,* No tumor is seen in fundus on conventional single contrast study. *B,* With greater gaseous distention of fundus, ulcerated lesion *(arrows)* is clearly seen adjacent to cardia on double contrast view. (From Glass, G.B.J. [ed.]: Progress in Gastroenterology, vol. 3. New York, Grune & Stratton, 1977, with permission.)

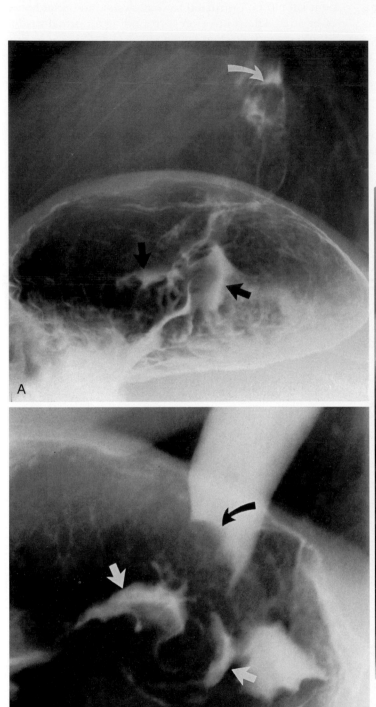

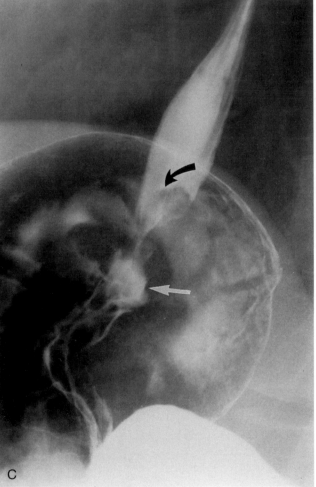

FIGURE 8–31. Three examples (*A* to *C*) of cardiac carcinoma in which normal anatomic landmarks at cardia have been obliterated and replaced by irregular areas of ulceration *(straight arrows).* In all three cases, note polypoid extension of tumor into distal esophagus *(curved arrows).* (*A*, From Levine, M.S., et al.: Carcinoma of the gastric cardia in young people. AJR Am. J. Roentgenol. *140*:69–72, 1983, with permission, © by American Roentgen Ray Society.)

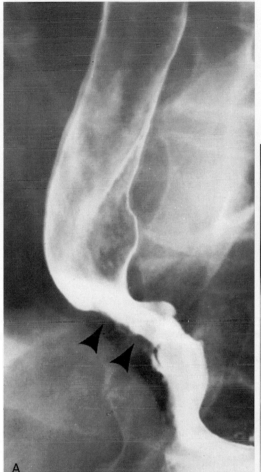

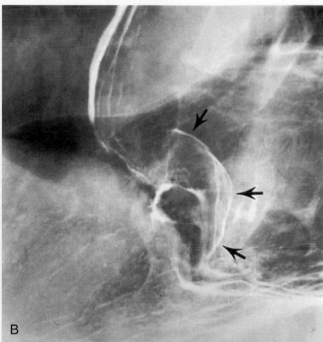

FIGURE 8–32. Carcinoma of the cardia causing dysphagia. *A,* Upright view of esophagus shows minimal irregularity along one wall of distal esophagus *(arrowheads). B,* Right posterior oblique view of fundus shows relatively flat polypoid lesion *(arrows)* surrounding cardia. *C,* Right lateral view of fundus also shows polypoid lesion *(arrowheads)* at cardia. Note small areas of ulceration in tumor.

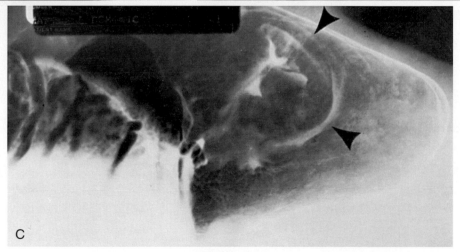

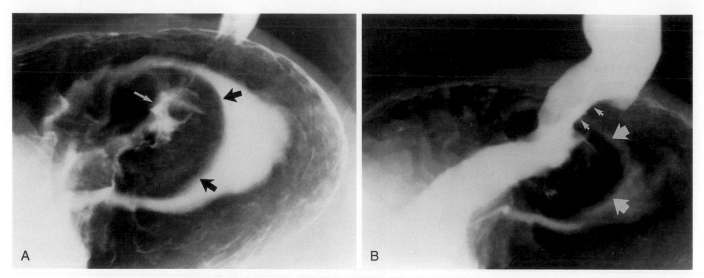

FIGURE 8–33. Carcinoma of the cardia. *A,* Smooth polypoid mass *(black arrows)* is seen surrounding cardia. Note central ulceration *(white arrow)* in mass. This lesion could be mistaken for cardiac rosette with hooding fold. *B,* Repeat view as patient swallows additional barium shows how mass persists *(large arrows)* even as cardia opens. Also note eccentric flattening *(small arrows)* of distal esophagus due to spread of tumor from cardia.

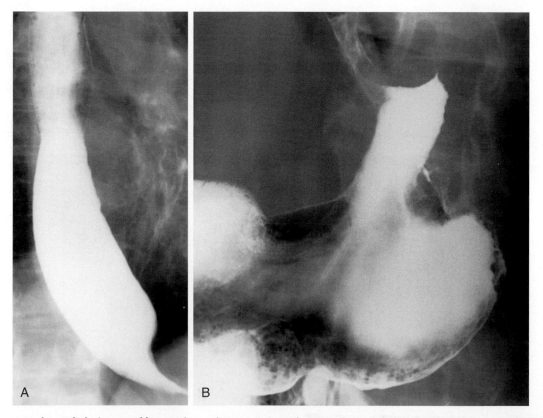

FIGURE 8–34. Secondary achalasia caused by gastric carcinoma. *A,* Smooth, tapered narrowing of distal esophagus, producing classic "bird-beak" appearance of achalasia. *B,* However, radiograph of stomach shows advanced, infiltrating carcinoma of gastric cardia and fundus invading distal esophagus. (From Levine, M.S.: Radiology of the Esophagus, Philadelphia, W.B. Saunders, 1989, p. 179, with permission.)

When a suspicious lesion is detected at the cardia, endoscopy should be performed for a definitive diagnosis. Nevertheless, radiographically diagnosed lesions at the cardia occasionally can be missed on endoscopic examination.[43] The barium study therefore should be repeated, despite a negative endoscopy, if the initial examination suggests a malignant lesion. Rarely, some patients with continuing radiologic evidence of malignancy may require surgery without preoperative histologic confirmation.

Postoperative Carcinoma

In patients who undergo partial gastrectomy for gastric carcinoma, the carcinoma may recur in the gastric remnant. However, patients who undergo partial gastrectomy for ulcer disease or other benign conditions are at increased risk for primary carcinoma of the gastric "stump" developing 5 years or more after the original surgery.[44] These stump carcinomas tend to be located in the distal portion of the gastric remnant near the gastrojejunal anastomosis. Both recurrent carcinomas and stump carcinomas may be manifested on double contrast studies by plaquelike, polypoid, ulcerated, or even scirrhous tumors that encase the gastric remnant, producing a linitis plastica appearance (Fig. 8–35). Endoscopy and

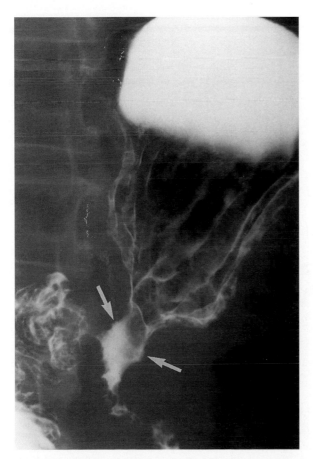

FIGURE 8–35. Recurrent carcinoma in gastric remnant. This patient has undergone a Billroth II partial gastrectomy for gastric carcinoma. Note marked narrowing and irregularity of distal portion of gastric remnant *(arrows)* due to encasement by recurrent tumor.

biopsy should be performed whenever recurrent carcinoma or gastric stump carcinoma is suspected on the basis of the radiographic findings.

Lymphoma

Gastric lymphoma accounts for about 50% of all gastrointestinal lymphomas.[45] The majority of patients have primary gastric lymphoma with disease confined to the stomach and regional lymph nodes, whereas the remainder have generalized lymphoma with associated gastric involvement. Histologically, 90% to 95% of patients have non-Hodgkin's lymphoma, and the remaining 5% to 10% have Hodgkin's disease involving the stomach.[45]

Mucosa-Associated Lymphoid Tissue Lymphoma

Most non-Hodgkin's gastrointestinal lymphomas are of B-cell origin.[46] Many of these B-cell gastrointestinal lymphomas are thought to arise from mucosa-associated lymphoid tissue (MALT) and therefore are classified as MALT lymphomas.[47,48] Paradoxically, low-grade MALT lymphomas often involve the stomach, which normally contains little lymphoid tissue.[47,48] However, chronic infection of the stomach by *Helicobacter pylori* is known to be associated with the development of lymphoid follicles and aggregates in the gastric mucosa.[49,50] In fact, most patients with gastric MALT lymphomas have been shown to have underlying *H. pylori* gastritis.[47,48] It therefore has been postulated that chronic *H. pylori* infection causes proliferation of lymphoid tissue in the gastric mucosa, which predisposes the patient to the development of gastric MALT lymphoma. Unlike high-grade gastric lymphomas, these low-grade MALT lymphomas may undergo complete regression after *H. pylori* has been eradicated from the stomach with antibiotics.[51,52] Thus, low-grade MALT lymphomas are curable lesions. Nevertheless, recent data suggest that untreated MALT lymphomas may undergo transformation to more advanced forms of gastric lymphoma.[53]

Gastric MALT lymphomas may be manifested on double contrast studies by varying-sized, rounded, often confluent nodules in the stomach (Figs. 8–36 to 8–38).[54] In some cases, this mucosal nodularity may be difficult to differentiate from enlarged areae gastricae, a finding also known to be associated with *H. pylori* gastritis.[55] However, areae gastricae tend to be more uniform in size, producing a sharply marginated reticular network (see Fig. 7–4). When gastric MALT lymphoma is suspected on the basis of the radiographic findings, endoscopy and biopsy should be performed for a definitive diagnosis. Although some patients may prove to have gastritis due to *H. pylori* or other causes, it seems reasonable to accept a certain percentage of false-positive diagnoses because of the importance of detecting these low-grade MALT lymphomas before they progress to intermediate or high-grade lymphomas. Radiologists therefore need to be aware of the findings associated with gastric MALT lymphoma because of the opportunity to diagnosis this curable form of gastric lymphoma on double contrast examinations.

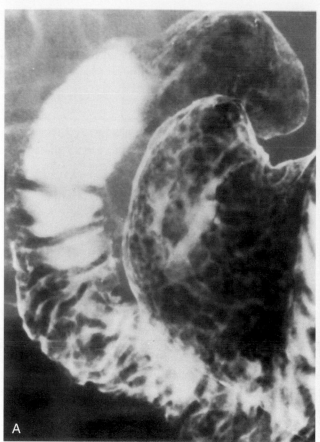

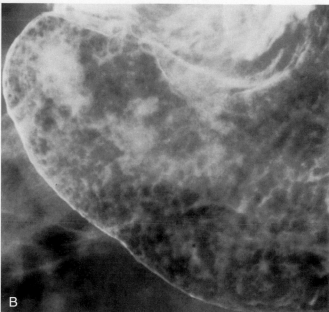

FIGURE 8–36. Two examples (*A* and *B*) of low-grade gastric MALT lymphoma. In both cases, note multiple confluent nodules of varying sizes in gastric antrum. These nodules could be mistaken for enlarged areae gastricae due to *H. pylori* gastritis. (*A* and *B*, From Yoo, C.C., Levine, M.S., Furth, E.E., et al.: Gastric mucosa–associated lymphoid tissue lymphoma: Radiographic findings in six patients. Radiology *208:*239, 1998, with permission.)

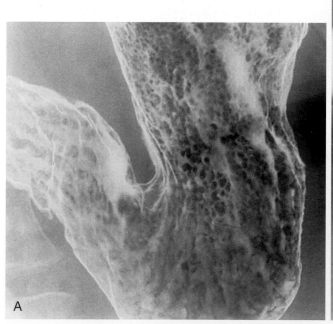

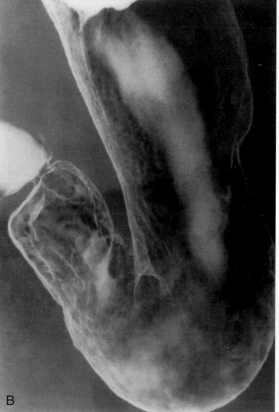

FIGURE 8–37. Low-grade gastric MALT lymphoma. *A,* Varying-sized, confluent nodules are seen in gastric body. *B,* Follow-up study 2 years later shows marked regression of tumor after treatment with antibiotics and chemotherapy. (*A* and *B,* From Yoo, C.C., Levine, M.S., Furth, E.E., et al.: Gastric mucosa–associated lymphoid tissue lymphoma: Radiographic findings in six patients. Radiology *208:*239, 1998, with permission.)

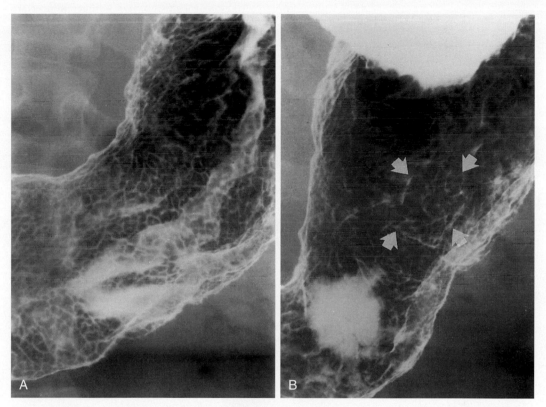

FIGURE 8–38. Development of low-grade gastric MALT lymphoma. *A,* Close-up of gastric body shows enlarged areae gastricae. Although no endoscopic biopsy specimens were obtained, this finding was presumably caused by *H. pylori* gastritis. *B,* Repeat study 6 years later shows focal area of confluent nodularity *(arrows)* superimposed on background of enlarged areae gastricae. Endoscopic biopsy specimens revealed low-grade gastric MALT lymphoma. (*B,* From Yoo, C.C., Levine, M.S., Furth, F.F., et al.: Gastric mucosa–associated lymphoid tissue lymphoma: Radiographic findings in six patients. Radiology *208:*239, 1998, with permission.)

Advanced Lymphoma

Depending on their gross morphology, advanced gastric lymphomas may appear radiographically as infiltrating, polypoid, nodular, or ulcerated lesions (Figs. 8–39 to 8–41), or they may be manifested by thickened folds (Fig. 8–42).[56–60] Occasionally, one or more submucosal masses that are centrally ulcerated may have a characteristic "bull's-eye" or "target" appearance (Fig. 8–43). However, many lesions have mixed morphologic features, so that considerable overlap exists in the radiologic classification of these tumors. The radiologist may not suggest the diagnosis of lymphoma because it is often indistinguishable from adenocarcinoma, a much more common malignant neoplasm in the stomach. Classically, the presence of grossly enlarged rugal folds in a stomach that retains its normal distensibility should suggest the possibility of gastric lymphoma (see Fig. 8–42).[56–60] Occasionally, however, gastric lymphoma may be manifested on double contrast studies by a linitis plastica appearance indistinguishable from a primary scirrhous carcinoma of the stomach (Fig. 8–44).[61] The radiologic findings apparently result from dense infiltrates of lymphomatous cells in the gastric wall without associated fibrosis.[61] Although non-Hodgkin's lymphoma is an unusual cause of linitis plastica, the diagnosis should be suspected in patients who have a history

of lymphoma or evidence of generalized lymphoma at the time of presentation.

Gastric lymphoma has a much better prognosis than gastric carcinoma, with 5-year survival rates approaching 60%.[62,63] As a result, the failure to obtain biopsy specimens from an advanced lesion that is assumed to be inoperable gastric cancer may deprive the patient of the opportunity for cure or long-term palliation. When the radiographic findings suggest a malignant tumor in the stomach, a histologic diagnosis therefore should be obtained because of the possibility of lymphoma. However, deep endoscopic biopsies are usually required for a definite pathologic diagnosis because the lymphomatous tissue tends to infiltrate the gastric wall beneath an intact mucosa. With adequate cytologic and histologic specimens, the endoscopic sensitivity in diagnosing gastric lymphoma may be as high as 90%.[64,65]

Proper staging of gastric lymphoma by CT or other diagnostic tests is important, so that a rational treatment decision can be made about the need for surgery, radiation, or chemotherapy. With the increasing use of systemic chemotherapy for advanced disease, follow-up double contrast studies may also be helpful for documenting the response to treatment and for evaluating abdominal pain or gastrointestinal bleeding after the initiation of systemic

FIGURE 8–39. Infiltrating gastric lymphomas involving antrum *(A)* and fundus *(B)* of stomach.

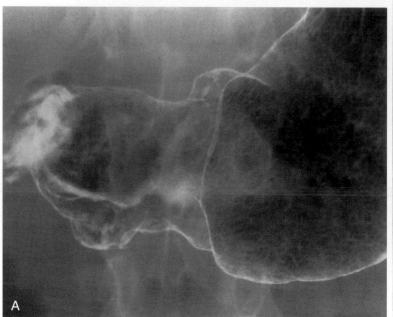

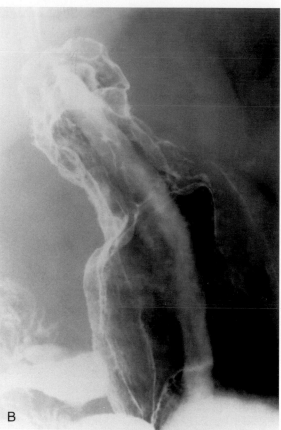

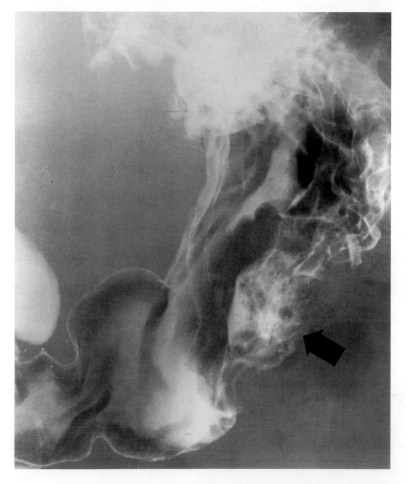

FIGURE 8–40. Gastric lymphoma manifested by polypoid mass on greater curvature with central area of ulceration *(arrow).*

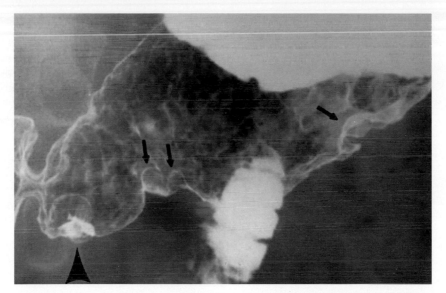

FIGURE 8–41. Gastric lymphoma with multiple small submucosal masses *(arrows).* The most distal mass is ulcerated *(arrowhead).*

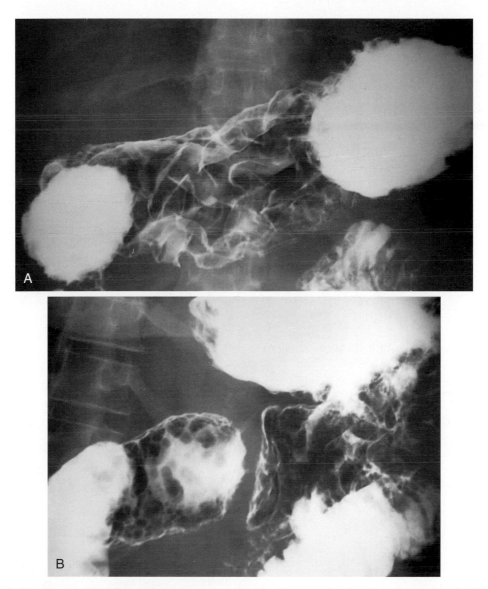

FIGURE 8–42. Gastric lymphoma with diffuse enlargement of rugal folds. Also note duodenal involvement in *B.* (Courtesy of Alec Megibow, M.D., and Patricia Redmond, M.D., New York, New York.)

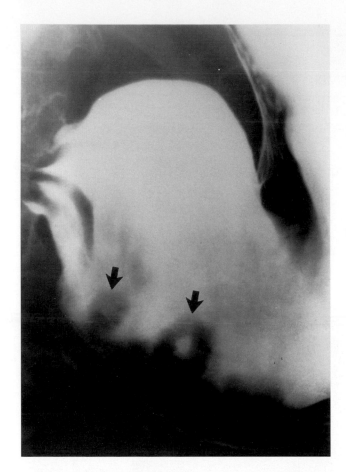

FIGURE 8–43. Gastric lymphoma with centrally ulcerated submucosal masses or bull's-eye lesions *(arrows)* in antrum.

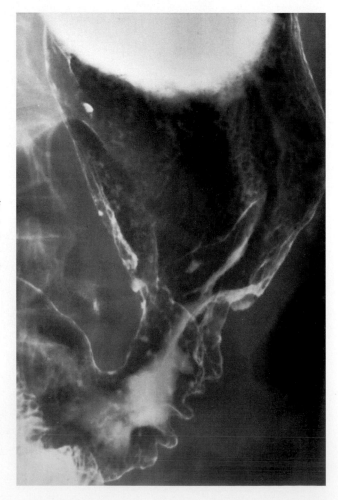

FIGURE 8–44. Gastric lymphoma with linitis plastica. Narrowing of gastric body is marked, with nodularity, ulceration, and sacculation of adjacent greater curvature. Primary scirrhous adenocarcinoma of stomach would be more likely to produce these findings. (From Levine, M.S., Pantongrag-Brown, L, Aguilera, N.S., et al.: Non-Hodgkin lymphoma of the stomach: A cause of linitis plastica. Radiology *201*:375, 1996, with permission.)

chemotherapy. In some patients, chemotherapy may lead to dramatic regression of ulcerated plaques or mass lesions with the development of a benign-appearing ulcer or ulcer scar at the site of the previous lesion (Figs. 8–45A and C).[66] However, chemotherapy may also lead to ulceration or perforation of these lymphomatous lesions with the development of massive upper gastrointestinal bleeding or peritonitis (Fig. 8–45B). These complications may necessitate discontinuation of chemotherapy, resulting in treatment failure.[67]

Metastatic Disease

Hematogenous or blood-borne metastases to the stomach may be manifested radiographically by one or more discrete submucosal masses (Fig. 8–46). As they out-grow their blood supply, these submucosal masses often undergo central necrosis and ulceration, producing characteristic "bull's-eye" or "target" lesions (Fig. 8–47).[68,69] Bull's-eye lesions are frequently seen in patients with metastatic melanoma, but the differential diagnosis includes other metastatic lesions, lymphoma, and, most recently, Kaposi's sarcoma in patients with AIDS (Fig. 8–48).[70–72] Less frequently, hematogenous metastases to the stomach may undergo excavation, producing giant, cavitated lesions (Fig. 8–49).[69] Gastric lymphoma, leiomyosarcoma, and, rarely, adenocarcinoma may produce similar findings. Metastatic breast cancer involving the stomach may also produce a linitis plastica appearance indistinguishable from that of a primary scirrhous carcinoma (see Figs. 8–25A, 8–26, and 8–29; see earlier discussion Scirrhous Tumors).[68,73]

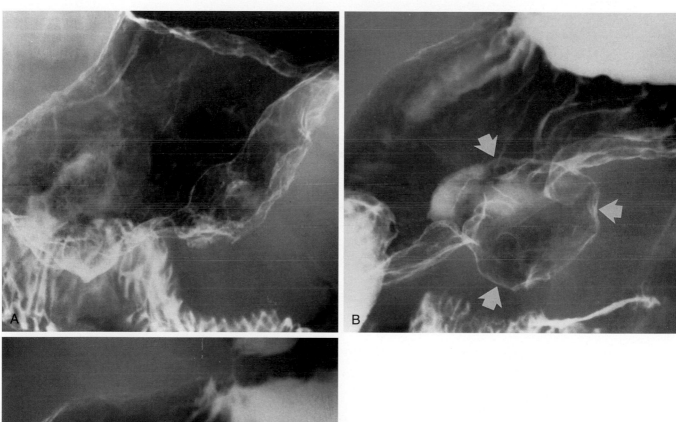

FIGURE 8–45. Response of gastric lymphoma to chemotherapy. *A,* Initial study shows thickened, irregular folds in gastric body due to lymphoma. *B,* After treatment with chemotherapy, follow-up study 6 months later shows regression of lymphoma with large area of cavitation *(arrows)* adjacent to posterior wall of stomach. *C,* Another follow-up study 1 year later shows further regression of lymphoma with radiating folds and tiny, benign-appearing residual ulcer *(arrow)* at site of previous excavation.

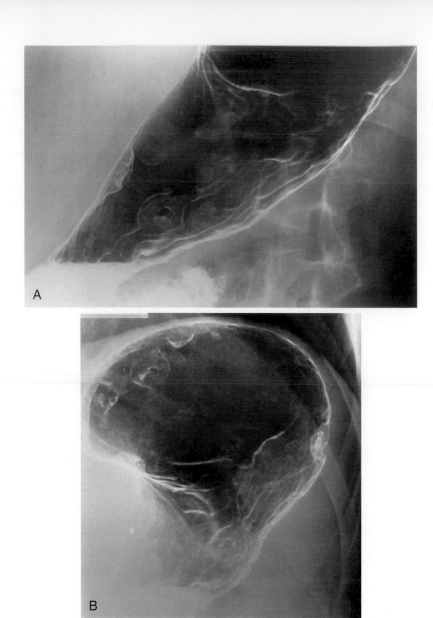

FIGURE 8–46. Multiple small submucosal lesions in stomach due to metastatic melanoma. (Courtesy of Herbert Y. Kressel, M.D., Philadelphia, Pennsylvania.)

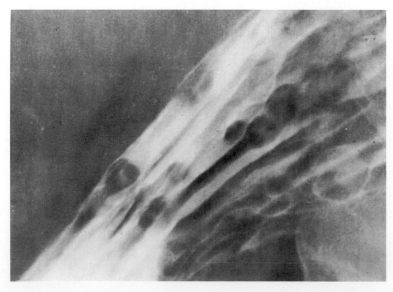

FIGURE 8–47. Multiple ulcerated metastases or bull's-eye lesions in stomach due to adenocarcinoma of unknown origin.

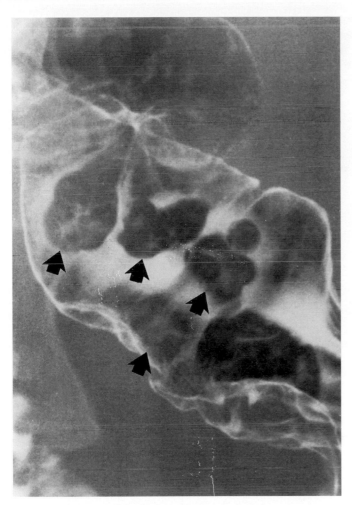

FIGURE **8–48.** **Kaposi's sarcoma involving stomach.** Multiple centrally ulcerated submucosal masses or bull's-eye lesions *(arrows)* are seen in gastric antrum.

The stomach may be directly invaded by malignant tumors arising in neighboring structures such as the esophagus and pancreas. Adenocarcinomas arising in Barrett's esophagus have a particular tendency to invade the gastric cardia and fundus.[74] These lesions may be indistinguishable radiographically from primary carcinomas of the cardia or fundus invading the esophagus (see Fig. 6–29). Depending on their location, carcinomas arising in the head, body, or tail of the pancreas may also invade the stomach, causing mass effect, nodularity, or spiculation of the greater curvature of the antrum or posterior wall of the body and fundus (Fig. 8–50).

The stomach may also be involved by direct extension of colonic or pancreatic carcinoma along mesenteric reflections such as the gastrocolic ligament or transverse mesocolon or by contiguous spread of tumor along the greater omentum (Fig. 8–51). Bulky omental metastases or "omental cakes" are a relatively common finding in patients with disseminated ovarian cancer or other gynecologic or gastrointestinal malignancies. These omental metastases may spread superiorly via the proximal por-

tion of the greater omentum, or gastrocolic ligament, to the greater curvature of the stomach, producing mass effect, nodularity, flattening, or spiculated, tethered mucosal folds on the greater curvature of the gastric antrum or body (Figs. 8–52 and 8–53*A*).[75] Carcinoma of the transverse colon invading the stomach via the gastrocolic ligament may produce identical radiographic findings.[68,76] However, patients with omental metastases involving the stomach almost always have associated colonic involvement, manifested by mass effect, nodularity, or spiculated folds on the superior border of the transverse colon or, in advanced cases, circumferential narrowing of the bowel (Fig. 8–53*B*).[75,77] Thus, a barium enema examination should differentiate omental metastases to the stomach from gastric invasion by carcinoma of the transverse colon. When gastric involvement by omental metastases is suspected on barium studies, CT should be performed to better delineate the nature and extent of metastatic tumor (Fig. 8–54).

Squamous cell carcinoma of the pharynx or esophagus may also spread to the stomach via submucosal esophageal lymphatic vessels that extend subdiaphragmatically to paracardiac, lesser curvature, or celiac nodes. These squamous cell metastases to the stomach usually appear radiographically as discrete submucosal masses in the gastric fundus at a considerable distance from the primary tumor.[78,79] The lesions may be quite large and often contain central areas of ulceration, so that they can be mis-

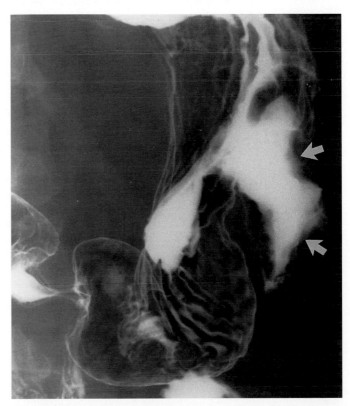

FIGURE **8–49.** Metastatic breast cancer with giant, cavitated lesion *(arrows)* in stomach.

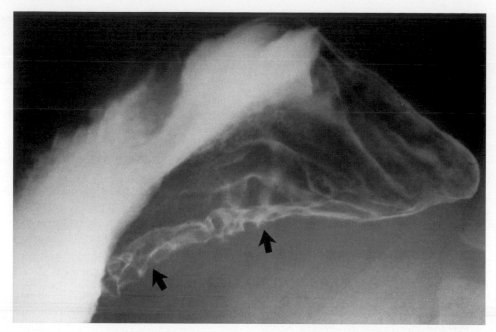

FIGURE 8–50. Carcinoma of tail of pancreas invading stomach with mass effect and spiculation of posterior wall of fundus *(arrows)*.

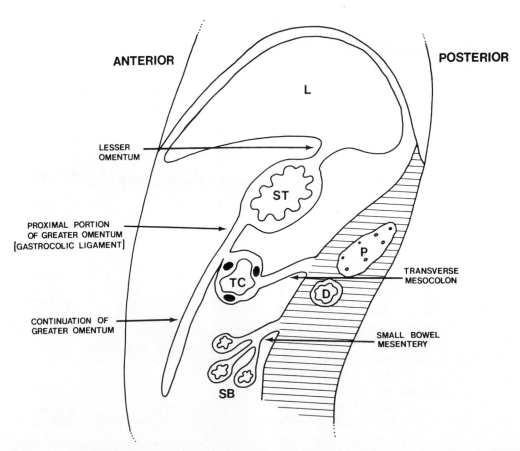

FIGURE 8–51. Sagittal diagram showing mesenteric attachments of stomach, small bowel, and colon. Because proximal portion of greater omentum or gastrocolic ligament inserts along greater curvature of stomach, contiguous spread of tumor from transverse colon or greater omentum primarily affects this region. (From Rubesin, S.E., and Levine, M.S.: Omental cakes: Colonic involvement by omental metastases. Radiology *154*:593–596, 1985, with permission.)

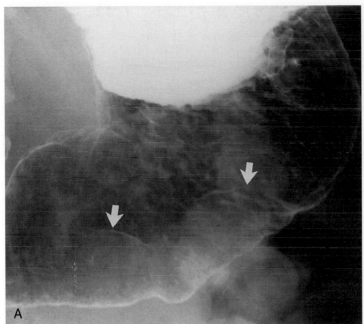

FIGURE 8–52. Gastric involvement by omental metastases from ovarian carcinoma. *A,* Oblique view of stomach shows slight flattening and irregularity of greater curvature due to contiguous spread of tumor from greater omentum. Also note curvilinear defects *(arrows)* caused by extension of tumor anteriorly. *B,* Steep oblique view better delineates metastases to anterior gastric wall *(arrows).* (From Rubesin, S.E., et al.: Gastric involvement by omental cakes: Radiographic findings. Gastrointest. Radiol. *11*:223, 1986, with permission.)

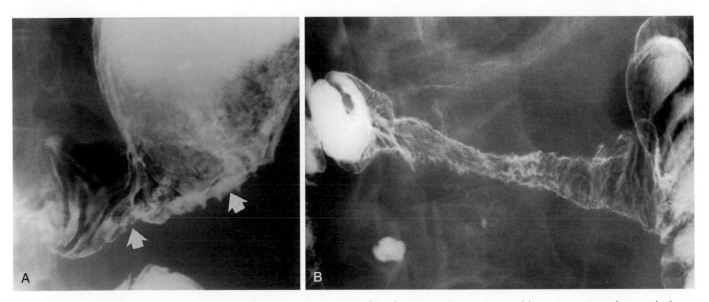

FIGURE 8–53. Gastric and colonic involvement by omental metastases from breast carcinoma. *A,* Double contrast view of stomach shows tethered, spiculated mucosal folds on greater curvature *(arrows)* due to direct extension of omental tumor. *B,* Close-up view from double contrast barium enema shows circumferential narrowing and fixation of transverse colon with severely distorted mucosal folds due to simultaneous colonic involvement by omental tumor. (From Rubesin, S.E., et al.: Gastric involvement by omental cakes: Radiographic findings. Gastrointest. Radiol. *11*:223, 1986, with permission.)

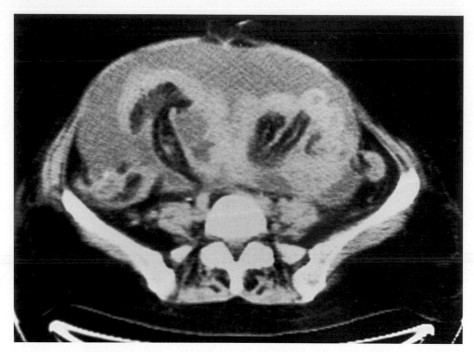

FIGURE 8–54. CT scan showing characteristic appearance of bulky omental metastases or "omental cake" in anterior portion of abdomen.

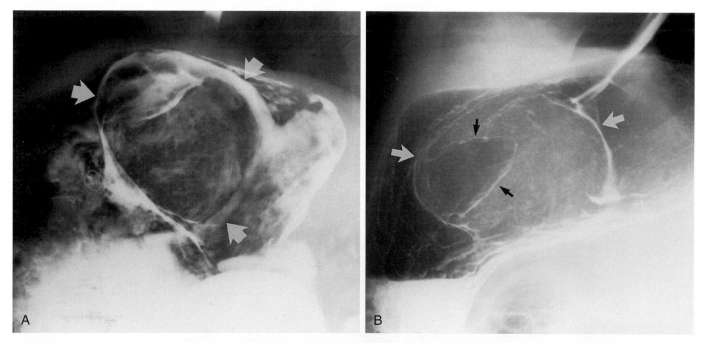

FIGURE 8–55. Squamous cell metastases to gastric cardia manifested by giant submucosal masses *(white arrows)* that could be mistaken for leiomyomas or leiomyosarcomas. Note triangular area of ulceration *(black arrows)* in B. (A, From Glick, S.N., et al.: Squamous cell metastases to the gastric cardia. Gastrointest. Radiol. *10*:339, 1985, with permission.)

taken for ulcerated leiomyomas or leiomyosarcomas (Fig. 8–55). Because the treatment for esophageal cancer depends on the stage of the tumor at the time of diagnosis, the gastric cardia and fundus should be carefully evaluated radiographically in all patients with esophageal cancer to rule out unsuspected metastases to the stomach.

REFERENCES

1. Gordon, R., Laufer, I., and Kressel, H.Y.: Gastric polyps found on routine double-contrast examination of the stomach. Radiology 134:27, 1980.
2. Feczko, P.J., Halpert, R.D., and Ackerman, L.V.: Gastric polyps: Radiologic evaluation and clinical significance. Radiology 155:581, 1985.
3. Op den Orth, J.O., and Ploem, S.: The stalactite phenomenon on double contrast studies of the stomach. Radiology 117:523, 1975.
4. Aronchick, J., Laufer, I., and Glick, S.N.: Barium stalactites: Observations on their nature and significance. Radiology 149:588, 1983.
5. Ming, S.C., and Goldman, H.: Gastric polyps: A histogenetic classification and its relation to carcinoma. Cancer 18:721, 1965.
6. Tomosulo, J.: Gastric polyps: Histologic types and their relationship to gastric carcinoma. Cancer 27:1346, 1971.
7. Ming, S.-C.: The adenoma-carcinoma sequence in the stomach and colon. II. Malignant potential of gastric polyps. Gastrointest. Radiol. 1:121, 1976.
8. Op den Orth, J.O., and Dekker, W.: Gastric adenomas. Radiology 141:289, 1981.
9. Delikaris, P., Golematis, B., Missitzis, G., et al.: Smooth muscle neoplasms of the stomach. South. Med. J. 76:440, 1983.
10. Hoare, A.M., and Elkington, S.G.: Gastric lesions in generalized neurofibromatosis. Br. J. Surg. 63:449, 1976.
11. Culver, G.J., and Toffolo, R.R.: Criteria for roentgen diagnosis of submucosal gastric lipoma. Radiology 82:254, 1964.
12. Heiken, J.P., Forde, K.A., and Gold, R.P.: Computed tomography as a definitive method for diagnosing gastrointestinal lipomas. Radiology 142:409, 1982.
13. Imoto, T., Nobe, T., Koga, M., et al.: Computed tomography of gastric lipomas. Gastrointest. Radiol. 8:129, 1983.
14. O'Riordan, D., Levine, M.S., and Yeager, B.A.: Complete healing of ulceration within a gastric leiomyoma. Gastrointest. Radiol. 10:47, 1985.
15. Kilman, W.J., and Berk, R.N.: The spectrum of radiographic features of aberrant pancreatic rests involving the stomach. Radiology 123:291, 1977.
16. Thoeni, R.F., and Gedgaudas, R.K.: Ectopic pancreas: Usual and unusual features. Gastrointest. Radiol. 5:37, 1980.
17. Herlinger, H.: The recognition of exogastric tumors: Report of six cases. Br. J. Radiol. 39:25, 1966.
18. Low, V.H.S., Levine, M.S., Rubesin, S.E., et al.: Diagnosis of gastric carcinoma: Sensitivity of double-contrast barium studies. AJR Am. J. Roentgenol. 162:329, 1994.
19. Llanos, O, Guzman, S, Duarte, I.: Accuracy of the first endoscopic procedure in the differential diagnosis of gastric lesions. Ann. Surg. 195:224, 1982.
20. Graham, D.Y., Schwartz, J.T., Cain, G.D., et al.: Prospective evaluation of biopsy number in the diagnosis of esophageal and gastric carcinoma. Gastroenterology 82:228, 1982.
21. Tatsuta, M., Iishi, H., Okuda, S., et al.: Prospective evaluation of diagnostic accuracy of gastrofibroscopic biopsy in diagnosis of gastric cancer. Cancer 63:1415, 1989.
22. Shirakabe, H., Nishizawa, M., Maruyama, M., et al.: Atlas of X-ray Diagnosis of Early Gastric Cancer, pp. 1–18. New York, Igaku-Shoin Ltd, 1982.
23. Kaneko, E., Nakamura, T., Umeda, N., et al.: Outcome of gastric carcinoma detected by gastric mass survey in Japan. Gut 18:626, 1977.
24. Montesi, A., Graziani, L., Pesaresi, A., et al.: Radiologic diagnosis of early gastric cancer by routine double-contrast examination. Gastrointest. Radiol. 7:205, 1982.
25. Gold, R.P., Greene, P.H., O'Toole, K.M., et al.: Early gastric cancer: Radiographic experience. Radiology 152:283, 1984.
26. White, R.M., Levine, M.S., Enterline, H.T., et al.: Early gastric cancer: Recent experience. Radiology 155:25, 1985.
27. Flerst, S.M.: Carcinoma of the cardia and fundus of the stomach. Am. J. Gastroenterol. 57:403, 1972.
28. Winawer, S.J., Posner, G., Lightdale, C.J., et al.: Endoscopic diagnosis of advanced gastric cancer: Factors influencing yield. Gastroenterology 69:1183, 1975.
29. Levine, M.S., Kong, V., Rubesin, S.E., et al.: Scirrhous carcinoma of the stomach: Radiologic and endoscopic diagnosis. Radiology 175:151, 1990.
30. Balthazar, E.J., Rosenberg, H., and Davidian, M.M.: Scirrhous carcinoma of the pyloric channel and distal antrum. AJR Am. J. Roentgenol. 134:669, 1980.
31. Evans, E., Harris, O., Dickey, D., et al.: Difficulties in the endoscopic diagnosis of gastric and oesophageal cancer. Aust. NZ J. Surg. 55:541, 1985.
32. Cady, B, Ramsden, D.A., Stein, A., et al.: Gastric cancer: Contemporary aspects. Am. J. Surg. 133:423, 1977.
33. Antonioli, D.A., and Goldman, H.: Changes in the location and type of gastric adenocarcinoma. Cancer 50:775, 1982.
34. Meyers, W.C., Damiano, R.J., Rotolo, F.S., et al.: Adenocarcinoma of the stomach: Changing patterns over the last 4 decades. Ann. Surg. 205:1, 1987.
35. Levine, M.S., Laufer, I., and Thompson, J.J.: Carcinoma of the gastric cardia in young people. AJR Am. J. Roentgenol. 140:69, 1983.
36. Freeny, P.C.: Double-contrast gastrography of the fundus and cardia: Normal landmarks and their pathologic changes. AJR Am. J. Roentgenol. 133:481, 1979.
37. Herlinger, H., Grossman, R., Laufer, I., et al.: The gastric cardia in double-contrast study: Its dynamic image. AJR Am. J. Roentgenol. 135:21, 1980.
38. Kobayashi, S., Yamada, A., Kawai, B., et al.: Study on early cancer of the cardiac region: X-ray findings of the surrounding area of the oesophago-gastric junction. Australas. Radiol. 16:258, 1972.
39. Freeny, P.C., and Marks, W.M.: Adenocarcinoma of the gastroesophageal junction: Barium and CT examination. AJR Am. J. Roentgenol. 138:1077, 1982.
40. Balthazar, E.J., Goldfine, S., and Davidian, N.M.: Carcinoma of the esophagogastric junction. Am. J. Gastroenterol. 74:237, 1980.
41. Lawson, T.L., and Dodds, W.J.: Infiltrating carcinoma simulating achalasia. Gastrointest. Radiol. 1:245, 1976.
42. Seaman, W.B., Wells, J., and Flood, C.A.: Diagnostic problems of esophageal cancer: Relationship to achalasia and hiatus hernia. AJR Am. J. Roentgenol. 90:778, 1963.
43. Milnes, J.P., Hine, K.R., Holmes, G.K.T., et al.: Limitations of endoscopy in the diagnosis of carcinoma of the cardia of the stomach. Br. J. Radiol. 55:593, 1982.
44. Feldman, F., and Seaman, W.B.: Primary gastric stump carcinoma. AJR Am. J. Roentgenol. 115:257, 1972.
45. Brady, L.W.: Malignant lymphoma of the gastrointestinal tract. Radiology 137:291, 1980.
46. Papadimitriou, C.S., Papacharalampous, N.X., and Kittas, C.: Primary gastrointestinal lymphoma: A morphologic and immunohistochemical study. Cancer 55:870, 1985.
47. Wotherspoon, A.C., Ortiz-Hidalgo, C., Falzon, M. R., et al.: *Helicobacter pylori*–associated gastritis and primary B-cell gastric lymphoma. Lancet 338:1175, 1991.
48. Eidt, S., Stolte, M., and Fischer, R.: *Helicobacter pylori* gastritis and primary gastric non-Hodgkin's lymphomas. J. Clin. Pathol. 47:436, 1994.
49. Eidt, S., and Stolte, M.: Prevalence of lymphoid follicles and aggregates in *Helicobacter pylori* gastritis in antral and body mucosa. J. Clin. Pathol. 46:832, 1993.
50. Genta, A.M., Hamner, H.W., and Graham, D.Y.: Gastric lymphoid follicles in *Helicobacter pylori* infection: Frequency, distribution, and response to triple therapy. Hum. Pathol. 24:577, 1994.
51. Wotherspoon, A.C., Doglioni, C., Diss, T.C., et al: Regression of primary low-grade B-cell gastric lymphoma of mucosa-associated lymphoid tissue type after eradication of *Helicobacter pylori*. Lancet 342:575, 1993.
52. Bayerdorffer, E., Neubaeur, A., Rudolph, B., et al.: Regression of primary gastric lymphoma of mucosa-associated lymphoid tissue type after cure of *Helicobacter pylori* infection. Lancet 345:1591, 1995.
53. Chan, J.K.C., Ng, C.S., and Isaacson, P.G.: Relationship between high-grade lymphoma and low-grade B-cell mucosa-associated lymphoid tissue lymphoma (MALToma) of the stomach. Am. J. Pathol. 136:1153, 1990.

54. Yoo, C.C., Levine, M.S., Furth, E.E., et al.: Gastric mucosa-associated lymphoid tissue lymphoma: Radiographic findings in six patients. Radiology *208*:239, 1998.

55. Sohn, J., Levine, M.S., Furth, E.E., et al.: *Helicobacter pylori* gastritis: Radiographic findings. Radiology *195*:763, 1995.

56. Menuck, L.S.: Gastric lymphoma: A radiologic diagnosis. Gastrointest. Radiol. *1*:157, 1976.

57. Privette, J.T.J., Davies, E.R., and Roylance, J.: The radiologic features of gastric lymphoma. Clin. Radiol. *28*:457, 1977.

58. Zornoza, J., and Dodd, G.D.: Lymphoma of the gastrointestinal tract. Semin. Roentgenol. *15*:272, 1980.

59. Fork, F.T., Ekberg, O., and Haglund, U.: Radiology in primary gastric lymphoma. Acta Radiol. Diagn. *25*:481, 1984.

60. Levine, M.S., Rubesin, S.E., Pantongrag-Brown, L., et al.: Non-Hodgkin's lymphoma of the gastrointestinal tract: Radiographic findings. AJR Am. J. Roentgenol. *168*:165, 1997.

61. Levine, M.S., Pantongrag-Brown, L, Aguilera, N.S., et al.: Non-Hodgkin lymphoma of the stomach: A cause of linitis plastica. Radiology *201*:375, 1996.

62. Lim, F.E., Hartman, A.S., Tan, E.G.C., et al.: Factors in the prognosis of gastric lymphoma. Cancer *39*:1715, 1977.

63. Mittal, B., Wasserman, T.H., and Griffith, R.C.: Non-Hodgkin's lymphoma of the stomach. Am. J. Gastroenterol. *78*:780, 1983.

64. Cabre-Fiol, V., and Vilardell, F.: Progress in the cytological diagnosis of gastric lymphoma. Cancer *41*:1456, 1978.

65. Spinelli, P., Gullo, C.L., and Pizzetti, P.: Endoscopic diagnosis of gastric lymphomas. Endoscopy *12*:211, 1980.

66. Fox, E.R., Laufer, I., and Levine, M.S.: Response of gastric lymphoma to chemotherapy: Radiologic appearance. AJR Am. J. Roentgenol. *142*:711, 1984.

67. Rosenfelt, F., and Rosenberg, S.A.: Diffuse histiocytic lymphoma presenting with gastrointestinal tract lesions. Cancer *45*:2188, 1980.

68. Meyers, M.A., and McSweeney, J.: Secondary neoplasms of the bowel. Radiology *105*:1, 1972.

69. Libshitz, H.I., Lindell, M.M., and Dodd, G.D.: Metastases to the hollow viscera. Radiol. Clin. North Am. *20*:487, 1982.

70. Goldstein, H.M., Beydoun, M.T., and Dodd, G.D.: Radiologic spectrum of melanoma metastatic to the gastrointestinal tract. AJR Am. J. Roentgenol. *129*:605, 1977.

71. Dunnick, R., Harell, G.S., and Parker, B.R.: Multiple bull's eye lesions in gastric lymphoma. AJR Am. J. Roentgenol. *126*:965, 1976.

72. Rose, H.S., Balthazar, E.J., Megibow, A.J., et al.: Alimentary tract involvement in Kaposi sarcoma: Radiographic and endoscopic findings in 25 homosexual men. AJR Am. J. Roentgenol. *139*:661, 1982.

73. Joffe, N.: Metastatic involvement of the stomach secondary to breast carcinoma. AJR Am. J. Roentgenol. *123*:512, 1975.

74. Levine, M.S., Caroline, D., Thompson, J.J., et al.: Adenocarcinoma of the esophagus: Relationship to Barrett mucosa. Radiology *150*:305, 1984.

75. Rubesin, S.E., Levine, M.S., and Glick, S.N.: Gastric involvement by omental cakes: Radiographic findings. Gastrointest. Radiol. *11*:223, 1986.

76. Bachman, A.L.: Roentgen appearance of gastric invasion from carcinoma of the colon. Radiology *63*:814, 1954.

77. Rubesin, S.E., and Levine, M.S.: Omental cakes: Colonic involvement by omental metastases. Radiology *154*:593, 1985.

78. Glick, S.N., Teplick, S.K., and Levine, M.S.: Squamous cell metastases to the gastric cardia. Gastrointest. Radiol. *10*:339, 1985.

79. Glick, S.N., Teplick, S.K., and Levine, M.S.: Gastric cardia metastasis in esophageal carcinoma. Radiology *160*:627, 1986.

9

Duodenum

MARC S. LEVINE
IGOR LAUFER
GILES STEVENSON

Fiberoptic endoscopy has exposed the limitations of conventional single contrast radiography in evaluating the duodenum, as 20% to 35% of lesions may be missed with single contrast technique.[1,2] However, the double contrast study has increased our radiologic sensitivity in this area to more than 90%.[3-5] Most false-negative results occur with examinations that the radiologist can recognize and report as less than ideal. The first part of this chapter therefore is devoted to some aspects of technique and anatomy that may help radiologists to indicate with confidence that the duodenum is normal. The finding of a normal duodenum depends upon the clear demonstration of normal anatomic landmarks in this region. The second part of the chapter deals with some of the common abnormalities found in and around the duodenum.

TECHNIQUE

In the past, double contrast duodenography was performed as a selective technique, utilizing a duodenal tube and hypotonia for evaluation of suspected pancreaticoduodenal disorders.[6,7] However, it is possible to perform "tubeless" hypotonic duodenography by using an effervescent agent to introduce gas into the stomach and duodenum.[8,9] With appropriate positioning of the patient, double contrast views of the duodenum can be readily

obtained. The modified technique of double contrast hypotonic duodenography described in this chapter is included in our routine upper gastrointestinal examination.

Routine Study

In ideal circumstances, radiologic examination of the duodenum would include meticulous fluoroscopic observation, single contrast films with low-density barium, compression spot films, mucosal relief films, and double contrast films with high-density barium. However, it is not feasible to use all these techniques in a single examination. We therefore rely primarily on double contrast technique for examining the duodenum. At the same time, it is important to recognize that overreliance on double contrast technique may result in errors, particularly if mucosal coating is inadequate or if lesions are suspected on the anterior wall of the duodenum. Instead, the study should be performed as a biphasic examination that includes double contrast views of the duodenum with high-density barium and single contrast prone or upright compression views of the duodenum with low-density barium.

The materials and techniques for performing a double contrast examination of the upper gastrointestinal tract are described in detail in Chapter 3. Hypotonic agents are particularly important for optimal delineation of the normal anatomic landmarks in the duodenum. A standard dose of 0.1 mg of glucagon or 20 mg of Busco-pan (hyoscine *N*-butyl bromide) is routinely administered at the beginning of the study to produce adequate hypotonia of the stomach and duodenum.[10] By the time double contrast views of the stomach have been obtained, barium usually has emptied into the duodenum. The patient is then turned to the left posterior oblique (LPO) position for 4-on-1 spot films of the duodenal bulb and vertically split 2-on-1 spot films of the descending duodenum (Fig. 9–1*A*). Even with a hypotonic agent and proper positioning of the patient, the duodenum may collapse intermittently during the fluoroscopic examination. It therefore is important to time the exposures to obtain views of the duodenum when it is optimally distended. The use of digital fluoroscopic equipment affords the radiologist a larger window of opportunity for imaging the duodenum because of the capability for rapid image acquisition.[11]

In some patients, gaseous distention of the stomach creates difficulties by rotating the duodenum more posteriorly. This problem can be overcome by turning the patient to the right posterior oblique (RPO) position (Fig. 9–1*B*) or to a steep LPO (Fig. 9–1*C*), left lateral (Fig.

9–1*D*), or even semiprone left anterior oblique (LAO) position (Fig. 9–1*E*), so that the duodenal bulb and descending duodenum are seen through the gas-filled stomach. If, despite these maneuvers, the bulb is inadequately distended with gas or obscured by barium, it may be necessary to elevate the table to a semiupright or fully upright position. This causes barium to pool in the antrum or descending duodenum and gas to rise into the duodenal bulb, which tends to assume a vertical configuration, so that adequate double contrast views of the bulb can be obtained (Fig. 9–1*F*). However, mucosal coating may deteriorate rapidly in the upright position, so that superficial lesions can sometimes be missed on these views.

When the double contrast portion of the examination is completed, the patient drinks a low-density barium suspension, and additional 4-on-1 prone or right anterior oblique (RAO) spot films of the duodenum are obtained with varying degrees of compression using an inflatable balloon or other prone compression device positioned beneath the patient's abdomen. These views are particularly helpful for showing depressed or protruded lesions on the anterior wall of the duodenum. In other patients, it may also be helpful to obtain upright 4-on-1 spot films

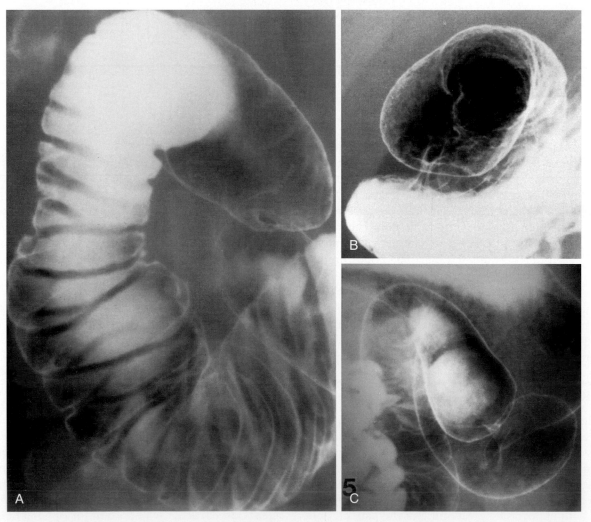

FIGURE 9–1. Normal duodenum. *A,* Ideal visualization of duodenum in LPO projection. Note smooth, featureless appearance of bulb. *B,* Duodenal bulb in RPO projection. *C,* Steep LPO view, projecting duodenum between stomach and jejunum.

of the duodenum with varying degrees of compression. The single contrast phase of the examination becomes even more important when the double contrast phase is suboptimal.

Selective Hypotonic Duodenography

The technique just described is suitable for evaluating the duodenum during routine double contrast upper gastrointestinal examinations. If there is a high clinical suspicion of disease in the duodenum or if the routine examination is equivocal, however, a modified technique for hypotonic duodenography can be used to obtain a more detailed examination of the duodenum. For this technique, the patient is given the effervescent agent and then asked to drink the high-density barium suspension while lying on the right side. In this position, barium should empty rapidly into the duodenum. As soon as the duodenum is seen to fill with barium, a larger dose of hypotonic agent (usually 1 mg of glucagon) is given intravenously to relax the duodenum. The patient is then turned to the left to allow gas to enter the duodenum and achieve adequate duodenal distention. If this technique is unsuccessful, hypotonic duodenography may be performed with a duodenal tube as a last resort.[6,7]

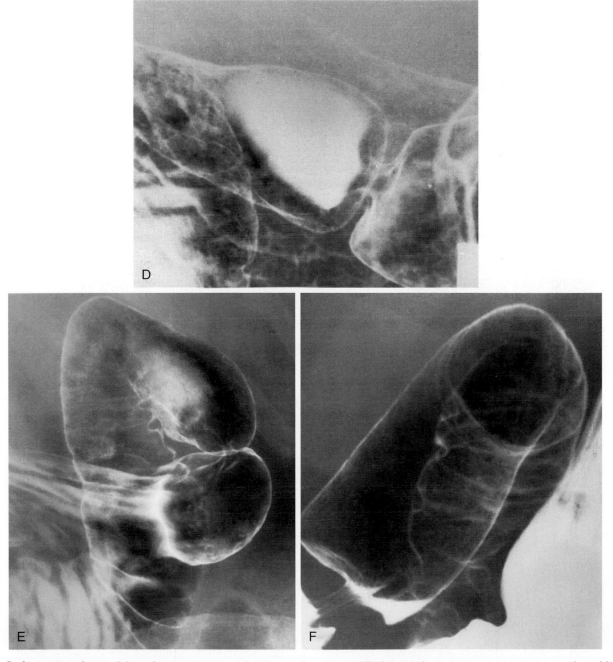

FIGURE 9–1 *Continued* *D,* Left lateral view, projecting duodenum through gas-filled stomach. *E,* Semiprone LAO view with pad between patient's abdomen and table to show bulb clear of stomach. *F,* Upright RPO view of bulb.

NORMAL APPEARANCES

Duodenal Bulb

With intravenous administration of glucagon or Buscopan, the pylorus is frequently seen as a circular ring with a diameter varying from a few millimeters to more than 1 cm (Fig. 9–2A). It normally has a central location at the base of the duodenal bulb. An eccentric location of the pylorus in relation to the stomach and duodenum may indicate scarring from peptic ulcer disease (Fig. 9–2B).

The duodenal bulb usually has a smooth, featureless appearance on double contrast studies (see Fig. 9–1). In about 5% to 10% of patients, however, a lacy, reticular mucosal pattern may be observed in the duodenum as a normal variation (Fig. 9–3).[12] This appearance results from tiny, interlacing circles of barium surrounding 1 to 2 mm lucencies that represent normal villous structures on the duodenal mucosa (Fig. 9–4).[12,13] Occasionally, these surface elevations may be larger and more irregular (Fig. 9–5). In patients with a coarsely nodular mucosa, the findings can be confused with pathologic conditions such as duodenitis, Brunner's gland hyperplasia, and benign lymphoid hyperplasia (see later sections, "Duodenitis" and "Duodenal Tumors"). In other patients, punctate collections of barium may be observed in the duodenum both en face and in profile as a result of trapping of barium in normal mucosal pits (Fig. 9–6).[12,13] This finding should not be mistaken for erosive duodenitis (see later discussion, Duodenitis).

Heaped-up areas of redundant mucosa are sometimes identified as a normal finding on the inner aspect of the superior duodenal flexure between the duodenal bulb and the proximal descending duodenum.[14,15] In some projections this finding can mimic a polyp, ulcer, or even ulcerated submucosal mass in the duodenum (Fig. 9–7). As a result, it has been described as the "flexural pseudolesion" or "flexural fallacy."[14,15] However, this redundant mucosal fold can be differentiated from true pathologic lesions by its characteristic location and changeable appearance at fluoroscopy.

Duodenal Loop

The major landmarks of the duodenal sweep are the circular valvulae conniventes and the papillae.[16] The ampulla of Vater usually lies on the medial aspect of the second portion of the duodenum and is approximately 5 mm in diameter (Fig. 9–8). Its position may vary from the midpoint of the second portion of the duodenum to as far distally as the third portion. Endoscopic analysis of the ampulla has revealed three common types: hemispheric, flat, and papillary (Fig. 9–9). The ampulla is often recognized radiographically by its associated mucosal folds (Fig. 9–10). A distal longitudinal fold and hooding fold are present in approximately 90% of patients. A proximal longitudinal fold and oblique folds are identified less frequently.

The minor or accessory papilla is located adjacent to the orifice of the minor pancreatic duct or Santorini's duct and usually is not patent. It seldom has a distal longitudinal fold, and even the hooding fold is rarely prominent. The minor papilla lies approximately 1 cm proximal to the major papilla and 30 to 45 degrees anterior to it. Thus, in the supine LPO position, the major papilla can often be seen posteriorly in the second portion of the duodenum, whereas the minor papilla, when identifiable, is seen tangentially on the medial wall of the duodenum (see Fig. 9–8A). Conversely, in the prone position, the major papilla can often be identified on the medial aspect of the second portion of the duodenum, whereas the minor papilla is seen anteriorly a short distance proximal to the major papilla (see Fig. 9–8B). This relationship between the major and minor papillae is amazingly constant. However, the minor papilla varies greatly in size and is sometimes as large as the major papilla (Fig. 9–11A).

Text continues on page 248

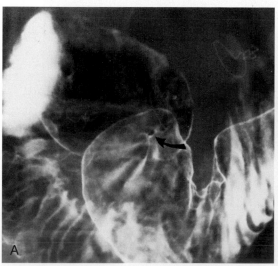
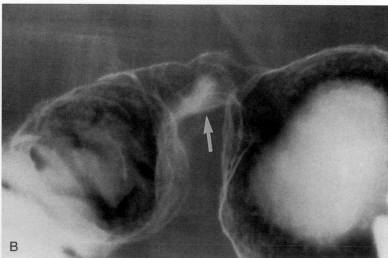

FIGURE 9–2. The pylorus. *A,* Normal pylorus seen as circular lucency *(arrow)* with folds radiating to this site. *B,* Widened, eccentric pylorus *(arrow)* due to scarring from peptic ulcer disease.

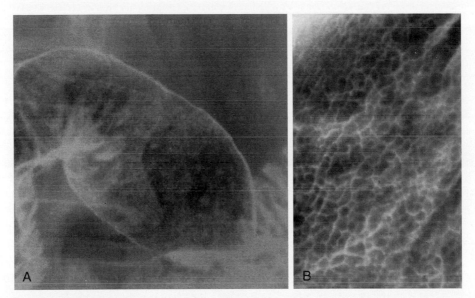

FIGURE 9–3. Normal mucosal surface pattern of duodenum. *A,* Fine villous pattern seen in duodenal bulb as normal variation. *B,* In contrast, much coarser surface pattern (i.e., the areae gastricae) is seen in stomach.

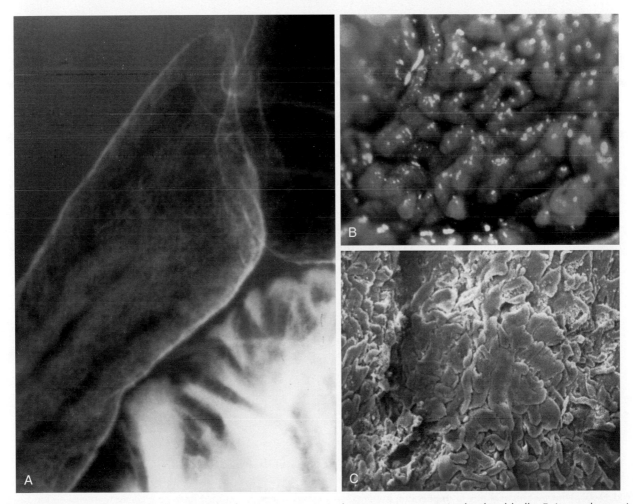

FIGURE 9–4. Normal mucosal surface pattern of duodenum. *A,* Lacy reticular pattern is present in duodenal bulb. *B,* In another patient, photograph of mucosal surface of bulb with dissecting microscope (× 10) shows tiny villous structures with sulci in between. *C,* Scanning electron microscopy at low power (× 20) shows numerous villi surrounded by tiny sulci. Trapping of barium in these sulci or grooves presumably accounts for the fine reticular pattern seen on double contrast studies. (*B* and *C,* From Bova, J.G., et al.: The normal mucosal surface pattern of the duodenal bulb: Radiologic-histologic correlation. AJR Am. J. Roentgenol. *145:*735–738, 1985, with permission, © by American Roentgen Ray Society.)

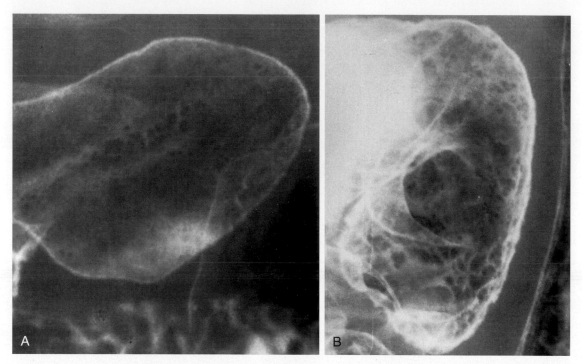

FIGURE 9–5. Larger, more irregular surface elevations in bulb. In both cases, endoscopic biopsy specimens revealed normal duodenal mucosa.

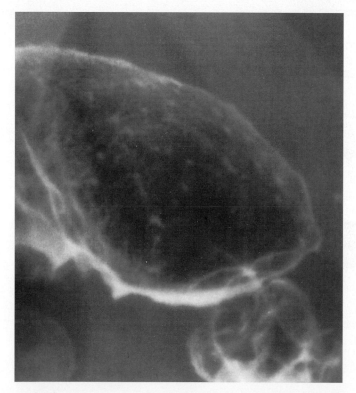

FIGURE 9–6. Normal mucosal pits in duodenum. Punctate collections of barium trapped in these pits can be mistaken for duodenal erosions. (From Bova, J.G., et al.: The normal mucosal surface pattern of the duodenal bulb: Radiologic-histologic correlation. AJR Am. J. Roentgenol. *145:*735–738, 1985, with permission, © by American Roentgen Ray Society.)

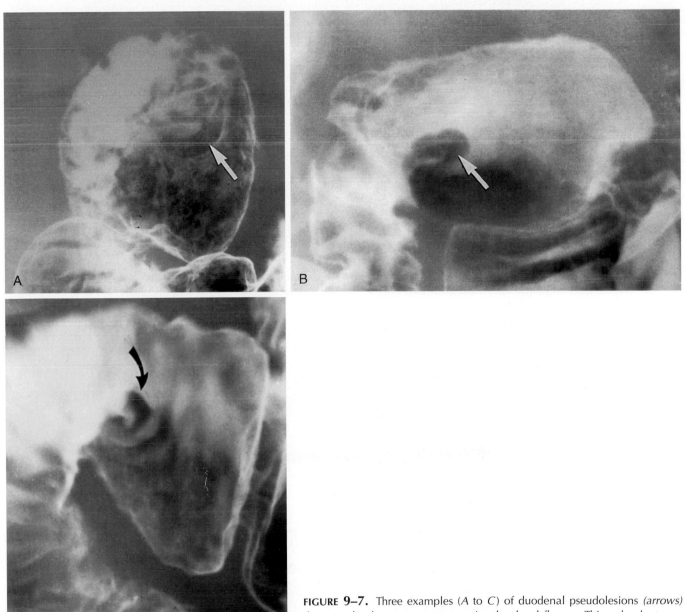

FIGURE 9–7. Three examples (*A* to *C*) of duodenal pseudolesions *(arrows)* due to redundant mucosa at superior duodenal flexure. This redundant mucosa sometimes can simulate polyps or ulcers.

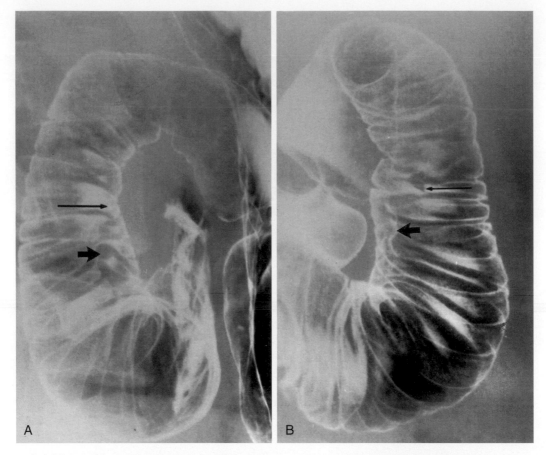

FIGURE 9–8. Duodenal loop with major and minor papillae. *A,* Supine LPO view shows major papilla *(short arrow)* on posterior wall of descending duodenum with minor papilla *(long arrow)* seen tangentially on medial wall 1 to 2 cm proximal to major papilla. *B,* Prone view shows major papilla *(short arrow)* on medial wall of descending duodenum with minor papilla *(long arrow)* seen anteriorly above this level.

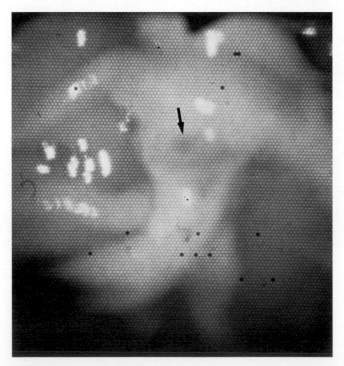

FIGURE 9–9. Endoscopic appearance of normal papilla. Note flat papilla with dark central area *(arrow)* representing the orifice. Hooding fold, distal longitudinal fold, and oblique folds are all clearly visible (see text).

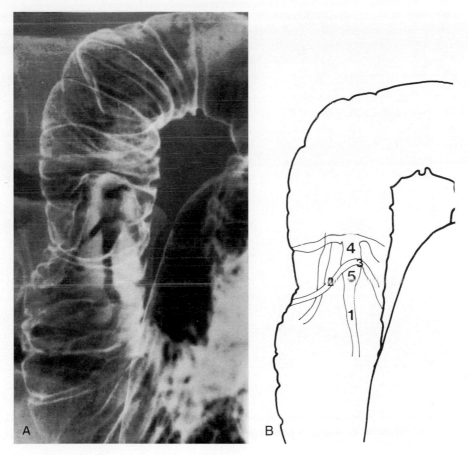

FIGURE 9–10. The ampulla of Vater and its associated folds. *1,* Distal longitudinal fold, present in most patients. *2,* Oblique folds—variable. *3,* Hooding fold, also present in most patients. *4,* Proximal longitudinal fold—variable. *5,* Ampulla of Vater.

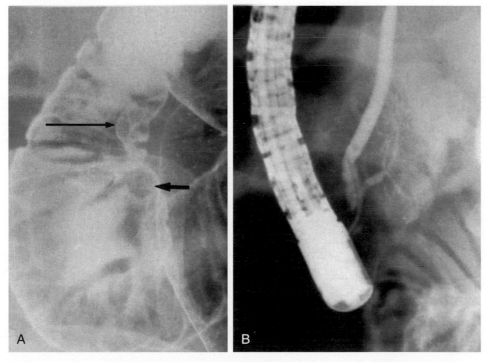

FIGURE 9–11. Unusually large minor papilla in patient with pancreas divisum. *A,* Major papilla *(short arrow)* and unusually large minor papilla *(long arrow)* are seen in descending duodenum. *B,* Injection of major papilla at endoscopic retrograde cholangiopancreatography (ERCP) shows filling of common bile duct and small dorsal pancreatic duct system in head of pancreas. No communication is seen with major portion of pancreatic duct, which must be draining through the enlarged minor papilla in this patient with pancreas divisum.

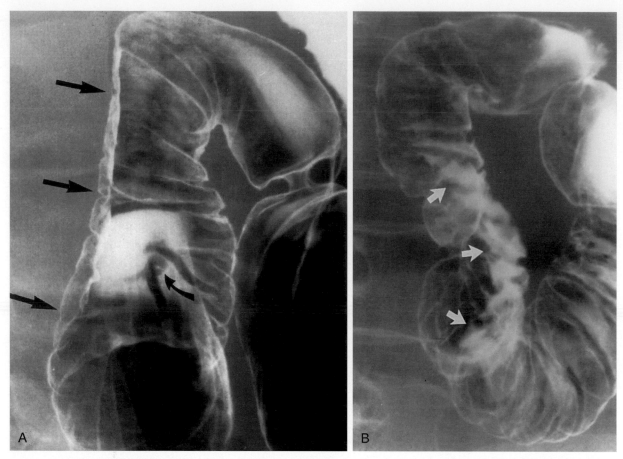

FIGURE 9–12. Extrinsic impressions on descending duodenum. *A,* Normal impression *(arrows)* along lateral aspect of descending duodenum from right kidney. *B,* More lobulated area of extrinsic mass effect *(arrows)* on duodenum from renal cell carcinoma.

The minor papilla may be patent and draining a significant portion of the pancreas, particularly in patients with pancreas divisum (Fig. 9–11*B*).

Demonstration of the major or minor papilla or the normal villous surface pattern of the duodenal bulb is seldom important. However, clear delineation of these anatomic landmarks indicates that the examination has been technically satisfactory and therefore increases the reliability of the radiologic diagnosis of a normal duodenum.

Extrinsic Impressions

Neighboring structures may produce a variety of extrinsic impressions on the gas-filled duodenum, particularly in thin patients. A smooth indentation may be observed on the superolateral border of the duodenal bulb from the gallbladder or on the posterolateral border of the descending duodenum from the right kidney (Fig. 9–12*A*). An enlarged kidney or polycystic kidney occasionally may produce a more prominent or lobulated area of mass effect posteriorly or laterally on the duodenum (Fig. 9–12*B*). Although the pancreas normally may cause some flattening of the medial border of the descending duodenum, significant compression or effacement of the duodenum in this region should suggest pancreatic disease (see later discussion, Pancreatic Diseases).

DUODENAL ULCERS

During the past two decades, it has become increasingly clear that *Helicobacter pylori* infection of the stomach is a major factor in the development of duodenal ulcers. In various studies, the prevalence of *H. pylori* gastritis has ranged from 90% to 100% in patients with duodenal ulcers.[17] These patients often have evidence of gastric metaplasia at the border of the ulcers and *H. pylori* infection of the metaplastic epithelium.[18] The infected mucosa therefore may be more susceptible to ulceration. Other studies have shown that treatment of duodenal ulcers with a combination of histamine-receptor antagonists (H_2 blockers) and antibiotics leads to higher rates of ulcer healing and lower rates of ulcer recurrence than treatment with H_2 blockers alone.[19,20] As a result, a National Institutes of Health consensus panel concluded that all patients with *H. pylori* who have duodenal ulcers should receive antibiotics and conventional antiulcer agents to accelerate healing of ulcers and decrease the rate of ulcer recurrence.[21]

Duodenal ulcers, unlike gastric ulcers, are virtually always benign. When these ulcers are detected on double contrast studies, endoscopy therefore is no longer required to differentiate benign and malignant lesions. However, a significant percentage of duodenal ulcers is

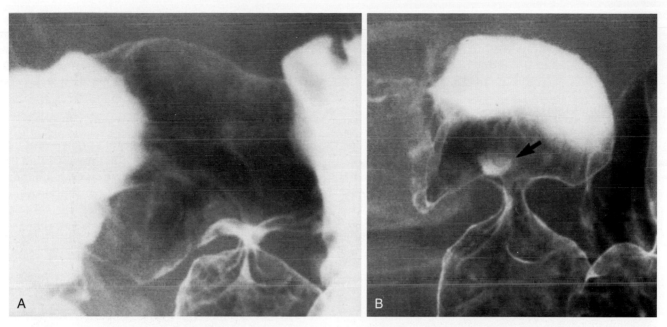

FIGURE 9–13. Importance of mucosal coating for demonstrating duodenal ulcers. *A,* Well-distended but poorly coated duodenal bulb. No ulcer is seen. *B,* With better mucosal coating, ulcer crater *(arrow)* is now clearly visible at base of bulb.

located on the anterior wall of the duodenal bulb, so that a definitive diagnosis is best made during the compression phase of the examination. Furthermore, duodenal ulcers may be obscured by edema, spasm, or scarring of the bulb. Radiologists therefore should be aware of the limitations of double contrast studies for diagnosing duodenal ulcers and of the need for performing a biphasic examination in these patients.

Technical Considerations

Adequate mucosal coating is essential for the detection of duodenal ulcers because an ulcer crater can easily be missed in a poorly coated bulb (Fig. 9–13). Duodenal spasm and deformity can also mask an ulcer crater, so that hypotonic agents such as glucagon are used to facilitate detection of ulcers by relaxing the duodenum (Fig. 9–14). Finally, the radiologic examination should include prone

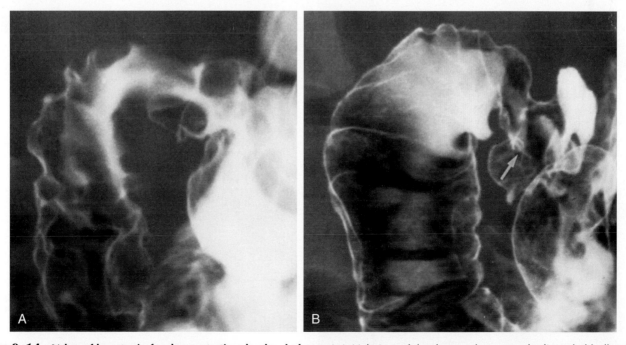

FIGURE 9–14. Value of hypotonia for demonstrating duodenal ulcers. *A,* Initial view of duodenum shows poorly distended bulb without definite ulcer. *B,* After intravenous glucagon, distention of duodenum is much better. As a result, the deformed bulb and ulcer crater *(arrow)* can now be recognized.

or upright compression views of the duodenum with low-density barium to detect ulcers on the anterior wall of the bulb (see following section).[22] Thus, double contrast technique complements but in no way replaces conventional techniques for the diagnosis of duodenal ulcers.

Features of Duodenal Ulcers
Location

About 95% of duodenal ulcers are located in the duodenal bulb and the remaining 5% in the postbulbar duodenum.[23] Bulbar ulcers may involve the apex, central portion, or base of the bulb (Fig. 9–15). Unlike gastric ulcers,

which rarely occur on the anterior wall, as many as 50% of duodenal ulcers are located on the anterior wall of the bulb.[2,24] When they occur, postbulbar ulcers usually are located in the proximal descending duodenum above the papilla of Vater (see later discussion, Postbulbar Ulcers).

Size

Most duodenal ulcers diagnosed on double contrast studies are less than 1 cm. A major advantage of double contrast technique is its ability to demonstrate small duodenal ulcers, frequently no more than several millimeters in diameter (Fig. 9–16). Conversely, giant ulcers (ulcers

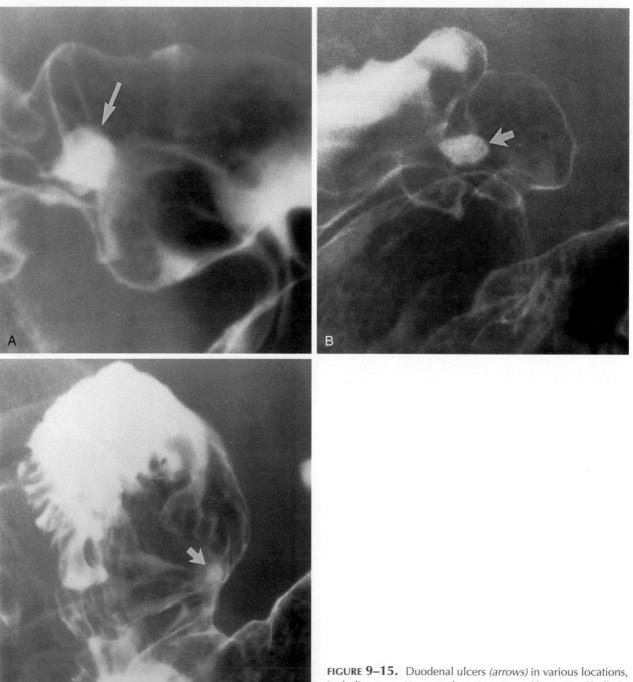

FIGURE 9–15. Duodenal ulcers *(arrows)* in various locations, including apex *(A)*, central portion *(B)*, and base *(C)* of bulb. In all cases, note folds radiating toward ulcer crater.

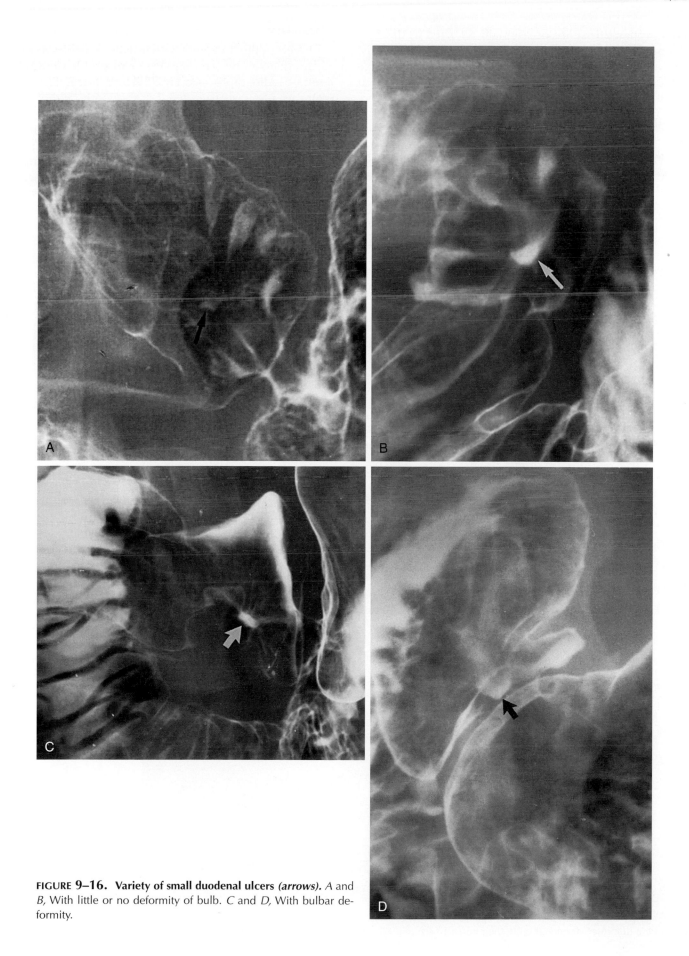

FIGURE 9–16. **Variety of small duodenal ulcers** *(arrows).* *A* and *B,* With little or no deformity of bulb. *C* and *D,* With bulbar deformity.

greater than 2 cm) are occasionally detected in the duodenum.[25] These ulcers can be so large that they replace virtually the entire duodenal bulb (Fig. 9–17). Paradoxically, giant ulcers can be mistaken for a normal or scarred bulb. However, their constant size and shape at fluoroscopy should help to differentiate these lesions from the changing appearance of the bulb.[25]

Shape

Most duodenal ulcers appear radiographically as round or ovoid barium collections. However, about 5% of duodenal ulcers have a linear configuration (Fig. 9–18).[26,27] These linear ulcers may be located near the base of the duodenal bulb, and they sometimes have a transverse orientation in relation to the bulb (see Fig. 9–18A).[27] As in the stomach, linear ulcers are thought to represent a stage of ulcer healing.[27,28] In fact, they may be indistinguishable from linear ulcer scars.

Morphology

Ulcers in the duodenal bulb usually appear as discrete niches that can be seen en face or in profile on double contrast radiographs (see Figs. 9–13 to 9–18). The ulcer crater is often surrounded by a smooth, radiolucent mound of edematous mucosa. Bulbar ulcers also tend to be associated with radiating folds that converge centrally at the edge of the crater (Fig. 9–19; see Figs. 9–15 and 9–16). In patients with shallow ulcers or small, healing ulcers the ulcer crater may be visible only with optimal radiographic technique. Thus, the presence of radiating folds should prompt a careful search for an active ulcer at the site of fold convergence before attributing these folds to an ulcer scar.

As in the stomach, ulcers on the anterior wall of the duodenal bulb may be difficult to detect on routine double contrast views (Fig. 9–20A). Other anterior wall (nondependent) ulcers may be manifested by a ring shadow

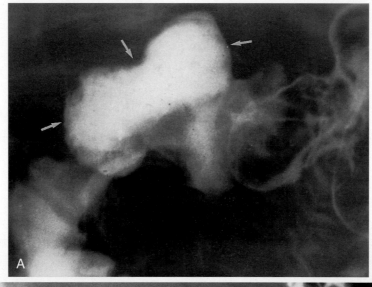

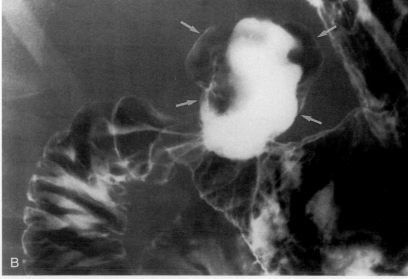

FIGURE 9–17. Two examples (*A* and *B*) of giant duodenal ulcers *(arrows)* replacing duodenal bulb. Although these ulcers could be mistaken for a deformed duodenal bulb, their constant size and shape at fluoroscopy should help differentiate giant ulcers from a scarred bulb.

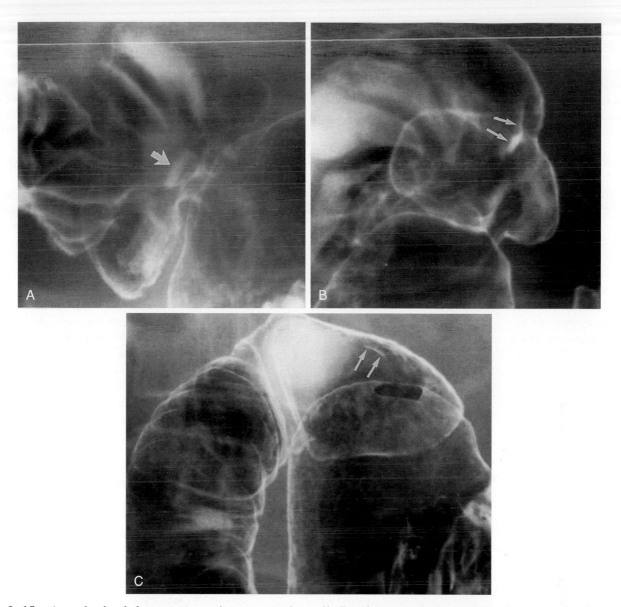

FIGURE 9–18. Linear duodenal ulcers. *A,* Linear ulcer *(arrow)* at base of bulb with transverse orientation in relation to bulb. Also note folds radiating toward ulcer crater. *B* and *C,* Two patients with linear ulcers *(arrows)* near apex of bulb.

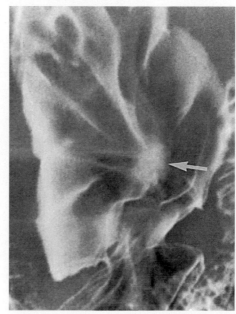

FIGURE 9–19. Duodenal ulcer *(arrow)* with radiating folds.

due to barium coating the rim of the unfilled ulcer crater (Fig. 9–21*A*).[29] These anterior wall ulcers can be demonstrated by turning the patient into the prone position or by compressing the bulb in either the prone or upright positions to fill the crater with barium (Figs. 9–20*B* and 9–21*B*).

Duodenal ulcers are often associated with significant deformity of the bulb because of edema and spasm accompanying the ulcer or scarring from a previous ulcer (Fig. 9–22; see Figs. 9–16*C* and 9–16*D*).[22] This deformity sometimes can obscure small ulcers in the bulb. Conversely, barium trapped in the crevices of a deformed bulb occasionally can be mistaken for an active ulcer crater. Thus, it is important to recognize the limitations of the radiologic diagnosis of duodenal ulcers in the presence of a deformed bulb. Although a confident diagnosis of "peptic ulcer disease" can be made in patients with bulbar deformity, it is often unclear whether an active ulcer is present. Nevertheless, because of the high risk of ulcer disease, symptomatic patients with a deformed bulb on barium studies probably should be treated for an active duodenal ulcer regardless of whether an ulcer is demonstrated with certainty.

Multiplicity

About 15% of patients with duodenal ulcers have multiple ulcers.[30] Most of these ulcers are located in the duodenal bulb.

Ulcer Healing

Duodenal ulcers usually heal rapidly during treatment with antisecretory agents. Ulcer healing is often associated with the development of an ulcer scar, manifested by radiating folds or bulbar deformity. When radiating folds are present, they almost always converge at the site of the previous ulcer (Fig. 9–23). In some patients, a residual depression in the central portion of the scar may simulate an active ulcer crater.

Bulbar deformity results from asymmetric scarring of the bulb. Uninvolved segments of the bulb may balloon out between areas of fibrosis, producing one or more pseudodiverticula. These pseudodiverticula usually can be differentiated from ulcers by their tendency to change in size and shape at fluoroscopy. When multiple pseudodiverticula are present, the duodenal bulb may have a classic "cloverleaf" appearance (Fig. 9–24).

Postbulbar Ulcers

Postbulbar ulcers are usually located on the medial wall of the proximal descending duodenum above the papilla of Vater (Fig. 9–25*A* and 9–26*A*).[23,31] These ulcers are notoriously difficult to demonstrate on barium studies, presumably because of severe edema and spasm accompanying the ulcer that prevent visualization of the ulcer crater. This edema and spasm often results in a smooth, rounded indentation on the lateral wall of the proximal descending duodenum opposite the crater (Fig. 9–25*A*).[31] Subsequently, these patients may develop a "ring stricture," with eccentric narrowing of the postbulbar duodenum due to scarring and fibrosis from previous ulcers in this region (Fig. 9–25*B* and 9–26*B*).[32] Hypotonic duodenography may be performed to better delineate postbulbar ulcers when these lesions are suspected on routine studies (see earlier discussion, Technique).

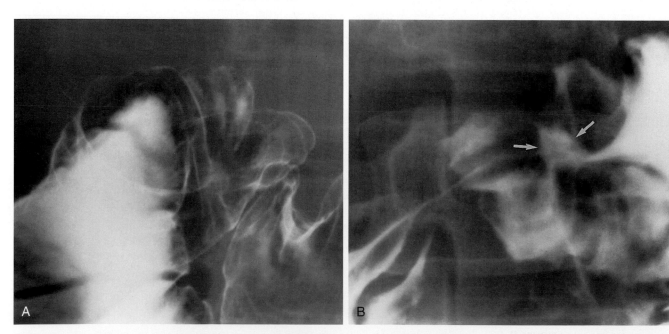

FIGURE 9–20. Value of prone compression for demonstrating anterior wall duodenal ulcers. *A,* Double contrast view of duodenum shows deformity of bulb and radiating folds without definite ulcer. *B,* Prone compression view shows filling of anterior wall ulcer *(arrows).*

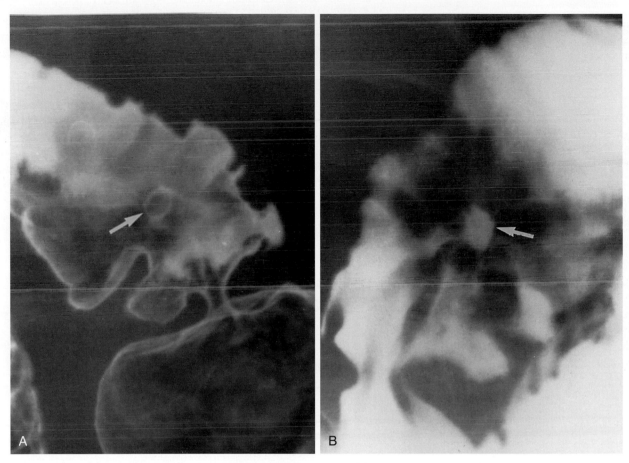

FIGURE 9–21. Ring shadow in duodenum due to anterior wall ulcer. *A,* Double contrast view of duodenum shows ring shadow *(arrow)* in bulb due to barium coating rim of unfilled ulcer on nondependent surface. *B,* Prone compression view shows filling of anterior wall ulcer *(arrow).*

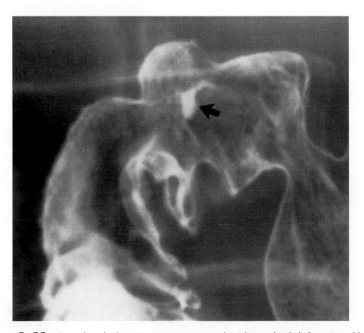

FIGURE 9–22. Duodenal ulcer *(arrow)* associated with marked deformity of bulb.

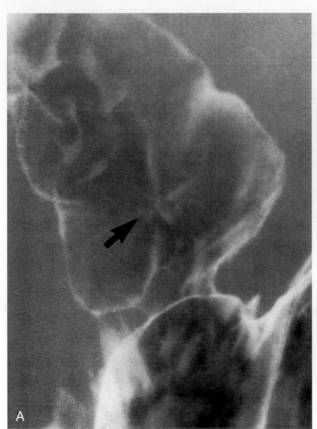

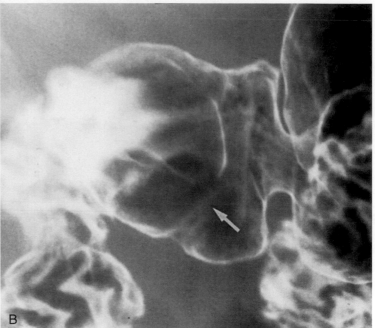

FIGURE 9–23. Two examples (*A* and *B*) of ulcer scars *(arrows)* in duodenum with folds radiating to site of previous ulcer.

FIGURE 9–24. Two examples (*A* and *B*) of scarred duodenal bulb with multiple pseudodiverticula, producing "cloverleaf" appearance.

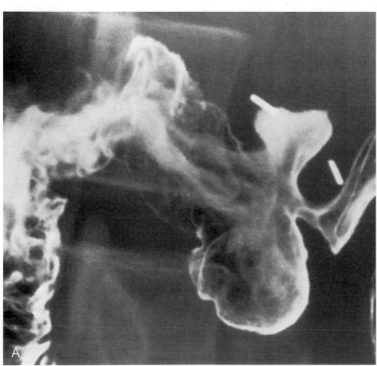

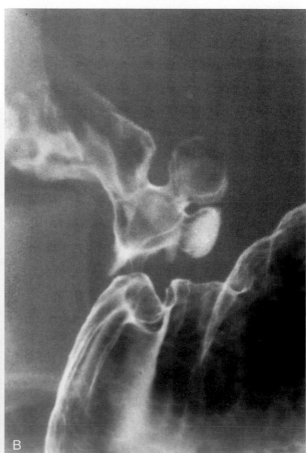

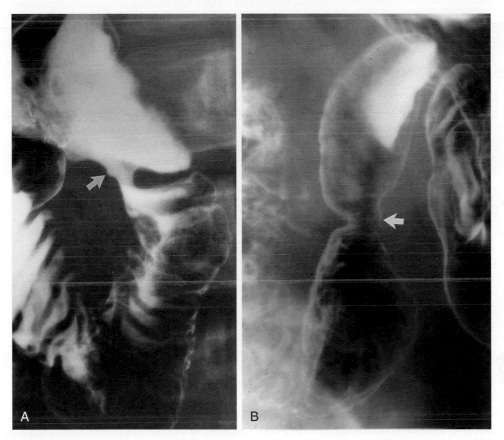

FIGURE 9–25. Postbulbar ulcers. *A,* Postbulbar ulcer *(arrow)* on medial wall of proximal descending duodenum with smooth, rounded indentation of opposite wall. *B,* Different patient with postbulbar "ring stricture" *(arrow)* but no definite ulcer.

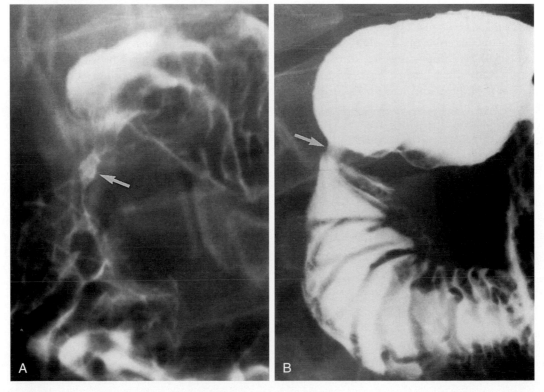

FIGURE 9–26. Postbulbar ulcer with scarring. *A,* Ulcer *(arrow)* on medial wall of proximal descending duodenum. Note narrowing of duodenum due to edema and spasm associated with ulcer. *B,* Follow-up study 6 months later shows healing of ulcer with development of "ring stricture" *(arrow)* due to focal scarring and fibrosis in this region.

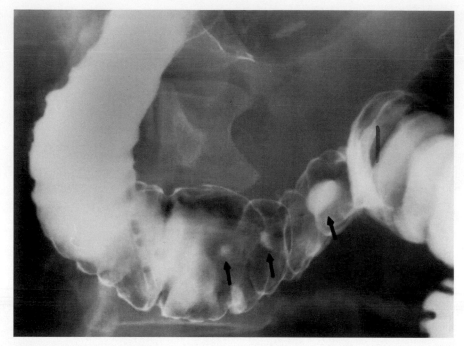

FIGURE 9–27. Multiple postbulbar duodenal ulcers *(arrows)* in patient with Zollinger-Ellison syndrome. Note how ulcers are located distal to papilla. (Courtesy of Wylie J. Dodds, M.D., Milwaukee, Wisconsin.)

Because most postbulbar ulcers are located above the papilla of Vater, the presence of one or more ulcers distal to the papilla should suggest the possibility of Zollinger-Ellison syndrome (Fig. 9–27).[33]

Approach to Duodenal Ulcers

When a duodenal ulcer is diagnosed on double contrast studies, a decision must be made about whether to treat these patients with antibiotics as well as antisecretory agents. Endoscopy and biopsy could be performed to look for *H. pylori,* but other noninvasive tests for this organism, such as a urea breath test and serum antibody test, have been shown to be highly accurate for diagnosing *H. pylori* gastritis.[34–36] Because these tests have become widely available, clinicians now have at their disposal a safe, relatively inexpensive means for the detection of *H. pylori* gastritis without need for endoscopy. Alternatively, patients with duodenal ulcers could be treated empirically with antibiotics (as well as conventional antiulcer medication) because of the high prevalence (90% to 100%) of *H. pylori* infection in these individuals.[17]

DUODENITIS

It is unclear whether duodenitis represents part of the spectrum of peptic ulcer disease or a separate pathologic entity. The clinical significance of duodenitis has also been a subject of controversy. However, many investigators believe that it is a major cause of dyspepsia in the adult population.[37,38] Less frequently, erosive duodenitis may be associated with upper gastrointestinal bleeding. In some patients, hemorrhagic duodenitis may occur as a complication of myocardial infarction or congestive heart failure.[39] Occasionally, the site of bleeding in the duodenum can be documented by angiography.[40,41]

The diagnosis of duodenitis may be suggested radiographically in patients who have a spastic, irritable duodenal bulb or thickened, nodular folds in the proximal duodenum (Fig. 9–28A).[42] For reasons that are unclear, patients with chronic renal failure who are on dialysis often have enlarged duodenal folds to a degree rarely encountered in other patients with duodenitis (Fig. 9–28B).[43,44] In most cases, however, thickened folds and spasm are nonspecific findings, so that the upper gastrointestinal examination generally has not been considered to be an accurate technique for diagnosing duodenitis.

With double contrast technique, it is possible to demonstrate more subtle signs of inflammatory disease in the duodenum.[11,45–47] This inflammation may be manifested by mucosal nodules or nodular folds (Fig. 9–29) or by diffuse coarsening of the mucosal surface pattern of the bulb with lucent areas surrounded by barium-filled grooves that resemble the areae gastricae (Fig. 9–30).[12,46,47] With double contrast technique, it is also possible to diagnose erosive duodenitis, a condition previously thought to be solely in the domain of the endoscopist.[45–47] These erosions may be found in the duodenal bulb or, less frequently, in the descending duodenum. As in the stomach, incomplete erosions in the duodenum appear as tiny flecks of barium (Fig. 9–31A), whereas complete or varioliform erosions appear as central barium collections surrounded by radiolucent halos of edematous mucosa (Fig. 9–31B).[45] False-positive radiologic diagnoses occasionally may result from normal mucosal pits in the duodenum that are mistaken

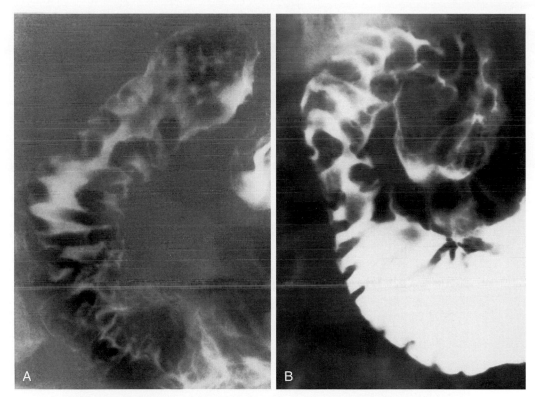

FIGURE 9–28. Duodenitis with thickened folds. *A,* Thickened, nodular folds are seen in descending duodenum. Also note erosions in bulb. *B,* Another patient with grossly thickened, polypoid folds associated with chronic renal failure.

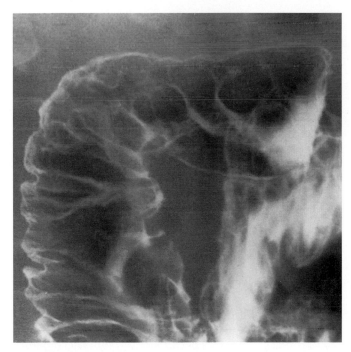

FIGURE 9–29. Duodenitis with nodular mucosa in proximal duodenum.

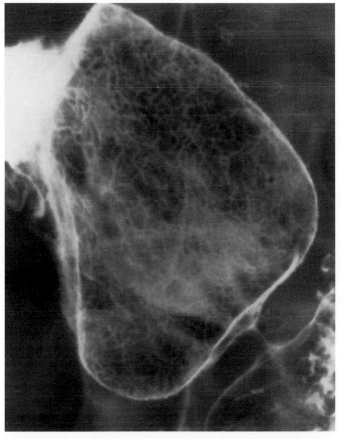

FIGURE 9–30. Duodenitis with coarse reticular pattern in bulb. This patient had Crohn's disease.

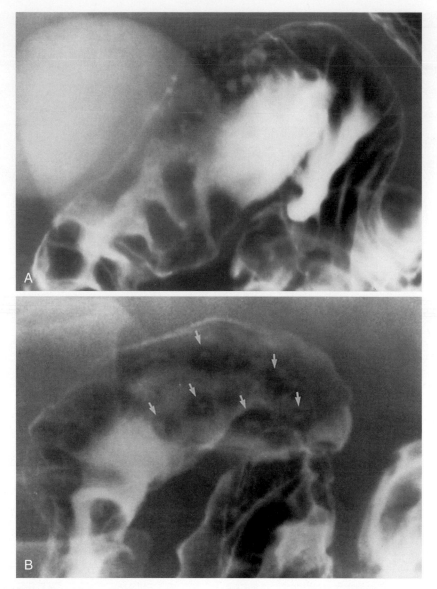

FIGURE 9–31. **Erosive duodenitis.** *A,* Incomplete erosions in bulb manifested by tiny flecks of barium seen both en face and in profile. (Note contrast in gallbladder adjacent to duodenum.) *B,* Complete erosions *(arrows)* appearing as central barium collections with surrounding mounds of edema. (*B,* From Levine, M.S., et al.: Double-contrast upper gastrointestinal examination: Technique and interpretation. Radiology *168*:593, 1988, with permission.)

for incomplete erosions on double contrast studies (Fig. 9–32).[13,47] Barium precipitates may also resemble incomplete erosions. Thus, a confident diagnosis of erosive duodenitis can be only made when true varioliform erosions are demonstrated.

CROHN'S DISEASE

Only 1% to 3% of patients with Crohn's disease have evidence of upper gastrointestinal involvement on conventional single contrast barium studies.[48,49] These patients usually have advanced disease in the stomach and duodenum, manifested by thickened folds, ulcers, narrowing, and scarring.[48–50] In our experience, however, early signs of gastroduodenal Crohn's disease may be detected on double contrast studies in more than 20% of

patients with granulomatous ileocolitis. Occasionally, the onset of upper gastrointestinal involvement may coincide with or even precede the onset of ileal or colonic involvement, so that these patients do not necessarily have known Crohn's disease when they seek medical attention. Endoscopic biopsy specimens from the duodenum may fail to reveal granulomas because of the superficial nature of the biopsy specimens and the patchy distribution of the disease.[51] Thus, the absence of definitive histologic findings should not discourage a diagnosis of duodenal Crohn's disease if the clinical and radiographic findings suggest this condition.

The earliest lesions of duodenal Crohn's disease are "aphthous ulcers" similar to those found elsewhere in the gastrointestinal tract in this disease.[52–54] Although these lesions may be indistinguishable from duodenal

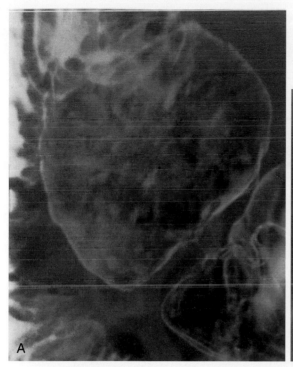

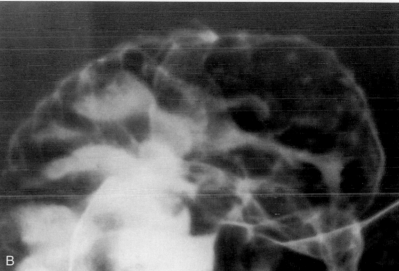

FIGURE 9–32. Two examples (*A* and *B*) of normal mucosal pits in duodenal bulb simulating erosions. In both cases, endoscopic biopsy specimens revealed normal duodenal mucosa. (*B*, From Levine, M.S., et al.: Double-contrast upper gastrointestinal examination: Technique and interpretation. Radiology *168*:593, 1988, with permission.)

erosions associated with peptic duodenitis (see previous discussion, Duodenitis), the latter condition typically involves the duodenal bulb, whereas the aphthous ulcers of Crohn's disease may be located anywhere in the duodenum from the bulb to the ligament of Treitz (Fig. 9–33). Most patients with duodenal Crohn's disease have concomitant involvement of the small bowel or colon, so that a small bowel follow-through or barium enema should be performed when duodenal involvement is suspected.

More advanced duodenal Crohn's disease may be manifested radiographically by thickened folds (Fig. 9–34*A*), "cobblestoning" of the mucosa (Fig. 9–34*B*), ulceration (Fig. 9–34*C*), or strictures (Fig. 9–34*D*).[40] At this stage of disease, most patients have contiguous involvement of the gastric antrum, pylorus, and duodenum. Duodenal strictures often appear as smooth, tapered areas of narrowing involving the apical portion of the duodenal bulb and adjacent segment of the postbulbar duodenum (Fig. 9–34*D*).[49] Severe duodenal disease is almost always associated with Crohn's disease involving the small bowel or colon.

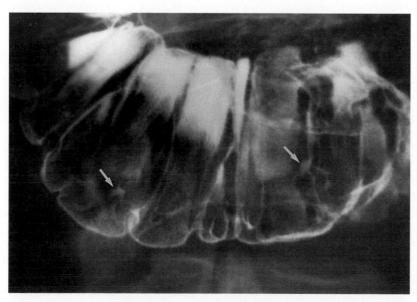

FIGURE 9–33. Duodenal Crohn's disease with discrete aphthous ulcers (*arrows*) in distal duodenum near ligament of Treitz. (Courtesy of Louis Engelholm, M.D., Brussels, Belgium. From Levine, M.S.: Crohn's disease of the upper gastrointestinal tract. Radiol. Clin. North Am. *25*:79, 1987, with permission.)

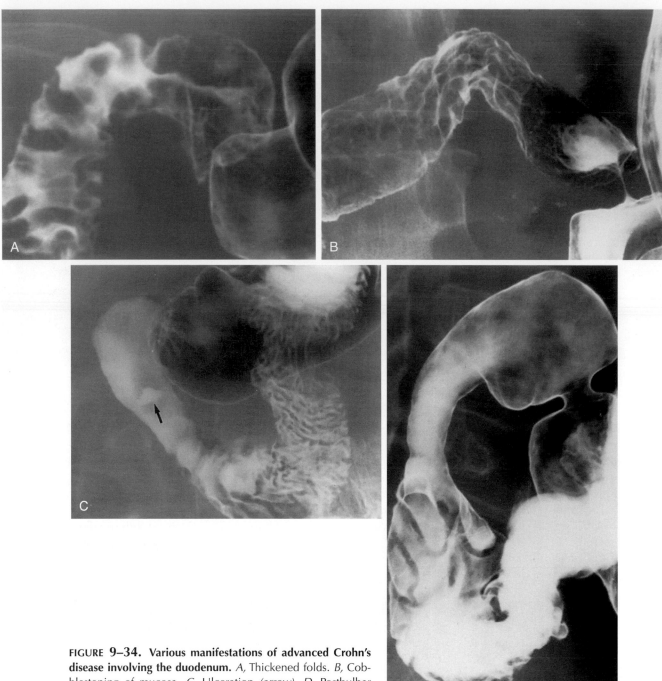

FIGURE **9–34. Various manifestations of advanced Crohn's disease involving the duodenum.** *A,* Thickened folds. *B,* Cobblestoning of mucosa. *C,* Ulceration *(arrow). D,* Postbulbar stricture.

CELIAC DISEASE

Celiac disease (nontropical sprue) typically involves the jejunum and ileum (see Chapter 10). However, it may also produce striking abnormalities in the duodenum. Some patients may have small (1 to 4 mm), hexagonal filling defects in the duodenal bulb, producing a distinctive mosaic pattern or "bubbly" bulb (Fig. 9–35).[55] Unlike heterotopic gastric mucosa, which predominantly affects the juxtapyloric region of the bulb (see later discussion, Masslike Lesions), these nodules tend to be located more diffusely throughout the bulb. They may reflect the underlying changes of celiac disease in the duodenum or Brunner's gland hyperplasia due to associated peptic duodenitis.[55] Other patients with celiac disease may have thickened folds or nodular mucosa in the descending duodenum (Fig. 9–36).[56] Thus the presence of a bubbly bulb or thickened duodenal folds in patients with malabsorption should suggest the possibility of celiac disease. A small bowel enema or small bowel biopsy may be required for a more definitive diagnosis (see Chapter 10).

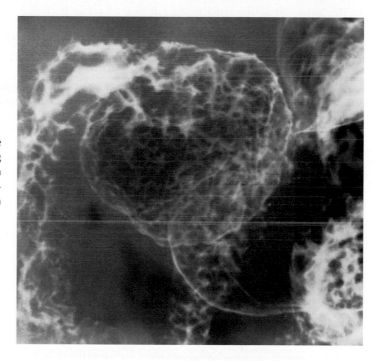

FIGURE 9–35. Celiac disease with "bubbly" bulb. Note multiple hexagonal filling defects in bulb and thickened folds in descending duodenum. (From Jones, B., et al.: "Bubbly" duodenal bulb in celiac disease: Radiologic-pathologic correlation. AJR Am. J. Roentgenol. *142:*119, 1984, with permission, © by American Roentgen Ray Society.)

FIGURE 9–36. Celiac disease with duodenitis. *A,* Thickened, nodular folds are seen in distal descending duodenum. *B,* Close-up view of this region shows polypoid folds and coarse nodularity of mucosa.

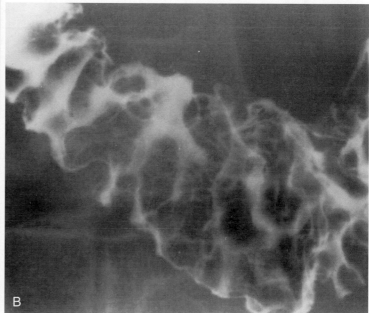

DUODENAL TUMORS

Polyps are much less common in the duodenum than in the stomach. They tend to be adenomatous or hyperplastic lesions. The vast majority cause no symptoms, so that duodenal polyps are almost always detected as incidental findings on radiologic or endoscopic examinations. They usually appear as smooth, sessile filling defects or ring shadows in the first or second portions of the duodenum (Fig. 9–37). Most duodenal polyps occur as solitary lesions, but multiple adenomatous, hyperplastic, or inflammatory polyps may be found in the duodenum as part of a diffuse polyposis syndrome.

Brunner's gland hyperplasia is another condition that may be manifested by multiple rounded nodules in the duodenal bulb and proximal duodenum, producing a characteristic "Swiss cheese" appearance (Fig. 9–38).[57] Benign lymphoid hyperplasia may also produce multiple nodular elevations in the duodenum, but the lesions tend to be smaller (1 to 2 mm) and more uniform in size (Fig. 9–39).[58] These patients often have generalized lymphoid hyperplasia of the small bowel or colon due to an under-

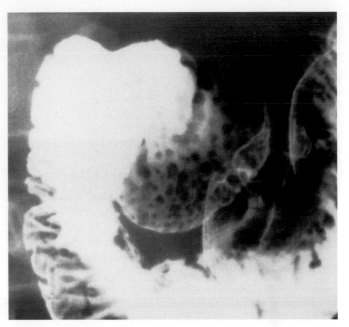

FIGURE 9–38. Brunner's gland hyperplasia with multiple round nodules in duodenal bulb, producing "Swiss cheese" appearance.

lying immunologic disorder. Both conditions should be differentiated from heterotopic gastric mucosa in the duodenal bulb (see next discussion, Masslike Lesions).

Although villous tumors are typically found in the colon, they also have a predilection for the duodenum, most frequently near the papilla of Vater. These villous tumors may have a reticular or "soap bubble" appearance due to barium trapped in multiple clefts between the frondlike projections of the tumor (Fig. 9–40 and 9–41).[59,60] Because these lesions may be obscured by superimposed mucosal folds, optimal distention of the duodenum is often required for their detection. As in the colon, villous tumors in the duodenum should be resected because of the high risk of malignant degeneration as these lesions enlarge.[61]

Primary malignant tumors of the duodenum are uncommon lesions. When they occur, they tend to be located at or below the ampulla of Vater.[62-64] Rarely, however, carcinoma has been reported to occur in the duodenal bulb.[65] We recently encountered a patient with a slightly lobulated 1.3-cm polyp in the duodenal bulb, which was found at surgery to represent an early duodenal cancer (Fig. 9–42). Despite the rarity of these lesions, any duodenal polyp that is lobulated or is greater than 1 cm probably should be evaluated by endoscopy and biopsy to be certain that it is not an early carcinoma.

Advanced duodenal carcinoma or lymphoma may be manifested by a polypoid, ulcerated, or annular lesion (Figs. 9–43 and 9–44). Both carcinoma and lymphoma of the duodenum or small bowel may occur as complications of long-standing celiac disease.[66] Unfortunately, treatment with a gluten-free diet has not been effective in

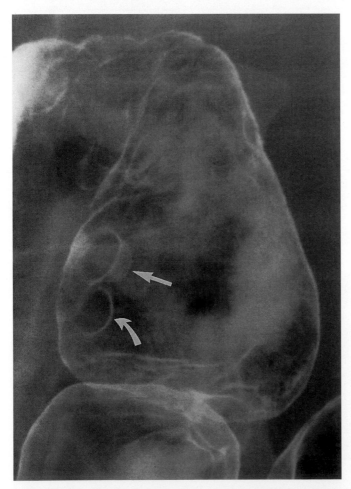

FIGURE 9–37. Duodenal polyps. Note that lower polyp appears as ring shadow *(curved arrow)*, whereas higher polyp can be recognized as bowler hat *(straight arrow)*.

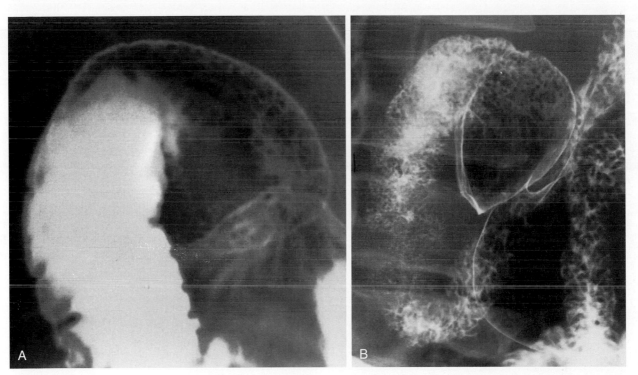

FIGURE 9–39. Two examples (*A* and *B*) of benign lymphoid hyperplasia with innumerable tiny nodules in duodenum. The patient in *B* had hypogammaglobulinemia.

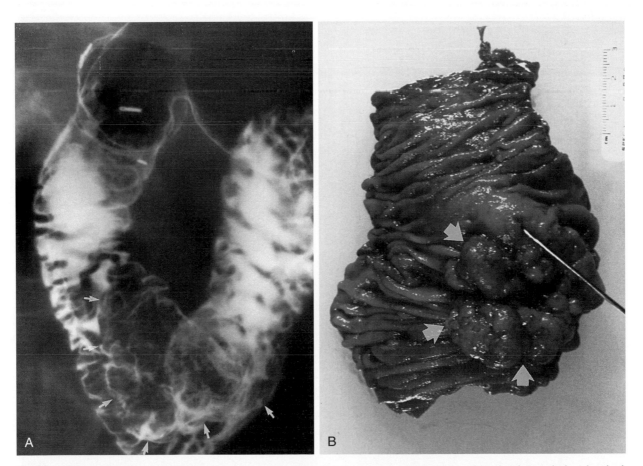

FIGURE 9–40. Villous adenoma in duodenum. *A,* Large polypoid lesion *(arrows)* is seen in descending duodenum below level of papilla. Note reticular appearance due to trapping of barium between frondlike projections of tumor. *B,* Photograph of gross specimen shows large villous adenoma *(arrows)* adjacent to papilla. (Note placement of probe with tip in orifice of papilla.)

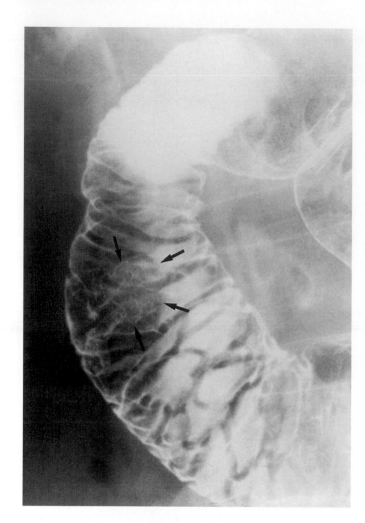

FIGURE 9–41. Villous adenoma in duodenum. Note small polypoid lesion *(arrows)* in descending duodenum. The fine nodularity and lobulation of lesion is typical of villous tumors.

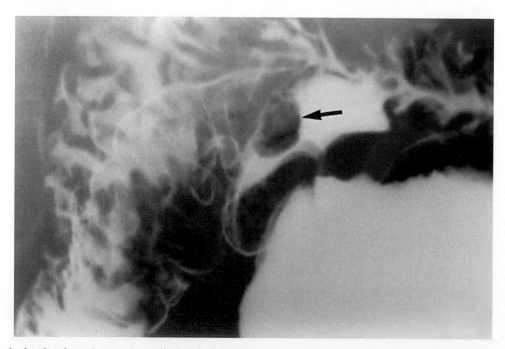

FIGURE 9–42. Early duodenal carcinoma. A small, slightly lobulated polyp *(arrow)* is seen near base of duodenal bulb. Duodenal cancer rarely occurs in the bulb.

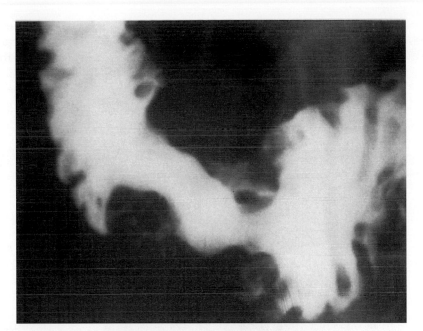

FIGURE 9–43. Annular carcinoma of distal duodenum. Note abrupt, shelflike borders of lesion.

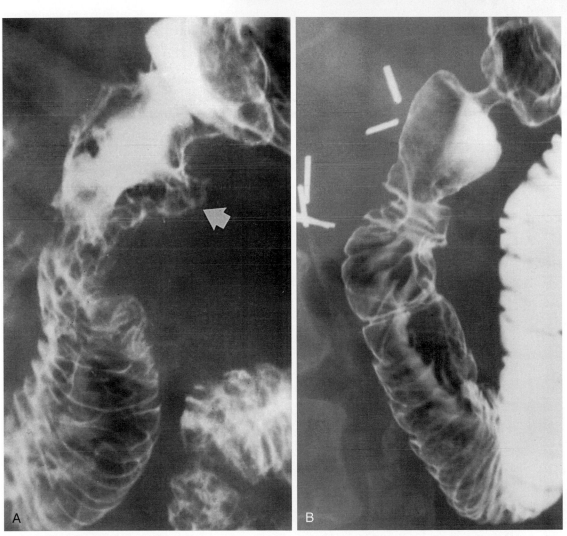

FIGURE 9–44. Duodenal lymphoma. *A,* Polypoid mass lesion is seen on medial wall of proximal descending duodenum. Note large area of ulceration *(arrow)* in lesion. At surgery this was found to be duodenal lymphoma. *B,* Follow-up study after radiation therapy shows regression of lesion with postbulbar scarring in region of previous ulcer. Note prominent longitudinal and oblique folds associated with duodenal papilla.

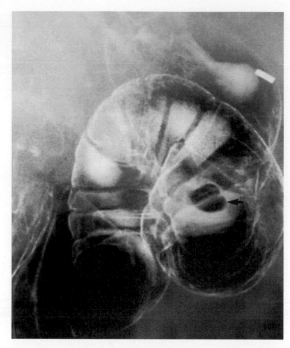

FIGURE 9–45. Small polypoid ampullary carcinoma *(arrow)* found in elderly man who presented with obstructive jaundice.

preventing the development of these tumors. Thus, radiologic surveillance of the small bowel has been advocated in patients with celiac disease to detect these lesions at the earliest possible stage.

Carcinoma of the ampulla of Vater may also involve the duodenum.[63] These tumors may appear as polypoid masses in the region of the papilla. Because of the location of these lesions, affected patients usually present with obstructive jaundice. However, some ampullary carcinomas may be quite small at the time of clinical presentation (Fig. 9–45). Even when the tumor itself is not visible, dilatation of the common bile duct may cause a broad impression on the medial aspect of the descending duodenum (Fig. 9–46).

MASSLIKE LESIONS

Duodenal tumors may be simulated by a variety of innocuous findings such as see-through artifacts (Fig. 9–47), surgical defects (Fig. 9–48), prolapsed gastric mucosa (Fig. 9–49), prolapsed gastric tumors (Fig. 9–50), and heterotopic gastric mucosa in the duodenum (Fig. 9–51). Occasionally, gastric mucosa that has prolapsed into the duodenum can be mistaken for a polypoid lesion (Fig. 9–49*A*). However, prolapsed gastric mucosa is usually characterized by a mushroom-shaped defect at the base of the bulb that is observed as a transient finding at fluoroscopy (Fig. 9–49*B*).[67] Apparent polypoid lesions in the duodenum may also represent gastric tumors that have prolapsed through the pylorus into the duodenal bulb (Fig. 9–50). Heterotopic gastric mucosa in the duodenum is another benign condition manifested by polygonal or angulated 1- to 5-mm nodules or plaques that tend to be clustered near the base of the duodenal bulb (Fig. 9–51).[68,69] Prolapsed gastric mucosa and heterotopic

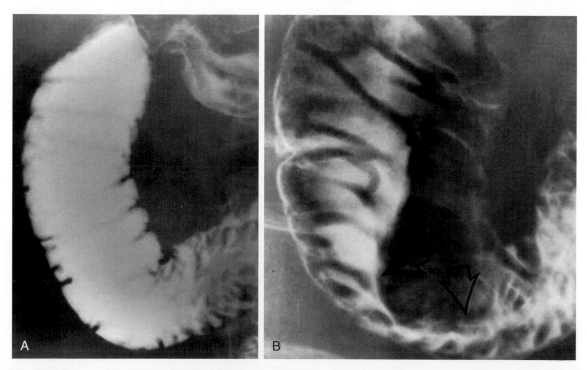

FIGURE 9–46. Ampullary carcinoma with dilated common bile duct. *A,* Barium-filled view of duodenum shows no abnormality. *B,* Hypotonic duodenography shows broad impression *(arrows)* on medial aspect of distal descending duodenum due to dilated common bile duct in patient with small ampullary carcinoma that was obstructing the duct. (From Laufer, I.: Double contrast radiology in the diagnosis of gastrointestinal cancer. *In* Glass, G.B.J. [ed.]: Progress in Gastroenterology, vol. 3. New York, Grune & Stratton, 1977, p. 643, with permission.)

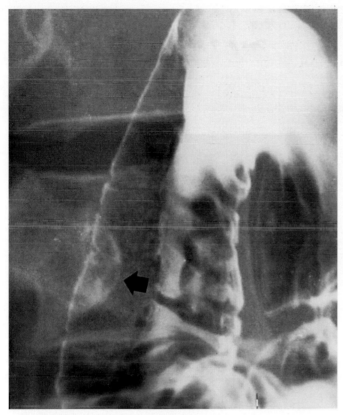

FIGURE 9–47. See-through artifact. Note vertebral pedicle *(arrow)* simulating polypoid lesion in descending duodenum.

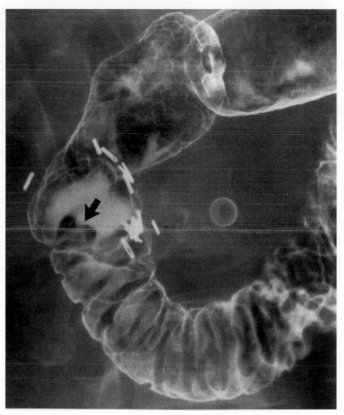

FIGURE 9–48. Surgical defect *(arrow)* appearing as small polypoid lesion in descending duodenum.

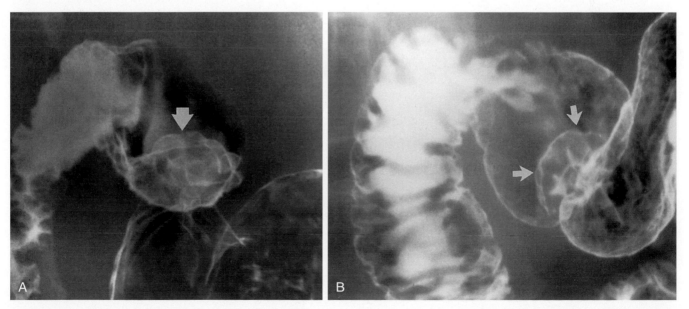

FIGURE 9–49. Prolapsed gastric mucosa. *A,* Prolapsed antral mucosa appearing as polypoid mass lesion *(arrow)* at base of bulb. *B,* More typical appearance of prolapsed gastric mucosa with mushroom-shaped defect *(arrows)* at base of bulb.

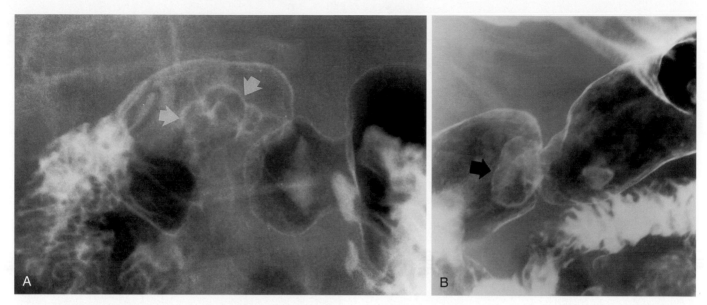

FIGURE 9–50. Prolapsed gastric tumors. *A,* Polypoid adenoma *(arrows)* prolapsed into duodenal bulb. *B,* Mass lesion *(arrow)* in bulb due to polypoid gastric carcinoma that has prolapsed into duodenum.

FIGURE 9–51. Two examples (*A* and *B*) of heterotopic gastric mucosa manifested by discrete, angulated filling defects near base of bulb. This appearance is so characteristic that a confident diagnosis can be made on double contrast studies without need for endoscopy. (*B,* From Levine, M.S., et al.: Double-contrast upper gastrointestinal examination: Technique and interpretation. Radiology *168*:593, 1988, with permission.)

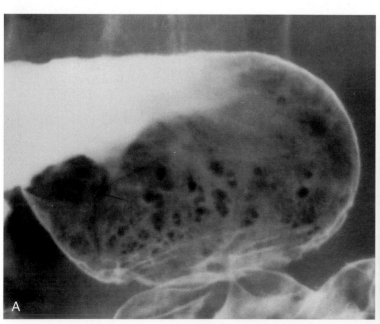

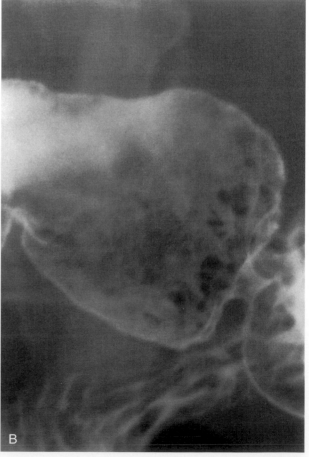

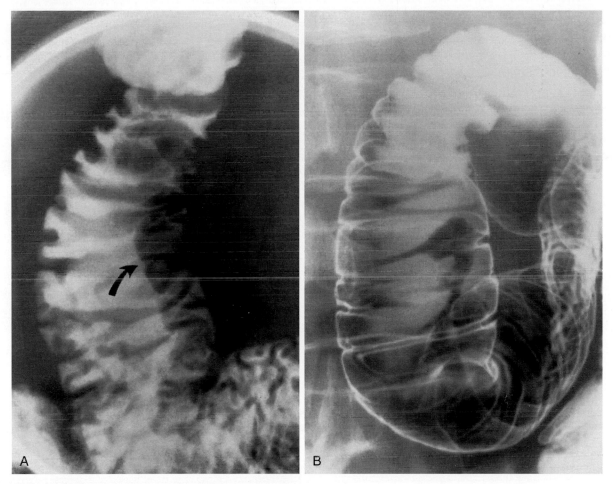

FIGURE 9–52. Prominent longitudinal fold mimicking mass lesion in duodenum. *A,* Initial view shows possible mass lesion *(arrow)* on medial wall of duodenum or head of pancreas. *B,* Hypotonic double contrast duodenography shows prominent longitudinal fold adjacent to major papilla without evidence of mass lesion. (Courtesy of Harvey M. Goldstein, M.D., San Antonio, Texas.)

gastric mucosa in the duodenum both have such characteristic findings on barium studies that endoscopy usually is unnecessary in these patients.

In patients with an impacted common duct stone or pancreatitis, the ampulla of Vater occasionally becomes large and edematous, simulating a duodenal tumor. A prominent longitudinal fold seen tangentially may also suggest an intrinsic or extrinsic mass lesion involving the medial aspect of the descending duodenum (Fig. 9–52A). By manipulating the barium pool in the proper projection, however, the true nature of this longitudinal fold can be recognized (Fig. 9–52B).

PANCREATIC DISEASES

Inflammatory or neoplastic diseases of the pancreas are best evaluated by cross-sectional imaging techniques such as computed tomography and ultrasonography. However, duodenal manifestations of pancreatic disease are sometimes seen on double contrast studies. In patients with acute or chronic pancreatitis, an enlarged head of the pancreas may cause widening of the duodenal sweep, compression of the medial aspect of the duodenum, or thickened, spiculated duodenal folds (Fig. 9–53). In other patients, pancreatitis may cause circumferential narrowing of the descending duodenum with varying degrees of obstruction. Pancreatic carcinoma may also result in compression and nodularity of the medial wall of the duodenum (Fig. 9–54A). As the tumor erodes into the bowel, ulceration eventually may occur (Fig. 9–54B). The reverse 3 sign is a classic sign of advanced pancreatic carcinoma involving the duodenum. However, this sign occasionally may be simulated by underfilling of the duodenum, particularly in the presence of a duodenal diverticulum (Fig. 9–55). Finally, annular pancreas is a congenital abnormality that occasionally may be manifested in adults by focal narrowing or obstruction of the descending duodenum.

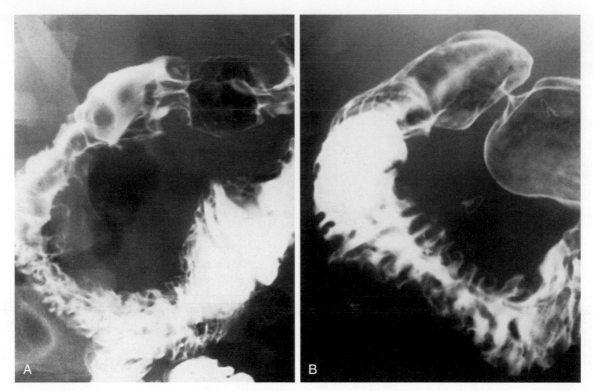

FIGURE 9–53. Acute pancreatitis involving duodenum. *A,* Widening of duodenal loop with compression of medial aspect of duodenum and thickened folds. *B,* Different patient with thickened, spiculated folds in descending duodenum.

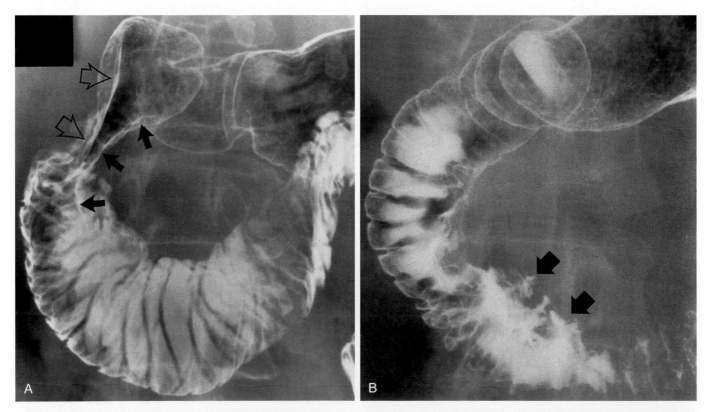

FIGURE 9–54. Pancreatic carcinoma involving duodenum. *A,* Area of mass effect *(closed arrows)* is seen on medial aspect of proximal descending duodenum. Lateral aspect of postbulbar duodenum is compressed by an enlarged gallbladder *(open arrows).* (Courtesy of Harvey M. Goldstein, M.D., San Antonio, Texas.) *B,* Different patient with irregular ulceration *(arrows)* of descending duodenum due to invasion by pancreatic carcinoma.

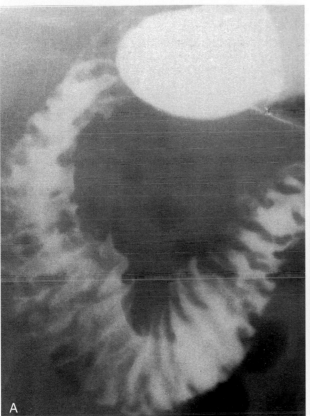

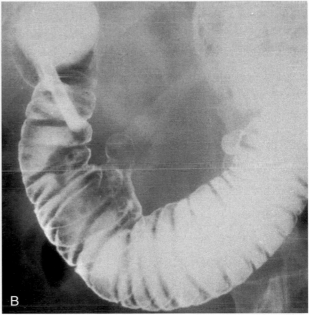

FIGURE 9–55. Spurious reverse 3 sign due to duodenal di verticulum. *A,* Initial view shows apparent compression of medial aspect of duodenum with reverse 3 sign. *B,* However, hypotonic duodenography with a tube shows a duodenal diverticulum without evidence of pancreatic or duodenal disease.

REFERENCES

1. Salmon, P.R., Brown, P., Htut, T., et al.: Endoscopic examination of the duodenal bulb; Clinical evaluation of forward- and side-viewing fibreoptic systems in 200 cases. Gut *13:*170, 1972.
2. Classen, M.: Endoscopy in benign peptic ulcer. Clin. Gastroenterol. *2:*315, 1973.
3. Herlinger, H., Glanville, J.N., and Kreel, L.: An evaluation of the double contrast barium meal (DCBM) against endoscopy. Clin. Radiol. *28:*307, 1977.
4. Laufer, I., Mullens, J.E., and Hamilton, J.: The diagnostic accuracy of barium studies of the stomach and duodenum: Correlation with endoscopy. Radiology *115:*569, 1975.
5. Laufer, I.: Assessment of the accuracy of double contrast gastroduodenal radiology. Gastroenterology *71:*874, 1976.
6. Bilbao, M.K., Frische, L.H., and Dotter, C.T.: Hypotonic duodenography. Radiology *89:*438, 1967.
7. Eaton, S.B., Benedict, K.T., Ferruci, J.T., et al.: Hypotonic duodenography. Radiol. Clin. North Am. *8:*125, 1970.
8. Martel, W., Scholtens, P.A., and Lim, L.W.: "Tubeless" hypotonic duodenography: Technique, value, and limitations. AJR Am. J. Roentgenol. *107:*119, 1969.
9. Sear, H.S., and Friedenberg, M.J.: Simplified technique for tubeless hypotonic duodenography. Radiology *103:*210, 1972.
10. Miller, R.E., Chernish, S.M., Greenman, G.F., et al.: Gastrointestinal response to minute doses of glucagon. Radiology *143:*317, 1982.
11. Levine, M.S., and Laufer, I.: The do's and don'ts of digital GI imaging. Radiology *207:*311, 1998.
12. Glick, S.N., Gohel, V.K., and Laufer, I.: Mucosal surface patterns of the duodenal bulb. Radiology *150:*317, 1984.
13. Bova, J.G., Kamath, V., Tio, F.O., et al.: The normal mucosal surface pattern of the duodenal bulb: Radiologic-histologic correlation. AJR Am. J. Roentgenol. *145:*735, 1985.
14. Nelson, J.A., Sheft, D.J., Minagi, H., et al.: Duodenal pseudopolyp: The flexural fallacy. AJR Am. J. Roentgenol. *123:*262, 1975.
15. Burrell, M., and Toffler, R.: Flexural pseudolesions of the duodenum. Radiology *120:*313, 1976.
16. Ferruci, J.T., Benedict, K.T., Page, D.L., et al.: The radiographic features of the normal hypotonic duodenogram. Radiology *96:*401, 1970.
17. Levine, M.S., and Rubesin, S.E.: The *Helicobacter pylori* revolution: Radiologic perspective. Radiology *195:*593, 1995.
18. Moss, S., and Calam, J.: *Helicobacter pylori* and peptic ulcers: The present position. Gut *33:*289, 1992.
19. Graham, D.Y., Lew, G.M., Klein, P.D., et al.: Effect of treatment of *Helicobacter pylori* infection on the long-term recurrence of gastric or duodenal ulcer. Ann. Intern. Med. *116:*705, 1992.
20. Hentschel, E., Brandstatter, G., Dragosics, B., et al.: Effect of ranitidine and amoxicillin plus metronidazole on the eradication of *Helicobacter pylori* and the recurrence of duodenal ulcer. N. Engl. J. Med. *328:*308, 1993.
21. NIH consensus conference: *Helicobacter pylori* in peptic ulcer disease. JAMA *272:*65, 1994.
22. Stein, G.N., Martin, R.D., Roy, R.H., et al.: Evaluation of conventional roentgenologic techniques for demonstration of duodenal ulcer craters. AJR Am. J. Roentgenol. *91:*801, 1964.
23. Rodriquez, H.P., Aston, J.K., and Richardson, C.T.: Ulcers in the descending duodenum: Postbulbar ulcers. AJR Am. J. Roentgenol. *119:*316, 1973.
24. Sheppard, M.C., Holmes, G.K.T., and Cockel, R.: Clinical picture of peptic ulceration diagnosed endoscopically. Gut *18:*524, 1977.
25. Eisenberg, R.L., Margulis, A.R., and Moss, A.A.: Giant duodenal ulcers. Gastrointest. Radiol. *2:*347, 1978.
26. Braver, J.M., Paul, R.E., Philipps, E., et al.: Roentgen diagnosis of linear ulcers. Radiology *132:*29, 1979.
27. de Roos, A., and Op den Orth, J.O.: Linear niches in the duodenal bulb. AJR Am. J. Roentgenol. *140:*941, 1983.
28. Poplack, W., Paul, R.E., Goldsmith, M., et al.: Linear and rod-shaped peptic ulcers. Radiology *122:*317, 1977.
29. Lubert, M., and Krause, G.R.: The "ring" shadow in the diagnosis of ulcer. AJR Am. J. Roentgenol. *90:*767, 1963.
30. Kawai, K., Ida, K., Misaki, F., et al.: Comparative study for duodenal ulcer by radiology and endoscopy. Endoscopy *5:*7, 1973.
31. Ball, R.P., Segal, A.L., and Golden, R.: Postbulbar ulcer of the duodenum. AJR Am. J. Roentgenol. *59:*90, 1948.

32. Bilbao, M.K., Frische, L.H., Rosch, J., et al.: Postbulbar duodenal ulcer and ring-stricture. Radiology *100*:27, 1971.

33. Nelson, S.W., and Christoforidis, A.J.: Roentgenologic features of the Zollinger-Ellison syndrome: Ulcerogenic tumor of the pancreas. Semin. Roentgenol. *3*:254, 1968.

34. Graham, D.Y.: Treatment of peptic ulcers caused by *Helicobacter pylori* (editorial). N. Engl. J. Med. *328*:349, 1993.

35. Talley, N.J., Kost, L., Haddad, A., et al.: Comparison of commercial serological tests for detection of *Helicobacter pylori* antibodies. J. Clin. Microbiol. *30*:3146, 1992.

36. Negrini, R., Zanella, I., Savio, A., et al.: Serodiagnosis of *Helicobacter pylori*–associated gastritis with a monoclonal antibody competitive enzyme-linked immunosorbent assay. Scand. J. Gastroenterol. *27*:599, 1992.

37. Thomson, W.O., Robertson, A.G., Imrie, C.W., et al.: Is duodenitis a dyspeptic myth? Lancet *1*:1197, 1977.

38. Greenlaw, R., Sheehan, D.G., DeLuca, V., et al.: Gastroduodenitis: A broader concept of peptic ulcer disease. Dig. Dis. Sci. *25*:660, 1980.

39. Katz, A.M.: Hemorrhagic duodenitis in myocardial infarction. Ann. Intern. Med. *51*:212, 1959.

40. Baum, S., Ward, S., and Nusbaum, M.: Stress bleeding from the mid-duodenum: An often unrecognized source of gastrointestinal hemorrhage. Radiology *95*:595, 1970.

41. Blakemore, W.S., Baum, S., and Nusbaum, M.: Diagnosis and management of massive hemorrhage from postoperative stress ulcers of the descending duodenum. Surg. Clin. North Am. *50*:979, 1970.

42. Fraser, G.M., Pitman, R.G., Lawrie, J.H., et al.: The significance of the radiological finding of coarse mucosal folds in the duodenum. Lancet *2*:979, 1964.

43. Wiener, S.N., Vertes, V., Shapiro, H.: The upper gastrointestinal tract in patients undergoing chronic dialysis. Radiology *92*:110, 1969.

44. Zukerman, G.R., Mills, B.A., Koehler, R.E., et al.: Nodular duodenitis: Pathologic and clinical characteristics in patients with end-stage renal disease. Dig. Dis. Sci. *11*:1018, 1983.

45. Catalano, D., and Pagliari, U.: Gastroduodenal erosions: Radiological findings. Gastrointest. Radiol. *7*:235, 1982.

46. Gelfand, D.W., Dale, W.J., Ott, D.J., et al.: Duodenitis: Endoscopic-radiologic correlation in 272 patients. Radiology *157*:577, 1985.

47. Levine, M.S., Turner, D., Ekberg, O., et al.: Duodenitis: A reliable radiologic diagnosis? Gastrointest. Radiol. *16*:99, 1991.

48. Legge, D.A., Carlson, H.C., and Judd, E.S.: Roentgenologic features of regional enteritis of the upper gastrointestinal tract. AJR Am. J. Roentgenol. *110*:355, 1970.

49. Thompson, W.M., Cockrill, H., and Rice, R.P.: Regional enteritis of the duodenum. AJR Am. J. Roentgenol. *123*:252, 1975.

50. Marshak, R.H., Maklansky, D., Kurzban, J.D., et al.: Crohn's disease of the stomach and duodenum. Am. J. Gastroenterol. *77*:340, 1982.

51. Danzi, J.T., Farmer, R.G., Sullivan, B.H., et al.: Endoscopic features of gastroduodenal Crohn's disease. Gastroenterology *70*:9, 1976.

52. Ariyama, J., Wehlin, L., Lindstrom, C.G., et al.: Gastroduodenal erosions in Crohn's disease. Gastrointest. Radiol. *5*:121, 1980.

53. Kelvin, F.M., and Gedgaudas, R.K.: Radiologic diagnosis of Crohn's disease (with emphasis on its early manifestations). Crit. Rev. Diagn. Imaging *16*:43, 1981.

54. Levine, M.S.: Crohn's disease of the upper gastrointestinal tract. Radiol. Clin. North Am. *25*:79, 1987.

55. Jones, B., Bayless, T.M., Hamilton, S.R., et al.: "Bubbly" duodenal bulb in celiac disease: Radiologic-pathologic correlation. AJR Am. J. Roentgenol. *142*:119, 1984.

56. Marn, C.S., Gore, R.M., and Ghahremani, G.G.: Duodenal manifestations of nontropical sprue. Gastrointest. Radiol. *11*:30, 1986.

57. Weinberg, P.E., and Levin, B.: Hyperplasia of Brunner's glands. Radiology *84*:259, 1965.

58. Govoni, A.F.: Benign lymphoid hyperplasia of the duodenal bulb. Gastrointest. Radiol. *1*:267, 1976.

59. Ring, E.J., Ferruci, J.T., Eaton, S.B., et al.: Villous adenoma of the duodenum. Radiology *104*:45, 1972.

60. Miller, J.H., Gisvold, J.J., Weiland, L.H., et al.: Upper gastrointestinal tract: Villous tumors. AJR Am. J. Roentgenol. *134*:933, 1980.

61. Spira, I.A., and Wolff, W.I.: Villous tumors of the duodenum. Am. J. Gastroenterol. *67*:63, 1977.

62. Bosse, G., and Neeley, J.A.: Roentgenologic findings in primary malignant tumors of the duodenum. AJR Am. J. Roentgenol. *170*:111, 1969.

63. Blumgart, L.H., and Kennedy, A.: Carcinoma of the ampulla of vater and duodenum. Br. J. Surg. *60*:33, 1973.

64. Balikian, J.P., Nassar, N.T., Shamma'a, M.H., et al.: Primary lymphomas of the small intestine including the duodenum. AJR Am. J. Roentgenol. *107*:131, 1969.

65. Barloon, T.J., Lu, C.H., Honda, H., et al.: Primary adenocarcinoma of the duodenal bulb: Radiographic and pathologic findings in two cases. Gastrointest. Radiol. *14*:223, 1989.

66. Collins, S.M., Hamilton, J.D., Lewis, T.D., et al.: Small bowel malabsorption and gastrointestinal malignancy. Radiology *126*:603, 1978.

67. Feldman, M., and Myers, P.: The roentgen diagnosis of prolapse of gastric mucosa into the duodenum. Gastroenterology *20*:90, 1952.

68. Langkemper, R., Hoek, A.C., Dekker, W., et al.: Elevated lesions in the duodenal bulb caused by heterotopic gastric mucosa. Radiology *137*:621, 1980.

69. Agha, F.P., Ghahremani, G.G., Tsang, T.K., et al.: Heterotopic gastric mucosa in the duodenum: Radiographic findings. AJR Am. J. Roentgenol. *150*:291, 1988.

Small Bowel

HANS HERLINGER

The small intestine, a winding tube of variable length and position within the abdomen, forms an environment that is potentially hostile to ingested barium suspensions. About 9 liters of fluid, two thirds of it secretions, pour into the small bowel daily. These secretions contain protein, fat and electrolytes, gastric juice, bile salts, mucus, and about 250 g of shed epithelial cells every day.[1] Almost 8 of the 9 liters are absorbed by the small bowel, the remainder enter the colon. In the fasting state this out-pouring diminishes considerably, although there is still a daily outflow that includes 10 to 25 ml of fat,[2] most of it reabsorbed. A mucous layer covers the entire surface of the small bowel mucosa. In this environment even flocculation-resistant barium may occasionally flocculate in patients whose fecal fat levels are normal.[3]

Normal variation of bowel tone and transit time[4] can affect the radiologic appearance, showing the valvulae conniventes either as circular bands surrounding a wider lumen or as a feathery pattern in collapsed small bowel. The variable appearance of the normal surface of the small bowel, coating difficulties due to gut contents and technical factors, the unpredictable transit time, and problems caused by overlap of loops have made it difficult for the radiologist to be confident of either normality or of early changes in disease. Moreover, even the most carefully done small bowel studies produce a very low yield of organic disease. It is not surprising that many radiologists show a low level of interest in the small bowel and that clinicians have often been induced to accept, as sufficient radiodiagnostic effort, follow-through examinations based mostly on overview radiographs of barium-filled loops with the assurance that major pathology had not been revealed.

The purpose of this chapter is to describe an intubation-based method that produces a multiphasic form of lumen delineation, which changes from single contrast through developing into completed double contrast. However, not every patient requires such an intubation-based technique. An alternative method, the fluoroscopic follow-through, will be described with reference to its technique, indications, and limitations. Because the investigation of the duodenum forms part of the upper gastrointestinal barium routine, the term *small intestine* in the context of this chapter refers to the jejunum and ileum only. This chapter is concerned primarily with the examination of adolescents and adults. However, early recognition of small bowel disease is of great importance in children because of the danger of retarded development. A modified technique for enteroclysis in children will, therefore, be briefly described.[5]

TECHNIQUES
Fluoroscopic Follow-Through

Reliance on overhead films of barium-filled and overlapping loops of small bowel has been shown to result in missed lesions.[6] Transit acceleration and type and quantity of barium used are important factors for success.

Metoclopramide accelerates gastric emptying and shortens transit time through the intestine. It can be administered as two 10-mg tablets about 20 minutes before the barium.[7] At least 500 ml of barium at 40% w/v, such as Entero-H diluted with an equal volume of water (E-Z-EM Co., Westbury, NY 11590), should be ingested by the patient. The upper gastrointestinal tract can be examined in single contrast, but the emphasis of this examination and of its clinical indications should be on the small bowel. It is essential that repeated spot films guided by fluoroscopy are taken with abdominal compression and in suitable degrees of obliquity of the patient. Such fluoroscopic sessions need to be repeated at intervals, depending on the rate of transit and the need to outline and image all bowel loops when optimally distended. Attention should be paid to the mobility and pliability response of bowel loops to abdominal palpation. Overhead

views of the abdomen can be taken at intervals but serve mainly for orientation. Most examinations can be completed in 90 minutes.

Distal segments of ileum are often suboptimally shown by this method. The peroral pneumocolon can then usefully supplement the examination.

Limitations

Acceleration of small bowel transit is associated with a reduction of the lumen diameter. This method cannot, therefore, test the distensibility of the small intestine. In the absence of lumen distention and the associated straightening of mucosal folds, this method cannot provide a confident diagnosis of morphologic normality.

Indications

The fact that intubation is not required constitutes the major advantage of the fluoroscopic follow-through over the small bowel enema or enteroclysis. The fluoroscopic study may be used in the routine follow-up of known Crohn's disease, in the demonstration of any lesions (with peroral pneumocolon) suspected to be situated in the ileocecal area, and in the assessment of diseases that resist lumen widening and extend over longer segments of intestine, such as radiation enteritis.

Peroral Pneumocolon

Peroral pneumocolon (PNC) technique[8-10] can significantly improve detail and information quality in the distal ileum, cecum, and right colon. It follows the peroral barium examination of the small bowel and is used after

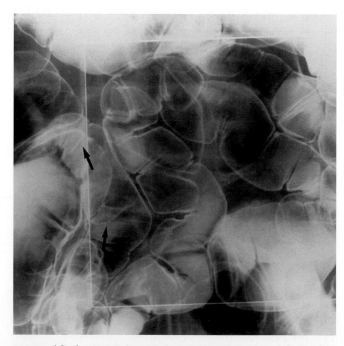

FIGURE 10–1. Normal peroral pneumocolon. The peroral pneumocolon outlines the normal terminal ileum *(arrows)* and distal ileum in excellent double contrast.

the ileum and cecum have become opacified. An intravenous injection of 1 mg of glucagon is given. A small rectal catheter is then inserted, an insufflator is attached, and air is introduced with the patient supine. The patient is then turned to the left to fill the right colon with air. To get air into the terminal ileum, it may be necessary to turn the patient further into a prone or semiprone position. After good distention has been achieved, compression spot films are taken of the areas of interest (Fig. 10–1).

Double Contrast Enema

Excellent double contrast views of the terminal ileum can also be obtained during the course of the double contrast enema. Reflux of air and barium into the terminal ileum is promoted by the use of intravenous glucagon. These views are particularly valuable for the diagnosis of early changes of Crohn's disease.

SMALL BOWEL ENEMA (ENTEROCLYSIS)

A catheter, passed into the distal duodenum or first loop of jejunum, makes possible the introduction of contrast materials directly into the small bowel, bypassing the delaying and limiting action of the pylorus. The rate of injection influences both speed of transit and distention. The barium suspension, which is introduced first and is then propelled further by the infusion of methylcellulose (MC), forms the single contrast phase. Gradually, the MC produces the required double contrast against a persistent barium coating of the mucosal surface.

Historical Note

The development of intubation techniques for the examination of the small bowel has been based on early work done and reported by Cole,[11] Einhorn,[12] Pribram and Kleiber,[13] Pesquera,[14] Gershon-Cohen and Shay,[15] Schatzki,[16] and Lura.[17]

Initially Einhorn duodenal tubes were used, later followed by Scott-Harden's coaxial tube system.[18] The Einhorn tube was replaced by the more easily managed tube described by Bilbao and coworkers.[19] Intubation was further facilitated by Gianturco's application of a modified Volkswagen speedometer cable as a guide in a duodenal tube described by Bilbao and coworkers.[20]

The small bowel enema came of age with the publications of Sellink.[21-23] His method essentially consisted of the infusion of barium by gravity through a nasoduodenal tube. The density of the suspension was adjusted to the patient's body thickness, the whole small bowel was filled with an uninterrupted column, and the examination could be completed with the injection of water for time-limited double contrast in the proximal small bowel.

Most publications concerning the intubation examination of the small bowel have come from innovators and enthusiasts who have not critically questioned the clinical value of this more complex procedure. Fleckenstein and

Pedersen[21] in 1975 were the first to report a series of enteroclyses and follow-through examinations carried out in the same patients. In 52 evaluation pairs they considered the enema to be superior in the jejunum and upper ileum but found no significant difference in the terminal ileum. Sanders and Ho[25] were able to compare the conventional small bowel examination with the small bowel enema (SBE) in 26 patients; the latter gave relevant additional information in 50% of their patients. In a comparison of the oral technique with the double contrast SBE in 43 patients with Crohn's disease, intubation was found to demonstrate pathology more clearly and to delineate the proximal extension of disease more accurately.[26] Fistulae were shown equally well by both modalities. A more recent prospective comparison study confirmed the significantly greater accuracy of intubation-based examinations over peroral methods.[27]

Technical Considerations
Distention

Distention is an integral part of the SBE and is associated with a few disadvantages that are greatly outweighed by its benefits. Disadvantages are that dilatation is rendered less obvious as a sign of disease and that the small bowel crowding in the peritoneal cavity increases. The advantages are that distention causes small bowel folds to straighten so that they can be assessed and measured. Misinterpretations can be avoided (Fig. 10–2); tiny surface alterations become visible (Fig. 10–3); and by testing distensibility, attention is drawn to even mildly narrowed or rigid segments (Fig. 10–4).

Transradiancy of Loops

Small bowel loops normally overlap within the abdominal cavity. This situation is aggravated with loop distention. When distended loops are filled with high-density barium, mucosal detail will be inadequate even when abdominal compression is applied. Transradiancy can be achieved by the use of barium of lower density together with a high kilovolt technique. This forms the basis of single contrast enteroclysis as described by Sellink[23] and Nolan.[28] The double contrast method combines transradiancy, distention, and the demonstration of mucosal surface detail by barium coating even at sites of overlapping bowel loops (Fig. 10–5).

Double Contrast Agents

The double contrast effect requires that the barium mucosal coating be highlighted against a distending agent of lower density. Water and air[13] were in use as double contrast agents before methylcellulose.

Air

Air should be the ideal double contrast medium because its density difference against barium is maximal and diffusion between them can never be a problem. Although well proved in the esophagus, stomach, and colon, air

FIGURE **10–2. Value of distention.** *A,* Before infusion of MC a false impression of nodularity is produced by the intersection of superimposed folds in contracted loops. *B,* Distention and double contrast demonstrate normal folds without nodules.

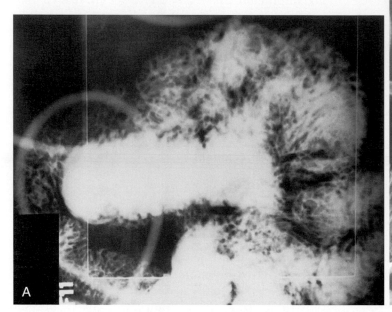

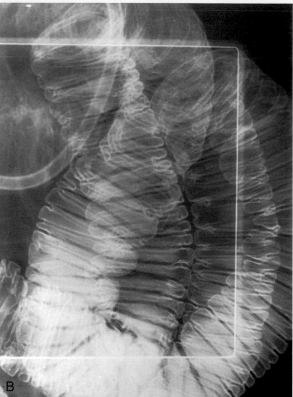

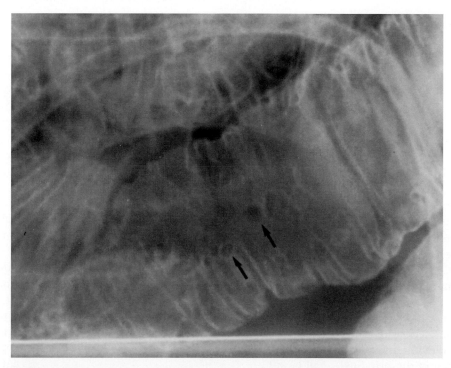

FIGURE **10–3. Value of double contrast.** Several small inflammatory polyps *(arrows)* are shown together with an interruption of mucosal folds. These are features of early Crohn's disease.

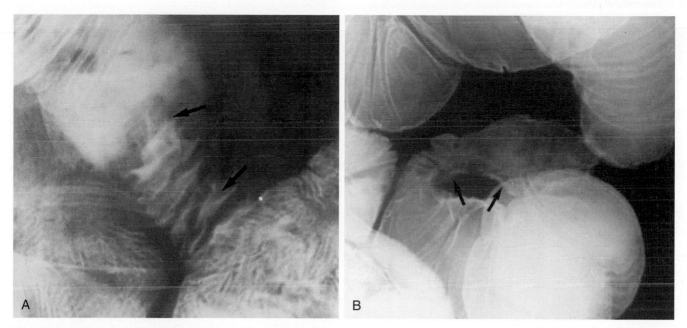

FIGURE 10–4. Two short skip lesions of early Crohn's disease in the lower jejunum present a nondistensible lumen. *A,* Segment with swollen folds is readily identified against the distended bowel above. *B,* A short skip lesion, a miniature representation of mesenteric border ulceration *(arrows)* and antimesenteric redundancy. Such lesions might not be recognized in most follow-through examinations.

double contrast for the small bowel has presented problems in our hands.

1. Air does not propel barium through the small bowel. Rather, air percolates through the small bowel loops without advancing the barium, which tends to collect in dependent pools.
2. As could be shown in the colon, a vertical x-ray beam may fail to demonstrate lesions submerged in

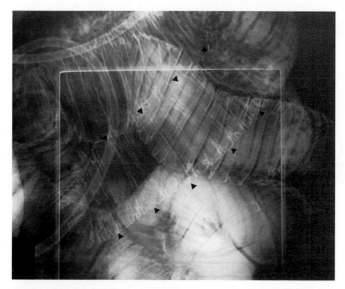

FIGURE 10–5. Importance of transradiancy. Two superimposed segments of jejunum are seen in double contrast *(arrowheads* outline one of the segments). Mucosal fold detail of both segments can be clearly seen. Compression spot film.

a barium pool or may show them inadequately against a background of pooled barium. In the colon this can be corrected by taking opposing lateral decubitus views with a horizontal beam. This cannot be usefully applied to the small bowel, where the lateral decubitus position causes dependent loop crowding with alteration of loop distribution in response to position change. This renders orientation between decubitus film pairs an impossible task.

Nevertheless, the air double contrast method can produce the most subtle surface detail. This method is the best way to image the terminal ileum, whether air is introduced as part of a barium enema or as part of the peroral pneumocolon method. It has been developed into a highly accurate technique by Japanese gastroenterologists.[29,30]

Methylcellulose

Historical Review. Having found the "water flush" method[31,32] diluted barium too much in the ileum, Trickey and coworkers[33] searched for a "flush" that would not readily mix with barium, that would be able to propel the barium toward the colon, and that would distend the lumen while rendering it radiolucent. They introduced a 0.7% solution of water containing hydroxyethylcellulose with a wetting agent, a proprietary preparation no longer available. A 1% suspension of methylcellulose (MC) in water had been used as a contrast agent for barium enemas,[34] with the claim that removal of barium coating from the bowel wall was minimized in this way. For their method of double contrast SBE, Gmündner and Wirth[35] used a "flush" of 2 tsp of MC in 900 ml of water, following

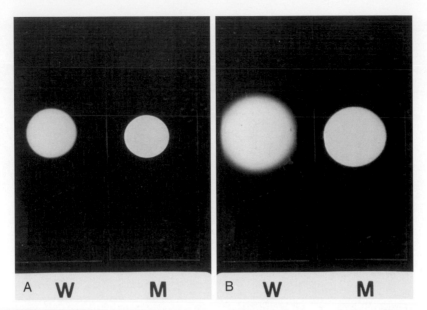

FIGURE 10–6. Diffusivity experiment. A drop of a barium suspension has been placed in the center of a slide covered in water and another drop into a slide covered with 0.5% MC solution. Images taken at 1 minute *(A)* and at 5 minutes *(B)* show diffusion with unsharp margins developing in water but continued sharp margination in MC.

the injection of only 50 ml of Micropaque (Nicholas Laboratories, Slough, England).

Methylcellulose for the Small Bowel Enema. A 0.5% solution of MC in water is used as a double contrast agent for the enteroclysis for the following reasons:

1. Used with compatible barium suspensions, such as Entero-H (E-Z-EM Co., Westbury, NY 11590), Micropaque liquid (Nicholas Laboratories, Slough, England), or Micropaque reconstituted powder (Picker Co., Cleveland, OH 44143), the MC solution shows a very low degree of diffusivity (Fig. 10–6).

2. The MC solution efficiently propels an unbroken though gradually diluting barium column toward the cecum while maintaining an uninterrupted barium coating of the mucosal surface. Although the density difference from barium to MC cannot approach that of barium to air, the MC method can produce excellent surface detail without interference from barium pools.

3. Small bowel loops distended with MC tend to remain in a state of relaxation or low activity and retain their double contrast for 15 to 25 minutes (Fig. 10–7).[36]

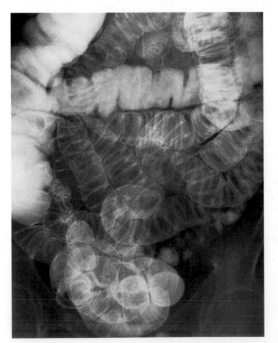

FIGURE 10–7. Effect of MC on the small bowel. An overhead film taken 20 minutes after the infusion of barium and MC shows a relaxed, still barium-coated small bowel even though barium has progressed to fill the colon.

4. The combination of compatible barium and 0.5% MC has been shown to resist unacceptable degrees of flocculation long enough for the examination to be completed, even in severe cases of malabsorption.

5. On entry into the colon the desiccation-resistant MC and barium mixture provoke more complete evacuation.

Entrocel, a concentrated solution of MC (Lafayette Pharmaceuticals, Lafayette, IN 47904), should be diluted with water to make 1900 ml of a 0.5% solution.

Barium Flocculation

Commercial barium preparations are held in suspension by additives that provide a protective coating to individual particles preventing particle-to-particle contact.[36] Nevertheless, even protected particles may flocculate in the presence of mucin or secretion from an inflamed mucosa. Flocculated barium does not provide a reliable image of the mucosal surface. A mild degree of flocculation appears as a granular pattern, whereas severe degrees of flocculation present patterns that reflect the physical chemical change in the barium rather than the pattern of the mucosal surface ("segmentation," "moulage").

A direct relationship could be demonstrated in vitro among the degree of flocculation, the relative quantity of interacting fluids, and the duration of exposure to them. The comparatively small quantities of barium intermittently leaving the stomach in a follow-through examination and passing rather slowly through the small intestine are readily overwhelmed by abnormal small bowel contents. Enteroclysis, with larger amounts of barium introduced almost as a bolus, is usually able to coat the mucosa and produce images before flocculation develops.[37] Although flocculation eventually occurs in the presence of abnormal fluid material, it tends to be less pronounced and may be delayed long enough for adequate imaging of the small bowel to be possible in most adverse circumstances.

Patient Preparation

We agree that a clean right colon is important.[14,22] The presence of feces in the right colon is often associated with the presence of similar material in the terminal ileum and tends to retard the passage of barium. It increases the amount of barium required for the examination because the distal ileum has to be cleared of debris before it can be shown in useful double contrast.[22] This is usually achieved by having the patient take four bisacodyl (Dulcolax) tablets with 2 glasses of water in the afternoon before the day of the examination. No further food or fluid is allowed until the examination has been completed. Drugs that decrease bowel activity should be discontinued until after the examination.

Except in cases of higher grade small bowel obstruction, we ask the patient to take 20 mg of metoclopramide (two 10-mg tablets) 20 minutes before starting the SBE.[38]

Low-level conscious sedation should ideally be part of an enteroclysis. However, this requires nurse-assisted monitoring of pulse oximetry and of pulse and blood pressure recordings. Midazolam (Versed), 1 to 5 mg intravenously, is injected very slowly, the amount related to the patient's response. Occasionally, fentanyl may have to be added for greater sedative-analgesic effect.[39]

Intubation

Local anesthesia is given either to the throat as a 20% benzocaine spray (for peroral intubation) or to the nasal passages as 2% lidocaine viscous gel (for transnasal intubation). We prefer to use a 13F catheter with a balloon and side holes distal to it (Maglinte type catheter, E-Z-EM Co., Westbury, NY 11590). A Teflon-coated, rotationally rigid guide wire with a curved tip can be advanced to the closed end of the catheter. The balloon can be inflated with up to 25 ml of air and serves to control reflux from the jejunum or duodenum. Before use, the catheter system should be lubricated inside and out with a silicone spray. The integrity of the balloon should be tested before introduction. A sharp bend is made in the outer end of the guide wire for turning of the tip during introduction.

With the patient sitting on the x-ray examination table, the catheter is introduced with the guide wire about 7.5 cm away from the tip. When the fundus or body of the stomach is believed to have been reached, the patient is then placed supine and the position of the catheter is checked by fluoroscopy. A routine method of intubation is described and illustrated below.

We generally aim to position the balloon of the tube beyond the duodenojejunal junction. Several problems may be encountered during the course of intubation:

Catheter Coiled in the Fundus (Fig. 10–8). The tube is withdrawn until its tip lies at the cardia. The patient is turned to the right, which greatly reduces the depth of the fundal recess. Reintroduction of the tube now usually takes it into the antrum.

Catheter Doubled Back in the Antrum (Fig. 10–9). When advancing the catheter toward the pylorus, the guide is held back about 7.5 cm. Turning the patient toward the left may reveal the duodenal bulb outlined by air. More importantly, it also shifts the stomach toward the left, straightens the approach to the bulb, and widens the proximal duodenal flexure. Occasionally the catheter doubles back within the antrum. This is corrected by the "double-back maneuver": The catheter is withdrawn slowly while the guide is advanced until the end of the tube flicks forward again.

Catheter Held Up at the Pylorus (Fig. 10–10). Rarely will entry into the duodenal bulb fail with the patient turned left and the operator patiently persevering. It may then be necessary to withdraw the wire and inject a bolus of air or a sufficient amount of barium to outline the passage and exclude a possible abnormality as the cause.

Catheter Stopped at the Inferior Duodenal Flexure. If possible, the guide is advanced beyond the superior flexure. Pressure by the gloved hand helps the end of the catheter round the retroperitoneally fixed inferior flexure.

Catheter Through the Duodenojejunal Junction (Fig. 10–11). After the catheter has reached the expected position of the duodenojejunal junction, the patient is turned on the left side and then slightly semiprone. This makes the mobile jejunum fall away from the retroperitoneal termination of the duodenum and widens the flexure. The patient is also asked to take deep breaths and to cough while the tube is slowly advanced with the guide wire held back at the upper or lower duodenal flexure. If this fails, it may be that the flexure is directed toward the right and that the patient may have to turn right for successful catheter passage. The patient may be turned supine to ascertain the correct position of the tube, after which the balloon can be inflated (Fig. 10–12). If transit into the jejunum has failed after two or three attempts, it is best to give up and leave the catheter as near to the end of the duodenum as possible.

Catheter Arrested at Unexpected Level. It is absolutely essential not to force the advance of the catheter. It may be arrested in a Zenker's diverticulum, by a duodenal tumor, or by a stricture. Always remove the wire and inject barium. The catheter may also try to take an unexpected turn. If it does, there is usually a good reason for it, for example, a right paraduodenal hernia or a simple case of nonrotation. (For a more detailed description of intubation with its problems and their solutions, see reference 40.)

Barium Injection

We use 60-ml syringes for the injection of the barium suspension, either Entero-H at 80% w/v or Micropaque at 85% w/v. A total of 180 to 200 ml is normally injected, somewhat less when the patient is very thin or has had a small bowel resection, more when the patient is stout or when the diagnostic problem relates to the distal ileum. Considerably more barium may have to be given (up to 400 ml) if there is small bowel dilatation with fluid excess (Fig. 10–13).

Barium should not be injected at a rate that will cause undue jejunal distention because this may delay or arrest forward flow. The aim is to achieve forward movement of an uninterrupted column of barium. We normally turn patients halfway to the left during barium injection to delay the entry into ileal loops. If the barium column stops advancing, the patient may be turned prone because peristaltic activity usually improves in this position.

Patients with bowel atony due to neuromuscular disease or prolonged obstruction are a special problem. Overinjection and overdistention of the jejunum are to be avoided. Instead, careful turning of the patient may promote onward flow of the heavier barium even through fluid-filled loops.

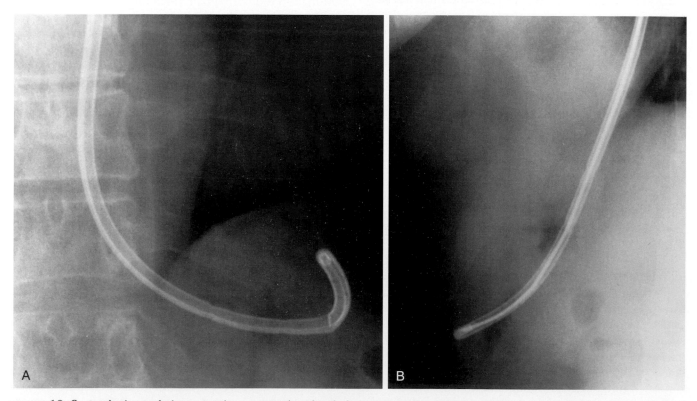

FIGURE 10–8. Intubation technique. *A,* Tube was introduced with the patient sitting. Patient recumbent, tube is found to have coiled into the fundus. *B,* The patient is turned sharply to the right, the tube is pulled back to the cardia, and the wire is advanced and its tip rotated toward the body of the stomach. Tube and wire can then be introduced further.

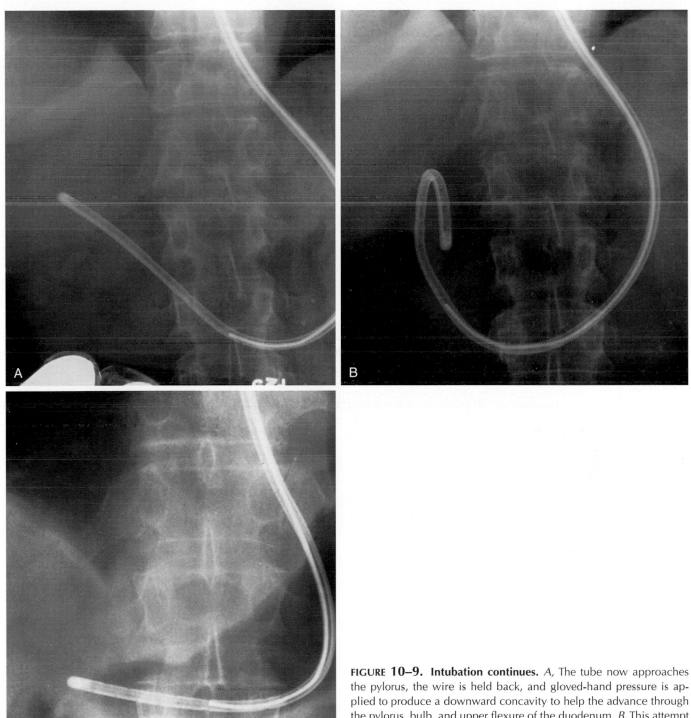

FIGURE 10–9. Intubation continues. *A,* The tube now approaches the pylorus, the wire is held back, and gloved-hand pressure is applied to produce a downward concavity to help the advance through the pylorus, bulb, and upper flexure of the duodenum. *B,* This attempt failed, and the tube has folded back into the antrum. *C,* The catheter was withdrawn somewhat while the wire was advanced to straighten the tube again.

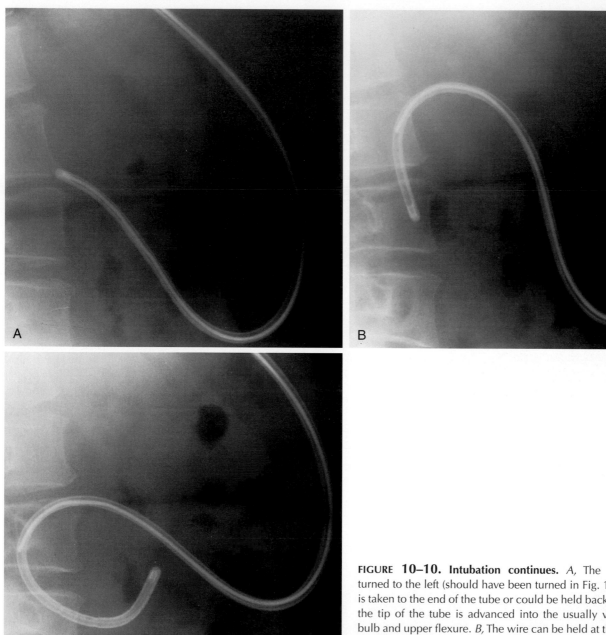

FIGURE 10–10. Intubation continues. *A,* The patient is now turned to the left (should have been turned in Fig. 10–9*A*), the wire is taken to the end of the tube or could be held back somewhat, and the tip of the tube is advanced into the usually visible duodenal bulb and upper flexure. *B,* The wire can be held at the flexure to advance the catheter over it. *C,* The tube moves into the ascending duodenum but may need to be helped by hand pressure through the distal duodenal flexure.

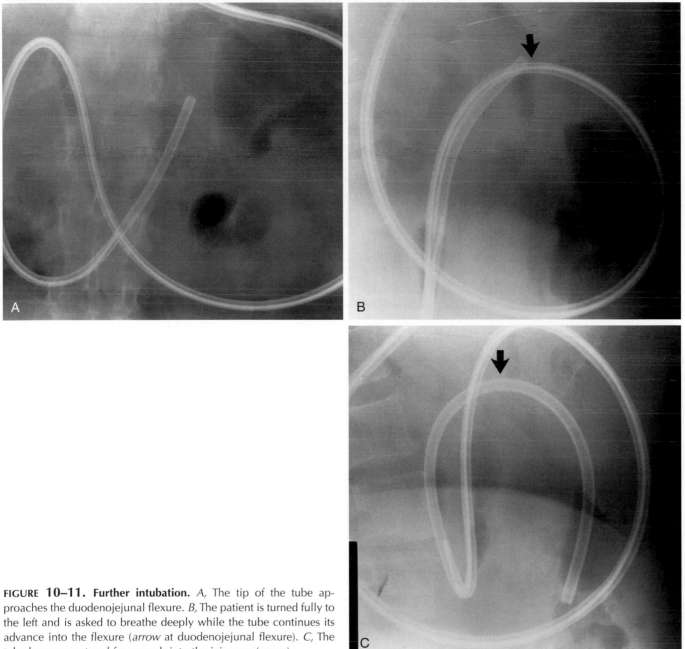

FIGURE 10–11. Further intubation. *A,* The tip of the tube approaches the duodenojejunal flexure. *B,* The patient is turned fully to the left and is asked to breathe deeply while the tube continues its advance into the flexure *(arrow* at duodenojejunal flexure). *C,* The tube has now entered far enough into the jejunum *(arrow).*

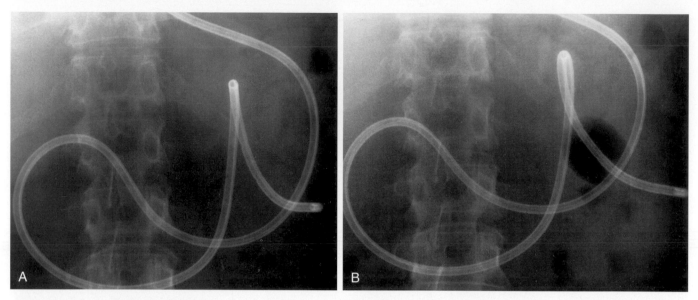

FIGURE 10–12. Intubation completed. *A,* The patient is placed supine to confirm the correct position of the tube. *B,* The balloon of the catheter is now inflated with 20 ml of air. The balloon is situated beyond the ligament of Treitz.

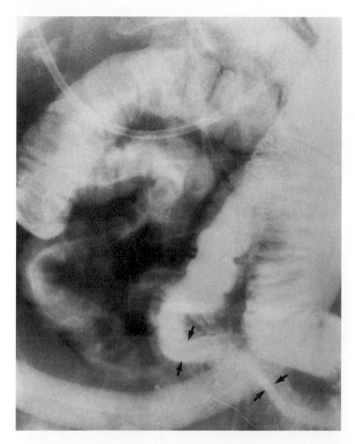

FIGURE 10–13. Evidence of excess fluid. Streaming of barium *(arrows)* and increasing barium dilution indicate excess fluid. A larger than usual amount of barium is required in such cases.

Methylcellulose Infusion

The 0.5% solution of MC is best infused by an electric pump, which ensures a steady inflow at an accurately adjustable rate, usually between 60 and 100 ml/min. This is continued until sufficient transradiancy and distention have been achieved in the distal and terminal ileum. If progress is too rapid and distention is inadequate, the rate of inflow of MC should be increased to cause proximal jejunal distention, which also slows movement through more distal bowel loops.

Normally up to 2 liters of MC is injected. If barium reaches the sigmoid and rectum before adequate transradiancy has been attained in the distal small bowel (rapid transit into the colon), a barium enema catheter may be inserted into the rectum and its contents gradually siphoned into an attached empty enema bag.

The balloon of the catheter must be deflated before it is withdrawn. In certain circumstances, such as occult bleeding, we withdraw the catheter into the duodenum, reinflate the balloon and inject barium followed by boluses of air. It is also possible to take the catheter back into the stomach and carry out a limited double contrast study of the stomach and duodenum, although barium in the transverse colon often interferes with this examination.

Imaging

Although we observe the progress and appearance of the barium column by intermittent fluoroscopy with abdominal compression—the single contrast phase—we do not usually record images unless an abnormality is seen or suspected. More frequent films are taken in the phase of developing double contrast, usually with compression. It is, however, important to compress and release compression gradually to avoid forcible mixing of barium and MC, which would negate the double contrast result. The patient should also be instructed to turn slowly or slide gently when changing position.

The proximal and distal jejunum are usually best shown with the patient turned slightly to the right (Fig. 10–14A–D), and the proximal and mid-ileum with the patient turned toward the left (Fig. 10–14E, F). The demonstration of the distal and terminal ileum can be a problem. Because the accumulation of barium in the cecum may interfere with its visualization, it may be important to film the terminal ileum during the passage of the first bolus. Later on, the terminal ileum should be imaged in double contrast (Fig. 10–14G, H); it may be necessary to inject glucagon, 0.5 mg IV, to achieve satisfactory double contrast in the terminal ileum.

A valuable part of the examination can be the observation of peristaltic activity, best seen before distention with MC. It is also important to carefully palpate all accessible loops. We particularly evaluate the mobility of loops to identify any adhesive processes and their pliability, that is, the ability to change shape in response to compression. Mural infiltration and inflammation stiffen loops and reduce or abolish pliability.

A prone overhead view on a 14/17 film (Fig. 10–15) is taken at the end of the fluoroscopic examination. In cases of obstruction or in adynamic states, it may be necessary to follow up with later spot and overhead films. Such an examination may have to continue intermittently for as long as 24 hours. In fact, in all cases of high-grade obstruction or prolonged obstruction with aperistalsis, enteroclysis is the wrong examination and should be replaced by CT scanning.

A successful SBE presents the whole of the small bowel in double contrast, with the density difference between barium on the mucosa and the MC in the lumen often showing a gradual but slight decrease in the distal ileum. It provides strong evidence of normality or of disease.

Problems of Examination

Misjudged Quantities. If *too little barium* has been introduced, visualization of the distal ileum suffers and MC may actually overtake the barium column. If recognized earlier, it is still possible to salvage the study by injecting additional barium and then resuming the infusion of MC. If *too much barium* has been given, filling of the colon may occur before double contrast has extended into the distal ileum. Barium in the rectosigmoid may then have to be evacuated as suggested earlier. If in doubt regarding the amount of barium to be given, it is better to give too much than too little.

Reflux into the Stomach. Reflux of MC was a more serious problem before balloon catheters became available. Occasionally reflux may still occur even with an inflated balloon, especially when the balloon has been inflated in the duodenum. The rate of injection of MC must then be reduced and the patient turned well to the left during injection. However, slowing the injection of MC necessarily causes less adequate distention of bowel loops and compromises the quality of the examination. Massive reflux can be dangerous to older or enfeebled patients because aspiration into the lung may follow. It is important to watch out for this complication, stop the examination, and aspirate stomach contents if it has occurred.

Ileal Loops in the Pelvis. Patients ought to be advised not to empty the bladder immediately before the examination. Not infrequently, however, especially after hysterectomy, ileal loops can be found lying deep in the pelvis, inaccessible to compression. For a successful examination it is then necessary to extend double contrast throughout these ileal loops and to take spot films of the pelvis with the patient in lateral or off-lateral positions (Fig. 10–16A). A prone view with the tube angled 30 degrees caudad is also helpful (Fig. 10–16B).

Inadequate Double Contrast Distention in Distal/ Terminal Ileum. As already mentioned, an IV injection of 0.5 mg glucagon produces hypotonia with lumen widening and better double contrast. Careful compression is needed, at times with the patient prone and balloon paddle compression from underneath.

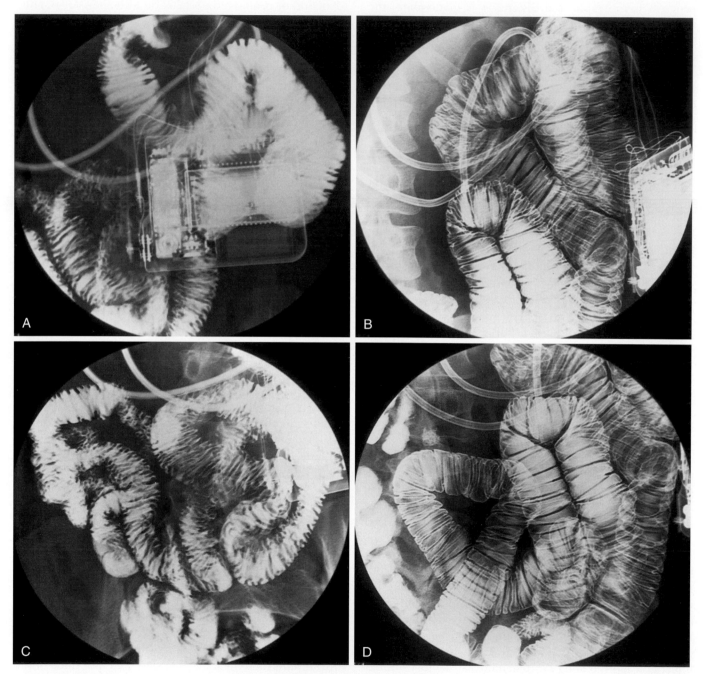

FIGURE 10–14. Development of single contrast into double contrast enteroclysis. *Proximal jejunum: A,* In single contrast. *B,* Into double contrast after infusion of MC. *Midjejunum: C,* In single contrast. *D,* Into double contrast.

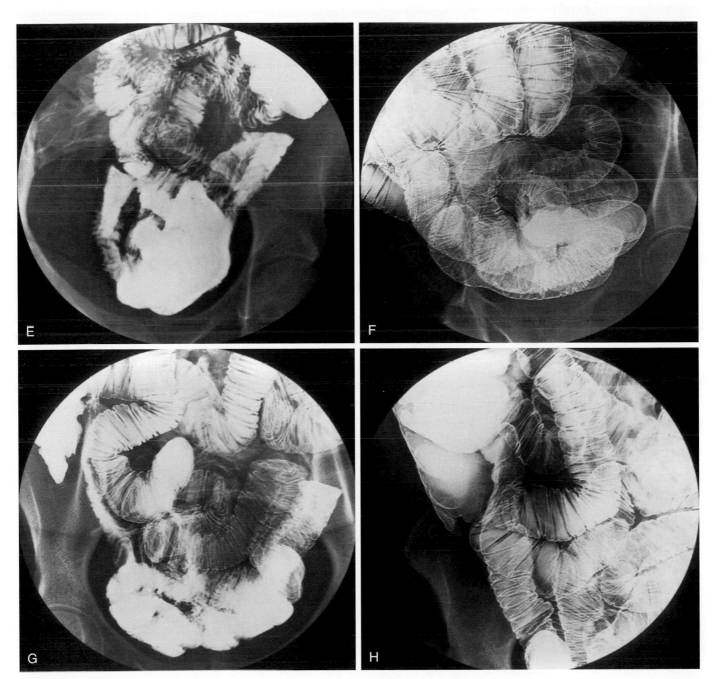

FIGURE 10–14 *Continued* *Distal ileum: E,* In single contrast. *F,* Into double contrast. *Area of terminal ileum: G,* In single contrast. *H,* Into double contrast.

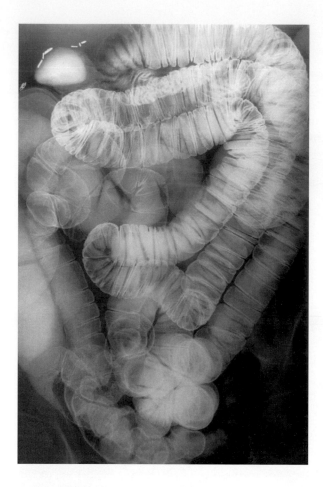

FIGURE 10–15. Completion of fluoroscopic examination. A final prone overhead image is obtained.

FIGURE 10–16. Problem of bowel loops prolapsed deep into the pelvis. *A,* Good mucosal detail is obtained by taking a lateral or off-lateral view of pelvis after full double contrast development in prolapsed bowel loops. *B,* A 30 degree caudad angled prone film can be useful.

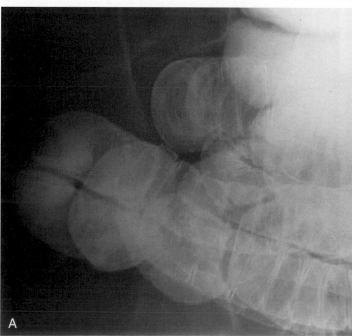

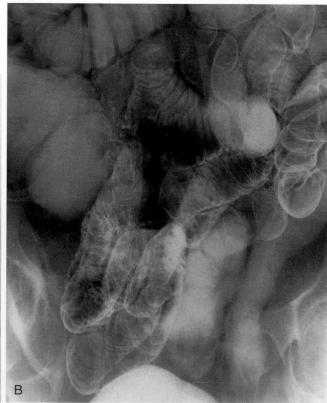

Small Bowel Enema Through a Long Intestinal Tube

Patients in whom a long intestinal tube, such as a Miller-Abbott (MA) tube, has been inserted in the clinical management of small bowel obstruction may require a barium study to demonstrate the level, degree, and cause of the obstructing lesion. The MA tube can be used for the introduction of contrast material provided that attention is given to the following points.

1. The tip of the tube should reach fairly close to the expected level of obstruction. At the very least it must reach 15 cm into the jejunum to ensure that all its side holes are beyond the ligament of Treitz.
2. Whenever possible, enough barium should be introduced to reach the site of obstruction. A maximum amount of 400 ml should not be exceeded.
3. MC infusion is begun only after barium has reached the obstructing lesion or after as much as 400 ml of barium has failed to get to that level (however, see an earlier note on the careful introduction of barium in patients with bowel atony). In the absence of bowel atony an infusion of MC can be started to try to propel the barium onward. Whenever possible, the object is to produce double contrast at the obstruction site and reach a more accurate diagnosis of the nature of the obstructing lesion. In the presence of excessive amounts of retained fluid in distended bowel loops, as indicated on the plain film of the abdomen, an enteroclysis should not be done. (For further reading on all aspects of the SBE technique, see reference 40).

Features of Small Bowel Normality

The combination of distention, double contrast, and abdominal compression makes it possible to study the shape of folds and to measure further parameters.

Fold Shape. Valvulae conniventes are found throughout the small bowel but can be less pronounced or absent in the ileum. With the bowel distended, these folds run fairly straight across the long axis, their sides parallel, joining the bowel wall in the form of "rounded corners" (Fig. 10–17A).[23] At times, more often in the ileum, a few of the folds crowd together on the concave side of a bend in a bowel loop. Such triangular fold patterns can be found even in straight segments of ileum, when their direction of convergence is seen to alternate (Fig. 10–17B).

Fold Thickness. Folds are normally slightly thicker in the nondistended bowel and become thinner with distention. In distended loops, jejunal folds are normally up to 2 mm thick, and ileal folds are up to 1 mm thick (Fig. 10–17A, C). Fold thickness is considered pathologic when it exceeds 2.5 mm in the distended jejunum and 2 mm in the distended ileum.

Number of Folds. In the more distended, possibly somewhat elongated, small bowel as seen in this form of SBE, the number of circular folds per inch of length was found to be less than previously reported by Sellink.[23] We have found four to seven folds per inch in the distended proximal jejunum (Fig. 10–17D) and two to four folds per inch in the more distal ileum (Fig. 10–17E). In the occasional patient in whom small bowel tone appears to be increased, particularly in young persons, a greater number of folds was seen in what appeared to be shortened bowel.

Fold Height. Jejunum and ileum also differ in the height of folds, which usually varies from 3 to 7 mm in the jejunum (Fig. 10–17D) and from 1.5 to 2.5 mm in the ileum (Fig. 10–17F). The decrease in height occurs gradually in a caudad direction (Fig. 10–17F). However, fold height may vary considerably within the same segment of bowel.

Lumen Diameter. Because of the lumen distention characteristic for the enteroclysis, diameters for the proximal jejunum are from 3 to 4 cm, from 2.5 to 3.5 cm in the lower jejunum, and from 2 to 2.8 cm in the ileum (Fig. 10–17A, B). Diameters are considered abnormal when they exceed 4.5 cm in the upper jejunum, 4 cm in the mid-small bowel, and 3 cm in the ileum. Diameters should not be measured in front of a wave of contraction.

Wall Thickness. Wall thickness can be measured if two barium-coated luminal surfaces are seen to be parallel over at least 4 cm on a film taken with abdominal compression. We then consider the loops to lie in the same plane and regard the distance between the two mucosal surfaces to represent the combined thickness of the two bowel walls. Half this measurement then gives the thickness of a single bowel loop (Fig. 10–17D). Of normal patients, 75% showed a wall thickness of 1 to 1.5 mm, 12.5% showed a thickness of 1.5 to 2 mm, and 12.5% showed a thickness less than 1 mm. This measurement was found to be the same throughout the small bowel. A wall thickness greater than 2 mm is considered abnormal.

Length of the Small Bowel. No accurate estimate can be made of this three-dimensional reality on the basis of its two-dimensional x-ray film representation. There is no doubt that the length of bowel varies greatly with the height and weight of the individual. Muscle tone may also be a factor. Withdrawing an MA tube under x-ray control has shown that approximately two thirds of it can be pulled back through an increasingly telescoping gut before the tip of the tube even begins to move.

Variations and Developmental Anomalies of the Small Bowel

Malrotation. Malrotation is the most common anomaly occurring in the second stage of reentry into the abdominal cavity. This process can be arrested at any stage. With *nonrotation,* the mesenteric small bowel is situated on the right side of the abdomen. Symptoms may then be produced by bands extending from the medially placed cecum or right colon to the right lateral abdominal wall. These are Ladd's bands, which may cause compression of the duodenum.

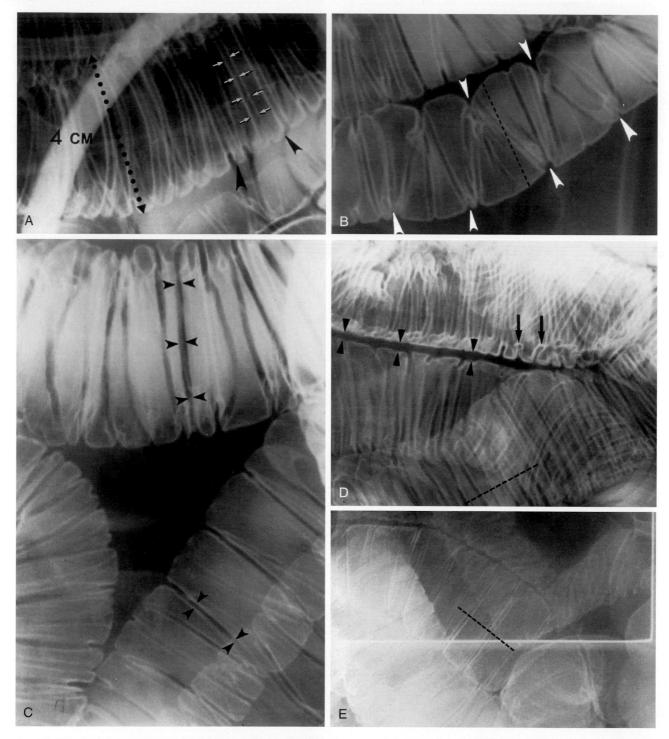

FIGURE 10–17. Normal appearances: Kerkring's folds and wall thickness. *A,* Straightened mucosal folds form slightly rounded corners at their junctions with the bowel wall *(arrowheads).* Normal lumen diameter of the proximal jejunum (4 cm) is indicated by *dots,* and normal thickness of straight folds (2 mm), by *arrows. B,* Triangular fold patterns in parts of a normal ileum *(arrowheads). C,* Comparison of the greater thickness of jejunal folds above with that of ileal folds below (between *arrowheads*). *D,* Height of jejunal folds (5 to 7 mm) *(arrows).* Number of folds per 2.5 cm of length (as crossed by *interrupted line*) = five to eight folds in jejunum. Combined wall thickness between adjacent and parallel mucosal surfaces *(arrowheads)* = 2 to 3 mm (i.e., single bowel wall thickness = 1 to 1.5 mm). *E,* Number of folds per 2.5 cm length *(interrupted line)* of ileum = 2 to 4.

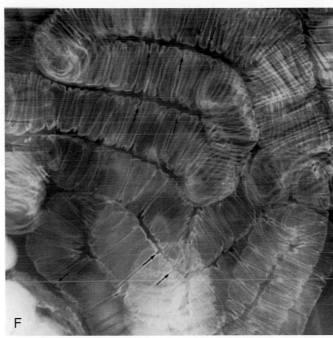

FIGURE **10–17** *Continued* F, Close-up view of a segment of jejunum above and proximal ileum below illustrates the gradual change in fold thickness and height. Fold heights seen in profile are indicated by arrows.

Anomalies of Fixation. Premature fixation of the cecum in the right upper quadrant occurs not infrequently. More commonly, there is a freely mobile cecum with its own mesentery. It may be found folded upward, in which case the terminal ileum appears to enter from below and from the right. Such a cecum may also prolapse into the pelvis, where it fills with barium and obscures the terminal ileum.

Lymph Follicles. Numerous 2- to 3-mm rounded, often umbilicated elevations scattered over an otherwise normal mucosa can be found in the terminal ileum (Fig. 10–18); these elevations extend further proximal in children and in some adults. These elevations become particularly prominent in those patients with immune deficiency.

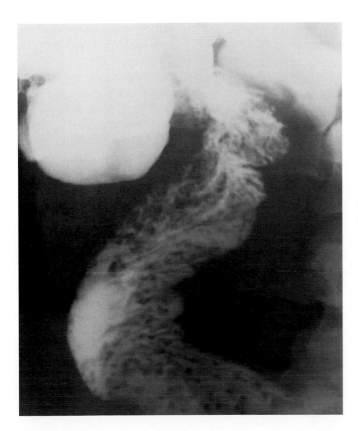

FIGURE **10–18.** **Lymph follicles in the terminal ileum.** The elevations, each 2 to 3 mm in diameter, are distributed fairly evenly against a background of normal mucosa. This may be a normal finding.

SMALL BOWEL ENEMA IN DISEASE

Examples rather than complete descriptions of disease processes are presented here. The purpose is to show the versatility and increased accuracy of the double contrast method and its relevance to clinical management.

Meckel's Diverticulum

Meckel's diverticulum is found in 1% to 3% of autopsies. It is a true diverticulum arising from the antimesenteric border of the ileum within 90 cm of the ileocecal valve. Its demonstration by follow-through barium examination has been infrequent. The SBE is the most reliable method for its demonstration in the adult.[41–43] The fold at the base of the diverticulum usually forms a triangle with the ileal folds in its immediate vicinity (Fig. 10–19).

Malabsorption States

The term *malabsorption* is frequently applied to a combination of maldigestion and mucosal malabsorption of food substances. Occasionally there may be a postmucosal element of malassimilation. Most generalized small

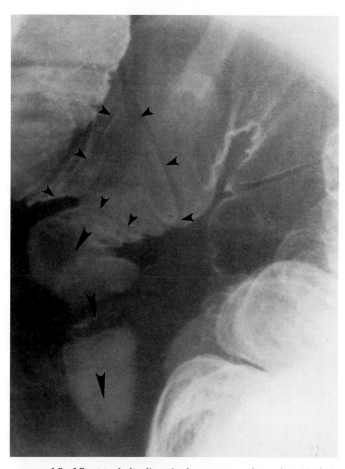

FIGURE 10–19. Meckel's diverticulum. A 5-cm long diverticulum *(large arrowheads)* arises at the antimesenteric aspect of a loop of distal ileum. A triangular fold pattern (between small *arrowheads)* outlines a mucosal plateau at the origin of the diverticulum.

bowel diseases are accompanied by a degree of malabsorption, which may be accentuated by actual loss of nutrients in increased secretions. The disturbance of absorption is usually multifactorial, although in mild forms of even generalized small bowel disease it may be limited to selected materials. More localized disease affects only substances that are normally absorbed at those levels. In most conditions, steatorrhea, the disturbance of fat absorption, is the distinctive clinical marker of malabsorption. Secondary immunodeficiencies may accompany malabsorption states.

Pattern recognition–based x-ray diagnosis is not often possible in the small bowel, and is even less likely in malabsorption states. It is, therefore, necessary to be aware of and be able to interpret a patient's clinical presentation to evaluate x-ray findings against this background.

Clinical Diagnosis

The amount of fat excreted is expressed as grams per day. Reported upper limits of normality vary between 5 and 12 g.[44,45] The fact that fecal fat content varies with the amount of dietary fat ingested may explain this considerable difference. According to Losowsky and coworkers,[1] a fat excretion of 7% of intake would express the upper limit of normality more accurately. However, quantitative fecal fat analyses are now not often requested, and a qualitative fecal fat test is often used instead. More widely used in patients believed to have impairment of fat absorption is the ^{14}C-triolein breath analysis. A positive test does not, however, give information as to the cause or site of the underlying abnormality. A positive D-xylose absorption test would indicate more proximal intestinal mucosal disease as a cause for steatorrhea. The same test would also be useful in patients with intestinal bacterial overgrowth when it may also be supplemented by a hydrogen breath test.

Mucosal biopsies are the most important method for positive diagnosis in many conditions presenting with malabsorption. Until recently, perorally passed tubes using a suction technique had been the standard method for obtaining biopsy specimens. Endoscopic sampling has now largely replaced it and has the added advantage of direct visualization of the biopsy site. However, endoscopic biopsy specimens are mostly taken in the duodenum rather than the proximal jejunum, which is the predominant site of most of the pathologies.

To simplify radiologic diagnosis, several authors have presented lists of x-ray findings in steatorrhea.[46,47] The list presented here is based on the increased imaging accuracy of enteroclysis (Table 10–1).

Role of Radiology

Clinical awareness that a state of malabsorption exists should precede referral for an SBE. The purpose of radiology is to demonstrate or at least suggest a cause for malabsorption. It is important to defer the possible onset of flocculation so that mucosal surfaces can be imaged in

TABLE 10–1. *Small Bowel Enema in Malabsorption States*

X-ray Feature	No Fluid Increase	Fluid Increase
Folds of normal thickness	Maldigestion—pancreatic enzyme or bile salt deficiency; gastric surgery; alactasia	Adult celiac disease or dermatitis herpetiformis (fold separation in proximal jejunum)
Dilatation of lumen	Scleroderma (hide-bound bowel sign); dermatomyositis; amyloidosis	Celiac disease; obstruction; pseudo-obstruction; jejunal diverticulosis (fluid in diverticula)
Folds, thickened, straight	Radiation enteropathy; eosinophilic enteritis; macroglobulinemia	Edema (e.g., due to hypoalbuminemia); Zollinger-Ellison syndrome (duodenum mostly); abetalipoproteinemia; giardiasis (increased irritability)
Folds, unevenly thickened, nodular	Amyloidosis AL; lymphoma; extensive Crohn's disease (ulceration); mastocytosis (gastric antrum)	Crohn's disease, ischemia
Micronodularity (nodules 1–3 mm size)	Whipple's disease (1–3 mm nodules); amyloidosis AA; macroglobulinemia; IgA deficiency	Lymphangiectasia (1–3 mm grouped nodules); giardiasis (if associated IgA deficiency); *Mycobacterium avium* in AIDS
Structural lesions		Stasis and bacterial overgrowth associated with strictures, blind loop, blind pouch; pseudo-obstruction; diverticulosis

sufficient detail. The technique of the SBE needs to be slightly modified:

1. The balloon of the catheter should be inflated in the fourth part of the duodenum to include the entire duodenojejunal flexure in the imaging process.
2. More barium is infused at a slightly higher rate of flow.
3. Compression spot films are taken early during the infusion of MC, without waiting for fully developed double contrast.

It should be a rare event for radiology to suggest the presence of a clinically unsuspected malabsorption state on the basis of flocculation of barium, a most unreliable sign.

Celiac Disease
Clinical Diagnosis

The clinical diagnosis of celiac disease can be difficult because not every patient presents with steatorrhea. In fact, most patients show atypical or minimal features, such as only hematologic abnormalities in 38% of diagnosed cases.[48] Essential to definitive diagnosis is the demonstration of subtotal villous atrophy in the jejunum or, somewhat less adequately, in the duodenum. A return to clinical normality (but not necessarily histologic normality) after a period of gluten withdrawal confirms the diagnosis of celiac disease, which requires lifelong avoidance of gluten-containing foods.

Radiologic Findings

The SBE can play an important diagnostic function, especially in cases with atypical clinical presentation. In 75% of patients with adult celiac disease, the separation of mucosal folds in the distended proximal jejunum is wider than normal. A finding of three or fewer folds over the length of 1 inch is highly diagnostic of celiac disease (Fig. 10–20A), whereas the presence of five or more folds per inch strongly refutes this diagnosis. The demonstration of four folds per inch of proximal jejunum would be equivocal.[49] A further SBE feature aiding the diagnosis of celiac disease is the presence of an increased number of slightly thickened folds in the ileum (jejunization) (Fig. 10–20B), a feature of adaptation to the reduced absorptive capacity of the diseased jejunum.[50] Combining the celiac disease features of the jejunum and ileum, a positive identification by enteroclysis increases to 84% of cases.

It is a not infrequent misconception that mucosal folds are thickened in uncomplicated celiac disease. It is true that apparent fold thickening may develop in the course of the SBE and is due to an increased output of secretions, a pseudofold thickening now hardly ever seen.[51] However, real fold thickening may occur and be due to edema caused by malabsorption-related hypoalbuminemia.[52]

Transient intussusceptions are commonly seen during follow-through fluoroscopy in patients with celiac disease.[53] They are not seen with the SBE. Dilatation can be a feature of celiac disease but is more difficult to appreciate by enteroclysis.

Complications

Ulcerative Jejunoileitis. Patients with prolonged celiac disease may occasionally present with strictures, probably a result of prior ulcerative jejunoileitis. A more acute form of ulcerative jejunoileitis has been described in patients with celiac disease. It involves a segment of variable length and causes thickening of its wall and of its folds, with shallow ulceration. It not only resembles lym-

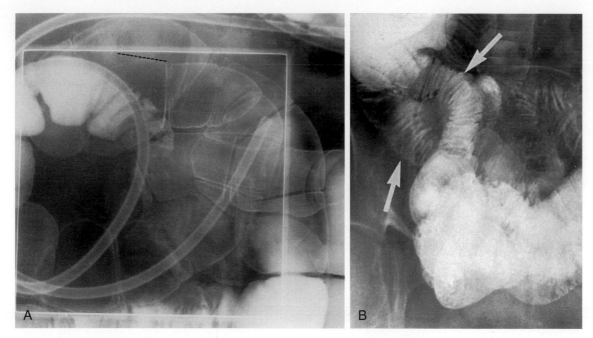

FIGURE 10–20. Celiac disease. *A,* Separation of folds in the distended jejunum. The 2.5 cm *interrupted line* touches only one fold. Two folds, at most, would be crossed if the line had been placed elsewhere. This finding is highly characteristic of adult celiac disease. *B,* Ileal folds are crowded and slightly thicker than those normally seen in the ileum *(arrows).* This appearance has been termed "jejunization" of the ileum.

phoma but may also be its precursor. It rarely has been encountered in patients without celiac disease.

Carcinoma. The relationship of celiac disease to gastrointestinal malignancy has been well documented.[54,55] A significantly increased incidence of esophageal, gastric, and rectal carcinoma and to a lesser degree of small bowel carcinoma occurs in patients with long-established celiac disease. Men are particularly at risk.

Enteropathy-associated T-cell Lymphoma (EATCL). Lymphoma has long been known to complicate celiac disease, and its prevalence does not seem to be affected by gluten abstention or the lack of it. It has been suggested that depression of cell-mediated immunity may relate to this increased risk. T-cell lymphoma seems to predominate and progress rapidly. Its radiologic features can be subtle, a mere nodular thickening of folds over a limited length of bowel (Fig. 10–21*A*), or atypical, an ulcerated stricture with "shouldering" (Fig. 10–21*B*). Other patients with celiac-related lymphoma may show the more typical findings of larger nodules and of endoenteric or exoenteric masses. However, the exact relationship of this lymphoma to celiac disease is not as clear-cut as previously believed. The lymphoma may occur in patients after years of fully documented celiac disease. But it may also occur at a time when the diagnosis of celiac disease had not yet been made or it may precede a diagnosis of celiac disease (EATCL).[56–58]

Hyposplenism. Hyposplenism tends to accompany long-standing celiac disease. A reduced size of the spleen expresses the degree of hyposplenism. Spleen size can be adequately measured by CT scans. The cavitary lymph node syndrome can be a late complication of hyposplenism.

Dermatitis Herpetiformis

Dermatitis herpetiformis is associated with the small bowel abnormalities of celiac disease. Clinically, this may vary from asymptomatic villous atrophy to florid celiac disease. The radiologic appearances are indistinguishable from those of celiac disease, and the symptoms and small bowel abnormalities respond to gluten withdrawal.[1]

Tropical Sprue

Jejunal or duodenal biopsy findings may resemble those in celiac disease, but a completely flat mucosa is not seen. This is a totally different disease from celiac sprue, a result of usually prolonged contamination of the small bowel with toxigenic strains of coliform bacteria. Improvement follows the administration of folic acid. Radiologic findings are nonspecific.

Malabsorption States with Lumen Dilatation
Progressive Systemic Sclerosis

Systemic sclerosis affects multiple systems, including skin, joints, lungs, and kidneys. The esophagus is commonly involved with changes caused by the replacement of muscularis by collagen. In more than 40% of cases the small bowel is similarly involved. Dilatation, atony, and delayed emptying are most likely to be found in the duodenum and upper jejunum. Malabsorption develops in a small number of patients and may be due to stasis with

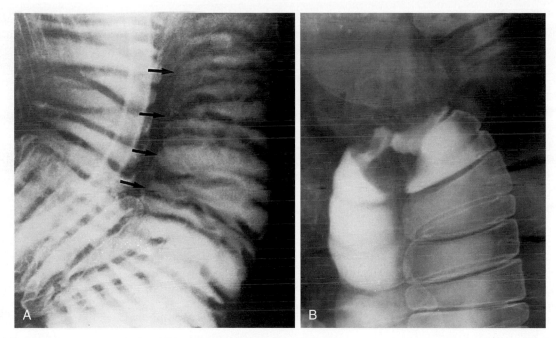

FIGURE 10–21. Enteropathy-associated T-cell lymphoma. *A,* Changes are somewhat subtle in this patient in whom a diagnosis of underlying celiac disease was made at the same time as that of enteropathy-associated T-cell lymphoma. Jejunal folds are generally increased in thickness. One segment *(arrows)* shows irregular nodularity of the folds. *B,* An atypical presentation of enteropathy-associated T-cell lymphoma, one of three similar lesions showing "shouldering" and likely ulceration.

bacterial overgrowth or to the accumulation of collagen around small vessels in the submucosa.

Dilated loops may show sacculation (Fig. 10–22A). Highly characteristic for systemic sclerosis is the "hidebound" small bowel sign,[59] tightly packed folds of normal thickness within a dilated segment (Fig. 10–22B). It occurs in more than 60% of cases and is most helpful in differentiating progressive systemic sclerosis (PSS) from other conditions that present with small bowel atony.

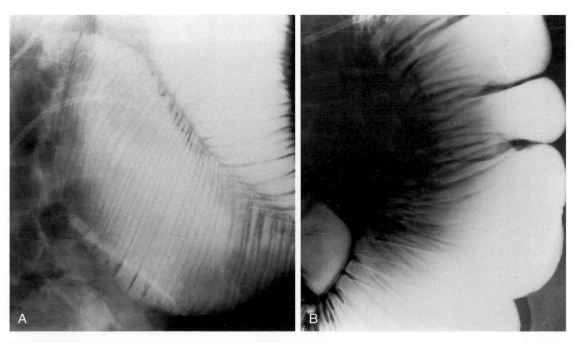

FIGURE 10–22. Two features of systemic sclerosis. *A,* The "hidebound" small bowel sign, a combination of lumen dilatation and crowding of normal folds is characteristic of systemic sclerosis. *B,* Crowding of folds is seen along the mesenteric border and sacculation on the antimesenteric side. Sacculation is infrequently seen in the small bowel and is more often found in the colon.

Dermatomyositis

In patients with dermatomyositis the smooth and striated muscles are gradually replaced by collagen. The esophagus is involved over its entire length; stomach, small bowel, and colon are affected. Radiologic findings in the small bowel are indistinguishable from PSS.

Chronic Intestinal Pseudo-obstruction

Pseudo-obstruction is a condition with clinical manifestations of small bowel obstruction in the absence of a mechanical obstruction. If this condition is suspected, peroral barium should be avoided, whether in the form of a follow-through or an enteroclysis. CT scans are a better option.

Chronic intestinal pseudo-obstruction may be the expression of numerous underlying pathologies. These are the collagen diseases, amyloidosis, endocrine and neurologic disorders, and the effects of drugs.[60] An idiopathic subgroup includes rare cases with neuropathy or myopathy and those without demonstrated pathology.[61]

Malabsorption States with Thickened Folds
Amyloidosis

Gastrointestinal tract involvement is common in the primary (AL) as well as the secondary (AA) forms of amyloidosis.[62] Yet, malabsorption is unusual. The small bowel, if affected, may present a normal enteroclysis appearance or may show a variety of changes. Uniform fold thickening affecting most of the small bowel does occur but is not the frequent finding it was once reported to be. *AL amyloidosis* may present with nodularities in the 5- to 10-mm size, or the lumen may be contracted with thickening of its wall and folds, or there may be decreased motor activity presenting as pseudo-obstruction. Rectal or gingival biopsy can confirm the diagnosis. *Secondary amyloidosis* may be one of the few conditions presenting with micronodules in the 1- to 3-mm size, an expression of lamina propria involvement causing distention of villi.[63,64]

Abetalipoproteinemia

Abetalipoproteinemia is a rare inherited disease that combines steatorrhea with acanthocytosis, retinal abnormalities, and central nervous system damage. Betalipoproteins are absent from the plasma.[1] More likely to require enteroclysis for diagnosis is the variant disease *hypobetalipoproteinemia*,[65] which may affect older children and young adults and is not associated with retinal and central nervous system lesions. The SBE has shown dilatation, fluid increase, fold thickening, and a fine granular pattern. Appreciation of the clinical background is essential for the inclusion of this diagnosis among the differential diagnoses.

IgA Deficiency and Giardiasis

IgA deficiency is not a rare condition but may be masked by a compensatory increase of secretory IgM.[66] Nodular lymphoid hyperplasia may be the only radiologic presentation of IgA deficiency.[67] If there is associated infection with *Giardia lamblia,* fold thickening and increased irritability are found in the duodenum and proximal jejunum.[68] Giardiasis can also occur in the absence of immunodeficiency.

Mastocytosis

Mastocytosis is a rare systemic disorder, not necessarily associated with urticaria pigmentosa. Acid peptic disease with gastric acid hypersecretion occurs in about 50% of patients. Malabsorption is common but of mild degree.[69]

Segments of the small intestine may show fold thickening with scattered nodules. Thickening of the bowel wall may also be seen.[70] Peptic ulceration and inflammatory changes may be demonstrated in the stomach and duodenum. Endoscopic biopsy can establish the diagnosis by demonstrating an excess of mast cells in the lamina propria and submucosa. Mostly osteoblastic bone lesions are seen in almost 70% of cases.

Zollinger-Ellison Syndrome

Maximum secretion of gastric acid is stimulated by a usually malignant gastrin-secreting tumor located in the pancreas or duodenal wall. The highly acidic gastric hypersecretion is responsible for duodenitis and for reflux esophagitis in about 60% of patients with Zollinger-Ellison syndrome.[71]

In addition to gastric hyperrugosity and fluid increase, single or multiple peptic ulcers are usually present and are often postbulbar. The widened descending duodenum may show characteristically thickened folds, often with erosions and nodularities.[72] Fold thickening extends into the proximal jejunum.

Eosinophilic Gastroenteritis

An eosinophilic infiltrate of the mucosa and submucosa may be associated with periodic diarrhea, abdominal pain, and protein loss with mild steatorrhea. The gastric antrum is involved as well and is the best site for diagnostic biopsy. In this rare disease peripheral eosinophilia is absent in about a quarter of the patients.

Enteroclysis demonstrates segmental or extensive thickening of straight mucosal folds and of the bowel wall (Fig. 10–23).[73] The disease may also involve the colon. Mucosal nodularity is seen in the gastric antrum.[74] Return to a normal appearance either spontaneously or after corticosteroid therapy supports the diagnosis.

Malabsorption States with Mucosal Micronodularity
Whipple's Disease

Whipple's disease is a rare multisystem disease mostly affecting white males, with preferential involvement of joint capsules, the small bowel and its regional nodes, heart valves, and the central nervous system.[75] With small bowel involvement, steatorrhea is usually present, and characteristic Whipple's bacilli can be found in the lamina propria, usually within macrophages. Villi are distended by macrophages filled with periodic acid–Schiff–positive material derived from the capsules of the bacilli.

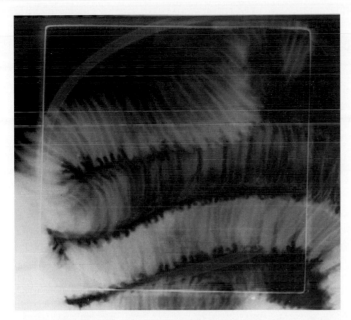

FIGURE 10–23. Recurrence of eosinophilic gastroenteritis in a young physician. Enteroclysis demonstrates mildly thickened, straightened folds throughout much of the jejunum and proximal ileum. Good response to steroids.

Mesenteric nodal masses may contain bacilli and abundant fatty material. An immunodeficiency of limited degree may be part of the clinical picture.

A successful SBE shows extensive 1- to 2-mm surface micronodulation representing the distended villi. Folds tend to be of normal thickness (Fig. 10–24A).[76] CT may show low attenuation of fat-containing nodal masses in the mesentery (Fig. 10–24B); ultrasonography shows these masses to be highly echogenic.[77] Diagnosis should not be unduly delayed because specific but prolonged treatment with tetracycline is available for this otherwise fatal disease. Radiology can suggest the diagnosis if SBE findings are evaluated against the patient's clinical background.

Intestinal Lymphangiectasia

Intestinal lymphangiectasia is a rare but important condition, with protein loss into the gut resulting in hypoalbuminemia and hypogammaglobulinemia. It is usually due to a congenital malformation of intestinal and mesenteric lymphatics. Milroy's disease, lymphedema of the lower extremities, may be another expression of the lymphatic malformation. A secondary immune deficiency is generally present, resulting from the loss of B and T lymphocytes into the gut lumen.[78]

The valvulae conniventes are extensively thickened. There is considerable fluid increase. It is important to avoid premature flocculation of barium, and the SBE needs to be modified in the way described earlier. With enteroclysis it may be possible to outline a patchy distribution of 1- to 2-mm micronodules representing villi distended by engorged lymphatics (Fig. 10–25).[79] Associated lymphatic changes in the mesentery may cause submucosal edema with thickening of folds.

In cases in which lymphangiectasia is secondary to an obstructing, usually malignant process, CT may demonstrate mesenteric nodal enlargement or other masses.

Waldenström's Macroglobulinemia

The principal clinical features of Waldenström's macroglobulinemia are monoclonal IgM protein peaks in plasma, hepatosplenomegaly, lymphadenopathy, and anemia. Small bowel involvement is rare and associated steatorrhea is rarer still. Macroglobulin deposition in villi and secondary lymphangiectasia due to lymphatic blockage by IgM monoclonal protein can produce an enteroclysis picture of widespread surface micronodulation with fold thickening.[80] These changes can also be recognized in the duodenum, where biopsy specimens may be obtained.[81] The condition is likely to progress to lymphomatous change in bowel and mesentery.

Malabsorption Associated with Structural Lesions

Structural lesions are mostly the result of surgery or inflammation. The formation of a blind loop with stasis of intestinal contents allows for bacterial overgrowth and malabsorption. If the structural abnormality cannot be corrected, treatment with antibiotics provides symptomatic relief. Other structural abnormalities associated with stasis and malabsorption can be strictures, a blind pouch, duplications, and bypassed bowel loops.

Jejunal Diverticulosis

Jejunal diverticula are acquired herniations of mucosa through the mesenteric border of the bowel at the entry sites of mesenteric vessel. These atonic sacs can result in significant metabolic abnormalities, even when few or solitary.[82] The reported incidence of jejunal diverticulosis varies between 0.06% and 1.3% in autopsy series and between 0.02% and 0.042% in diagnoses by radiology.[83]

Supine images taken in the course of the SBE readily show characteristic rounded barium-filled structures devoid of fold patterns, having a narrow neck at their passage through the bowel wall (Fig. 10–26). They are pseudodiverticula, not being formed by the full thickness of the bowel wall. Erect views occasionally show them more convincingly, containing fluid levels between barium and MC. Malabsorption may develop because of stasis and bacterial overgrowth. Motility disturbance is common and may amount to acute or repeated pseudo-obstruction in more than 10% of patients.[83] Bleeding and diverticulitis with perforation are among the possible but rare complications.

Short Bowel Syndrome

Significant loss of small bowel length reduces the area available for absorption of nutrients. To a limited extent the loss of jejunum can be compensated by ileal adaptation. The loss of more than 100 cm of distal ileum leads

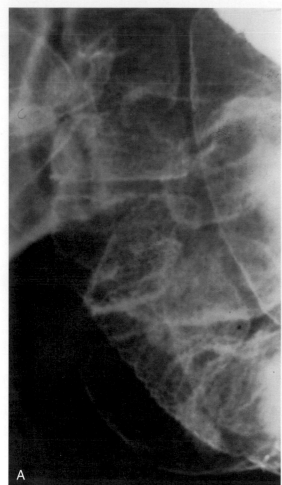

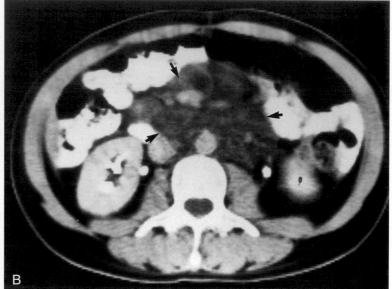

FIGURE 10–24. Whipple's disease. *A,* The mucosal surface shows crowded micronodularity (individual nodules 1 to 2 mm in diameter). Folds are usually of normal thickness. The disease distends the lamina propria of the mucosa, which forms the core of each villus and enlarges it. (Courtesy of E. Salomonowitz, M.D., St. Pölten, Austria). *B,* A mass of matted fat containing lymph nodes *(arrows)* is shown by CT in another case of Whipple's disease.

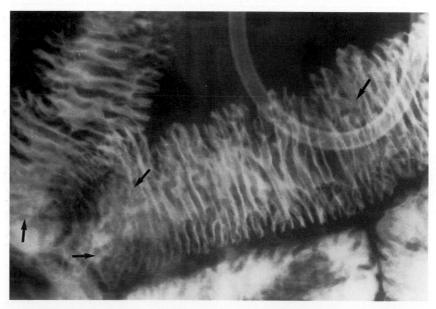

FIGURE 10–25. Primary intestinal lymphangiectasia. Folds are extensively thickened. Grouped micronodules (some indicated by *arrows*) are due to distention of villi by engorged lymphatic vessels.

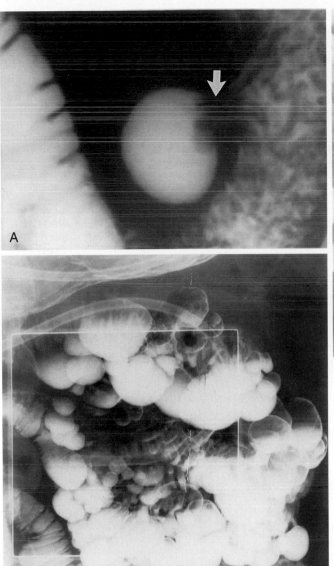

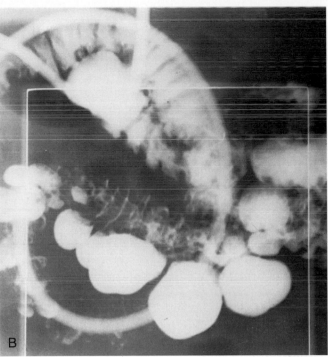

FIGURE 10–26. Jejunal diverticulosis. *A,* Jejunal diverticula represent a protrusion of mucosa with some muscularis mucosae through vascular transit points along the mesenteric border, hence the neck *(arrow)* of the "pseudodiverticulum." *B,* Supine film in the single contrast phase of an enteroclysis. Diverticula are beginning to opacify. *C,* Erect view in the fully distended double contrast phase. A large number of diverticula are now visible, showing fluid levels between barium and MC solution.

FIGURE 10–27. Short bowel syndrome. About 3 m of mid-small bowel has been resected. Although sufficient jejunum remains above the enteroenteric anastomosis *(arrow),* the ileum shows recurrent Crohn's disease *(smaller arrows),* which will adversely affect the outcome (jejunal diverticula are also present).

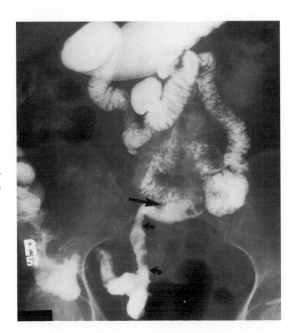

to uncompensated reduction of the circulating bile salt pool and to fat malabsorption.

Barium studies of the short bowel provide an estimate of the extent and type of bowel loss, provide an estimate of the developing adaptation process (increase in number and thickness of folds, lumen widening), and may demonstrate a possible recurrence of the underlying pathology, for example, ischemia, further Peutz-Jegher's polyposis, or Crohn's disease (Fig. 10–27).[84,85]

INFLAMMATORY DISEASES

Crohn's Disease

A chronic nonspecific granulomatous process, Crohn's disease, when fully developed, involves and thickens the entire wall of a small bowel segment together with its mesentery and lymph nodes. Segments with established disease can be readily identified by the fluoroscopic follow-through because they stand away from one another and from noninvolved, closely folded loops of bowel. However, the SBE has distinctly useful applications in Crohn's disease:

1. It is more accurate in showing the proximal limit of the disease process. This is particularly relevant in patients in whom surgery is contemplated.
2. In addition to the obvious disease, at least 1 in 10 patients have additional, more proximal skip lesions with the disease usually at an earlier stage of development (Fig. 10–4). The enteroclysis can

show these more subtle lesions, thus providing valuable information for planning of surgery.

3. Features of early Crohn's disease are best demonstrated by the SBE (see below). In patients with an uncertain history of Crohn's disease the SBE is capable of either ruling out or confirming this diagnosis.
4. At least one third of patients with Crohn's disease have some degree of steatorrhea and malabsorption.[1] Its causation is multifactorial: loss of absorptive surface by disease, resection, or bypass; stagnation in loops with abnormal bacterial flora; and increased gastrointestinal loss of nutrients.[86] As explained earlier, SBE is the method of choice for barium imaging in malabsorption states.
5. Testing the distensibility of strictures by the lumen-distending SBE can be relevant to surgical management.
6. Crohn's disease of proximal distribution occurs in 2% to 3% of cases. The SBE may demonstrate such diseased segments in the presence of normal distal small bowel.

Early Changes

A coarse granular pattern due to thickened and fused villi is frequently present in Crohn's disease (Fig. 10–28A).[87] However, this pattern may also occur in other inflammatory conditions and in ischemia or radiation enteropathy. However, if associated with fold thickening and aphthous ulcers (Fig. 10–28B), a definite diagnosis of

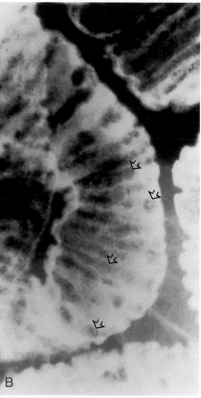
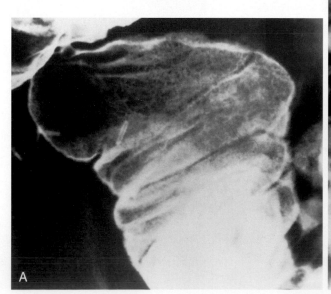

FIGURE 10–28. Crohn's disease of the terminal ileum: early changes. *A,* Follow-through study shows a coarse villous surface pattern, not in itself specific for Crohn's disease. *B,* In another patient the coarse villous pattern is associated with fold thickening and numerous aphthoid ulcers (*open arrows* to some). This combination is diagnostic for as yet not transmural Crohn's disease. (Courtesy of O. Ekberg, M.D., Malmo, Sweden.)

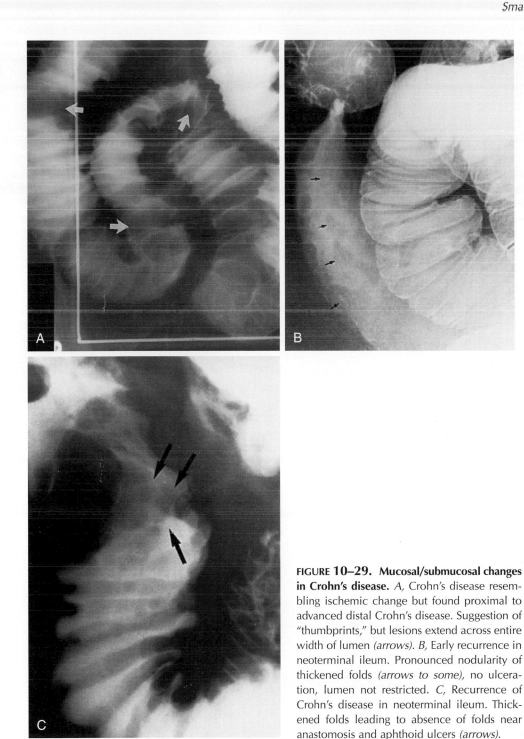

FIGURE 10–29. Mucosal/submucosal changes in Crohn's disease. *A,* Crohn's disease resembling ischemic change but found proximal to advanced distal Crohn's disease. Suggestion of "thumbprints," but lesions extend across entire width of lumen *(arrows). B,* Early recurrence in neoterminal ileum. Pronounced nodularity of thickened folds *(arrows to some),* no ulceration, lumen not restricted. *C,* Recurrence of Crohn's disease in neoterminal ileum. Thickened folds leading to absence of folds near anastomosis and aphthoid ulcers *(arrows).*

Crohn's disease can be made. Crohn's disease that is not yet transmural can present with thick folds, at times resembling ischemic bowel or lymphoma (Fig. 10–29*A*). Thickened folds are also an early feature of Crohn's recurrence in the neoterminal ileum; this may be associated with aphthous ulcers or a nodular outline of the thick folds (Fig. 10–29*B, C*). Slightly more advanced disease can take the form of a nodular pattern in which inflamed, swollen mucosal nodules are demarcated by curving barium channels; in this presentation there are as yet no linear ulcers and the bowel lumen is not narrowed (Fig. 10–30). Mucosal folds may be found to be

not only thickened but also distorted, fused, interrupted, or even absent; this may be seen during a period of quiescence (Fig. 10–31). Aphthous ulcers are an early feature of Crohn's disease in the small bowel and colon. However, follow-up of some cases that presented with aphthous lesions in the terminal ileum did not progress to established Crohn's disease.[88] Nodules, representing inflammatory polyps, are less common than in the colon. Uncommon in the small bowel are also postinflammatory polyps,[89] some of them filiform and associated with interruption of changes to mucosal folds (Fig. 10–31).

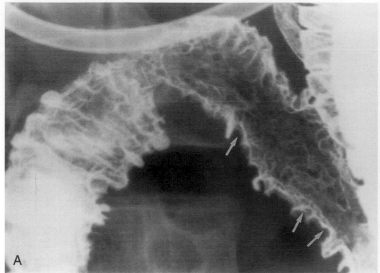

FIGURE 10–30. Nodular patterns in Crohn's disease. *A,* Segment of mid-small bowel showing a crowded pattern of inflammatory nodules, which are separated by curving, barium-filled grooves. Profile view of nodules at edge of segment *(arrows)*. *B,* Crohn's disease of terminal ileum with irregular mucosal elevations surrounded by curving barium outlines. Incipient mesenteric border ulceration.

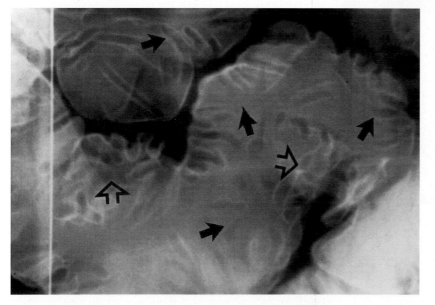

FIGURE 10–31. Fold changes in quiescent Crohn's disease. Segment of ileum showing interrupted, displaced, fused folds *(arrows)* with only few folds in the center of dilated portions. Few groups of filiform polyps are seen with their usually adherent tips *(open arrows).*

Ulcerative Changes

Characteristic for small bowel Crohn's disease are linear ulcers extending along the mesenteric border,[90] often accentuated by an ulcer-collar-like margin formed by the fusion of thickened transverse folds (Fig. 10–32*A*).[91] The linear ulcers and an associated fibrosis of the mesentery cause shortening and straightening of the mesenteric border and, therefore, redundancy of the yet uninvolved antimesenteric side (Fig. 10–32*B*).[90] Antimesenteric sac-

culation or folding continues until the disease process gradually extends transaxially to produce uniformly narrowed, ulcerated segments (Fig. 10–32*C*). Occasionally, a few saccules survive uninvolved as part of a transaxially ulcerated, narrow segment (Fig. 10–32*D*).

Cleftlike linear ulcers are the hallmark of the transmural stage of Crohn's disease. An ulceronodular or "cobblestone" pattern is produced by extensive linear ul-

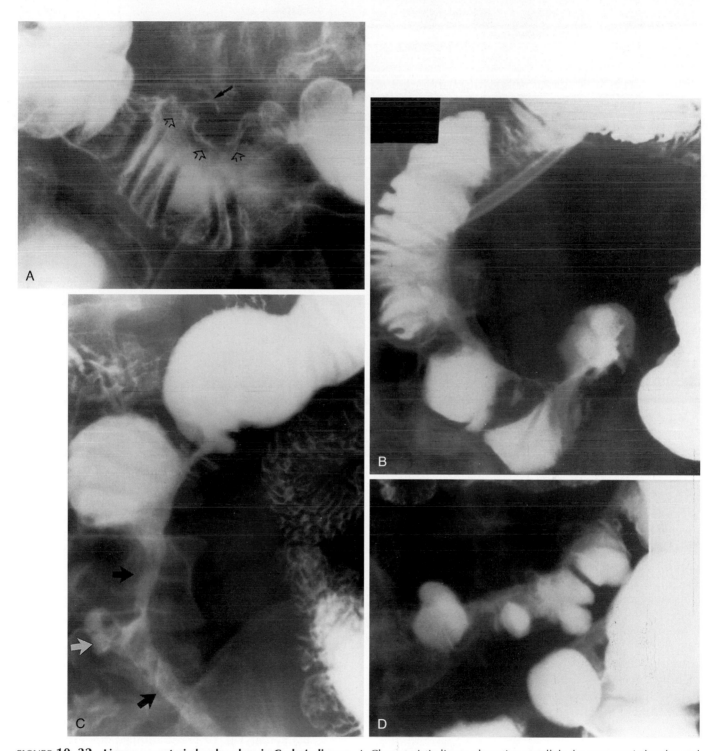

FIGURE 10–32. Linear mesenteric border ulcer in Crohn's disease. *A,* Characteristic linear ulceration parallels the mesenteric border and may extend into the mesentery *(arrow).* The ulcer is accentuated by an elevation *(open arrows)* at its luminal aspect that represents fusion of thickened folds extending from the antimesenteric side. Shortening of the mesenteric border causes antimesenteric redundancy expressed as pleating (as here) or sacculation. *B,* Linear mesenteric border ulceration indicated by shortening and straightening of its border with antimesenteric sacculation. *C,* In lesions as shown in *B* there is a tendency for disease to advance in caudad direction. Transaxial extension of the ulcerative process involves and almost eliminates one saccule *(white arrow).* Beyond it is advanced stenotic disease. *D,* Some saccules may survive within the advanced stenotic disease.

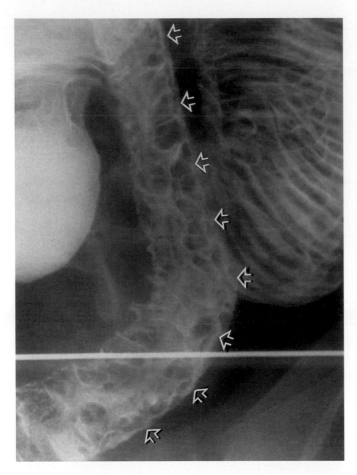

FIGURE **10–33.** Ulceronodular "cobblestone" pattern in Crohn's disease. The cobblestone appearance is caused by crossing linear ulcers separated by elevated islands of inflamed and residual mucosa (open arrows). Because of transmural extension of disease, the bowel segment is narrow and no longer distensible. Adjacent to the advanced disease is a dilated segment almost devoid of folds.

cerations that separate inflamed islands of surviving mucosa that is elevated by submucosal edema (Fig. 10–33).

Complications

The SBE, by testing distensibility, can distinguish fibrous strictures from ulcerated, stenotic disease (Fig. 10–34). It also unmasks the "string sign," an appearance caused by spasm related to surrounding inflammation (Fig. 10–35).[89,92] Fistulae are well outlined, including those that lead to the sigmoid colon or the duodenum, in which only nonspecific focal changes are produced at the entry site of the fistulae (Fig. 10–36).[93] Enteroclysis may identify abscesses by outlining communicating tracts with barium but extrinsic inflammatory changes are best demonstrated by CT.

Yersinia Ileitis

Yersinia ileitis is a self-limited, benign disease. The diagnosis is based on positive bacteriology or serology for *Yersinia enterocolitica*. In adults the more severe disease may affect the colon. The radiologic features are wall and fold thickening with mucosal nodularity (Fig. 10–37); ulcers may be seen in the acute stage of the disease but are usually healed by the time radiology is requested.[94]

Ileocecal Tuberculosis

A rare condition in developed countries, ileocecal tuberculosis is an important and frequent health problem throughout much of the world, where Crohn's disease is an unusual diagnosis. Only a minority of patients with abdominal tuberculosis show features of active pulmonary infection.[95]

The diagnosis should be based on a demonstration of *Mycobacterium tuberculosis* of typical histology. In North America and Europe the main issue is to differentiate an occasional intestinal tuberculosis from Crohn's disease. Radiologic features that suggest tuberculosis rather than Crohn's disease are the following[96,97]:

1. The terminal ileum may be ulcerated with individual ulcers often broad and transaxially directed; cecal involvement tends to exceed that of the terminal ileum (Fig. 10–38*A*); annular strictures can be a late result.
2. Cephalad retraction of the cecum leads to straightening of the ileocecal junction angle (Fig. 10–38*B*).
3. A fairly abrupt change from normality to disease is usual; inflammatory exudate is usually seen in the diseased portion.
4. Mesenteric adenopathy on CT scans may be more pronounced than in Crohn's disease; ascites of increased CT attenuation may be present.

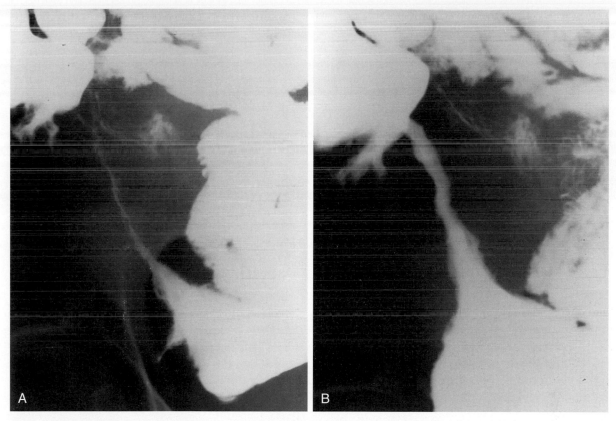

FIGURE 10–34. Fibrous stricture in the terminal ileum in Crohn's disease. *A,* Early stage of the single contrast phase of an SBE shows a thin, frayed 6-cm-long narrowed segment. *B,* The distensibility of the stricture is tested by the infusion of MC. There is only minimal widening without pattern change, typical for a fibrous stricture.

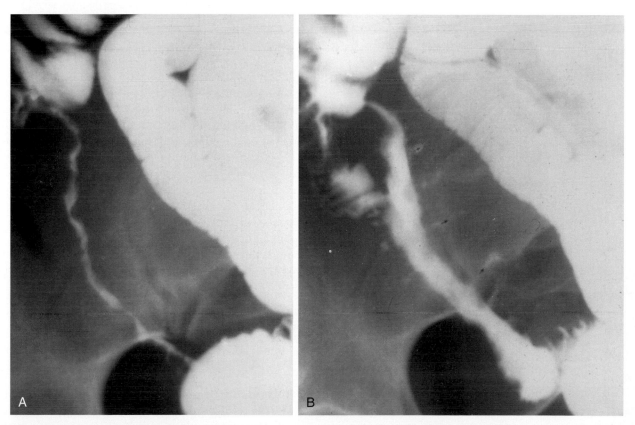

FIGURE 10–35. The "string sign" in Crohn's disease. *A,* In the single contrast phase the terminal ileum has the appearance of an irregularly frayed string. *B,* After infusion of MC, significant widening of the lumen and numerous tracks extending into an inflammatory mass are seen. The distention achieved by MC proves that this lesion is not a fibrous stricture. CT is now indicated.

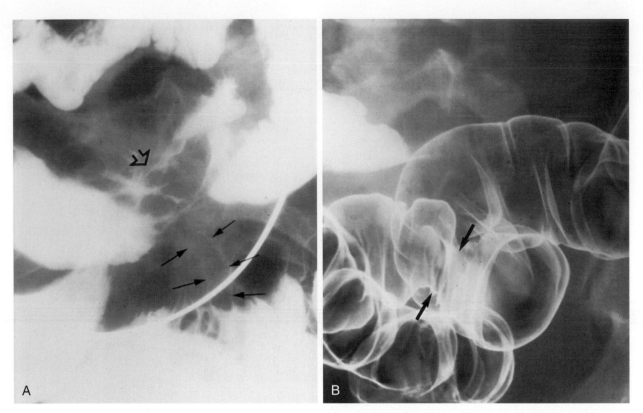

FIGURE 10–36. Ileosigmoid fistulae. *A,* From an area of ileum affected by Crohn's disease *(open arrow)* at least two fistulae *(arrows)* lead to and penetrate the wall of the sigmoid colon, where there seems to be fold thickening. *B,* Double contrast barium enema shows a short segment of sigmoid with limited distensibility and slight thickening of folds, marking the site of entry of the Crohn's fistula *(arrows).* There is no evidence of sigmoid Crohn's disease. The sigmoid colon returned to a normal appearance after resection of the diseased ileum and of the fistula.

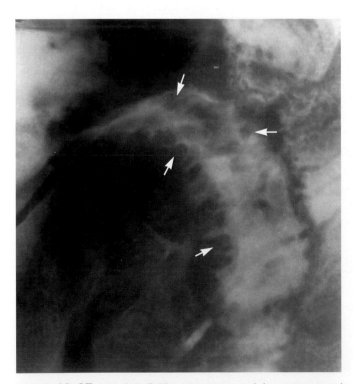

FIGURE 10–37. *Yersinia* ileitis. Numerous nodules *(arrows)* and thickened folds are seen. Normal width of lumen, no ulcers demonstrated. Return to a normal appearance within 6 weeks.

Appendix Abscess

An appendiceal abscess may affect the adjacent terminal ileum.[93] The folds of the terminal ileum may be thickened by edema on the side that is displaced and compressed by the adjacent inflammatory mass (Figs. 10–39). The cecum is frequently indented at its lower pole, and the appendix does not opacify. However, appendicitis may affect only the distal aspects, and part of the appendix may be visualized in such cases. Graded compression ultrasonography is a preferred alternative to barium studies in patients with suspected acute appendicitis.[98] The main differential diagnosis is the distinction from a tubo-ovarian abscess and occasionally terminal ileal diverticulitis or Crohn's disease.

TUMORS

Small bowel tumors are rare. They account for between 1% and 5% of all tumors of the gastrointestinal tract.

Benign Tumors[99]

Leiomyomas, lipomas, adenomas, and hamartomas are the more common benign tumors of the small bowel. Only about half cause symptoms. Pain is usually due to intussusception, more often intermittent than lasting.

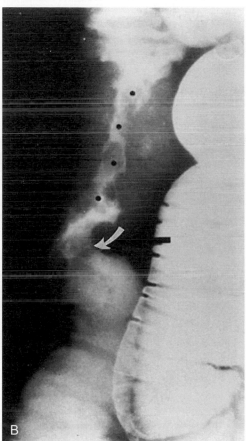

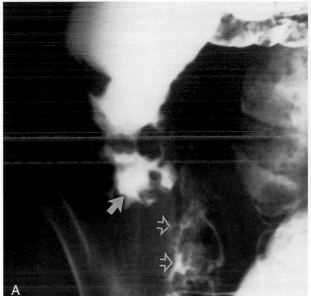

FIGURE **10–38. Ileocecal tuberculosis.** *A,* Ulcers are demonstrated in the terminal ileum *(open arrows)* and in the contracted cecum *(arrow). B,* Gaping ileocecal valve *(arrow)* with slightly dilated but otherwise normal appearing terminal ileum. The cecum is totally contracted. The extensively ulcerated ascending colon *(dots)* seems to be in direct continuation with the terminal ileum

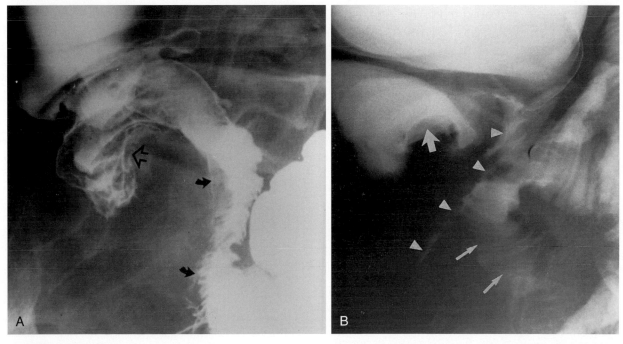

FIGURE **10–39. Appendix abscess, two examples.** *A,* Terminal ileum displaced and compressed *(short arrows)* and cecum indented *(open arrow)* by an extrinsic mass with nonfilling of appendix. *B,* Terminal ileum with thickened folds distally and compressed folds more proximally *(arrowheads).* An adjacent segment of ileum shows fold thickening *(arrows).* The medial border of the cecum is indented *(thick arrow),* and the appendix has not been opacified.

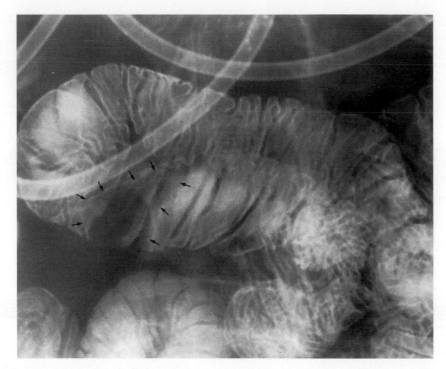

FIGURE 10–40. Jejunal lipoma. A broad-based, 3-cm polyp *(arrows)* was found in a patient who complained of intermittent crampy abdominal pain. The polyp could be slightly flattened by compression. It had also been demonstrated by enteroclysis 2 years before and had grown very little. A lipoma was later resected.

Bleeding is the other likely presentation. The tumors are fairly evenly distributed throughout the small bowel. Lipomas protrude into the lumen and may be shown to be soft and compressible, at times with a pseudopedicle (Fig. 10–40). CT scan can confirm their fat composition.[100] Adenomatous polyps may be found in the duodenum of patients with polyposis coli and may extend into the jejunum (Fig. 10–41).

An antegrade barium demonstration of an intussuscepting lipoma shows the dilated lumen narrowing abruptly to a beaklike shape. Barium passing through this obstruction outlines the lumen beyond, possibly demonstrating the leading tumor at the apex of the intussusceptum. The "coiled-spring" appearance of stretched folds is faintly visible after retrograde entry of barium into the space between intussusceptum and intussuscipiens (Fig. 10–42). CT can clearly demonstrate an intussusception in longitudinal and cross sections and demonstrates the entering mesenteric vessels surrounded by fat.[101] In institutions where ultrasonography tends to be the primary radiologic study in patients with abdominal symptoms, this method has been reported to be able to identify small bowel tumors with increasing accuracy.[102]

Peutz-Jeghers Syndrome

Peutz-Jeghers syndrome is an important cause of abdominal pain and bleeding in adolescents. Multiple lobulated hamartomatous tumors occur mostly in the jejunum and intussuscept intermittently (Fig. 10–43). Malignant degeneration is rare.[103]

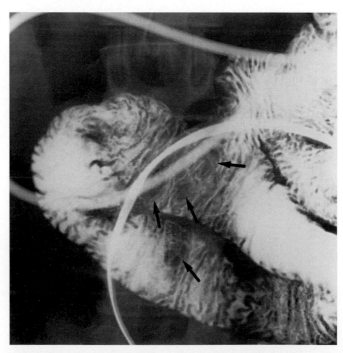

FIGURE 10–41. Adenomatous polyps. In a patient with polyposis coli, enteroclysis demonstrated several jejunal adenomatous polyps *(arrows).*

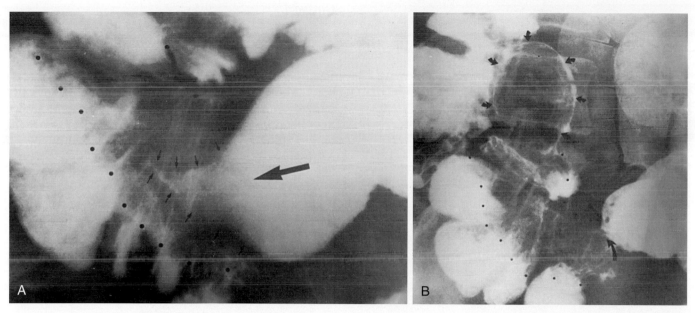

FIGURE 10–42. Intussusception of a lipoma of terminal ileum. *A,* Beak-shaped narrowing at entry into the intussusception *(arrows).* Barium flowing back from beyond the intussusception outlines its soft tissue mass *(dots),* which includes the related mesentery and faintly shows the stretched "coiled spring" pattern of folds. *B,* A lipoma coated with barium forms the leading point of the intussusception *(small arrows).*

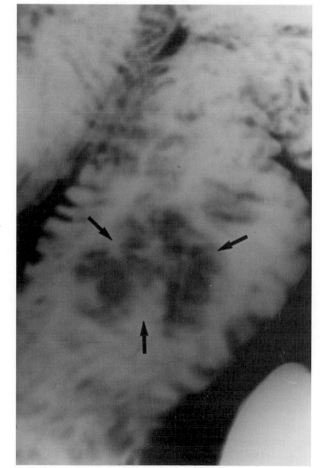

FIGURE 10–43. Peutz-Jeghers syndrome with jejunal hamartoma. (Courtesy of Grant Saunders, M.D., Winnipeg, Manitoba.)

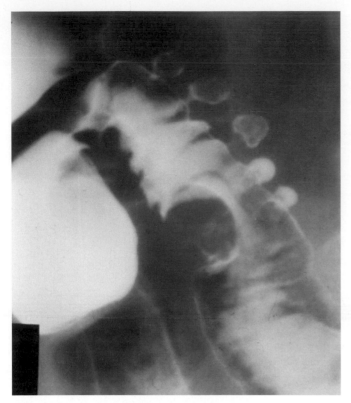

FIGURE 10–44. Asymptomatic carcinoid. A 1.2-cm polyplike tumor apparently of mucosal origin (angle against surrounding base less than 90 degrees) is a chance finding in an enteroclysis done to exclude bowel obstruction. Surgery confirmed the radiologic suspicion of carcinoid. Terminal ileal diverticula are present.

Malignant Tumors
Carcinoid

The carcinoid is a common small bowel neoplasm that occurs more frequently in the distal and terminal ileum and is seen twice as often in men than in women. Carcinoids are multiple in 30% of cases. Ileal carcinoids tend to grow through the bowel wall and invade the mesentery, where they form masses that become larger than the primary tumor. Hormonal substances produced by the primary tumor and its mesenteric deposits cause an intense, focal desmoplastic process. This can be well demonstrated by SBE with regard to the primary tumor and by CT for the mesenteric metastases. A CT examination is mandatory whenever barium studies show lesions that might represent a carcinoid. Hormonally active liver metastases develop in only 10% of patients and produce the carcinoid syndrome of flushing, diarrhea, and bronchospasm.

A smoothly rounded polyp seen in the terminal ileum should always be considered a probable carcinoid. Such tumors may be asymptomatic at this early stage (Fig. 10–44). At a somewhat later stage the SBE shows carcinoid-related desmoplastic changes affecting mucosal folds and the bowel wall (Fig. 10–45A). By this time CT may demonstrate a frequently calcium-containing mesenteric mass that, by desmoplastic constriction of mesenteric vessels together with a further reaching elastic sclerosis, can cause significant bowel ischemia expressed as wall thickening (Fig. 10–45B).[104,105] CT may also demonstrate a double halo sign in an ischemic bowel wall[104] and also widespread metasta-

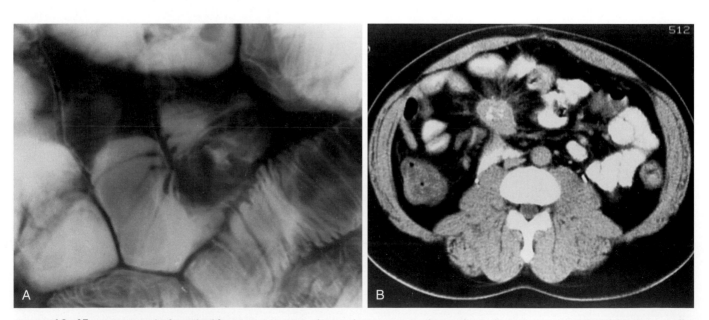

FIGURE 10–45. A more typical carcinoid tumor. *A,* A 2-cm ulcerated tumor causes desmoplastic changes to surrounding folds. Two smaller tumors were seen in the distal ileum. Carcinoid was the likely diagnosis but required CT to demonstrate likely mesenteric changes that would confirm the diagnosis. *B,* CT outlined a calcium-containing mesenteric mass surrounded by pronounced lines of retraction. Adjacent small bowel loops have slightly thickened walls.

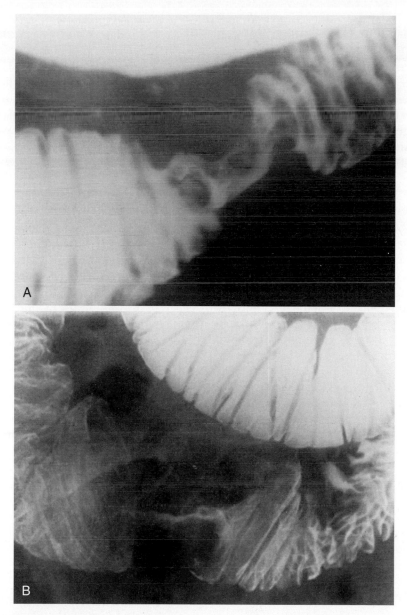

FIGURE 10–46. **Adenocarcinoma.** *A,* An annular carcinoma. Remnants of a fold pattern are still visible in the lumen of the tumor. *B,* More advanced, typical "apple core" carcinoma without identifiable folds in the constricted segment. NOTE low degree of obstruction, mostly due to the fluid content of the small bowel.

tic deposits in the peritoneal cavity and omentum, often with ascites. CT or MRI identify liver metastases, usually associated with the carcinoid syndrome.

Adenocarcinoma

Most carcinomas are found in the proximal jejunum. They soon encircle the gut to produce "applecore" lesions (Fig. 10–46). Because gut contents are fluid, obstruction is usually low grade in less advanced cases. The presenting features are pain, anemia, occult blood, and weight loss.

It is important to recognize adenocarcinomas by radi-

ology, and enteroclysis is the best method for this purpose. It should be possible, if clinical referral has not been unduly delayed, to make this diagnosis before mesenteric nodal metastases have developed.[106] An increased incidence of second malignancies has been observed, most having occurred before the small bowel adenocarcinoma.[107]

Non-Hodgkin's Lymphoma[108,109]

Lymphomas involving the small bowel are non-Hodgkin's lymphoma (NHL). NHL affecting the small intestine can be grouped in the following way.

1. *Disseminated NHL,* usually already widespread, may involve the small bowel together with the stomach and duodenum. This may take the form of frequently ulcerated nodules (Fig. 10–47).

2. *Mesenteric nodal lymphoma with secondary involvement of small bowel.* A mesenteric nodal mass may develop as primary tumor or as part of nodal dissemination. As the mass enlarges, it first displaces and then surrounds bowel but eventually infiltrates adjacent bowel loops (Fig. 10–48).

3. *Primary small bowel lymphoma* may present as infiltrating or cavitary NHL. *Infiltrating* NHL affects a limited, sharply demarcated segment with thickening and later obliteration of mucosal folds. Gradual replacement of muscularis by lymphoma may cause lumen widening most pronounced in the central portion of the lesion (Fig. 10–49). These primary lymphoma infiltrates can affect more than a single segment. *Cavitary* NHL occurs when, either because of ulceration or leakage through a tumor-replaced bowel wall, barium and other contents extend into the mesentery to form an exoenteric collection surrounded by a usually thin rim of lymphoma (Fig. 10–50). It is possible for this exoenteric collection to extend into a space between the leaves of the mesentery.

4. *Multiple lymphomatous polyposis* is a rare form of lymphoma, usually part of widespread nodal disease. Its typical histologic finding is a monoclonal infiltrate that surrounds germinal centers, and this form of the disease is now known as *mantle cell lymphoma.*[110] Polypoid changes are reported to be more pronounced in the distal ileum and may extend into the colon.

5. *Lymphoma associated with celiac disease* has already been described (see Fig. 10–27).

6. *Lymphoma associated with other diseases.* There is an increased incidence of NHL in patients with AIDS, lupus erythematosus, Waldenström's macroglobulinemia, and in organ transplant recipients. A special type of lymphoma, Mediterranean lymphoma, is associated with alpha heavy chain disease.

CT is an essential additional radiologic method that can provide a more complete diagnosis of NHL and can aid in the staging of the disease.

Seeded Carcinoma Metastases

Meyers[111] has shown that circulating ascitic fluid slows down and stagnates in certain areas of the peritoneal cavity, which become favorite sites for the deposition and implantation of cancer cells. Such areas include the ileocecal region, the ruffles of the mesentery, and the pelvic cavity. The most frequent primary sources for seeded metastases to the small bowel are the ovary and cervix in women and the colon, pancreas, and stomach in men.

SBE features of sufficiently developed metastases deposited on serosal surfaces of the small intestine are the following:

1. Initially, a rounded protrusion toward the lumen (Fig. 10–51*A*).

2. Later, signs of mural infiltration with tethering of the folds (Fig. 10–51*B*).[112] When viewed en face, this presents as mucosal folds that appear thickened or flattened or transaxially stretched or curved (Fig. 10–51*C*). When viewed in profile, the bowel lumen may show crowded fixation of folds at the side of the

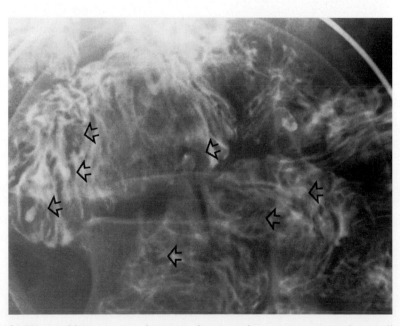

FIGURE 10–47. Disseminated NHL. In addition to target lesions in the stomach, numerous, somewhat smaller lesions of the same type are seen in the proximal jejunum *(arrows to some).*

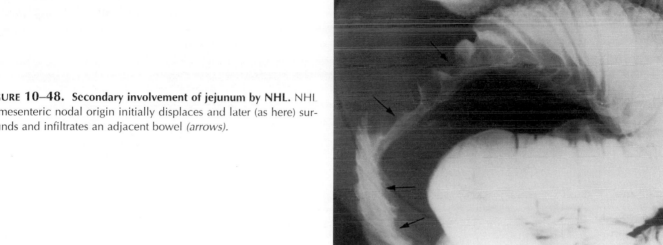

FIGURE 10–48. Secondary involvement of jejunum by NHL. NHL of mesenteric nodal origin initially displaces and later (as here) surrounds and infiltrates an adjacent bowel *(arrows).*

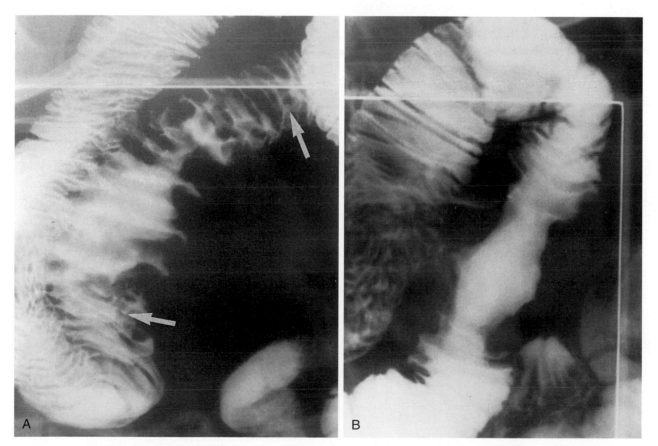

FIGURE 10–49. Infiltrating form of primary small bowel NHL. *A,* Well-demarcated segment shows irregular fold thickening that can progress to virtual absence of a fold pattern. *Arrows* demarcate extent of NHL involvement. *B,* This 8-cm segment of jejunum has complete fold effacement due to lymphoma having replaced much of the bowel wall. This replacement weakens the wall and here leads to widening of the lumen in the midportion. Primary lesions as shown above can be found simultaneously in two or three places.

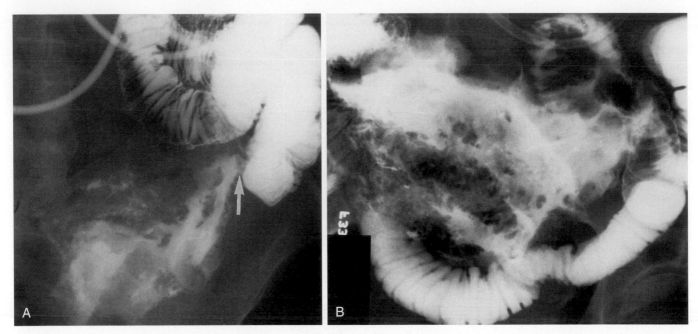

FIGURE 10–50. Cavitary form of primary small bowel NHL. *A,* Mesenteric border ulceration causes extravasation of barium from a segment of jejunum into a mesenteric space. *B,* Late film shows the extent of the cavity, which contains barium, debris, and air and is surrounded by lymphoma tissue. Extensive surgery was curative.

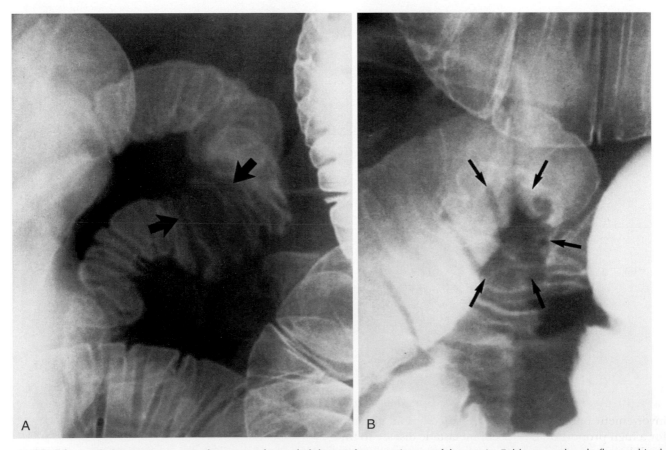

FIGURE 10–51. Seeded metastases. *A,* En face view of a seeded deposit from carcinoma of the cervix. Folds are unsharply flattened in this well-demarcated *(arrows)* lesion. *B,* Another lobulated metastasis *(arrows)* from carcinoma of the cervix causes partial obstruction and some tethering of folds distally.

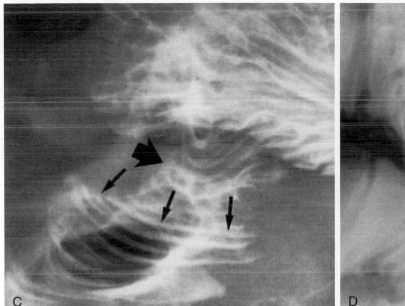

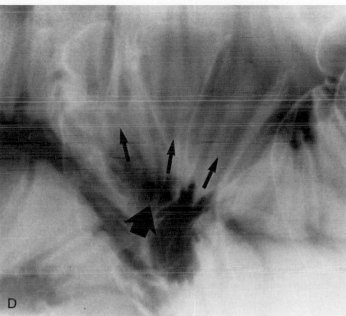

FIGURE 10–51 *Continued* *C,* En face view of a metastasis similar to *B* shows stretched, curving folds at the periphery of the deposit *(arrows to one side)* and tethered folds with narrowed lumen centrally *(broad arrow). D,* Profile view of a metastasis from endometrial carcinoma. Fixed and crowded mucosal folds at the site of infiltration *(broad arrow)* fan out toward the opposite, unaffected, and distensible side *(arrows);* note rounded soft tissue space next to infiltration.

implant and a normal separation of folds toward the opposite side; there is an increased space against adjacent bowel (Fig. 10–51D).[113]

3. Frequent desmoplastic changes with angulation, kinking, and stricture formation may cause high-grade small bowel obstruction (Fig. 10–52).

4. Seeded metastases, usually multiple, tend to be grouped as already described (Fig. 10–53); ascites is usually present.

5. Mesenteric carcinomatosis results from advanced and aggressive malignancy, often ovarian carcinoma; shortening of the mesentery then causes crowding of folds while, at the same time, the presence of interloop metastases causes separation of areas within these crowded loops.[114]

In addition to peritoneal seeding, carcinomas may involve the small bowel by hematogenous spread or by direct invasion.

Hematogenous Metastases

Hematogenous metastases occur less often than seeded metastases. Malignant melanoma shows a preference for small bowel localization. Carcinoma of the breast and lung show no particular predilection for small bowel involvement but, because they are so common, account for a high proportion of cases of metastatic disease to the small bowel.

Tumor emboli are mostly deposited at the antimesenteric aspect of small bowel loops (Fig. 10–54A). They are

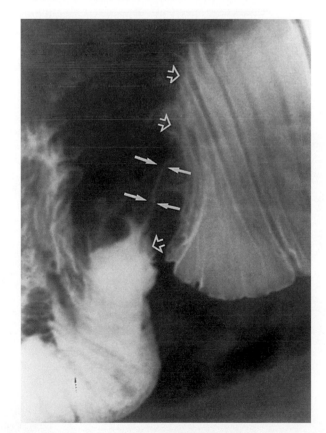

FIGURE 10–52. Obstructing annular metastasis. Metastasis from colon carcinoma severely narrows a short segment *(arrows),* which is at an angle against the long axis of the bowel above. Note the destruction of fold contours above and below the constriction *(open arrows).*

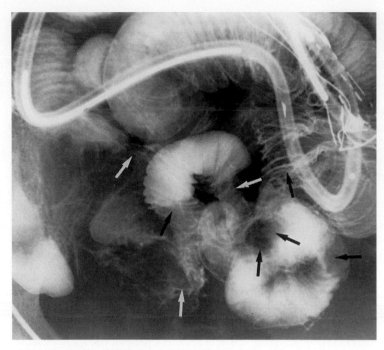

FIGURE 10–53. Partial small bowel obstruction due to multiple seeded metastases from carcinoma of the cervix grouped in the ileocecal area *(arrows),* the most favored site for tumor cell deposition.

typically multiple and grouped in stages of growth. Melanoma metastases tend to ulcerate in a stellate pattern and are soft and highly cellular.[115] These metastases often intussuscept but rarely obstruct (Fig. 10–54B). CT is a valuable addition to the investigation because it may draw attention to further metastases in the abdomen, such as in the liver, spleen, omentum, and mesentery.[116]

Bronchogenic metastases may cause desmoplastic changes and occasionally a localized extravasation. Breast metastases are more likely to involve the colon and the stomach and occasionally produce constricted segments in the small bowel.

Direct extension of a primary carcinoma may invade and constrict a segment of small bowel, usually the ileum.

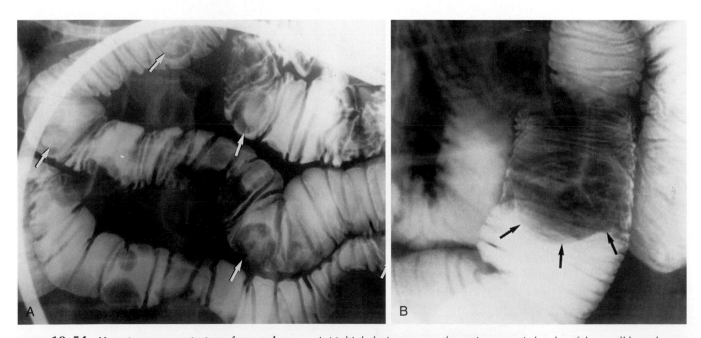

FIGURE 10–54. Hematogenous metastases from melanoma. *A,* Multiple lesions are on the antimesenteric border of the small bowel, many with a large, wheelspoke-like central ulceration *(arrows)* characteristic of metastatic melanoma. (Courtesy of L. Costopoulos, M.D., Edmonton, Alberta.) *B,* Intussusception of a metastatic melanoma *(arrows).* Such intussusceptions are usually transient and, because of the softness of the tumor, rarely produce small bowel obstruction.

VASCULAR LESIONS

Radiation Enteropathy

The small intestine is highly radiosensitive.[117] With higher radiation doses to the pelvis, the small intestine will escape injury only if, in the course of its normal position change, it escapes part of the direct x-ray radiation. Bowel tethered by previous surgery is likely to suffer damage from a dose as low as 5000 rad.

Chronic radiation damage makes its appearance 1 to 12 years after therapy and demonstrates recognizable changes on barium examination. The injury essentially involves endothelial cells of arterioles, leading to progressive ischemia of the mucosa and submucosa. The bowel wall becomes thickened by edema and fibrosis.

Enteroclysis demonstrates the associated radiologic changes. Folds are thicker than the compressed spaces between them (Figs. 10–55 and 10–56). The lumen shows limited distensibility and a degree of fixation after radiation-related serositis. At other times, severe damage may cause segments to become almost devoid of folds, matted, and encased by fibrosis, which allows very little peristaltic activity (Figs. 10–57A, B). More severe obstruction can be caused by a radiation stricture (Fig. 10–57C). There are occasions when distensibility is not yet lost altogether and the distention stage of double contrast enteroclysis makes it possible to distinguish what at first appears to be extension of malignancy from radiation-related narrowing and fixation (Fig. 10–58).[118] In most radiation enteropathies, however, follow-through barium studies can be almost as effective as an enteroclysis.

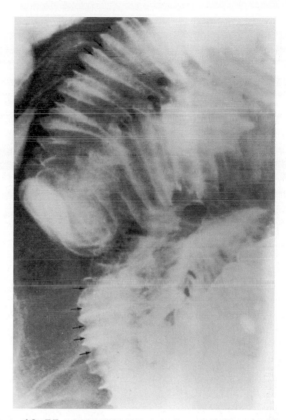

FIGURE 10–55. Radiation enteropathy. Ileal folds are thick, straight, and parallel. The spaces between folds are narrower than the diameter of the folds, a reversal from their normal appearance. Barium within these spaces is compressed by the thickened folds and produces short spiky protrusions (*arrows* outline thickened folds in profile view).

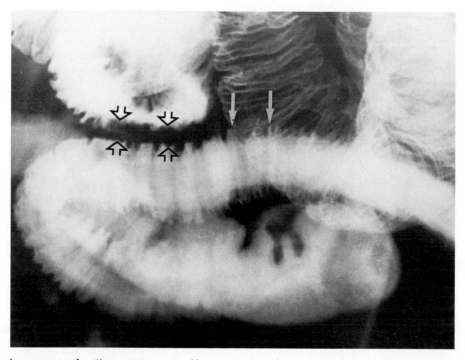

FIGURE 10–56. Radiation enteropathy. Sharp projections of barium (*arrows*) between thickened folds represent the interfold spaces compressed by the thickened folds. There is increased thickness of the combined walls (*open arrows*) of two adjacent bowel segments damaged by past radiation.

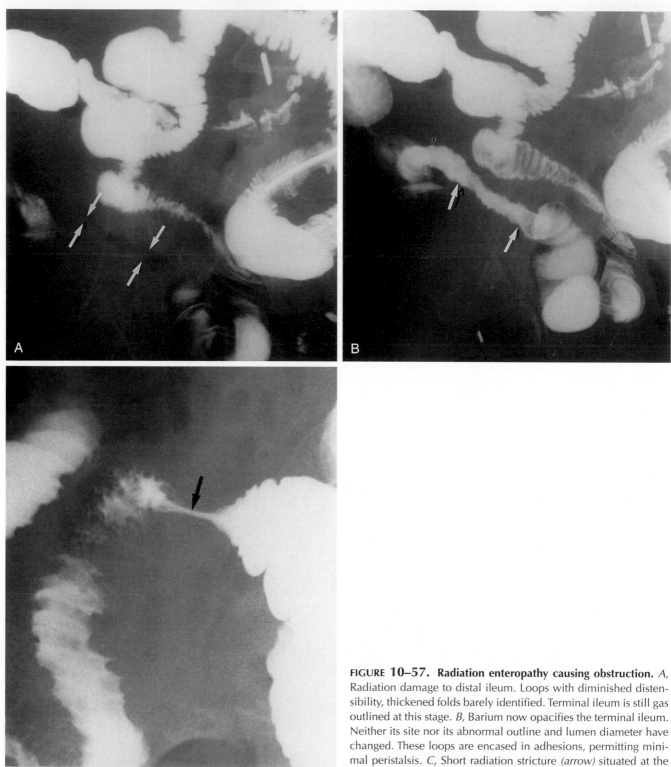

FIGURE 10–57. Radiation enteropathy causing obstruction. *A,* Radiation damage to distal ileum. Loops with diminished distensibility, thickened folds barely identified. Terminal ileum is still gas outlined at this stage. *B,* Barium now opacifies the terminal ileum. Neither its site nor its abnormal outline and lumen diameter have changed. These loops are encased in adhesions, permitting minimal peristalsis. *C,* Short radiation stricture *(arrow)* situated at the edge of the radiation portal causes partial small bowel obstruction. Thick folds are seen in the incompletely filled segment beyond the stricture.

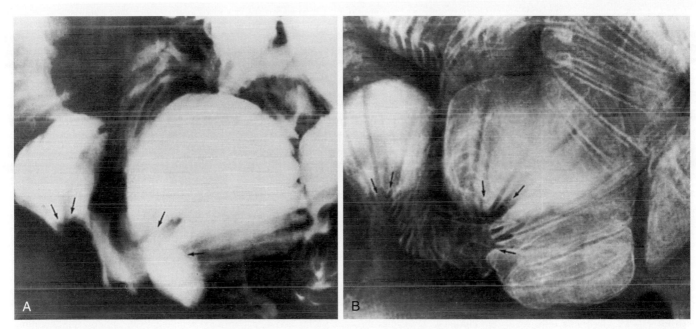

FIGURE 10–58. Radiation damage or malignancy? Previous surgery for carcinoma of the cervix with extensive resection was followed by radiotherapy. The patient later presented with malabsorption and intermittent bleeding. *A,* Fixed loop of ileum at pelvic inlet is shown in the single contrast phase (*arrows* to sites of possible metastases). Is the lesion benign or malignant? *B,* Fully developed double contrast with distention. Slightly thickened mucosal folds are demonstrated *(arrows),* with fixation caused by radiation-related adhesions and not to malignant infiltration.

Ischemia

Acute ischemic processes due to embolic or thrombotic occlusion of a major vessel are not normally referred for barium investigation. Subacute ischemia of a small bowel segment produces changes described as the "picket-fence" or "stacked-coin" appearance of straightened, thickened folds.[119] Contour defects (thumbprints) are often seen and occur mostly along the mesenteric border (Fig. 10–59A). These changes may best be shown in the single contrast phase of the SBE and may become less obvious during subsequent lumen distention. An important feature is the transient nature of these appearances, which may either progress to necrosis or stricture or, more often, return to a normal appearance within 2 to 3 weeks (Fig. 10–59B). Because this feature helps to distinguish ischemia from radiation enteropathy and some forms of inflammatory involvement, a repeat barium study approximately 3 weeks later should be recommended.

Intramural Hemorrhage

Intramural hemorrhage may develop spontaneously in patients taking anticoagulants or in patients who have a bleeding diathesis. Blunt trauma is another cause. The hemorrhage may be localized or diffuse. The former is likely to be caused by trauma and presents as a usually mesenteric border–related mass effect associated with thickening of folds. The more diffuse, often spontaneous intramural bleeding closely resembles an ischemic bowel segment (Fig. 10–60).

CT or MRI can be most useful in blunt trauma–related bowel injuries. Mural hematoma can be distinguished from injury to the mesentery, and exploratory laparotomy can often be avoided or hastened.[120]

Gastrointestinal Bleeding

Only patients with low-grade bleeding in whom upper and lower barium or endoscopic examinations have been unrewarding should be referred to enteroclysis.

Of lesions causing bleeding, 10% to 20% occur in the duodenum beyond the limit of the usual upper endoscopic examination. If enteroclysis has been negative, the catheter should be withdrawn into the proximal duodenum and the balloon reinflated. A barium and air double contrast study of the duodenum and the duodenojejunal flexure should then complete the examination. An approximately 20% positive diagnosis rate for enteroclysis in undiagnosed bleeding has now been reported.[121,122] Tumors, benign or malignant, primary or metastatic, accounted for most of the lesions. However, it is occasionally possible to demonstrate an arteriovenous malformation that has extended into the submucosal core of a fold to produce a scalloped filling defect (Fig. 10–61).[122]

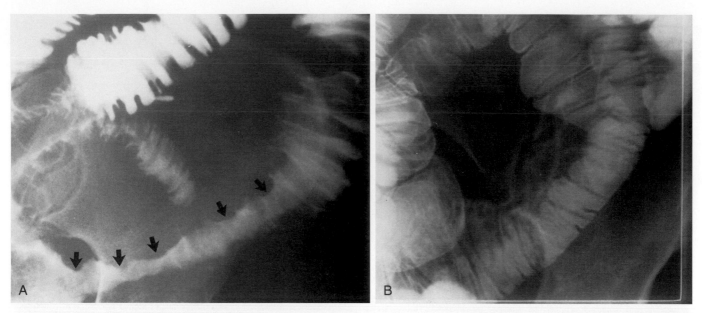

FIGURE 10–59. Ischemia with reversible changes. *A,* Beyond thickened folds above, a narrowed segment shows multiple indentations (thumbprints) of its mesenteric border *(arrows)* and barely identifiable outlines of very thick folds. *B,* An SBE 4 weeks later shows the same bowel segment now with a normal appearance.

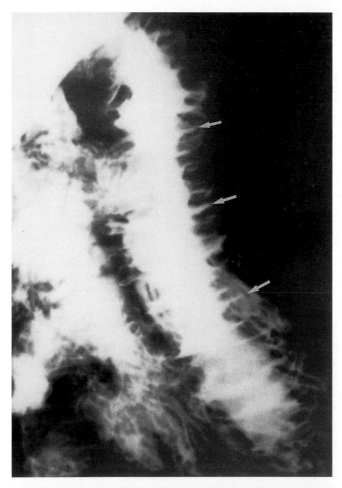

FIGURE 10–60. Superior mesenteric vein thrombosis. A typical "stacked-coin" appearance produced by thickened, straight folds with spiky compression of the spaces between them *(arrows)* is due to intramural bleeding and edema, a finding compatible with mesenteric vein thrombosis.

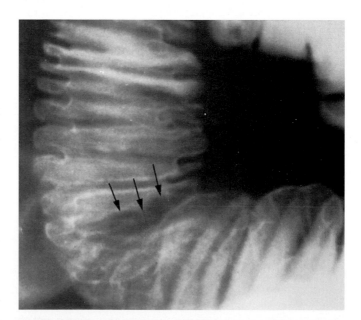

FIGURE 10–61. Arteriovenous malformation presenting with obscure bleeding. Enteroclysis demonstrates a lobulated widening of part of a fold in the proximal jejunum. Enteroscopy confirmed and fulgurized the lesion.

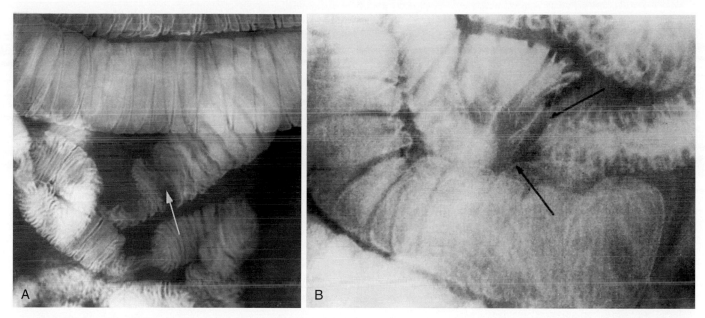

FIGURE 10–62. Adhesive band causing partial small bowel obstruction. *A,* There is an abrupt change of caliber at the site of compression by an adhesive band *(arrow).* Mucosal folds can be identified in the constricted segment and normal folds extend to the edge of the dilated proximal segment and in the nondistended segment beyond the constriction. *B,* The lumen-distending effect of enteroclysis makes it possible to identify a very-low-grade adhesive obstruction *(arrows)* at a time when the patient is free of symptoms.

SMALL BOWEL OBSTRUCTION

Small bowel obstruction (SBO) is no longer a major indication for enteroclysis. We prefer to use enteroclysis in patients with a history suggesting low-grade or intermittent obstructions or to rule out obstruction as cause of a patient's symptoms. We now consider the antegrade use of barium to be contraindicated in patients with complete or high-grade obstruction or patients with possible adynamic ileus. The possibility of vascular impairment by the obstruction also totally disallows antegrade barium. Not only would such barium studies take hours, even more than a day to complete, they would also negate a subsequent CT examination and would render early surgery difficult. CT is by far the best technique to replace enteroclysis.

In patients with lower grades of SBO, enteroclysis exceeds the sensitivity and specificity of CT (Fig. 10–62).[123] In a special category are patients with partial obstruction who have had a prior laparotomy for malignancy. CT and enteroclysis are equally successful in demonstrating a metastatic mass as a cause of obstruction. However, about 20% of patients in this group have their obstruction caused by adhesions, and some of them need to be surgically lysed even if metastases are present elsewhere. Enteroclysis is the best technique to positively identify adhesions versus metastases as cause of an obstruction (Fig. 10–63).[124]

Closed loop obstructions, implying compression of the afferent and efferent limbs of a loop of bowel protruding under an adhesive band, provided they are a cause of partial SBO, can be investigated by enteroclysis (Fig. 10–64).[125,126] CT replaces enteroclysis if vascular compromise is suspected.

Technique Modification

The SBE can be carried out by routine intubation or by using an already inserted long decompression tube. Depending on the quantity of retained fluid, an increased amount of barium will have to be infused. Whenever possible, barium should be taken close to the site of obstruction, usually identified as the site of an abrupt change from a dilated lumen proximally to a collapsed lumen beyond (the transition zone). MC is then infused for more detailed double contrast to identify the imprint of the causative lesion.

Adhesive Bands

With single adhesive band obstructions, dilated bowel with stretched mucosal folds is seen to extend to the edge of a sharply demarcated lumen reduction. A short, narrowed segment with compressed folds marks the site of the adhesive band (Fig. 10–62A).[124] The distention associated with the SBE can draw attention to minor degrees of band compression, even at a time when patients are asymptomatic (Fig. 10–62B).

Hernias

Small bowel obstruction due to external hernia is usually diagnosed by clinical examination. However, the SBE may be able to demonstrate clinically unsuspected hernial obstruction in obese patients.[127] Paraileostomy hernias (Fig. 10–65) and rarer forms of external and internal hernias may also be discovered by SBE.

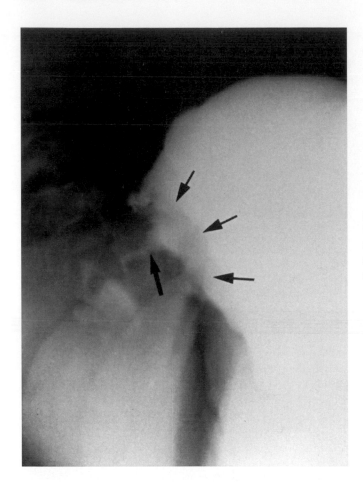

FIGURE 10–63. Metastatic lesion causing small bowel obstruction. The frayed outline of the narrow and angulated stricture *(single arrow)* and a pronounced irregularity of the rounded proximal contour *(multiple arrows)* favor a metastatic deposit. Past history of sigmoid colon carcinoma.

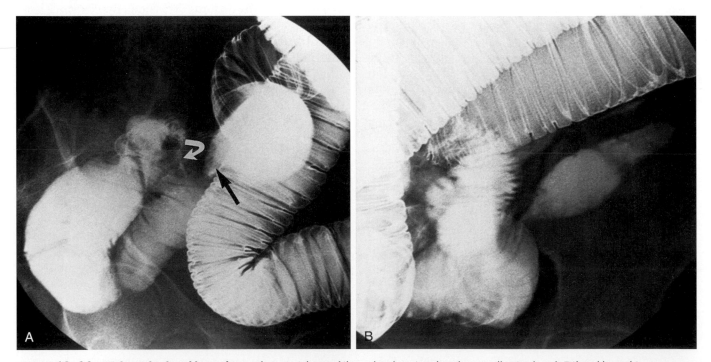

FIGURE 10–64. High-grade closed loop obstruction. *A,* A loop of ileum has herniated under an adhesive band. Dilated bowel is seen proximal to the entering limb *(arrow).* The adjacent exiting limb *(curved arrow)* is beak shaped, indicating torsion. No barium has yet passed beyond the closed loop. *B,* A delayed image records passage of a small amount of barium through the beak-shaped narrowing *(curved arrow).* Radiologic findings suggested ischemia. At surgery the slightly torsed bowel loop was considered to be still viable.

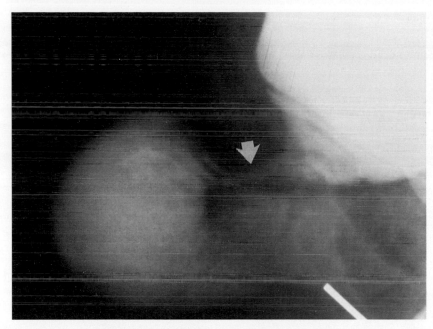

FIGURE 10–65. Paraileostomy hernia with partial obstruction. Such hernias may be overlooked at clinical examination. The entering limb of this hernia is compressed *(arrow)* and a dilated loop of ileum is seen proximal to it.

Whenever vascular impairment is suspected in cases of internal hernias, CT must replace enteroclysis.

MISCELLANEOUS DISORDERS

Edema

Edema is probably the most common abnormality of the small intestine. However, it is usually a secondary condition and submerged in the primary symptomatology of a patient and is not investigated radiologically as such. Hypoalbuminemia is the most common cause and may relate to protein-losing enteropathy, malabsorption, cirrhosis, or nephrosis. Edema may also be associated with congestive heart failure, constrictive pericarditis, and allergic states.

Interstitial fluid increase affects all layers of the bowel wall, but especially the submucosal space with its extensions into the core of the mucosal folds. Barium studies therefore show diffuse thickening of the folds with some degree of thickening and separation of loops (Fig. 10–66). Intraluminal fluid may be increased.

AIDS

AIDS is a disease of the immune system that can affect most organs of the body.[128] A significant proportion of secondary infections and neoplasms involves the abdomen, especially the gastrointestinal tract.

Cryptosporidiosis and *isosporiasis* are opportunistic infections by protozoa causing massive, cholera-like fluid loss into the gut. Barium studies show fluid increase and pronounced fold thickening, mostly in the proximal small bowel (Fig. 10–67).

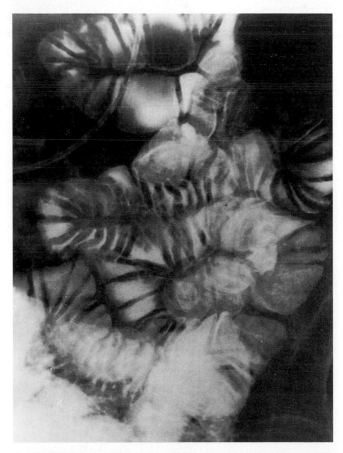

FIGURE 10–66. Small bowel edema. Patient with celiac disease and hypoalbuminemia. Folds are uniformly thickened, and slight wall thickening is evident. Folds in the distended proximal jejunum are widely separated, a sign typical of celiac disease. NOTE that folds are of normal thickness in uncomplicated celiac disease.

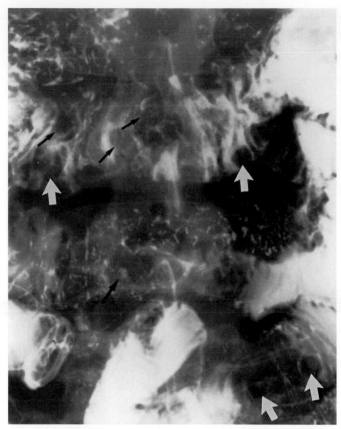

FIGURE 10–67. AIDS with cryptosporidiosis and Kaposi's sarcoma. Follow-through examination shows partly flocculated barium outlining thickened folds in the jejunum due to cryptosporidiosis. Several rounded filling defects, some with central ulceration *(arrows)*, were due to Kaposi's sarcoma, which was also present in the stomach and duodenum. (Courtesy of R. Goren, M.D., Philadelphia, Pennsylvania.)

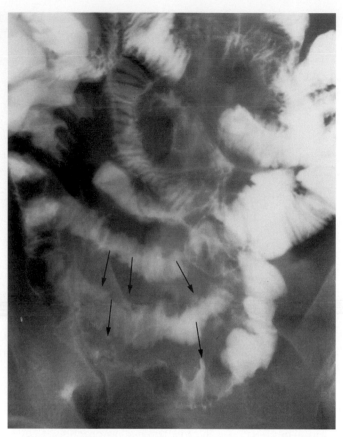

FIGURE 10–68. Cytomegalovirus enteritis in AIDS. Distal ileal loops show fold thickening and increased separation, indicating thickening of the bowel wall. In addition, several penetrating ulcers are seen in the distal ileum *(arrows).*

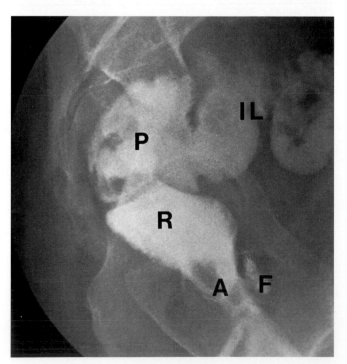

FIGURE 10–69. Ileoanal reservoir after colectomy for ulcerative colitis. Barium study before closure of diverting ileostomy. Barium introduced through the anus by soft catheter. Distal ileum *(IL)* continues into the "J" pouch *(P)*, which is inserted through the rectal cuff *(R)* (after mucosectomy) to be anastomosed to the dentate line of the anal canal *(A)*. From it arises a short fistula *(F)*. Closure of ileostomy will have to be delayed.

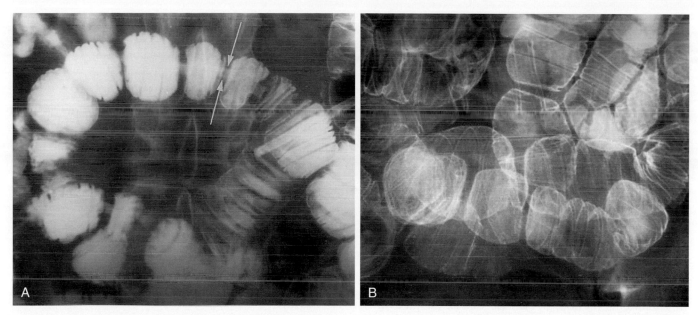

FIGURE 10–70. Prolonged medication with nonsteroidal anti-inflammatory drug, crampy abdominal pain. *A,* Enteroclysis in the stage of double contrast development demonstrates multiple diaphragms with central openings *(arrows). B,* Completed double contrast does not depict these diaphragms with the same clarity.

Cytomegalovirus, a member of the *Herpesvirus* group, can cause extensive intestinal and extraintestinal disease. Ulcers are a characteristic manifestation and may bleed or perforate (Fig. 10–68).

Mycobacterium avium intracellulare can infect most body systems. In the jejunum it can produce an appearance resembling Whipple's disease, with micronodules and enlarged, often matted, fat-containing mesenteric and retroperitoneal nodes.

Kaposi's sarcoma may be responsible for multiple cutaneous and visceral lesions, the latter showing a typical radiologic appearance of submucosal elevations with central umbilication (Fig. 10–66). There may be extensive lymph node enlargement.

AIDS-related lymphoma does not differ significantly from its usual small bowel localization. It affects younger patients and may involve the central nervous system.

Ileoanal Reservoir

Total colectomy for ulcerative colitis or familial polyposis coli can be combined with rectal mucosectomy, the formation of a distal ileal reservoir, and the introduction of its efferent segment through the rectal cuff for anastomosis at the dentate line. Continence is thus provided in a natural way by the anal sphincters.[129] A covering ileostomy is usually constructed and is closed after 6 to 8 weeks if no complications have occurred.

A barium examination should be done before closure of the ileostomy to ensure that a competent ileoanal anastomosis has been achieved (Fig. 10–69). For this purpose, a low-density barium suspension (30% to 40% w/v) can be injected antegrade through the ileostomy or retrograde through the anal canal by means of a soft catheter. These are not usually double contrast studies.

Nonsteroidal Anti-Inflammatory Drugs

Subacute small bowel obstructions have followed prolonged treatment with nonsteroidal anti-inflammatory drugs. In some cases multiple diaphragmlike strictures can be demonstrated by enteroclysis (Fig. 10–70).[130]

CONCLUSION

It is my belief that enteroclysis represents the most reliable method of investigating the small intestine and should be used whenever sound clinical indications exist. However, patient discomfort is associated with this method and should be mitigated by sedation and good technique. Only a high-quality study and a careful evaluation of its imaging result justify subjecting a patient to this examination.

In departments where small bowel examinations are undertaken on demand and for whatever reasons, the need to provide a follow-through examination remains. Even in these circumstances the follow-through should be a predominantly fluoroscopic examination and should be combined with a peroral pneumocolon if ileal pathology appears likely.

Enteroclysis can be expected to make a useful contribution to diagnosis in the following clinical circumstances.

1. All forms of *malabsorption*. Adult celiac disease, bacterial overgrowth syndrome, adult cystic fibrosis, Zollinger-Ellison syndrome, amyloidosis, Whipple's disease, lymphangiectasia, and the short bowel syndrome are among the causes of a malabsorption state in which characteristic findings can be demonstrated.

2. *Small bowel obstruction*. Whether done by routine intubation or through a decompression tube, the SBE can be accurate in determining the site and nature of the lesion responsible for obstruction. This can be of particular value in patients who have a history of laparotomy for malignancy. It is contraindicated in high-grade obstructions, adynamic ileus, or when ischemia appears to be a possible complication.

3. *Crohn's disease*. SBE is not always required to demonstrate Crohn's disease. The follow-through examination aided by the peroral pneumocolon is a satisfactory method in the follow-up of patients with known terminal ileal disease. The more accurate determination of the proximal extent of the disease, the exclusion or demonstration of early skip lesions, and the evaluation of strictures and fistulae are among the indications for enteroclysis to be performed.

4. *Tumors*. Benign or malignant tumors are more accurately demonstrated by SBE as long as both the single and double contrast phases of the examination are used. However, as in all cases, it makes good sense to stop the examination at the point of diagnosis. This may often be in the stage of double contrast development.

5. *Secondary malignancy and radiation damage*. The SBE is the most precise method available for differentiating between secondary malignancy and radiation damage, but careful and experienced evaluation is required.

6. *Occult blood loss* after studies of the upper and lower digestive tracts have been negative. It is a worthwhile diagnostic application but must be combined with duodenography.

7. *Determination of morphologic normality*. Only the SBE is capable of documenting those measurable parameters upon which a diagnosis of normality can be based.

Additional imaging methods, CT and increasingly MRI, can be of synergistic value. Their use is strongly recommended in tumors like carcinoids or lymphoma, with transmural extensions of inflammatory processes as in Crohn's disease, for higher grade obstructions, for the demonstration of nodal masses as in Whipple's disease, secondary lymphangiectasia, Kaposi's sarcoma, or mycobacterial infection, to mention only a few of these indications.

REFERENCES

1. Losowsky, M.S., Walker, B.E., and Kelleher, J.: Malabsorption in Clinical Practice. Edinburgh, Churchill-Livingstone, 1974.
2. Creamer, B.: The Small Intestine. London, William Heinemann, 1974.
3. Laws, J.W., Booth, C.C., Shawdon, H., et al.: Correlation of radiological and histological findings in idiopathic steatorrhoea. BMJ *1:*1311, 1963.
4. Kreel, L.: Pharmacoradiology in barium examinations with special reference to glucagon. Br. J. Radiol. *48:*691, 1975.
5. Ratcliffe, J.F.: The small bowel enema in children: A description of a technique. Clin. Radiol. *34:*287, 1983.
6. Maglinte, D.D.T., Burney, B.T., and Miller, R.E.: Lesions missed on small bowel follow-through: Analysis and recommendations. Radiology *144:*737, 1982.
7. Schulze-Delrieu, K.: Metoclopramide. *In* Koch-Weser, J. (ed.). Drug Therapy. N. Engl. J. Med. *305:*28, 1981.
8. Kelvin, F.M., Gedgaudas, R.K., Thompson, W.M., and Rice, R.P.: The peroral pneumocolon examination of the ileocecal region. AJR Am. J. Roentgenol. *39:*115, 1982.
9. Kressel, H.Y., Evers, K.A., Glick, S.N., et al.: Peroral pneumocolon examination: Technique and indications. Radiology *144:*414, 1982.
10. Fitzgerald, T.J., Thompson, G.T., Sommers, S.S., and Frank, S.S.: Pneumocolon as an aid to small bowel studies. Clin. Radiol. *36:*633, 1985.
11. Cole, L.G.: Artificial dilatation of the duodenum for radiographic examination. AJR Am. J. Roentgenol. *3:*204, 1911.
12. Einhorn, M.: The Duodenal Tube and Its Possibilities, (ed. 2). Philadelphia, F.A. Davis, 1926.
13. Pribram, B.O., and Kleiber, N.: Ein Neuer Weg zur roentgenologischen Darstellung des Duodenums (Pneumoduodenum). Fortschr. Geb. Roentgenstr. *36:*739, 1927.
14. Pesquera, G.S.: A method for the direct visualization of lesions in the small intestine. AJR Am. J. Roentgenol. *22:*254, 1929.
15. Gershon-Cohen, J., and Shay, H.: Barium enteroclysis. AJR Am. J. Roentgenol. *42:*456, 1939.
16. Schatzki, R.: Small intestine enema. AJR Am. J. Roentgenol. *30:*743, 1943.
17. Lura, A.: Enema of the small intestine with special emphasis on the diagnosis of tumors. Br. J. Radiol. *24:*264, 1951.
18. Scott-Harden, W.G.: Examination of the small bowel. *In* McLaren, J.W. (ed.): Modern Trends in Diagnostic Radiology, series 3. London, Butterworth & Company, 1960, pp. 84–87.
19. Bilbao, M.K., Frische, L.H., Dotter, C.T., et al.: Hypotonic duodenography. Radiology *89:*438, 1967.
20. Gianturco, C.: Rapid fluoroscopic duodenal intubation. Radiology *88:*1165, 1967.
21. Sellink, J.L.: Examination of a small intestine by duodenal intubation. Acta Radiol. *15:*318, 1974.
22. Sellink, J.L.: Examination of the small intestine by means of duodenal intubation. Leiden, HE, Stenfert Kroese, BV, 1971.
23. Sellink, J.L., and Miller, R.E.: Radiology of the small bowel. *In* Modern Enteroclysis Technique and Atlas. The Hague, Martinus Nijhoff, 1982.
24. Fleckenstein, P., and Pedersen, G.: The value of the duodenal intubation method (Sellink modification) for the radiological visualization of the small bowel. Scand. J. Gastroenterol. *10:*423, 1974.
25. Sanders, D.E., and Ho, C.S.: The small bowel enema: Experience with 150 examinations. AJR Am. J. Roentgenol. *127:*743, 1976.
26. Ekberg, O.: Crohn's disease of the small bowel examined by double contrast technique: A comparison with oral technique. Gastrointest. Radiol. *1:*355, 1977.
27. Taverne, P.P., and van der Jagt, E.J.: Small bowel radiography: A prospective comparison study of three techniques in 200 patients. Fortschr. Geb. Roentgenstr. *143:*293, 1985.
28. Nolan, D.J., and Traill, J.C.: The current role of the barium examination of the small bowel. Clin. Radiol. *52:*809–820, 1997.
29. Kobayashi, S., Nishizawa, M., Mizuno, K., et al.: Double contrast studies of the small bowel. Jpn. Clin. Radiol. *19:*619, 1974.
30. Nakamura, Y., Tani, K., Yao, T., et al.: X-ray examination of the small intestine by means of duodenal intubation—Double contrast of the small bowel. Stom. Intest. *9:*1461–1469, 1974.
31. Pigott, F., Street, D.F., Shellshear, M.F., et al.: Radiological investigation of the small intestine. Gut *1:*366, 1960.

32. Scott-Harden, W.G., Hamilton, H.A.R., and McCall-Smith, S.: Radiological investigation of the small intestine. Gut 2:316, 1961.

33. Trickey, S.F., Halls, J., and Hodson, C.J.: A further development of the small bowel enema. Proc. R. Soc. Med. 56:1070, 1963.

34. Sinclair, D.J., and Buist, T.A.S.: Water contrast barium enema technique using methyl cellulose in solution. Br. J. Radiol. 39:228, 1966.

35. Gmündner, U., and Wirth, W.: Dünndarmdoppelkontrastdarstellung. Schweiz. Med. Wochenschr. 100:1286, 1970.

36. Herlinger, H.: A modified technique for the double contrast small bowel enema. Gastrointest. Radiol. 3:201, 1987.

37. Maglinte, D.D.T., and Herlinger, H.: Enteroclysis catheters, intubation and infusion. *In* Herlinger, H., and Maglinte, D.D.T. (eds.): Clinical Radiology of the Small Intestine. Philadelphia, W.B. Saunders Co., 1989.

38. Christie, D.L., and Ament, M.E.: A double blind crossover study of metoclopramide versus placebo for facilitating passage of multipurpose biopsy tube. Gastroenterology 71:726, 1976.

39. Stevenson, G.W., and Malone, D.E.: Sedation and analgesia in abdominal imaging and intervention. Communication to the Society of Gastrointestinal Radiology Meeting 1998.

40. Maglinte, D.D.T., and Herlinger, H.: Single contrast and biphasic enteroclysis: the small bowel enema with methylcellulose. *In* Herlinger, H., and Maglinte, D.D.T. (eds.): Clinical Radiology of the Small Intestine. Philadelphia, W.B. Saunders Co., 1989.

41. Maglinte, D.D.T., and Herlinger, H.: Congenital and developmental anomalies in adolescents and adults. *In* Herlinger, H., and Maglinte, D.D.T. (eds.): Clinical Radiology of the Small Intestine. Philadelphia, W.B. Saunders Co., 1989.

42. Maglinte, D.D.T., Elmore, M.F., Isenberg, M., and Dolan, P.A.: Meckel's diverticulum: Radiologic demonstration by enteroclysis. AJR Am. J. Roentgenol. 134:925–932, 1969.

43. Ho, C.S., Shewchun, J., and Greenberg, J.R: Diagnosis of Meckel's diverticulum in adults. Mt. Sinai J. Med. 51:378–381, 1984.

44. Stewart, J.S., Pollock, D.J., Hoffbrand, A.V., et al.: A study of proximal and distal intestinal structure and absorptive function in idiopathic steatorrhea. Q. J. Med. 36:425, 1967.

45. Thaysen, T.E.H.: Absorption of Fat and Protein: Non-tropical Sprue. Copenhagen, Levin and Munksgaard, 1932.

46. Nelson, S.W.: Abnormal small bowel fold patterns. *In* Categorical Course on Gastrointestinal Radiology. Reston, VA, American Roentgen Ray Society, 1977.

47. Osborn, A.G., and Friedland, G.W.: A radiological approach to the diagnosis of small bowel disease. Clin. Radiol. 24:281, 1973.

48. Pare, P., Douville, P., Caron, D., and Lagace, R.: Adult celiac sprue: Changes in the pattern of clinical recognition. J. Clin. Gastroenterol. 10:395, 1988.

49. Herlinger, H., and Maglinte, D.D.T.: Jejunal fold separation in adult celiac diseases: Relevance of enteroclysis. Radiology 158:605, 1986.

50. Bova, J.G., Friedman, A.C., Weser, E., et al.: Adaptation of the ileum in nontropical sprue: reversal of the jejunoileal fold pattern. AJR Am. J. Roentgenol. 144:299, 1985.

51. Marshak, R.H., and Linder, A.E.: Malabsorption syndromes: Sprue. *In* Radiology of the Small Intestine, ed. 2. Philadelphia, W.B. Saunders Co., 1976.

52. Farthing, M.J., McLean, A.M., Bartram, C.I., et al.: Radiological features of the jejunum in hypoalbuminemia. AJR Am. J. Roentgenol. 136:883, 1981.

53. Cohen, M.D., and Lintott, D.J.: Transient small bowel intussusception in adult coeliac disease. Clin. Radiol. 29:529, 1978.

54. Collins, S.M., Hamilton, J.D., Lewis, T.D., et al.: Small bowel malabsorption and gastrointestinal malignancy. Radiology 126:603, 1978.

55. Bagos, C.D., Kuan, S., Dobbins, J., and Ravikumar, S.: Metachronous small-bowel adenocarcinoma in celiac sprue. J. Clin. Gastroenterol. 20:233–236, 1995.

56. Murray, A., Cuevas, E.C., Jones, D.B., and Wright, D.H.: Study of immunohistochemistry and T-cell clonality of enteropathy-associated T cell lymphoma. Am. J. Pathol. 146:509–519, 1995.

57. Murray, A., Slavin, G., Coles, E.C., and Booth, C.C.: Celiac disease and malignancy. Lancet 1:111–115, 1983.

58. Egan, L.J., Walsh, S.V., Stevens, F.M., et al.: Celiac-associated lymphoma. A single institution experience of 30 cases in the combination chemotherapy era. J. Clin. Gastroenterol. 21:123–129, 1995.

59. Horowitz, A.L., and Meyers, M.A.: The "hide-bound" small bowel of scleroderma: Characteristic mucosal fold pattern. AJR Am. J. Roentgenol. 119:332, 1973.

60. Golladay, L.S., and Byrne, W.J.: Intestinal pseudo-obstruction. Surg. Gynecol. Obstet. 153:257, 1981.

61. Rohrman, C.A., Jr., Ricci, M.T., Krisnamurthy, S., and Schuffler, M.D.: Radiologic and histologic differentiation of neuromuscular disorders of the gastrointestinal tract: Visceral myopathies, visceral neuropathies, and progressive systemic sclerosis. AJR Am. J. Roentgenol. 143:933, 1981.

62. Scott, P.P., Scott, W.W., and Siegelman, S.S.: Amyloidosis: An overview. Semin. Roentgenol. 21:103, 1986.

63. Tada, S., Iida, M., Matsui, T., et al.: Amyloidosis of the small intestine: Findings on double contrast radiographs. AJR Am. J. Roentgenol. 156:741–744, 1991.

64. Tada, S., Iida, M., Yao, T., et al.: Gastrointestinal amyloidosis. Radiologic features by chemical types. Radiology 190:37–42, 1994.

65. Lloyd, M.L., and Olsen, W.A.: Abetalipoproteinemia. *In* Yamada, T. (ed.): Textbook of Gastroenterology. Philadelphia, J.B. Lippincott, 1991, p. 1527.

66. Rosen, F.S., Cooper, M.D., and Wedgewood, R.J.P.: The primary immunodeficiencies. N. Engl. J. Med. 311:235, 1984.

67. Hermans, P.E.: Nodular lymphoid hyperplasia of the small intestine and hypogammaglobulinemia: Theoretical and practical considerations. Fed. Proc. 26:1606, 1967.

68. Brandon, J., Glick, S.N., and Teplick, S.K.: Intestinal giardiasis: Importance of serial filming. AJR Am. J. Roentgenol. 144:581, 1985.

69. Cherner, J.A., Jensen, R.T., Dubois, A., et al.: Gastrointestinal dysfunction in systemic mastocytosis. Gastroenterology 95:657–667, 1988.

70. Huang, T-Y, Yam, L.T., and Li, C-Y.: Radiological features of systemic mast-cell disease. Br. J. Radiol. 60:765–770, 1987.

71. Miller, L.S., Vinayek, R., Frucht, H., et al.: Reflux esophagitis in patients with Zöllinger-Ellison syndrome. Gastroenterology 98:341, 1990.

72. Matsui, T., Iida, M., Fujishima, M., et al.: Linear erosions on Kerkring's folds may be diagnostic of Zollinger-Ellison syndrome. J. Clin. Gastroenterol. 11:278, 1989.

73. Stallmeyer, M.J.B., and Chew, F.S.: Eosinophilic gastroenteritis. AJR Am. J. Roentgenol. 161:296, 1993.

74. Schulman, A., Morton, P.C.G., and Dietrich, P.E.: Eosinophilic gastroenteritis. Clin. Radiol. 31:101–104, 1980.

75. Dobbins, W.O. III: Current concepts of Whipple's disease [Editorial]. J. Clin. Gastroenterol. 4:205, 1982.

76. Herlinger, H.: Radiology in malabsorption [Editorial]. Clin. Radiol. 45:73–78, 1992.

77. Davis, S.J., and Patel, A.: Case report: Distinctive echogenic lymphadenopathy in Whipple's disease. Clin. Radiol. 42:60, 1990.

78. Heresbach, D., Raoul, J.L., Genetet, N., et al.: Immunological study in primary intestinal lymphangiectasia. Digestion 55:59–64, 1994.

79. Aoyagi, K., Iida, M., Yao, T., et al.: Intestinal lymphangiectasia: Value of double-contrast radiographic study. Clin. Radiol. 49:814–819, 1994.

80. Scully, R.E.: Case records of the Massachusetts General Hospital, Case 3-1990. N. Engl. J. Med. 322:183–192, 1990.

81. Gad, A., Willen, R., Carlen, B., et al.: Duodenal involvement in Waldenström's macroglobulinemia. J. Clin. Gastroenterol. 20:174–177, 1995.

82. Cooke, W.T., Cox, E.U., Fone, D.J., et al.: The clinical and metabolic significance of jejunal diverticula. Gut 4:115, 1963.

83. Scully, R.E. (ed.): Case records of the Massachusetts General Hospital, Case 25-1990. N. Engl. J. Med. 322:1796, 1990.

84. Stollman, N.H., Neustater, B.R., and Rogers, A.L.: Short bowel syndrome. Gastroenterologist 4:118–128, 1996.

85. Vanderhoof, J.A., and Langnas A.N.: Short bowel syndrome in children and adults. Gastroenterology 113:1767–1778, 1997.

86. Smith, A.N., and Balfour, T.W.: Malabsorption in Crohn's disease. Clin. Gastroenterol. 1:433 1972.

87. Glick, S.N., and Teplick, S.K.: Crohn's disease of the small intestine: Diffuse mucosal granularity. Radiology 154:313, 1985.

88. Ekberg, O., Baath, L., Sjostrom, B., and Linghagen, T.: Are super-

ficial lesions in the distal part of the ileum early indicators of Crohn's disease in adult patients with abdominal pain? A clinical and radiologic long-term investigation. Gut *25*:341, 1984.

89. Kelvin, M.F., and Herlinger, H.: Crohn's disease. *In* Herlinger, H., Maglinte, D.D.T., Birnbaum, B.A. (eds.): Clinical Imaging of the Small Intestine, ed. 2. New York, Springer Verlag, 1999.

90. Meyers, M.A.: Clinical involvement of mesenteric and antimesenteric borders of small bowel loops. Gastrointest. Radiol. *1*:49, 1976.

91. Herlinger, H., Rubesin, S.E., and Furth, E.E.: Mesenteric border linear ulcers in Crohn's disease: Historical, radiologic and pathologic perspectives. Abdom. Imaging *23*:122–126, 1998.

92. Nolan, D.J.: Radiology of Crohn's disease of the small intestine: A review. J. R. Soc. Med. *74*:294, 1981.

93. Herlinger, H., O'Riordan, D., Saul, S., and Levine, M.S.: Nonspecific involvement of bowel adjoining Crohn's disease. Radiology *159*:47, 1986.

94. Ekberg, O., Sjostrom, B., and Brahme, F.J.: Radiologic findings in *Yersinia* ileitis. Radiology *123*:15, 1977.

95. Palmer, K.R., Patil, D.H., Basran, G.S., et al.: Abdominal tuberculosis in urban Britain—A common disease. Gut *26*:1296, 1985.

96. Brombart, M., and Massion, J.: Radiologic differential diagnosis between ileocecal tuberculosis and Crohn's disease. Am. J. Dig. Dis. *6*:589, 1961.

97. Yao T.: Roentgenographic analysis of tuberculosis of the small intestine. Stom. Intest. *12*:1467, 1977.

98. Jeffrey, R.B., Laing, F.C., and Townsend, R.R.: Acute appendicitis: Sonographic criteria based on 250 cases. Radiology *167*:327, 1988.

99. Olmstead, W.W., Ros, P.R., Hjermstad, B.M., et al.: Tumors of the small intestine with little or no malignant predispositions: A review of the literature and report of 56 cases. Gastrointest. Radiol. *12*:231, 1987.

100. Megibow, A.J., Redman, P.E., Bosniak, M.A., and Horowitz, L.: Diagnosis of gastrointestinal lipomas by CT. AJR Am. J. Roentgenol. *133*:743, 1979.

101. Curcio, C.M., Feinstein, R.S., Humphrey, R.L., et al.: Computed tomography of enteroenteric intussusception. J. Comput. Assist. Tomogr. *6*:969, 1982.

102. Paivansalo, M., Siniluoto, T., and Jalovaara, P.: Radiological findings in small bowel tumors. Fortschr. Roentgenstr. *149*:615, 1988.

103. Linos, D.A., Dozios, R.R., Dahlin, D.C., and Bartholomew, L.G.: Does Peutz-Jegher's syndrome predispose to gastrointestinal malignancy? Arch. Surg. *116*:1182, 1981.

104. Payne-James, J.J., DeGaza, C.J., Lovill, D., et al.: Metastatic carcinoid tumour in association with small bowel ischaemia and infarction. J. R. Soc. Med. *63*:54, 1990.

105. Woodard, P.K., Feldman, J.M., Paine, S.S., and Baker, M.E.: Midgut carcinoid tumors: CT findings and biochemical profile. J. Comput. Assist. Tomogr. *19*:400, 1995.

106. Gore, R.M.: Small bowel cancer. Clinical and pathologic features [Review]. Radiol. Clin. North Am. *35*:351–360, 1997.

107. Ripley, D., and Weinerman, G.H.: Increased incidence of second malignancies associated with small bowel adenocarcinoma. Can. J. Gastroenterol. *11*:65–68, 1997.

108. Gilchrist, A.M., Herlinger, H., Carr, R.F., et al.: Small bowel lymphoma, a radiologic-pathologic correlation. *In* Herlinger, H., Megibow, A. (eds.): Gastrointestinal Radiology Review. New York, Marcel Dekker, 1990, p. 187.

109. Levine, M.S., Rubesin, S.E., Pantongrag-Brown, L., et al.: Non-Hodgkin's lymphoma of the gastrointestinal tract. Radiographic findings. AJR Am. J. Roentgenol. *168*:165, 1977.

110. Agaroff, L.H., Connors, J.M., Klasa, R.J., et al.: Mantle cell lymphoma: A clinicopathologic study of 80 cases. Blood *69*:2067, 1997.

111. Meyers, M.A.: Dynamic Radiology of the Abdomen: Normal and Pathologic Anatomy, ed. 3. New York, Springer-Verlag, 1988.

112. Marshak, R.H., Khilnani, M.T., Eliasoph, J., and Wolf, B.S.: Metastatic carcinoma of the small bowel. AJR Am. J. Roentgenol. *94*:385, 1965.

113. Maglinte, D.D.T., Birnbaum, B.A., and Herlinger, H.: Neoplasms. *In* Clinical Imaging of the Small Intestine, ed. 2. New York: Springer Verlag, 1998.

114. Wittich, G., Salomonowitz, E., Szepesi, T., et al.: Small bowel double contrast enema in stage III ovarian cancer. AJR Am. J. Roentgenol. *142*:299, 1994.

115. Goldstein, H.M., Beydoun, M.T., and Dodd, G.D.: Radiologic spectrum of melanoma metastatic to the gastrointestinal tract. AJR Am. J. Roentgenol. *129*:605, 1977.

116. Fishman, E.K., Kuhlman, J.E., Schucter, L.M., et al.: CT of malignant melanoma in the chest, abdomen and musculoskeletal system. Radiographics *10*:603, 1990.

117. Mason, G.R., Dietrich, P., Friedland, G.W., et al.: The radiologic findings in radiation-induced enteritis and colitis: A review of 30 cases. Clin. Radiol. *21*:232, 1970.

118. Morgenstern L., Hart M., Lugo D., and Friedman, M.B.: Changing aspects of radiation enteropathy. Arch. Surg. *120*:1225, 1985.

119. Marshak, R.H., Linder, A.E., and Maklansky, D.: Ischemia of the small intestine. Am. J. Gastroenterol. *66*:390, 1976.

120. Rizzo, M.J., Federle, M.P., and Griffiths, G.B.: Bowel and mesenteric injury following blunt abdominal trauma: Evaluation with CT. Radiology *173*:143, 1989.

121. Rex, D.K., Lappas, J.C., Maglinte, D.D.T., et al.: Enteroclysis in the evaluation of suspected small intestinal bleeding. Gastroenterology *97*:58, 1989.

122. Moch, A., Herlinger, H., Kochman, M.L., et al.: Enteroclysis in the evaluation of obscure gastrointestinal bleeding. AJR Am. J. Roentgenol. *163*:1381–1384, 1994.

123. Maglinte, D.D.T., Gage, S.N., Harmon, B.H., et al.: Obstruction of the small intestine: Accuracy and role of CT in diagnosis. Radiology *188*:61–64, 1993.

124. Caroline, D.F., Herlinger, H., Laufer, I., et al.: Small bowel enema in the diagnosis of adhesive obstruction. AJR Am. J. Roentgenol. *142*:1133, 1984.

125. Maglinte, D.D.T., Herlinger, H., and Nolan, D.J.: Radiologic features of closed loop obstruction: Analysis of 25 confirmed cases. Radiology *179*:383–387, 1991.

126. Price, J., and Nolan, D.J.: Closed loop obstruction: Diagnosis by enteroclysis. Gastrointest. Radiol. *14*:251, 1989.

127. Maglinte, D.D.T., and Birnbaum, B.A.: Obstruction. *In* Herlinger, H., Maglinte, D.D.T., Birnbaum, B.A. (eds.): Clinical Imaging of the Small Intestine. New York, Springer Verlag, 1998.

128. Megibow, A.J., Wall, S.D., Balthazar, E.J., and Rybak, B.J.: Gastrointestinal radiology in AIDS patients. *In* Federle, M.P., Megibow, A.J., Naidich, D.P. (eds.): Radiology of AIDS. New York, Raven Press, 1988.

129. Lycke, K.G.: Radiology of the ileal reservoirs. *In* Herlinger, H., and Megibow, A.J. (eds.): Advances in Gastrointestinal Radiology, vol. 1. Chicago, Mosby–Year Book, 1991.

130. Levi, S., deLacey, G., Price, A.B., et al.: "Diaphragm-like" strictures of the small bowel in patients treated with non-steroidal anti-inflammatory drugs. Br. J. Radiol. *6*:186, 1990.

11

Double Contrast Barium Enema: Technical Aspects

STEPHEN E. RUBESIN
IGOR LAUFER

CONTRAINDICATIONS

PATIENT PREPARATION
Bowel Cleansing

MATERIALS
Fluoroscope Pad
Hypotonic Drugs
Barium
Compression Devices

PROCEDURE
Preliminary Film
Insertion of the Rectal Tip
Barium Instillation
Spot Film Principles
Enema Tip Removal

SPOT FILM POSITIONS
Rectum
Rectosigmoid Junction
Sigmoid Colon
Erect Views
Splenic Flexure and Descending Colon
Mid-Transverse Colon
Hepatic Flexure
Ascending Colon
Cecum
Appendix and Terminal Ileum

OVERHEAD RADIOGRAPHS

VARIATIONS IN TECHNIQUE
Colostomy Study
Peroral Pneumocolon

PITFALLS
Prior Endoscopy
Colonic Spasm
Redundant Colon
Nonfilling of the Right Colon

COMPLICATIONS
Gas Pains
Perforation

NORMAL APPEARANCES
Surface Pattern
Transverse Folds
Lymph Follicles

ARTIFACTS

Early detection of colonic carcinoma or precursor adenomas by barium enema examination has a tremendous potential for saving lives,[1] as much as any radiologic study including mammography. Therefore radiologists must take interest in performing quality barium enema examinations.[2] The double contrast barium enema is our routine radiologic examination of the colon unless there are specific reasons for using an alternative technique. The double contrast barium enema is the primary radiologic investigative tool for the colon because of its ability to demonstrate small polypoid lesions and subtle surface alterations in the early stages of inflammatory bowel disease.

The indications for double contrast barium enema include rectal bleeding, diarrhea, abdominal pain, or screening for colorectal neoplasia. In patients with high-grade colonic obstruction or colonic fistula, either a single contrast barium or a barium enema using high-density barium may be performed. In patients with suspected Hirschsprung's disease, we prefer to use a single contrast barium enema. If the radiologist is ruling out a distal small bowel obstruction, a single contrast barium enema with reflux into the ileum may be used.

There are many ways to perform a double contrast barium enema. No set formula or cookbook approach exists, nor should there be one. Each barium enema is tailored to the clinical history, the patient's ability to perform the examination, and the fluoroscopic findings.[2] The radiologist interacts with the patient, the controls of the fluoroscope, and the radiographic findings on the television monitor to create images of the colon. Barium and air are the radiologist's artist materials; the colon is the canvas. The radiologist manipulates the barium pool to paint the mucosal surface, filling depressed lesions (Fig. 11–1) or coating elevated lesions (Fig. 11–2).

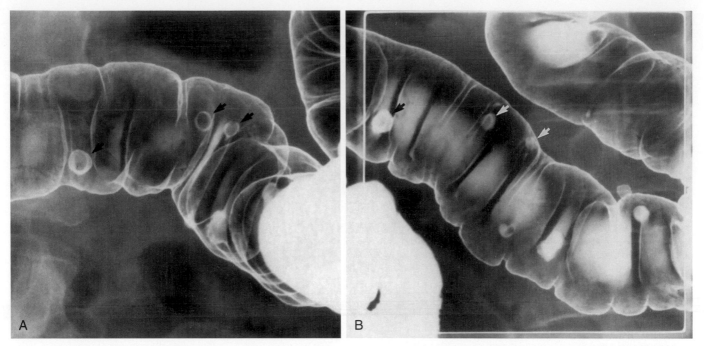

FIGURE 11–1. Manipulation of the barium pool. *A,* Barium filled-diverticula and ring shadows *(arrows)* are seen in the transverse colon. *B,* Barium is flowed across the posterior wall, filling three colonic diverticula *(arrows).*

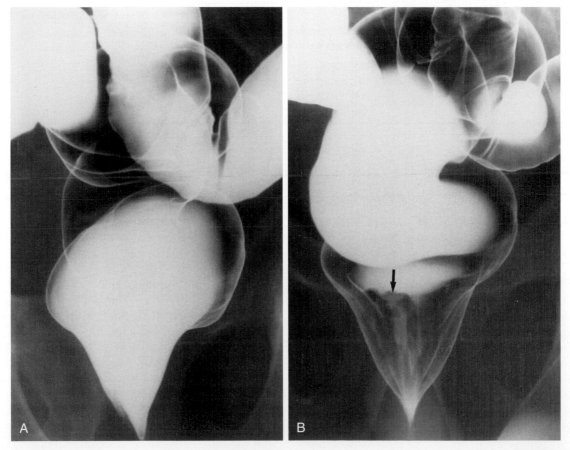

FIGURE 11–2. Changing patient position reveals tubulovillous adenoma. *A,* In the prone position, barium fills the distal rectum. *B,* In the supine position, air fills the distal rectum. A 1.2-cm lobulated polyp is now visible. A shallow barium pool coating the polyp fills a central umbilication *(arrow).* (*A* and *B* are photographed so the rectum is in the same anatomic orientation.)

CONTRAINDICATIONS

A double contrast barium enema is contraindicated in conditions that are also contraindications to the use of the single contrast enema. In patients with suspected colonic perforation, water-soluble contrast material is used. Toxic megacolon is a contraindication to barium study of the colon. Contrast studies of the colon should not be performed immediately after colonic biopsy through a rigid sigmoidoscope because large biopsy forceps may have perforated the colon, and barium could extravasate from the site of the colonic or rectal perforation if a barium enema is attempted. Contrast studies should also not be performed after snare polypectomy or a "hot" biopsy. Whenever the mucosa may have been breached, a delay of at least 6 days is advisable to allow the mucosa to heal. No such delay is required after endoscopic biopsy using fiberoptic instruments because the small forceps used during biopsy yield only a superficial bit of tissue.[3,4]

PATIENT PREPARATION

Bowel Cleansing

Adequate cleansing of the colon is equally critical for all types of colonic examination: single contrast enema, colonoscopy, and double contrast enema. A wide variety of preparations has been recommended.[5–7] The principal components of adequate preparation include a clear liquid diet, laxatives, and a suppository. Our current preparation consists of the following:

1. The day before the examination
   a. Clear liquids only by mouth
   b. At 5 PM: 10 to 16 oz magnesium citrate
   c. At 10 PM: 4 bisacodyl tablets
   d. Nothing by mouth after midnight
2. The morning of the examination: a bisacodyl suppository

This bowel cleansing preparation works reliably in most patients provided that the instructions are followed. Cleansing may be incomplete with this standard preparation in immobile or bedridden patients, patients with hypomotility disorders such as diabetes and hypothyroidism, postoperative patients, or in patients taking opiates or drugs with anticholinergic side effects. It is important to question patients upon arrival in the radiology department to determine whether the proper instructions were given and followed. If the patient reports that the last bowel movement was watery in nature, it is assumed that adequate preparation has been achieved. We no longer use cleansing enemas because they tend to leave residual fluid in the colon, which diminishes barium coating. Cleansing enemas also require that the patient wait approximately 1 hour before the study is performed, thus prolonging the patient's stay in the x-ray department. Rapid colonic lavage by the ingestion of electrolyte solution such as Go-lytely (Braintree Laboratories, Braintree, MA) or Colyte (Reed and Carnick, Piscataway, NJ) has been recommended for barium enema and colonoscopy.[8] However, we find that these solutions leave too much residual fluid in the colon, which degrades the quality of barium mucosal coating.[9]

Some patients have tremendous fear about undergoing a barium enema. This apprehension can be alleviated if the patient understands why the study is being ordered and what happens during the study. Our department provides a brief written description of the barium enema in the instruction sheet for colonic preparation.

MATERIALS

Fluoroscope Pad

The surface of a fluoroscopic table is firm, if not hard. Thin patients rolling around on this hard surface may be uncomfortable and occasionally bruise or tear their skin. Placing a washable pad and clean sheet on the top of the fluoroscopic table will alleviate some of the discomfort of turning on its hard surface. The fluoroscopic pad will help ease the pressure on bony protuberances such as the ribs or pelvis.

Hypotonic Drugs

We routinely use 1 mg glucagon given intravenously to induce colonic hypotonia. In other countries, Buscopan (hyoscine-N-butylbromide) may be used to decrease patient discomfort during double contrast barium enema. Glucagon is injected slowly over a 60-second period while the radiologist elicits additional clinical data from the patient. Although glucagon and Buscopan decrease patient discomfort,[10–12] we believe that they also improve diagnostic accuracy because they allow greater colonic distention (Fig. 11–3) and allow reflux of barium into the terminal ileum.

Other radiologists inject glucagon in selected patients only when the patient becomes very uncomfortable, with spasm resulting in pain, expulsion of barium, or diminished colonic distention.

Barium

A medium-density, medium-viscosity barium is used (such as Polibar+, E-Z-EM, Westbury, N.Y.). The barium must be of low enough viscosity to scrub the colonic mucus and residual feces into the barium pool. The barium must be viscous enough to adhere to the mucosal surface for a sufficient amount of time to take radiographs. The barium must be viscous enough to reabsorb residual water in the colon. The barium must not be too dense as to obscure lesions in the barium pool, but must be dense enough so that a thin layer of barium will be visible radiographically. Barium suspensions varying in concentration from 70% to 100% w/v concentration have been used.

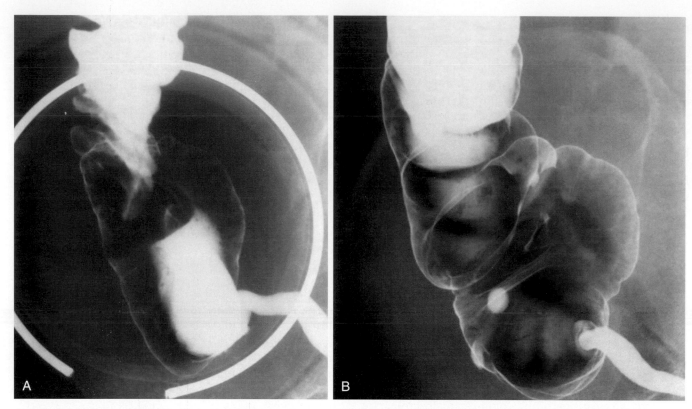

FIGURE 11–3. **Use of intravenous glucagon allowing greater colonic distention.** *A,* Spot radiograph of cecum before the use of intravenous glucagon shows spasm and lack of distention. *B,* Spot radiograph of cecum after the use of intravenous glucagon shows superior distention.

Compression Devices

We have found that colonic compression during barium enema helps splay apart loops and improves uniform exposure. Therefore various compression devices may be used to palpate patients' abdomens, including a soft rubber balloon or a gloved hand.

PROCEDURE

Preliminary Film

The preliminary or scout film of the abdomen has been shown to be of little value before a barium enema.[13] We therefore use it routinely only in hospitalized patients. We also obtain a preliminary film in ambulatory patients who have diarrhea, abdominal pain, or signs or symptoms of obstruction. We obtain this preliminary film in cases in which we are uncertain about the adequacy of colonic cleansing. If the preliminary film shows definite fecal material in the colon, the patient may return for an additional 24 hours of preparation with clear liquids and laxatives or, at some institutions, the patient may receive a cleansing enema.

Insertion of the Rectal Tip

A rectal examination performed before the insertion of the enema tip enables the radiologist to (1) determine the course of the anal canal, (2) check for hemorrhoids, inflammatory conditions, or unsuspected rectal masses

that would make enema tip insertion uncomfortable or dangerous, and (3) assess anal sphincter tone to help determine whether the balloon must be distended. A large amount of feces on the examiner's glove indicates the need for a second day of preparation. Anaphylactic reactions have been reported with the use of contaminated latex gloves.[14]

After spreading a thin layer of lubricant on the external surface of the anus and on the enema tip, the enema tip is inserted into the anal canal while the patient lies in a recumbent left-side down position. If the patient complains of any pain, the radiologist stops. If a digital examination of the rectum has not been performed previously, a rectal examination is now indicated. Once the catheter tip passes through the anal canal, the radiologist directs the tip posteriorly to parallel the course of the sacrum. A rectal tip pressed anteriorly will push against the prostate in a man or the vagina in a woman.

In patients with adequate rectal tone, distention of the balloon on the tip of the rectal catheter is usually not necessary. Encouraging the patient to hold the barium is usually sufficient. A distended enema-tipped balloon will make the examination more uncomfortable, and there is a small risk of distal rectal tear or perforation with the use of the balloon.[15] The balloon is insufflated in patients who are leaking barium or air out of the anal canal but not in patients who are apprehensive only about holding the barium. The balloon is inflated only after the rectum is outlined by barium and no abnormalities are seen. The balloon is distended minimally and retracted against the anal sphincter, producing a ball-valve effect. The balloon is distended only according to the manufacturer's recommendations.

Contraindications for inflating rectal balloons include suspected colitis, a history of pelvic radiation or colitis, solitary rectal ulcer syndrome, a large rectal mass, a suspected rectovaginal fistula, or perianal diseases such as Crohn's disease. If the anal canal is extremely tender during digital examination, a soft catheter such as a 24F Foley catheter will suffice for filling the colon first with barium then air.

Barium Instillation

Barium is slowly instilled into the colon while the patient lies in the prone position. Rapid filling of the rectum increases the patient's urge to defecate, and the physiologic sphincter at the rectosigmoid junction may go into spasm if the rectum is rapidly overdistended. Therefore the radiologist does not open the barium tube completely but only partially. Once a full column of barium has reached the descending colon, the tube is fully opened.

The length and caliber of the patient's colon determines the amount of barium administered. In general, to ensure that enough barium reaches the right colon, a full column of barium is instilled to the mid-transverse colon, so the contrast column passes just beyond the lumbar spine. The barium is then drained from the rectum by dropping the bag to the floor and using gravity. The goal of rectal draining is not to clear the entire rectosigmoid colon of barium but to empty the distal rectum so that when air is insufflated, bubbles are not created.

Spot Film Principles

A properly performed double contrast barium enema emphasizes the use of fluoroscopy and spot radiographs rather than overhead films. The radiologist obtains fluoroscopically guided images that show that the colonic mucosa is adequately coated with barium, the lumen is adequately distended by air, and a colonic segment is in a proper projection to eliminate overlapping bowel loops. Therefore the radiologist obtains spot films or digital spot films under fluoroscopic control to ensure adequate projection, distention, and coating. The overhead images that are of value are views the radiologist cannot obtain in fluoroscopy, including views in which the overhead tube is angled or the patient lies in a decubitus position.

Each segment of the colon should be seen in air contrast with the lumen etched in white by barium and the mucosal surface seen en face as a graduation from white to gray (Fig. 11–4). The radiologist turns the patient so that each surface is freshly scrubbed and coated with barium; then the radiologist turns the patient again to eliminate the barium pool from the area of interest, and finally a radiographic exposure is made. The colon should not be devoid of barium pools and only etched in white by barium.

Rather, approximately one third of the decubitus luminal diameter should be filled with barium. Without enough barium, adequate mucosal scrubbing is not possible; feces and mucus will not be washed into the barium pool.

The radiologist should not have a rigid order for obtaining exposures but should have a flexible approach based on the fluoroscopic appearance of the colon, any abnormality that is detected, and how the patient feels. Exposures of the sigmoid colon are first obtained before barium reaches the ascending colon. If barium reaches the right colon and refluxes through the ileocecal valve, the sigmoid colon may be partly obscured by barium in the distal ileum. Therefore after a full column of barium has reached the mid-transverse colon and crossed the spine, the first exposures that should be obtained are supine and right and left oblique views of the sigmoid colon. Repeat images of the sigmoid colon may be obtained at a later time after further turning of the patient has improved mucosal coating.

In general, barium is moved into the hepatic flexure by turning the patient onto the right side and then onto the back. Barium is moved into the descending colon and cecum by turning the patient to the left and, if necessary, semierect or erect. Barium drainage from the rectum may be repeated and facilitated by insufflation of air and by angulation of the enema tip.

The colon is distended by gentle air insufflation by squeezing the air bulb. Rapid air insufflation is very uncomfortable, inciting rectosigmoid spasm and possible air or barium evacuation. Therefore air is intermittently and

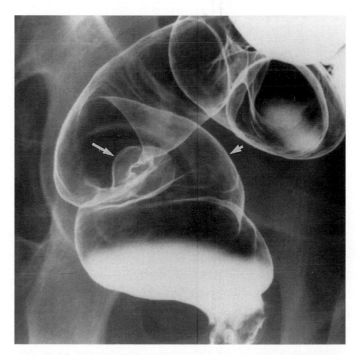

FIGURE 11–4. Mucosal coating. Spot radiograph of the rectum shows the colonic contour *(short arrow)* etched in white. The mucosal surface "fades to gray." A tubular adenoma is manifested as barium etched lines *(long arrow)* surrounding an area of increased radiopacity.

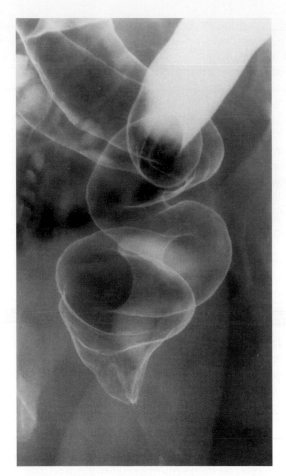

FIGURE 11–5. Spot radiograph of rectum with patient in supine position. The distal rectum is air filled.

SPOT FILM POSITIONS

Rectum

Views of the colon are named by describing the patient's position with respect to the fluoroscopic tabletop because in some fluoroscopes the x-ray tube is posterior to the tabletop and in other fluoroscopes the tube is anterior to the tabletop. The rectum is imaged early in the prone and lateral positions before the enema tip is removed. In the prone position the barium pool obscures the distal rectum and the enema tip. The distal rectum is visualized after the enema tip has been removed; spot films are obtained in the supine position (Fig. 11–5) with the distal rectum filled with air and in a lateral view of the rectum (Fig. 11–6) opposite to the one obtained previously with the enema tip in. Views of the distal rectum after tip removal are important because the distal rectum may be partially obscured by the enema tip (Fig. 11–7).

Rectosigmoid Junction

The rectosigmoid junction may be difficult to image because it is often obscured by overlapping sigmoid loops or filled with barium. The radiologist may try either a right side down lateral or a left side down lateral view to

slowly insufflated and the patient is turned in various positions to redistribute the air to the right colon. Depending on patient mobility, the patient is turned at least once 360 degrees to the left to coat the entire right colon. The patient may be repeatedly turned and placed in various positions to move the barium pool.

In general, spot films of the various segments of the colon are obtained in the following sequence: sigmoid colon, rectum, ascending colon, transverse colon, splenic and hepatic flexures, descending colon, and cecum, and erect views of the splenic and hepatic flexures and rectum.

Enema Tip Removal

Because the anorectal junction is an area of the colon that is sometimes difficult to view endoscopically, views of the anorectal junction with the tip out can be particularly useful.[16] Early enema tip removal will result in great physical and psychologic relief and allow better evaluation of the distal rectum.[16,17] Early removal of the enema tip is usually possible in young, healthy patients with good rectal tone. The enema tip may be left in place in patients who are expelling gas and in patients who may need additional air to visualize the terminal ileum (e.g., patients with Crohn's disease).

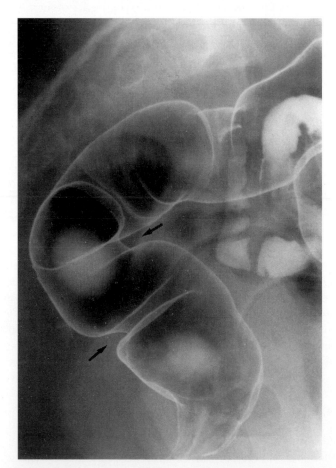

FIGURE 11–6. Spot radiograph of rectum with patient in left side down, lateral position, after enema tip is pulled. The valves of Houston are etched in white *(arrows).*

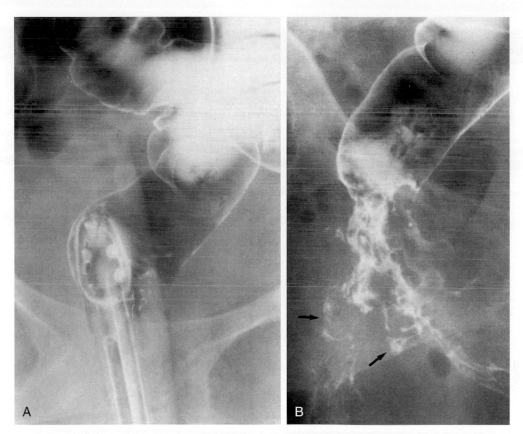

FIGURE 11–7. The value of enema tip removal. *A,* Spot radiograph of rectum before the enema tip has been removed. *B,* Spot radiograph after enema tip removal reveals that the distal rectum is diffusely narrowed, with a coarsely nodular mucosa. Numerous fissures and fistulous tracks *(arrows)* extend from the distal rectum and anal canal into the perirectal tissue and perineum. This patient had Crohn's disease.

demonstrate the rectosigmoid junction. The fluoroscopist should remember that the prone-angled overhead film of the sigmoid colon is tailored specifically to view the rectosigmoid junction. The prone-angled view may be the only image that shows a rectosigmoid junction mass.

Sigmoid Colon

The radiologist may have to use every trick of the trade to image the sigmoid colon, including compression, angulation of the overhead tube if in a remote-controlled room, and even prone compression. The distal sigmoid colon is often best imaged in the right or left posterior oblique (Fig. 11–8) or supine positions. The most inferior loop of the mid-sigmoid colon is often best air-filled in the prone (Fig. 11–9) or left side down lateral view. Placing the patient into a prone position and compressing with a balloon-tipped paddle may splay apart sigmoid loops (Fig. 11–10). The proximal sigmoid colon may be best imaged in the left posterior oblique position or even occasionally in the prone position.

Erect Views

Erect views are often helpful for imaging the hepatic and splenic flexures, the upper walls of the transverse colon, the upper portions of the ascending and descending colon, elevated loops of redundant sigmoid colon,

and even the rectum (Fig. 11–11). The radiologist carefully turns the patient into an erect position and watches for a vasovagal response. Early removal of the enema tip may prevent a vasovagal response. The fluoroscopic table and patient are slowly elevated to the erect position, stopping frequently to allow the patient to attain equilibrium. The radiologist makes sure that the patient's feet are flat against the platform of the fluoroscopic table. The radiologist may place his or her hand on the patient's shoulder to reassure the patient that they will not fall.

Splenic Flexure and Descending Colon

Views of the splenic flexure are obtained in the erect position with the patient turned so that the ascending and descending limbs of the splenic flexure are separated (Fig. 11–12A). Several views of the splenic flexure may be necessary. Lateral or recumbent oblique positions may be used (Fig. 11–12B). Women are instructed to manually elevate their left breast out of the radiation field, preventing radiation exposure to the breast and preventing the breast shadow from overlying the splenic flexure. Views of the proximal (upper) descending colon are often best obtained in the erect position (Fig. 11–13). The distal descending colon is often best imaged in the recumbent (Fig. 11–14) or semierect position and occasionally in the prone position.

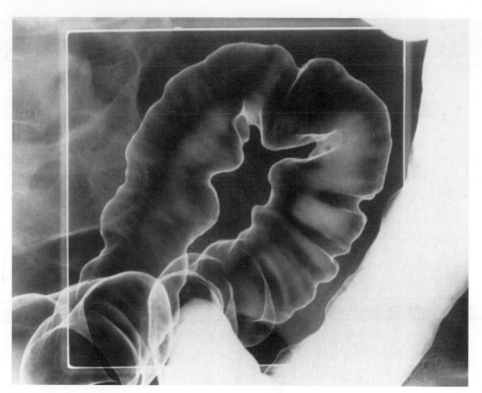

FIGURE 11–8. Distal sigmoid colon viewed with patient in left posterior oblique position, using compression.

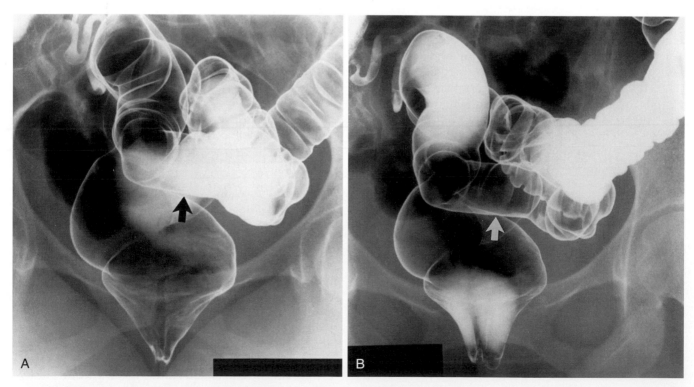

FIGURE 11–9. Value of the prone view of the sigmoid colon. *A,* Spot radiograph of rectum and sigmoid colon with the patient in the supine position shows barium filling the most dependent loop of the mid-sigmoid colon *(arrow). B,* When the patient is turned into the prone position, the mid-sigmoid colon is now seen in air contrast *(arrow).* This radiograph is displayed in the same anatomic position as in *A* to allow direct comparison of images. (Reproduced with permission from Rubesin, S.E., and Levine, M.S.: Principles of Performing a Double Contrast Barium Enema. Westbury, NY, E-Z-EM, Inc., 1998, pp. 1–33.)

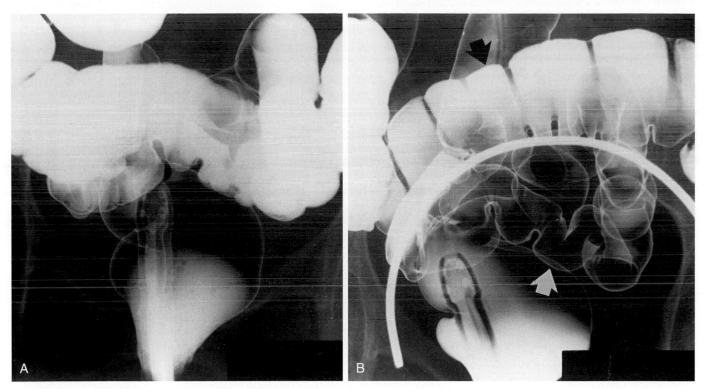

FIGURE 11–10. Value of compression. *A,* Spot radiograph of rectum with the patient in the prone position. The enema tip is placed too proximally. *B,* A compression balloon is placed underneath the patient in prone position. The transverse colon *(black arrow)* is pushed up, out of the pelvis. The mid-sigmoid colon *(white arrow)* is now visualized in air contrast. (Reproduced with permission from Rubesin, S.E., and Levine, M.S.: Principles of Performing a Double Contrast Barium Enema. Westbury, NY, E-Z-EM, Inc., 1998, pp. 1–33.)

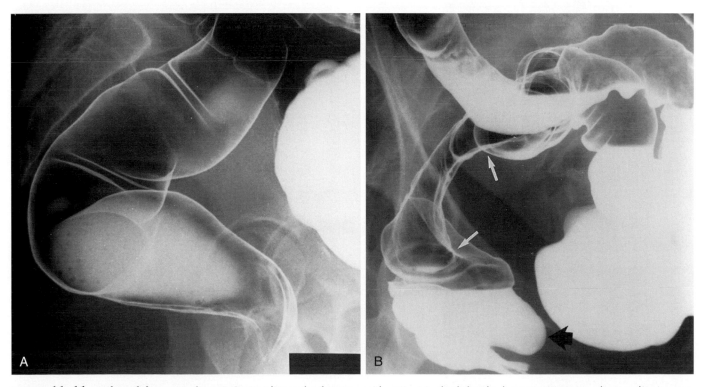

FIGURE 11–11. Value of the erect view. *A,* Spot radiograph of rectum with patient in the left side down position. No abnormality is seen. *B,* Spot radiograph of rectum with the patient standing in the erect, near-lateral position. Pelvic floor descent and a small anterior rectocele *(black arrow)* are present. An extrinsic mass effect upon the rectosigmoid junction *(white arrows)* is now demonstrated. This patient had an enlarged uterus filled with leiomyomata. (Reproduced with permission from Rubesin, S.E., and Levine, M.S.: Principles of Performing a Double Contrast Barium Enema. Westbury, NY, E-Z-EM, Inc., 1998, pp. 1–33.)

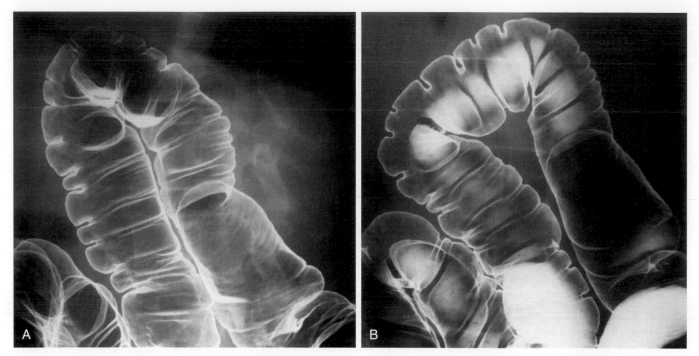

FIGURE 11–12. Splenic flexure. *A,* Spot radiograph of the splenic flexure with the patient in the erect, right posterior oblique position. The ascending and descending limbs of the splenic flexure are separated. *B,* Spot radiograph of the splenic flexure with the patient in the recumbent right posterior oblique position.

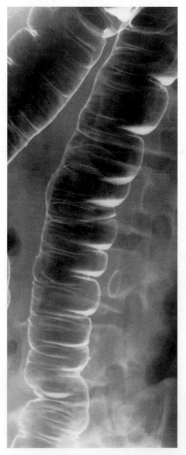

FIGURE 11–13. Spot radiograph of the proximal descending colon with the patient in the erect right posterior oblique position.

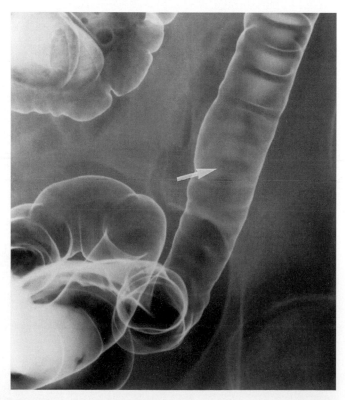

FIGURE 11–14. Spot radiograph of the distal descending colon *(arrow)* with the patient in the supine position.

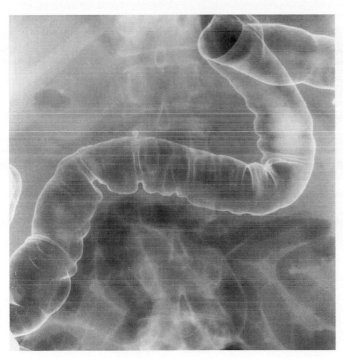

FIGURE 11–15. Spot radiograph of mid-transverse colon with patient in the supine position.

Mid-Transverse Colon

Both supine (Fig. 11–15) and erect (Fig. 11–16) views of the mid-transverse colon are valuable.

Hepatic Flexure

The hepatic flexure is often best seen in the erect left posterior oblique position (Fig. 11–17). Women are instructed to elevate their right breast out of the radiation field. Supine views may be of value, especially for the medial border of the proximal hepatic flexure.

Ascending Colon

If the medial wall of the ascending colon is not well coated, the patient is turned 360 degrees toward the left side down. Two-in-one vertically oriented spot films of the ascending colon are obtained, especially in the erect position (Fig. 11–18). The proximal ascending colon may be best distended with air in the prone or Trendelenburg left posterior oblique position.

Cecum

The cecum may be viewed in the supine, left posterior or right posterior oblique positions (Fig. 11–19). Compression is frequently used (Fig. 11–20). If too much barium is in the cecum, the patient may be rolled to the right in the Trendelenburg position, then quickly returned to the left. With this maneuver, barium will fall from the cecum into the ascending colon while air rises superiorly. If this maneuver fails, the patient may be rolled 360 degrees to the right in the Trendelenburg position. The radiologist should carefully evaluate the cecum in the prone position because the anterior wall of the cecum may be difficult to visualize en face in supine views. Therefore spot films of the cecum may include the left posterior oblique position for the lateral wall, the right posterior oblique position for the medial wall, and the prone position for the anterior wall.

Appendix and Terminal Ileum

Every effort should be made to fill the appendix (Fig. 11–21) in patients with right lower quadrant pain or the terminal ileum (Fig. 11–22) in patients with diarrhea.

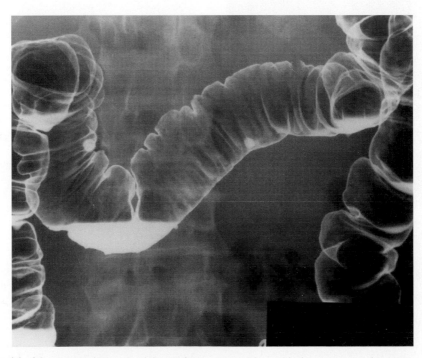

FIGURE 11–16. Spot radiograph of the mid-transverse colon with the patient in the erect position.

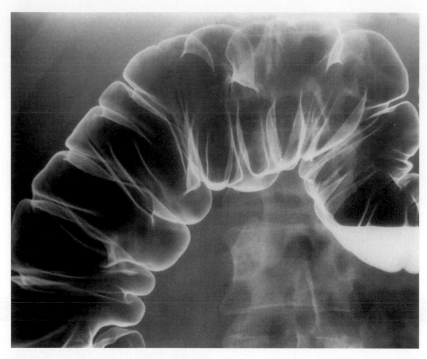

FIGURE 11–17. Spot radiograph of hepatic flexure with the patient in the erect position. (Reproduced with permission from Rubesin, S.E., and Levine, M.S.: Principles of Performing a Double Contrast Barium Enema. Westbury, NY, E-Z-EM, Inc., 1998, pp. 1–33.)

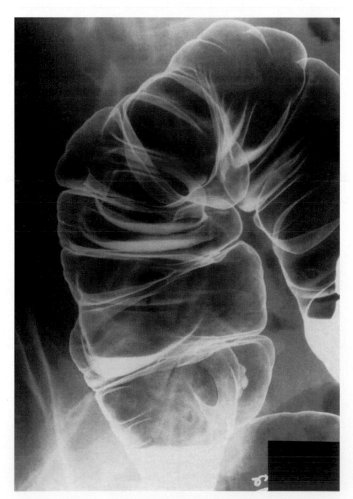

FIGURE 11–18. Spot radiograph of the ascending colon with the patient in the erect, left posterior oblique position.

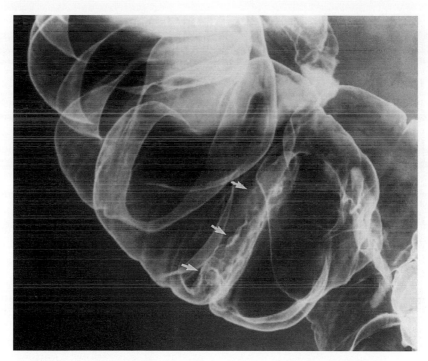

FIGURE 11–19. Spot radiograph of the cecum with the patient in the right posterior oblique position. A tubulovillous adenoma is manifested as lobulated lines along an interhaustral fold *(arrows)*.

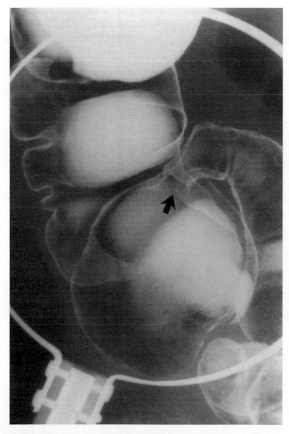

FIGURE 11–20. Spot radiograph of the cecum, using compression. The ileocecal valve is open *(arrow)*, and air refluxes into the normal terminal ileum.

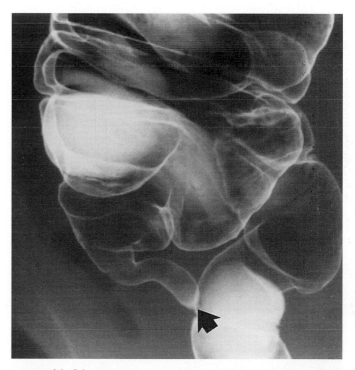

FIGURE 11–21. Spot radiograph of the cecum, appendix, and terminal ileum. The appendix is filled to its bulbous tip *(arrow)* and is therefore normal.

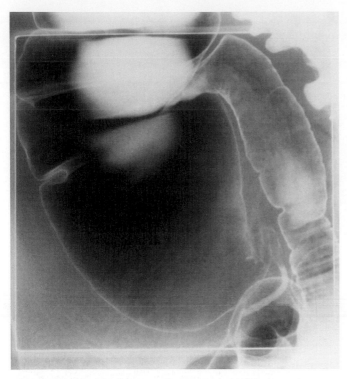

FIGURE 11–22. Spot radiograph of the terminal ileum and cecum.

These regions may be better filled with barium before complete gaseous distention of the right colon occurs, occluding the appendiceal orifice or the ileocecal valve. The radiologist may use compression to push barium into these areas, while the patient is placed in either the erect or recumbent left posterior oblique position. The terminal ileum may be best distended with air while the patient lies in a prone position, placing the ileocecal valve anteriorly, enabling air to rise into the terminal ileum.

OVERHEAD RADIOGRAPHS

The most important overheads are views that cannot be obtained with the standard fluoroscope: the left side down (Fig. 11–23) and the right side down (Fig. 11–24) decubitus views, and the prone-angled view of the rectosigmoid colon (Fig. 11–25). At our hospital, we add cross-table lateral views of the rectum (Fig. 11–26) and a prone view of the abdomen. Overhead films are not routinely obtained in the supine or the supine-oblique positions because the colon has been fluoroscopically evaluated in these positions. Limiting the number of overhead radiographs does not diminish the diagnostic accuracy provided that good spot films are obtained.[18] Postevacua-

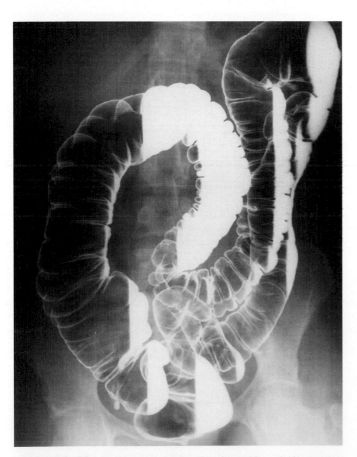

FIGURE 11–23. Cross-table overhead radiograph with the patient in the left side down decubitus position.

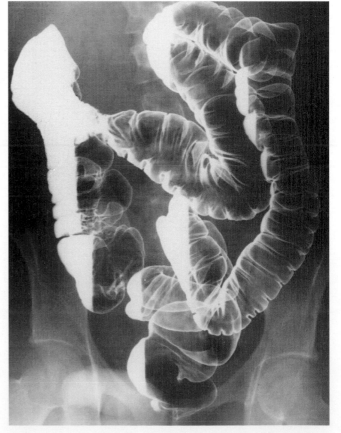

FIGURE 11–24. Cross-table overhead radiograph with the patient in the right side down decubitus position.

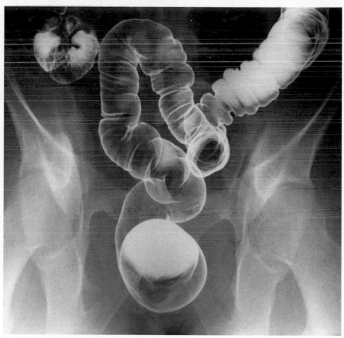

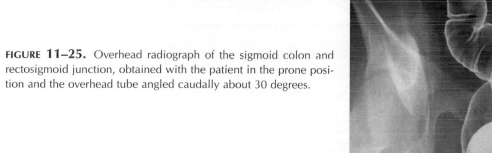

FIGURE 11–25. Overhead radiograph of the sigmoid colon and rectosigmoid junction, obtained with the patient in the prone position and the overhead tube angled caudally about 30 degrees.

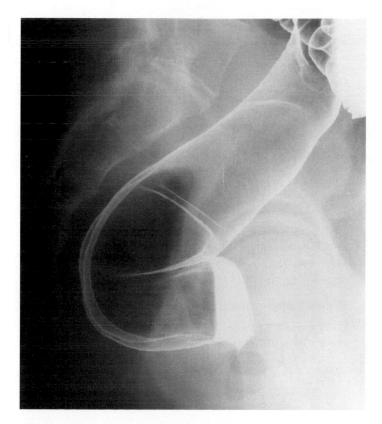

FIGURE 11–26. Cross-table lateral overhead radiograph of the rectum with the patient in the prone position.

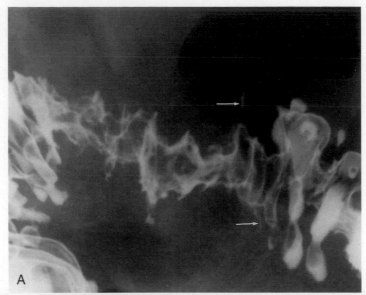

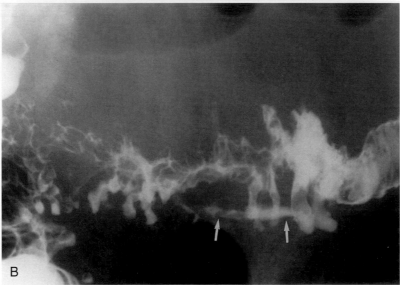

FIGURE 11–27. Value of postevacuation spot radiographs in evaluation of diverticulitis or fistulae. *A,* Spot radiograph of the sigmoid colon shows diffuse narrowing and deformed diverticula *(arrows). B,* A pericolic fistulous track *(arrows)* is demonstrated on a spot radiograph of the sigmoid colon obtained after the patient has evacuated. This confirms the preevacuation radiographic diagnosis of diverticulitis.

tion films are not included because these have little diagnostic value except to document appendiceal filling.[19] If it is important to fill the appendix or terminal ileum, postevacuation fluoroscopy is performed. Postevacuation fluoroscopic spot films are obtained in patients with suspected fistulas or extraluminal collections, especially associated with diverticulitis (Fig. 11–27).

VARIATIONS IN TECHNIQUE
Colostomy Study

A double contrast enema can be performed in patients with a colostomy (Fig. 11–28). Double contrast examination of the residual colon after colostomy may be

particularly important because of the increased incidence of metachronous carcinomas in patients with previous resection of colorectal carcinoma.[20]

Peroral Pneumocolon

A peroral pneumocolon examination is an air contrast study of the distal small bowel and right colon after a small bowel follow-through. The colon is cleansed with a barium enema–type preparation. A small bowel follow-through is performed in the usual fashion with barium sulfate, such as Enterobar (Lafayette Pharmacal, Lafayette, Ind.). After the terminal ileum and right colon are opacified with barium traversing to the mid-transverse colon, a small soft catheter is inserted in the rectum, and air is insufflated to obtain double contrast views (Fig. 11–29). If 1 mg

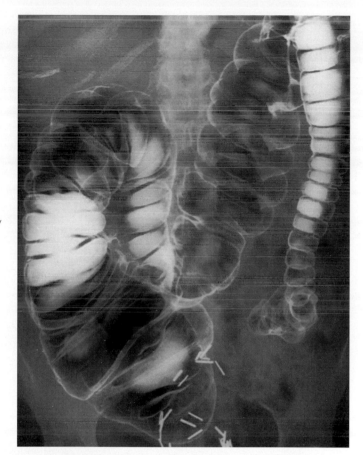

FIGURE 11–28. Overhead radiograph from double contrast colostomy enema.

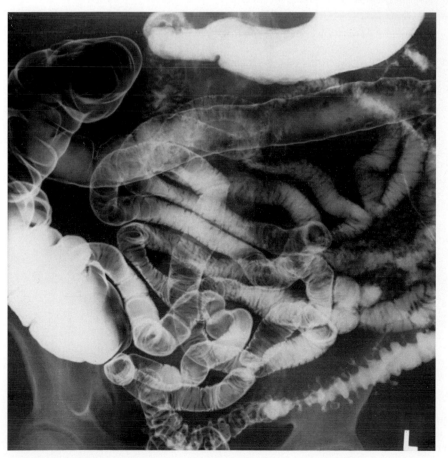

FIGURE 11–29. Overhead radiograph from peroral pneumocolon. The distal small intestine is demonstrated in air contrast.

glucagon is given intravenously, small bowel and colonic distention will improve and air will enter the terminal ileum. This examination is of value in patients with diarrhea and in patients in whom examination of the right colon has not been achieved because of retained fluid or feces or other technical reasons.

PITFALLS
Prior Endoscopy

There is continuing debate regarding the advisability of performing double contrast enemas immediately after sigmoidoscopy or colonoscopy. Prior endoscopy increases the amount of air in the colon.[21] This air makes the double contrast examination difficult, more uncomfortable, and results in less than optimal mucosal coating. Ideally, we prefer not to perform the barium enema immediately after endoscopy. However, as a matter of logistics and convenience for patients, barium enemas may be performed after endoscopic procedures. It is of critical importance, however, to ascertain whether a biopsy has been performed. Radiographic examination should not be performed immediately after sigmoidoscopic biopsy through a rigid sigmoidoscope or after a polypectomy. The barium enema should be performed at least 6 days after the mu-

cosa has been possibly breached by large forceps biopsy, cautery, or polypectomy.

Colonic Spasm

Colonic spasm may be either diffuse or focal, resulting in suboptimal visualization of a colonic loop or the entire colon. In most cases, colonic spasm is prevented or ameliorated by the use of intravenous glucagon or other hypotonic agents. Focal colonic spasm (Fig. 11–30) may prevent filling of the proximal colon or simulate an annular lesion. In most cases, focal colonic spasm responds to intravenous glucagon. In some patients, the colon may have to be refilled with single contrast barium to show that the focal colonic spasm changes and distends completely.[22]

Redundant Colon

The colon is of extremely variable length. Various portions of the colon (Fig. 11–31) or the entire colon (Fig. 11–32) may elongate. People with a diet containing nondigestible cellulose often have elongated colons. A redundant colon makes barium filling of the colon more difficult. It may be difficult to titrate the amount of barium needed to coat a redundant colon or to fill the right colon with barium. Overlapping, redundant loops may obscure lesions.

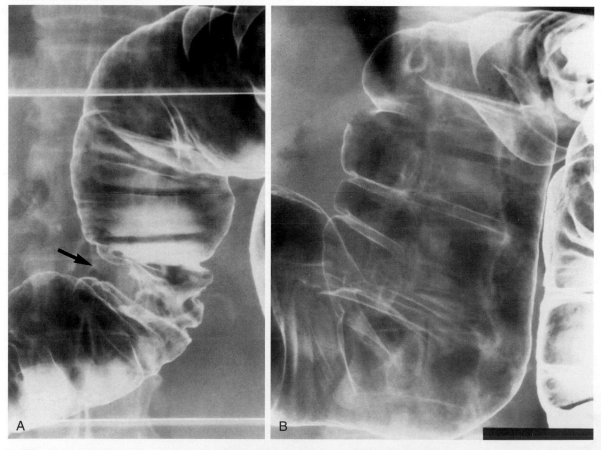

FIGURE 11–30. Focal colonic spasm. *A,* Spot radiograph of the distal transverse colon shows a focal, asymmetric area of narrowing *(arrow)* with preservation of mucosal folds. This area of spasm is known as a Cannon's point. *B,* Spot radiograph of the distal transverse colon obtained several minutes later demonstrates that the spasm has disappeared.

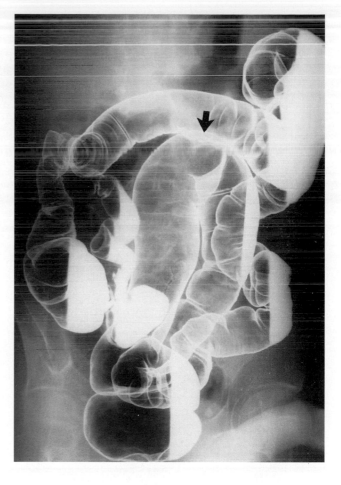

FIGURE 11–31. A redundant sigmoid colon is elevated superiorly out of the pelvis.

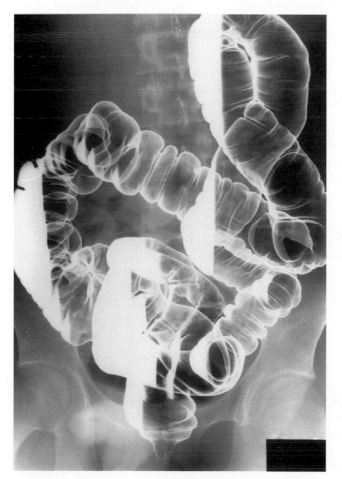

FIGURE 11–32. The transverse, descending, and sigmoid colon are redundant.

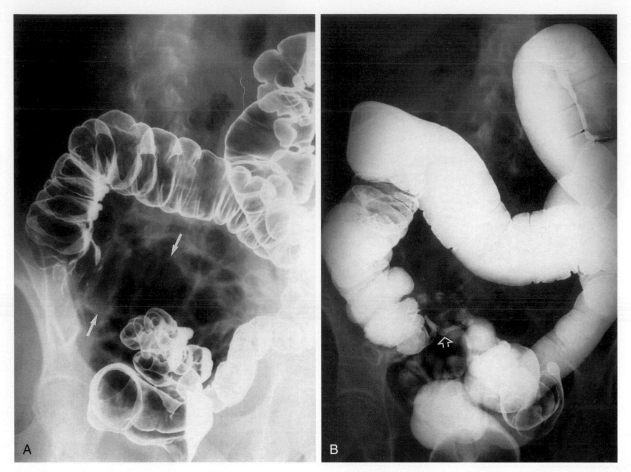

FIGURE 11–33. Incomplete visualization of right colon. *A,* Left side down decubitus view. An air-filled structure with interhaustral folds *(arrows)* demonstrates lack of barium filling of the right colon. Either the appendix, ileocecal valve, or terminal ileum must be demonstrated to prove that the right colon has been completely visualized. *B,* A single contrast barium enema performed immediately after *A* now demonstrates the entire right colon, appendix *(arrow),* and a part of the terminal ileum.

Nonfilling of the Right Colon

The right colon may not fill if an inadequate volume of high-density barium has been instilled into the transverse colon. If attempts to fill the right colon fail, we obtain radiographs of the coated and distended portions of the colon and hope that postevacuation films demonstrate filling of the right colon. In some patients the right colon may be filled by repeating the study using single contrast barium technique (Fig. 11–33) or single contrast barium may be used to push the high-density barium into the right colon.[23]

COMPLICATIONS
Gas Pains

Residual air within the colon after barium enema may result in abdominal pain. Up to 50% of patients will complain of discomfort and abdominal pain after double contrast barium enema.[24] To reduce the incidence of postbarium enema pain, some radiologists use carbon dioxide for gaseous distention instead of room air. Carbon dioxide is readily absorbed from the gastrointestinal tract and, therefore, produces less colonic distention after the examination. We have had difficulty distending the colon adequately during barium enema using carbon dioxide, however.

Perforation

The most serious complication of barium enema, either single or double contrast, is perforation.[25] There is no evidence that double contrast enemas have higher complication rates than single contrast studies. Similar intracolonic pressures are generated by both types of examinations.[26] Intraperitoneal rupture of the colon is almost always due to an underlying pathologic process that weakens the bowel wall. Intraperitoneal rupture is recognized fluoroscopically by barium outlining the external surfaces of bowel or barium flowing into the pericolic gutters (Fig. 11–34). Pneumoperitoneum, pneumoretroperitoneum, and even pneumomediastinum without barium extravasation has been reported with double contrast barium enema.[27,28] Extraluminal accumulation of air without perforation is more likely to occur in the presence of diverticulosis and surgery may not be necessary.

Rectal perforation or laceration results in extravasation of barium into the wall of the rectum, perirectal, or retroperitoneal tissues. Rectal laceration almost exclusively occurs when the retention balloon is inflated in patients with rectal pathology. Therefore, it is important to avoid insufflation of enema tip balloons in patients who have had a deep rectal biopsy, radiation proctitis, or other forms of proctitis. When rectal perforation occurs, streaks of barium are seen in the wall of the rectum or linear strands of barium are seen in the retroperitoneal tissue. Rarely, barium may enter the venous system and embolize to the liver or lungs.[14]

If air enters the bowel wall because of traumatic laceration or inflammatory or ischemic disease, air may gain access to the venous system and may enter the portal vein.[29,30]

Other complications related to various aspects of the double contrast enema are rare. Allergic reactions to barium or glucagon or the preparation have been reported.[31–33] Patients may undergo myocardial ischemia or infarction during the performance of a barium enema.[34]

Allergic reactions such as fatal anaphylaxis to the latex content of the retention balloon on enema tips or to la-

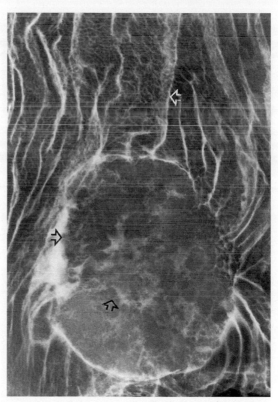

FIGURE 11–35. Innominate grooves. A radiograph of a barium-coated specimen shows the normal innominate groove pattern (representative area identified by *white arrow*) manifested as barium-filled clefts surrounding relatively uniform flat islands of mucosa similar to the areae gastricae of the stomach. In contrast, in the adjacent mucosa the surface pattern of a tubulovillous adenoma shows mucosal nodules of varying size (representative areas identified by *black arrows*). (Reproduced with permission from Rubesin, S.E., Furth, E.E., Rose, D., et al.: The effects of distention of the colon during air-contrast barium enema on colonic morphology: Anatomic correlation. AJR Am. J. Roentgenol. *164*:1387–1389, 1995. © American Roentgen Ray Society.)

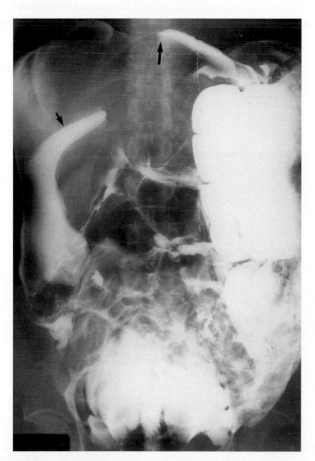

FIGURE 11–34. Perforation during barium enema. Overhead radiograph demonstrates barium in the peritoneal space, including filling of Morrison's pouch (hepatorenal fossa) *(short arrow)* and the coating of the cupola of the diaphragm *(long arrow)*.

tex exposure during digital examination have been reported. Retention balloons made of silicon rubber are now available.[14]

There is considerable debate about the need for antibiotic prophylaxis in certain patients undergoing barium enema. Evidence is conflicting regarding the occurrence of bacteremia in association with barium enema.[35,36] Endocarditis or septicemia as a complication of barium enema is rare. Therefore routine antibiotic prophylaxis is not recommended, except in patients with susceptible cardiac lesions who have a history of endocarditis or a prosthetic valve.

NORMAL APPEARANCES
Surface Pattern

The colonic mucosa is divided into a series of tufts separated by a network of grooves (Fig. 11–35), analogous to the areae gastricae of the stomach. These grooves

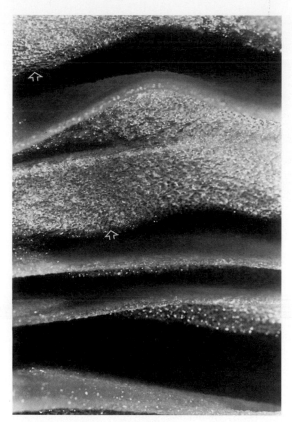

FIGURE 11–36. Innominate grooves. A photograph of a barium-coated specimen shows barium filling the innominate grooves (representative areas identified with *arrows*). (Reproduced with permission from Rubesin, S.E., Furth, E.E., Rose, D., et al.: The effects of distention of the colon during air-contrast barium enema on colonic morphology: Anatomic correlation. AJR Am. J. Roentgenol. *164:* 1387–1389, 1995. © American Roentgen Ray Society.)

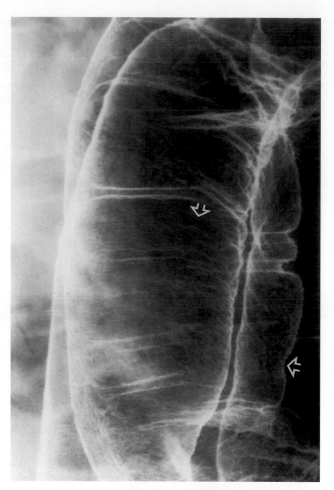

FIGURE 11–37. Innominate grooves *(arrows)* are seen during air-contrast barium enema.

are termed the innominate lines or innominate grooves (Fig. 11–36). The grooves are seen in up to 90% of double contrast barium enemas, when using a barium preparation of relatively low weight/volume and low viscosity (67% w/v) in contrast to the higher weight/volume and higher viscosity of standard American double contrast barium enema suspensions (100% w/v).[37,38] Only rarely are innominate grooves demonstrated with standard American double contrast suspensions, usually when the colon is collapsed. The distended colonic surface is usually smooth and featureless during double contrast barium enema. If demonstrated during double contrast barium enema, however, the innominate grooves appear as barium-etched lines arranged in a linear or reticular pattern (Figs. 11–37 and 11–38). Innominate grooves were originally described on single contrast barium studies as tiny V-shaped projections extending beyond the luminal contour called pseudoulcerations.[38,39]

Visualization of the innominate grooves in the normal colon is related primarily to the degree of colonic distention (Fig. 11–39) as well as to the density and viscosity of the barium suspension.[40] When colonic mucosa is stretched, a flat featureless surface is seen (Fig. 11–39A).

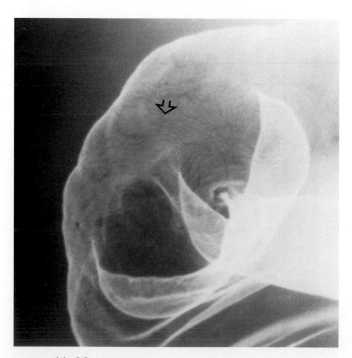

FIGURE 11–38. Innominate grooves *(arrow)* are seen in the hepatic flexure.

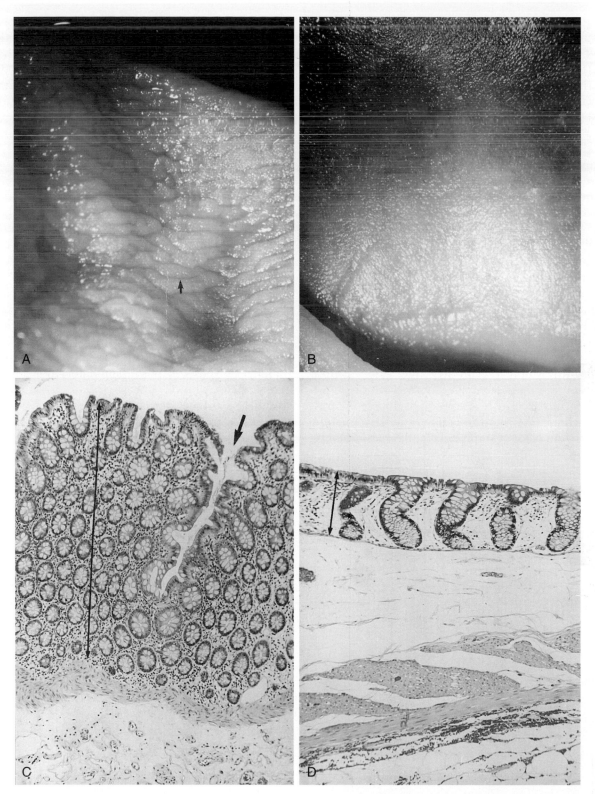

FIGURE 11–39. Appearance and disappearance of innominate grooves with varying degrees of colonic distention. *A,* Dissecting photomicrograph while the colon is in a contracted, unstretched state shows the innominate grooves surrounding tufts of mucosa (representative groove identified by *arrow*). *B,* Photograph of stretched colon at the same magnification as in *A* shows relatively smooth colonic mucosa. *C,* Low-power photomicrograph of unstretched colonic mucosa demonstrates a cleft *(arrow)* lined by surface epithelial cells and goblet cells, representing the pathologic correlate of the innominate groove. Note the thickness of the epithelial layer *(double arrow).* *D,* Photomicrograph of stretched colonic mucosa obtained at the same magnification as in *C* shows loss of colonic clefts, thinning of the epithelial layer *(double arrow),* and separation of crypts. (Reproduced with permission from Rubesin, S.E., Furth, E.E., Rose, D., et al.: The effects of distention of the colon during air-contrast barium enema on colonic morphology: Anatomic correlation. AJR Am. J. Roentgenol. *164*:1387–1389, 1995. © American Roentgen Ray Society.)

When the colon spontaneously contracts, the innominate grooves appear, creating a finely nodular surface (Fig. 11–39*B*). The innominate grooves represent clefts in the mucosa (Fig. 11–39*C*), which disappear with colonic distention (Fig. 11–39*D*). The clefts are created by redundancy in the colonic epithelial layer present in the contracted state.

Transverse Folds

The innominate grooves should not be confused with transverse folds that are tightly spaced circular folds (Figs. 11–40 and 11–41) seen as a transient phenomenon in contracted colon.

Lymph Follicles

Gastrointestinal-associated lymphoid tissue is present in the colon and in the small intestine. Lymphoid hyperplasia is particularly frequent in children, appearing radiographically as multiple, 1- to 2-mm smooth-surfaced hemispheric projections above the colonic surface (Fig. 11–42). Lymph follicles may represent a response to infection, allergy, or immunologic-deficient states.[41–45] In some cases the lymph follicles are larger and a central umbilication may be present. The normal lymphoid follicular pattern is seen in 13% to 63% of double contrast barium enemas.[44,45] Lymph follicles are most commonly seen in the right colon. Lymph follicles have also been reported in patients with lymphoma, Crohn's disease, polyposis syndromes, and in association with colonic carcinoma.[46,47] Lymphoid follicular hyperplasia may be associated with colonic carcinoma, both focally or diffusely. Whenever lymphoid follicles are seen diffusely throughout the colon in a patient older than 60, a careful search should be made for underlying colonic neoplasm.

ARTIFACTS

Although it is generally considered that a meticulously clean colon is a prerequisite for performing double contrast enema, double contrast technique is even more valuable in patients whose colon is imperfectly prepared.[48] Solid fecal material and other extraneous material can frequently be definitively diagnosed by virtue of their mobility on horizontal beam films. Although solid fecal material is usually easily differentiated from polyps, sometimes solid feces may mimic polyps. Smaller fecal residue and debris may adhere to the colonic mucosa and produce an appearance indistinguishable from that seen in familial polyposis or postinflammatory polyposis due to inflammatory bowel disease. Thick tenacious mucus strands occasionally form relatively solid polypoid masses. Strands of mucus may mimic a polyp (Fig. 11–43), the stalk of a polyp, or filiform polyps.

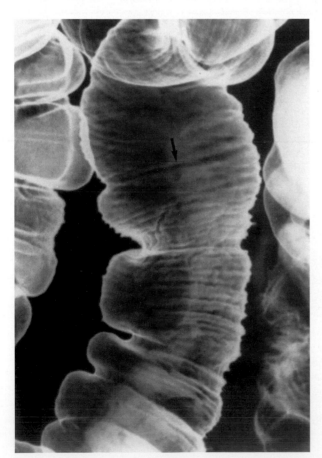

FIGURE 11–40. Thin, transverse folds cross the lumen of the mildly contracted colon. (Representative fold identified by *arrow*).

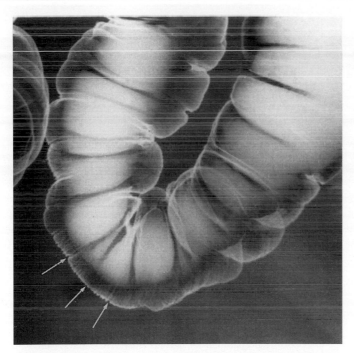

FIGURE 11–41. Thin, transverse folds are only seen in the portion of transverse colon that is contracted. Representative folds are identified by *arrows*.

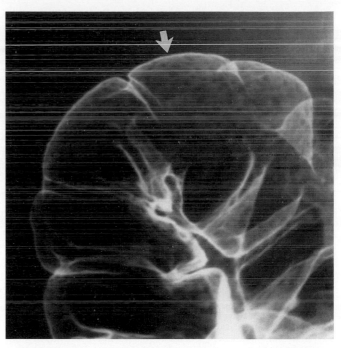

FIGURE 11–42. Numerous lymph follicles are seen in the hepatic flexure as 1- to 2-mm smooth-surfaced round to ovoid radiolucencies.

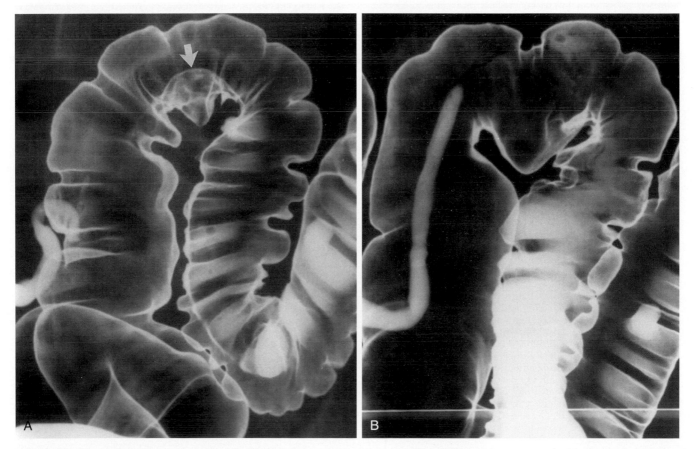

FIGURE 11–43. Conglomerate of mucus mimicking polyp. *A*, A barium-etched mound *(arrow)* projects intraluminally, mimicking a polyp in the mid-sigmoid colon. *B*, After further turning of the patient and manual compression, the mound of mucus disappears. A polyp was not seen during flexible sigmoidoscopy performed before this examination.

Objects seen through the air-filled colon may produce polypoid appearances on the double contrast enema. Shadows from the greater trochanter projected over the rectum, hemorrhoids, an inverted appendiceal stump, the tip of the appendix projected over the rectosigmoid, renal calculi, phleboliths, and calcified lymph nodes may produce confusing shadows that overlap the colon. Reference to a preliminary film and careful roentgen interpretation avoids potential errors.

REFERENCES

1. Rice, R.P.: Lowering death rates from colorectal cancer: Challenge for the 1990's. Radiology 176:297, 1990.
2. Rubesin, S.E., and Levine, M.S.: Principles of Performing a Double Contrast Barium Enema. Westbury, NY, E-Z-EM, Inc., 1998, p. 1.
3. Maglinte, D.D.T., Strong, R.C., Strate, R.W., et al.: Barium enema after colorectal biopsies: Experimental data. AJR Am. J. Roentgenol. 139:693, 1982.
4. Harned, R.K., Consigny, P.M., and Cooper, N.B.: Barium enema examination following biopsy of the rectum or colon. Radiology 145:11, 1982.
5. Gelfand, D.W., Chen, Y.M., and Ott, D.J.: Colonic cleansing for radiographic detection of neoplasia: Efficacy of the magnesium citrate-castor oil-cleansing enema regimen. AJR Am. J. Roentgenol. 151:705, 1988.
6. Gelfand, D.W., Chen, Y.M., and Ott, D.J.: Preparing the colon for the barium enema examination. Radiology 178:609, 1991.
7. Dodds, W.J., Scanlon, G.T., Shaw, D.K., et al.: An evaluation of colon cleansing regimens. AJR Am. J. Roentgenol. 128:57, 1977.
8. Chan, C.H., Diner, W.C., Fontenot, E., et al.: Randomized single-blind clinical trial of a rapid colonic lavage solution (Golytely) vs. standard preparation for barium enema and colonoscopy. Gastrointest. Radiol. 10:378, 1985.
9. Bakran, A., Bradley, J.A., Bresnihan, E., et al.: Whole gut irrigation: An inadequate preparation for double contrast barium enema examination. Gastroenterology 73:28, 1977.
10. Miller, R.E., Chernish, S.M., Skucas, J., et al.: Hypotonic colon examination with glucagon. Radiology 113:555, 1974.
11. Gohel, V.K., Dalinka, M.K., and Goren, G.S.: Hypotonic examination of the colon with glucagon. Radiology 115:1, 1975.
12. Lee, J.R.: Routine use of hyoscine N butylbromide (Buscopan) in double contrast barium enema examinations. Clin. Radiol. 33:273, 1982.
13. Eisenberg, R.L., and Hedgcock, M.W.: Preliminary radiograph for barium enema examination: Is it necessary? AJR Am. J. Roentgenol. 136:115, 1981.
14. Gelfand, D.W.: Barium enemas, latex balloons and anaphylactic reactions. AJR Am. J. Roentgenol. 156:1, 1991.
15. Dodds, W.J., Stewart, E.T., and Nelson, J.A.: Rectal balloon catheters and the barium enema examination. Gastrointest. Radiol. 5:227, 1989.
16. Kahn, S., Rubesin, S.E., Levine, M.S., et al.: Polypoid lesions at the anorectal junction: Barium enema findings. AJR Am. J. Roentgenol. 161:339, 1993.
17. Maglinte, D.D.T., Miller, R.E., Chernish, S.M., et al.: Early rectal tube removal for improved patient tolerance during double contrast barium enema examination. Radiology 155:525, 1985.
18. Feczko, P.J., and Halpert, R.D.: Limiting overhead views in double-contrast colon examinations does not affect diagnostic accuracy. Gastrointest. Radiol. 12:175, 1987.
19. Smith, C., and Gardiner, R.: Efficacy of postevacuation view after double-contrast enema. Gastrointest. Radiol. 12:268, 1987.
20. de Roos, A., Hermans, J., and Op den Orth, J.O.: Polypoid lesions of the sigmoid colon: A comparison of single-contrast, double-contrast, and biphasic examinations. Radiology 151:597, 1984.
21. Rodney, W.M., Randolph, J.F., and Peterson, D.W.: Cancellation rates and gas scores for air contrast barium enema immediately after 65-CM flexible sigmoidoscopy: A randomized clinical trial. J. Clin. Gastroenterol. 10:311, 1988.
22. Levine, M.S., and Gasparaitis, A.E.: Barium filling for glucagon-resistant spasm on double-contrast barium enema examinations. Radiology 160:264, 1986.
23. Maglinte, D.D.T., and Miller, R.E.: Salvaging the failed pneumocolon: A simple maneuver. AJR Am. J. Roentgenol. 142:719, 1984.
24. Coblentz, C.L., Frost, R.A., Molinaro, V., et al.: Pain after barium enema: Effect of CO_2 and air on double-contrast study. Radiology 157:35, 1985.
25. Gelfand, D.W.: Complications of gastrointestinal radiologic procedures: I. Complications of routine fluoroscopic studies. Gastrointest. Radiol. 5:293, 1980.
26. Diner, W.C., Patel, G., Texter, E.C., Jr., et al.: Intraluminal pressure measurements during barium enema: Full column vs. air contrast. AJR Am. J. Roentgenol. 137:217, 1981.
27. Gelfand, D.W., Ott, D.J., and Ramquist, N.A.: Pneumoperitoneum occurring during double-contrast enema. Gastrointest. Radiol. 4:307, 1979.
28. Beerman, P.J., Gelfand, D.W., and Ott, D.J.: Pneumomediastinum after double-contrast barium enema examination: A sign of colonic perforation. AJR Am. J. Roentgenol. 136:197, 1981.
29. Stein, M.G., Crues, J.V.I., and Hamlin, J.A.: Portal venous air associated with barium enema. AJR Am. J. Roentgenol. 140:1171, 1983.
30. Kees, C.J., and Hester, C.L.: Portal vein gas following barium enema examination. Radiology 102:525, 1972.
31. Galloway, D., Burns, H.J.G., Moffat, L.E.F., et al.: Faecal peritonitis after laxative preparation for barium enema. Br. Med. J. Clin. Res. Ed. 284:472, 1982.
32. Zeligman, B.E., Feinberg, L.E., and Johnson, E.D.: A complication of cleansing enema: Retained protective shield of the enema tip. Gastrointest. Radiol. 11:372, 1986.
33. Schwartz, E.E., Glick, S.N., Foggs, M.B., et al.: Hypersensitivity reactions after barium enema examination. AJR Am. J. Roentgenol. 143:103, 1984.
34. Smith, H.J.: Performance of barium examinations after acute myocardial infarction: report of a survey. AJR Am. J. Roentgenol. 149:63, 1987.
35. Butt, J., Hentges, D., Pelican, G., et al.: Bacteremia during barium enema study. AJR Am. J. Roentgenol. 130:715, 1978.
36. Schimmel, D.H., Hanelin, L.G., Cohen, S., et al.: Bacteremia and the barium enema. AJR Am. J. Roentgenol. 128:207, 1977.
37. Matsuura, K., Nakata, H., Takeda, N., et al.: Innominate lines of the colon. Radiology 123:581, 1977.
38. Williams, I.: Innominate grooves in the surface of the mucosa. Radiology 84:877, 1965.
39. Frank, D.F., Berk, R.N., and Goldstein, H.M.: Pseudoulcerations of the colon on barium enema examination. Gastrointest. Radiol. 2:129, 1977.
40. Rubesin, S.E., Furth, E.E., Rose, D., et al.: Pictorial essay. The effects of distention on colonic morphology: Barium radiography and anatomic correlation. AJR Am. J. Roentgenol. 164:1387, 1995.
41. Dukes, C., and Bussey, H.J.R.: The number of lymphoid follicles of the human large intestine. J. Pathol. Bacteriol. 29:111, 1926.
42. Laufer, I., and deSa, D.: The lymphoid follicular pattern: A normal feature of the pediatric colon. AJR Am. J. Roentgenol. 130:51, 1978.
43. Riddlesberger, M.M.J., and Lebenthal, E.: Nodular colonic mucosa of childhood: Normal or pathologic? Gastroenterology 79:265, 1980.
44. Kelvin, F.M., Max, R.J., Norton, G.A., et al.: Lymphoid follicular pattern of the colon in adults. AJR Am. J. Roentgenol. 133:821, 1979.
45. Watanabe, H., Margulis, A.R., and Harter, L.: The occurrence of lymphoid nodules in the colon of adults. J. Clin. Gastroenterol. 5:535, 1983.
46. Glick, S.N., Teplick, S.K., and Goren, R.A.: Small colonic nodularity and the double contrast barium enema. RadioGraphics 1:73, 1981.
47. Bronen, R.A., Glick, S.N., and Teplick, S.K.: Diffuse lymphoid follicles of the colon associated with colonic carcinoma. AJR Am. J. Roentgenol. 142:105, 1984.
48. Laufer, I.: The double contrast enema: Myths and misconceptions. Gastrointest. Radiol. 1:19, 1976.

12

Tumors of the Colon

STEPHEN E. RUBESIN
IGOR LAUFER

ADENOMAS AND ADENOCARCINOMA

Epidemiology

Colonic carcinoma is a major medical problem in industrialized nations. For example, in the United States, 134,000 new cases of colonic cancer are diagnosed each year.[1] Approximately 3% of all deaths in the United States (55,000 people) can be attributed to colonic cancer.[1] The lifetime risk of developing colonic cancer in the United States varies from 3% to 6.7%.[2,3] Even more sobering is that the incidence of colonic cancer is increasing.

Risk Factors

There is a wide variety of risk factors for the development of colonic carcinoma. The complex interaction of environmental and host factors is not understood. At the extreme end of the host factors is a subgroup of people with genetic disposition to colonic cancer. For example, colonic cancer will develop in nearly 100% of those patients with the autosomal-dominantly transmitted familial adenomatous polyposis syndrome (FAPS).[4] Patients with FAPS represent the extreme end of the adenoma to carcinoma sequence, with adenomas developing by an average age of 18 years and cancers developing by an average age of 39 years.[4,5] The mutated adenomatous polyposis gene (APC) is on chromosome 5q21.[4]

Another autosomal-dominantly transmitted form of colonic carcinoma is the hereditary nonpolyposis colorectal cancer syndrome (HNPCCS) or Lynch syndrome, which may account for 5% of colonic cancers.[6–8] In patients with the Lynch syndrome, colonic carcinomas develop at an earlier age. The colonic cancers are located in the right colon in 65% to 90% of patients,[7] a far greater right-sided cancer predominance than normally seen. Multiple primary colonic carcinomas are found in about 20% of patients with the Lynch syndrome compared with the usual 5% synchronous rate. Many patients have increased incidence of various other primary cancers, especially endometrial cancers in women.

At the lower end of the genetic predisposition to colonic cancer is a general familial risk. There is a threefold risk of colonic cancer developing in an individual if there is a history of colonic cancer in a first-degree relative.[9]

The impact of environmental factors in the development of colonic cancer is strong, although unknown. There is a wide geographic variation in the incidence of colonic cancer. People in industrialized nations of North America, Western Europe, and Australia are at greatest risk. People in industrialized Japan are at less risk. Populations that migrate from areas of low colon cancer incidence to areas of high colon cancer incidence develop increased risk for colonic carcinoma.

The complex role of diet in the development of colon cancer is also unknown. Patients with a high alcohol intake have a two to three times higher risk for development of adenomas.[10,11] Patients whose diet is high in beef, pork, or lamb fat have an increased incidence of colonic cancer.[12] With increased dietary fat, the colon is exposed to increased bile acids, which results in increased colonic epithelial cell proliferation.[12,13] The role of lack of dietary fiber in development of colonic carcinoma is unknown.

People with chronic inflammatory processes in the colon such as ulcerative colitis or schistosomiasis japonicum also have an increased incidence of colonic carcinoma.[14] The greater the extent or duration of inflammation in ulcerative colitis, the greater the risk for colonic cancer.[15] There is also an increased risk of colonic cancer in women who have been irradiated for pelvic malignancy.[16]

Most colonic adenocarcinomas arise in adenomatous polyps. At least 30% to 40% of people have adenomatous polyps at autopsy.[17,18] Although colonic cancer does not develop in most people with adenomas, those patients with adenomas greater than 1 cm are at a threefold greater risk for carcinoma.[19]

Screening for Colonic Cancer

Screening for colonic cancer is a controversial area that this chapter will only briefly visit. When patients undergo screening, cancers are found in 1 to 450 to 1000 patients.[20,21] Cancers are detected at an earlier stage with screening. Numerous precursor adenomas are also found.

Fecal Occult Blood Tests

Fecal occult blood tests (FOBTs) have frequently been used to screen for colorectal cancer because of their relatively low cost and noninvasive nature. There is conflicting evidence that FOBT screening lowers colorectal can-

cer mortality.[22–24] Most colorectal cancer bleeding arises in nonneoplastic sources.[25,26] Most cancers in asymptomatic patients and 95% of adenomas do not bleed because they do not ulcerate, so they are not detected by FOBT. Therefore the sensitivity and specificity of FOBT for colorectal neoplasia is low.

Endoscopy

There is clear evidence that screening by flexible sigmoidoscopy reduces colorectal cancer mortality.[22,27,28] In contrast to FOBT, flexible sigmoidoscopy detects early cancers and precursor adenomas. Screening for colorectal cancer by flexible sigmoidoscopy, however, is flawed because flexible sigmoidoscopy looks at only one half of the colon. About 40% to 50% of colonic cancers are located in the cecum, ascending colon, and transverse colon, areas that are not visualized by the flexible sigmoidoscope.[29] If synchronous rectosigmoid polyps are found at flexible sigmoidoscopy, a full colon examination may be performed. The problem with relying on the detection of polyps in the sigmoid colon as a marker for cancer in the right colon is that most right-sided colonic cancers are not associated with synchronous rectosigmoid polyps.[30,31]

Barium Enema

It is common sense that the entire colon should be examined if colorectal cancer screening is to be successful. This common sense belief that the entire colon should be screened has been confirmed by mathematical models. Eddy has shown that barium enema is the most cost-effective strategy for the detection of colorectal cancer when compared with FOBT, flexible sigmoidoscopy, or colonoscopy either alone or in combination.[32,33] Barium enemas have certain advantages and disadvantages compared with colonoscopy. Barium enemas are much safer than colonoscopy. The risk of perforation of barium enema is less than 1 in 10,000, whereas the risk of perforation at colonoscopy is approximately 1 in 1000. The risk of severe hemorrhage during colonoscopy is approximately 1 in 300. The mortality rate of colonoscopy is approximately 1 to 3 in 10,000. At colonoscopy, lesions can be biopsied and removed. Early detection and treatment of colonic adenomas by colonoscopy has proven to reduce the colorectal cancer incidence and mortality.[34] A case control study has never been attempted to show that barium enema reduces the incidence of morbidity and mortality due to colonic cancer.

Double contrast barium enema looks at the entire colon in almost all patients, whereas colonoscopy incompletely examines the colon in about 10% to 15% of patients.[35] Colonoscopy is far more sensitive than barium enema for detection of diminutive polyps less than 5 mm. Colonoscopy is also more sensitive than double contrast barium enema for polyps in the 5 to 10 mm range. Double contrast barium enema detects 50% to 90% of polyps 5 to 10 mm, whereas colonoscopy detects 85% to 95% of polyps 5 to 10 mm. Double contrast barium enema and colonoscopy are comparable for detection of polyps greater than 1 cm and for detection of colonic carcinoma. At our institution, in a study from 1991 using barium inferior to the barium we use today, barium enema was slightly better than colonoscopy at detecting colonic cancer. In our study of primarily symptomatic or bleeding patients, the smallest tumor was 1.5 cm. The principle to remember is that most colonic cancers are large, greater than 2 cm, and are easily detected by double contrast barium enema. The second principle is that most adenomas grow slowly. For example, in the extreme case of patients with FAPS, the average time from the appearance of adenomas to the development of colonic cancer is 23 years.[36]

The American Gastroenterological Association (AGA) has concluded that barium enema is an effective screening strategy for average risk patients and for patients with first-degree relatives with a history of polyps or colonic cancer. The AGA also concluded that colonoscopy should be performed in patients with FAPS, HNPCCS, and inflammatory bowel disease.[37]

Adenomas: Pathology

Adenomas of the colon are subdivided into three categories: tubular adenomas, tubulovillous adenomas, and villous adenomas, a classification based on the relationship of the proliferating epithelium to the stroma.[38] Tubular adenomas are composed of branching tubules embedded in lamina propria (Fig. 12–1).[39] Villous adenomas are composed of frondlike structures covered by adenomatous epithelium (Fig. 12–2). Tubulovillous adenomas have a mixture of tubular and villous elements.[38] A continuous spectrum between pure tubular and pure villous architecture is present. A villous component is seen in 35% to 75% of all adenomas larger than 1 cm.[40,41]

Despite macroscopic architectural differences, all adenomatous polyps are expressions of the same neoplastic process. Whether an adenoma is classified as a tubular adenoma, tubulovillous adenoma, or villous adenoma, the cytologic features are similar (Fig. 12–3). A villous component increases the risk of invasive cancer for the same size lesion. However, the major risk for malignant potential of adenomas is their size (Table 12–1). The larger the adenoma, the greater the chance of malignancy.[38,42]

Macroscopically, adenomas may be pedunculated (see Fig. 12–1), semisessile, or sessile. Rare flat adenomas will crawl along the surface of the colon (Fig. 12–4). Approximately 20% of patients have multiple synchronous adenomas.[43]

Most patients with adenomatous polyps are asymptomatic. Villous tumors are more likely to bleed because they more frequently ulcerate, are a larger size, and have an increased incidence of coexisting carcinoma. Only rarely do villous adenomas cause patients to exhibit massive fluid and electrolyte loss.[44]

Adenomas: Radiographic Findings
Surface Pattern

Radiographically, the surface of a polyp may be smooth, lobulated, finely granular, or reticular in nature. Tubular adenomas often have a flat surface (Fig. 12–5), but may be macroscopically divided into several lobules. Under a dissecting microscope, tubular adenomas are divided into one to three lobules.[45] Tubulovillous adenomas are divided into approximately 3 to 10 lobules (Fig. 12–6) as seen under a dissecting microscope.[45] Villous adenomas have innumerable tiny lobules corresponding to the fronds seen histologically. When barium enters the interstices between villous adenoma fronds, a delicate lacework of barium creates a finely nodular, reticular (Fig. 12–7), or granular pattern.[46,47] Approximately two thirds to three quarters of villous adenomas display the reticular or granular surface pattern.[48,49]

Pedunculated Polyps

The pedicle and head of a pedunculated polyp may be seen in profile (Fig. 12–8), especially on erect (Fig. 12–9) or decubitus views or when a polyp is in the barium pool (Fig. 12–10). A pedunculated polyp may be difficult to see if it is only etched in white by barium (Figs. 12–11 and 12–12). En face, a pedunculated polyp may be seen as two concentric ring shadows surrounding areas of increased density, described by Laufer as a "Mexican hat sign" (the "sombrero sign") (Fig. 12–13).

A polyp may resemble a hat (Fig. 12–14).[50] Two hemispheric lines are seen at right angles to each other. The brim of the hat parallels the colonic wall and represents barium trapped between the polyp and the colonic surface. The top of the hat represents the superior surface of

Text continues on page 365

TABLE **12–1.** *Malignant Potential of Adenomas Based on Size*

| | No. of Lesions Versus % Malignant | | |
Histologic Type	<1 cm	1–2 cm	>2 cm
Tubular adenoma	1382 (1%)	392 (10.2%)	101 (34.7%)
Tubulovillous adenoma	76 (3.9%)	149 (7.4%)	155 (45.8%)
Villous adenoma	21 (9.5%)	39 (10.3%)	174 (52.5%)

NOTE: The percentage numbers indicate the percent of tumors of that size that were malignant.
Modified from Muto, T., Bussey, H.J.R., and Morson, B.C.: The evolution of cancer of the colon and rectum. Cancer 36:2251, 1975. Copyright © 1975 American Cancer Society. Reprinted by permission of Wiley-Liss, Inc., a subsidiary of John Wiley & Sons, Inc.

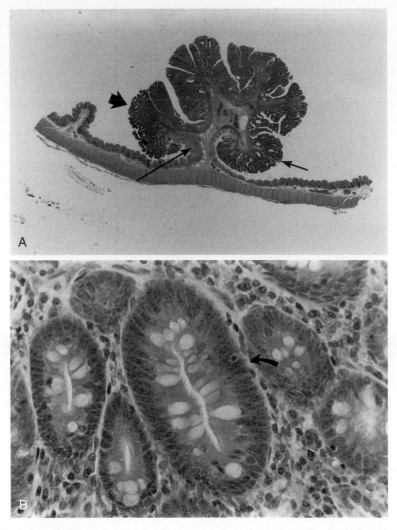

FIGURE 12–1. Pedunculated tubular adenoma. *A,* Low-power cross section of a pedunculated tubular adenoma shows that the tumor is composed of five lobules (representative lobule identified by *thick large arrow*). The lobules are composed of tubules *(short arrow)* of dysplastic cells embedded in stroma. The pedicle of the polyp *(long arrow)* is covered by normal colonic mucosa. *B,* Medium power photomicrograph of the lesion shows tubules (representative tubule identified by *arrow*) separated by normal lamina propria. The dysplastic epithelial cells have large, hyperchromatic nuclei. Mucin remains in some cells.

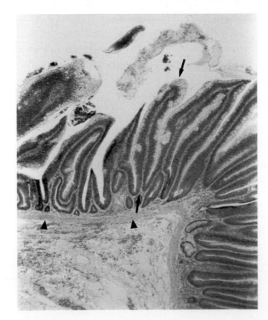

FIGURE 12–2. Villous adenoma. Large papillary fronds (representative frond identified by *arrows*) extend from the muscularis mucosae *(arrowheads)* to the surface of the adenoma.

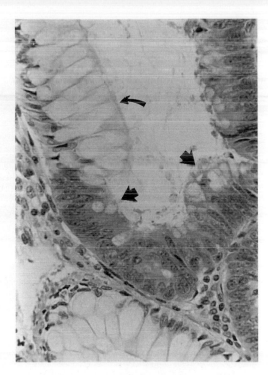

FIGURE 12–3. Adenomatous versus normal epithelium. Within a tubule both adenomatous *(straight arrows)* and normal epithelial *(curved arrow)* cells are seen. The dysplastic cells show enlarged, elongated, hyperchromatic nuclei. In comparison to the purely basal location of the nuclei in the normal epithelium, some nuclear stratification is seen. Much less mucin is seen in the cytoplasm of the dysplastic cells as compared with the normal cells.

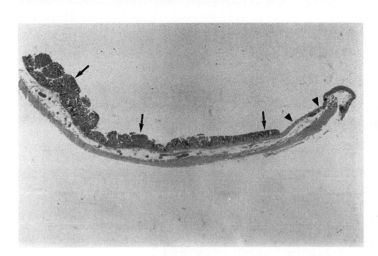

FIGURE 12–4. Flat adenoma. Adenomatous epithelium *(arrows)* crawls along the surface of the colon, without projecting much into the lumen. The height of the normal colonic epithelium *(arrowheads)* is identified for comparison purposes.

FIGURE 12–5. Pedunculated tubular adenoma, descending colon. The polyp's head *(large arrow)* has a smooth surface; the stalk *(small arrow)* is etched in white by barium.

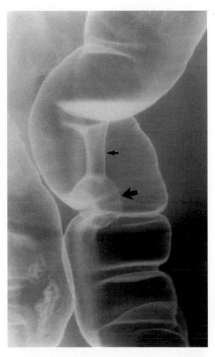

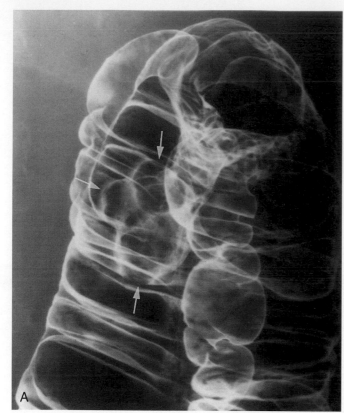

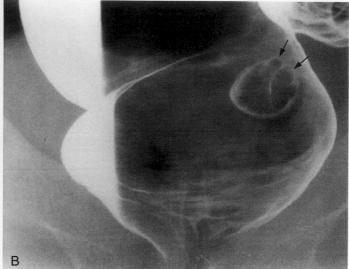

FIGURE 12–6. Tubulovillous adenoma. *A,* Tubulovillous adenoma, splenic flexure. Barium fills the interstices between coarse lobules. The contour is bosselated *(arrows). B,* Lobulated tubulovillous adenoma, rectum. Approximately eight lobules are etched by barium (two lobules are identified by *arrows*).

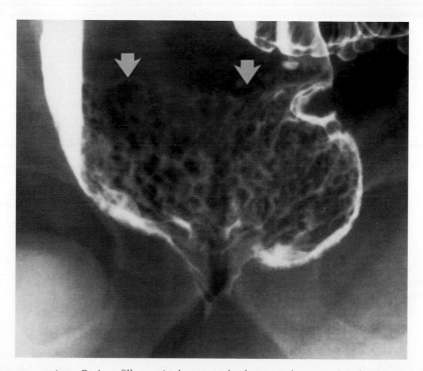

FIGURE 12–7. Villous adenoma, rectum. Barium fills a reticular network of grooves between fronds of tumor. Despite the circumferential nature of the tumor, the shape of the contour of the colon is relatively preserved, and tumor lobules are barely elevated above the colonic surface. The transition zone to normal epithelium is well demarcated *(arrows).* (From Rubesin, S.E., et al.: Carpet lesions of the colon. Radio-Graphics *5:*537–552, 1985, Fig. 1.)

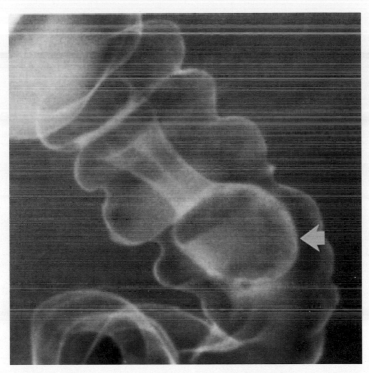

FIGURE 12–8. Tubular adenoma. The smooth-surfaced head of the polyp *(arrow)* is lined by adenomatous epithelium. Most of the stalk of the polyp is lined by normal columnar epithelium.

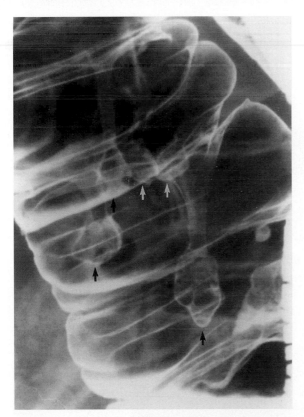

FIGURE 12–9. Cluster of pedunculated tubulovillous adenomas, ascending colon. The heads of the polyps *(arrows)* are lobulated, with barium filling interstices of the tumors. The polyps are hanging from their pedicles with this patient in the erect position.

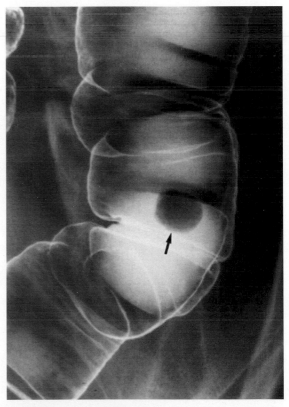

FIGURE 12–10. Tubulovillous adenoma in the barium pool. A slightly lobulated radiolucent filling defect *(arrow)* is seen in the barium pool of the descending colon.

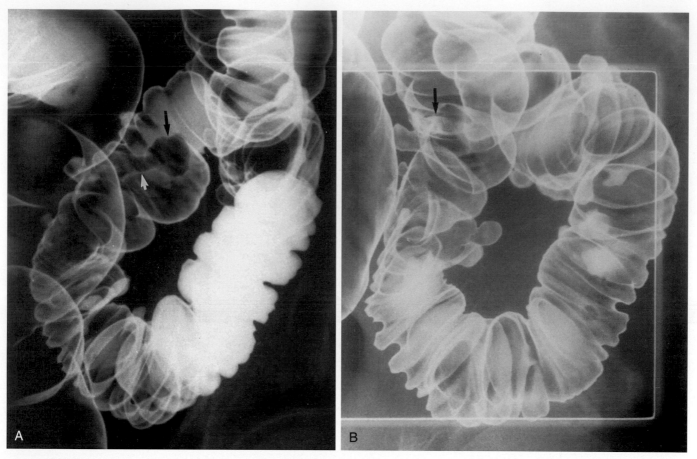

FIGURE 12–11. Tubulovillous adenoma best seen in barium pool. *A,* The head *(black arrow)* and stalk *(white arrow)* of a pedunculated polyp is seen primarily as a radiolucent filling defect in the barium pool. Part of the polyp is etched in white because the anterior wall lies above the barium pool. Diverticulosis of the sigmoid colon is present. *B,* When the sigmoid colon is devoid of the barium pool, the polyp *(arrow)* is difficult to identify.

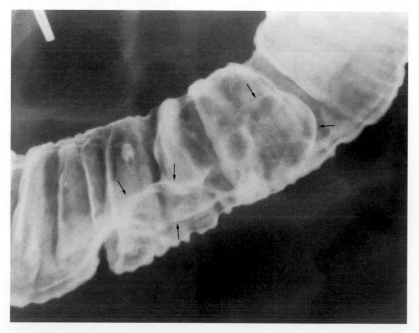

FIGURE 12–12. Difficult-to-identify pedunculated tubulovillous adenoma. Barium etches a large, pedunculated polyp *(arrows)* in the sigmoid colon.

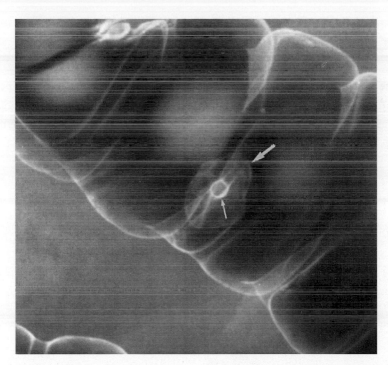

FIGURE **12–13.** The "sombrero" sign. A pedunculated polyp is seen en face. Two barium-etched concentric ring shadows are seen. The head of the polyp is manifested by the outer ring of barium *(large arrow)* surrounding an area of increased radiodensity in comparison to the adjacent air-filled lumen. The stalk of the polyp is seen en face as the inner ring shadow *(small arrow)* surrounding an area of even greater radiodensity. (From Rubesin, S.E., et al.: Tumors of the colon. Semin. Colon Rectal Surg. *4*:94–111, 1993, Fig. 5.)

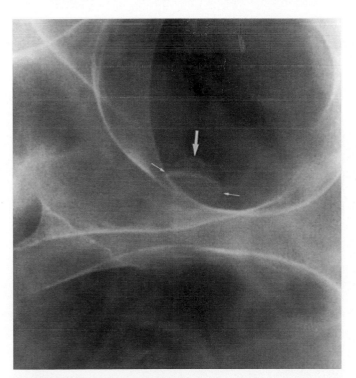

FIGURE **12–14.** "Bowler hat" polyp. The top of the polyp's head is an arc of barium *(long arrow)*. Barium trapped at the base of the head of the polyp retracted against the normal colonic surface appears as a hemispheric line *(small arrows)*. (From Miller, W.T., Levine, M.S., Rubesin, S.E., et al.: Bowler hats: A simple principle for differentiating polyps from diverticula. Radiology *173*:615–617, 1989, Fig. 2.)

the polyp. This sign has been described by Laufer as a "bowler hat." Both polyps and diverticula can resemble bowler hats. The direction that the dome of the bowler hat projects distinguishes most bowler hat polyps from diverticula.[51] If the dome of the bowler hat projects inwardly toward the longitudinal axis of the lumen of the bowel, the bowler hat represents a polyp (Figs. 12–15 and 12–16). Because diverticula protrude outside the expected luminal contour of the bowel, a bowler hat diverticulum will project away from the longitudinal axis of the bowel (see Figs. 12–14 to 12–16).[51]

Flat Adenomas (Carpet Lesions)

Some adenomas grow along the surface of the bowel, without much protrusion into the colonic lumen (Fig. 12–17). These flat adenomas are termed carpet lesions. Most carpet lesions are found in the cecum, ascending colon, or the rectum. Despite their relative large size, many carpet lesions are tubular adenomas and tubulovillous adenomas, not villous adenomas.[47] Only a small percent of carpet lesions harbor malignancy.[47] Whenever a contour defect is seen in a carpet lesion, however, malignancy should be suspected (Fig. 12–17D).

Polyps and the Radiographic Prediction of Malignancy

The size of the polyp is the most important predictor of malignancy[38] (Table 12–1). Almost all colonic cancers are greater than 1 cm in size. Only rarely does a colonic cancer arise in either a small polyp, a small umbilicated

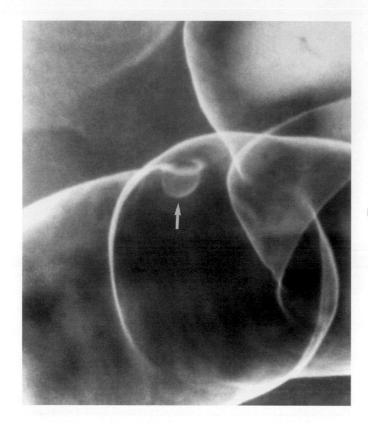

FIGURE 12–15. "Bowler hat" polyp *(arrow),* sigmoid.

FIGURE 12–16. "Bowler hat" tubular adenoma and pedunculated tubulovillous adenoma. A 3-mm bowler hat *(thick arrow)* is seen in the sigmoid colon. A pedunculated polyp *(thin arrows)* has a long, lobulated head and a long, smooth stalk. The pedunculated polyp hangs from the colonic wall while this patient is in a near-erect position. (From Rubesin, S.E., et al.: Tumors of the colon. Semin. Colon Rectal Surg. *4:*94–111, 1993, Fig. 4.)

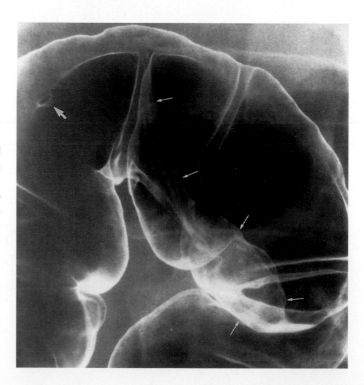

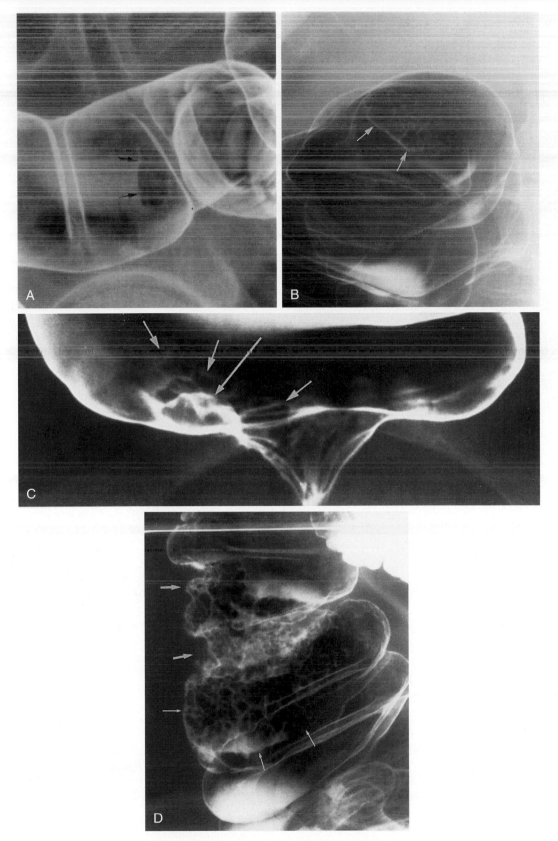

FIGURE 12–17. Carpet lesions of the colon. *A,* A tubulovillous adenoma is seen primarily as a radiolucent filling defect *(arrows)* in the shallow barium coating of the rectosigmoid junction. Barium barely opacifies the interstices of the tumor. *B,* Tubulovillous adenoma in the hepatic flexure. Barium within the interstices of the tumor *(arrows)* creates a focal reticular pattern. (From Rubesin, S.E., et al.: Tumors of the colon. Semin. Colon Rectal Surg. *4:*94–111, 1993, Fig. 9.) *C,* Tubulovillous adenoma, distal rectum. Part of the lesion is flat *(short arrows)* and part is elevated *(long arrow).* This lesion was not seen at endoscopy and was not felt by digital examination because of its soft nature. *D,* Adenocarcinoma arising in villous adenoma. A large carpet lesion *(thin arrows)* is manifest as a focal, reticular pattern. Indentation of the lateral contour of the ascending colon *(thick arrows)* indicates the site of adenocarcinoma. (From Rubesin, S.E., and Laufer, I.: Pictorial glossary of double contrast radiology. *In* Gore, R.M., Levine, M.S., and Laufer, I.: Textbook of Gastrointestinal Radiology. Philadelphia, W.B. Saunders Co., 1994, pp. 50–80, Fig. 5–10*B.*)

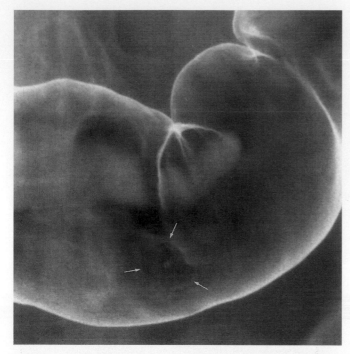

FIGURE 12–18. Early colon cancer. A centrally umbilicated, flat tumor is manifested primarily as a filling defect *(arrows)* disrupting the mucosal coating. This lesion was identified prospectively by barium enema. At polypectomy, carcinoma extended into the lamina propria.

flat lesion (Fig. 12–18), or a small depressed lesion.[52] Polyps greater than 0.5 to 1 cm should be examined histologically.[53,54]

Growth Rate

If a polyp grows quickly between consecutive studies, the polyp should be considered malignant and be removed.[55]

Pedicle

Adenocarcinomas may be present in a pedunculated polyp, but these are usually early cancers without deep invasion into the stalk.[56,57] Lymph node metastases are seen in approximately 7% to 10% of pedunculated tumors in which adenocarcinoma has invaded the submucosa but is not seen at the margins of the polypectomy stalk. If a cancer is deeply invasive into the stalk, the stalk usually appears short and thick. In one pathologic study, no cancers were found in polyps in which the stalk was greater than 3 mm long.[58]

Irregularity of the Polyp's Surface

With increasing nodularity of the polyp's surface, there is an increased chance that villous components are present and an increased chance of malignancy. A finely granular or reticular pattern (Fig. 12–19) therefore suggests the diagnosis of a villous tumor, which should be removed if larger than 5 mm.

Indentation of the Polyp's Base

Indentation, puckering, or irregularity of a sessile or semisessile polyp's base is not a reliable sign of malignancy, especially if the polyp is smaller than 1 cm (Fig. 12–20). Basal indentation is a function of a polyp's geometry rather than the true sign of malignancy.[59] Basal indentation is only worrisome in polyps larger than 1 cm,[60] but polyps larger than 1 cm should be removed by size criteria alone.

Polypoid Artifacts

A wide range of debris can resemble polyps. Strands of mucus may resemble a polyp's stalk (Fig. 12–21) but are often distinguished from polyps because mucus lacks a "head."[61] Feces is usually distinguished from polyps by its irregular contour, irregular coating, and mobility in the barium pool or on erect or decubitus views. Fecal-filled corn kernels and pills have characteristic shapes.[62] Normal variants such as the ileocecal valve or prominent haustral folds may be mistaken for polyps, especially when seen en face. The radiologist must not confuse calcified structures and skeletal structures when seen through the air-filled colon.

Adenocarcinoma
Distribution

The distribution of colonic carcinoma has shifted toward the right and transverse colon over the last several decades.[63–68] Approximately 40% to 50% or more of colonic cancers are out of reach of the flexible sigmoidoscope (Table 12–2).[29] There is an increased incidence of right colon cancers in African-Americans[69] and patients with Lynch syndrome. Synchronous colorectal carcinomas are found in 2% to 8% of patients.[63,64]

Symptoms

Most patients who present with symptoms related to colon cancer usually have advanced cancers. In our series of all patients with colorectal carcinomas detected from 1989 to 1991, nearly 72% of patients had symptoms referable to the tumors. In our series, 25% of the patients were

TABLE 12–2. Distribution of Colonic Cancers in 152 Patients

Location of Tumor	Percent of Colonic Cancers
Cecum	15
Ascending colon	12
Transverse colon	17
Descending colon	5
Sigmoid colon	30
Rectum	21

From McCarthy, P.A., Rubesin, S.E., Levine, M.S., et al.: Colon cancer: Morphology detected with barium enema examination versus histopathologic stage. Radiology *197*:683, 1995.

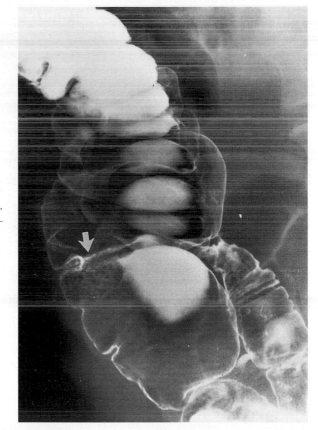

FIGURE 12 19. Tubulovillous adenoma, cecum. A focal reticular pattern *(arrow)* is seen on the lateral border of the cecum opposite the ileocecal valve. (From Rubesin, S.E., et al.: Carpet lesions of the colon. RadioGraphics 5:537–552, 1985, Fig. 10.)

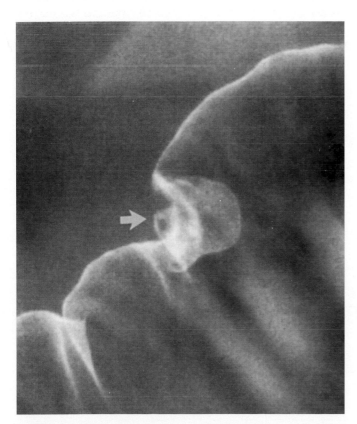

FIGURE 12–20. Tubular adenoma with irregular base. Indentation of the base of a polyp *(arrow)* less than 1 cm is not a reliable indicator of malignancy.

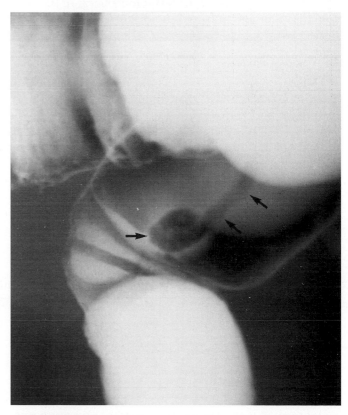

FIGURE 12–21. Coiled mucus strand *(arrows)* **mimics polyp.**

TABLE 12–3. *Morphology of Colonic Cancers in 152 Patients*

Morphology of Cancer	Percent of Cancers
Annular	47
Semiannular	6
Polyp >2 cm	32
Polyp <2 cm	5
Flat plaque or ulcerated	5
Carpet lesion	5

From McCarthy, P.A., Rubesin, S.E., Levine, M.S., et al.: Colon cancer: Morphology detected with barium enema examination versus histopathologic stage. Radiology *197*:683, 1995.

asymptomatic but had "risk" factors such as heme positivity, iron deficiency anemia, or family history of colonic cancer.[29] Less than 5% of our patients who had colonic cancers detected in 1989 to 1991 were studied for "screening."

Most patients with left-sided colon cancers have symptoms such as distention or pain related to obstruction by annular lesions in the relatively narrow sigmoid or descending colon. Bleeding or occult bleeding presenting as iron deficiency anemia or heme positivity is the more frequent presentation for polypoid tumors. Right-sided cancers less frequently cause symptoms because the right colon is wider and polypoid tumors are more frequent in this region.[29]

Radiographic Findings

Advanced colon cancers come in a large variety of gross morphologic shapes including annular, polypoid, plaquelike and carpetlike lesions (Table 12–3). Annular cancers (Fig. 12–22) are the most common form of advanced colonic cancer occurring in approximately one half of patients.[29] Annular cancers have a predilection for the transverse, descending, and sigmoid colon. Annular cancers represent the end stage of the polyp to carcinoma sequence. Small polypoid lesions spread laterally to form a semiannular tumor (Fig. 12–23). Continued spread

leads to circumferential tumor and the classic annular cancer. When an annular cancer is found, the chance of serosal invasion is approximately 98% and the chance of lymph node metastasis is approximately 50%.[29]

Radiographically, annular lesions have abrupt shelflike margins. The annular narrowing is frequently asymmetric, thicker at the site of the original spreading polypoid tumor. The mucosa is often nodular, irregular (Fig. 12–24), or focally ulcerated. In some cases, however, the surface of the tumor is smooth (Figs. 12–25 and 12–26). When seen in profile, semiannular cancers resemble a saddle (see Fig. 12–23). When seen en face, semiannular cancers may appear annular (see Fig. 12–23).

Polypoid cancers (Fig. 12–27) are the most common gross morphologic form of advanced colonic cancer in the rectum or cecum (Table 12–4).[29] By the time a polypoid adenoma has become a carcinoma, it is usually greater than 2 cm (Fig. 12–28).[29] The smallest polypoid cancer in our series was 1.5 cm without correction for radiographic magnification.[29] Patients with polypoid cancer have a better prognosis than patients with annular cancer. In our series of patients with polypoid cancers, 56% of patients had serosal invasion and 25% of patients had lymph node metastases. Cancer arising in pedunculated polyps usually behaves benignly. Polypoid cancers may appear sessile (Fig. 12–29) or semisessile (Fig. 12–30). When barium enters the interstices of a polypoid cancer, a coarsely lobulated or coarsely nodular surface pattern is seen (see Fig. 12–30). Loss of normal colonic contour and barium-etched lines within the lumen identify a lesion not in the barium pool (Fig. 12–31).

Carpetlike lesions of the colon are usually found in the cecum, ascending colon, and rectum (Table 12–4).[47,70] Cancers arising in carpet lesions are radiographically manifest in profile as disruption of the shape of the luminal contour (see Fig. 12–17D), either as a mass protruding into the lumen or as an ulcerated, depressed area. En face, a focal area that disrupts the relatively uniform granular, nodular, or reticular surface pattern should be viewed with suspicion for the presence of carcinoma. Despite the relatively large size of most carpet lesions, these tumors are usually benign adenomas. Their size and ma-

TABLE 12–4. *Location of Tumor Versus Morphology of Tumor in 152 Patients*

Location of Tumor	Lesion Morphology					
	Polyp <2 cm	Polyp ≥2 cm	Carpet	Plaque or Ulcer	Annular or Semiannular	Total
Cecum	1	16	1	1	3	22 (14%)
Other	6	17	0	4	71	98 (65%)
Rectum	1	16	6	2	7	32 (21%)
All locations	8 (5%)	49 (32%)	7 (5%)	7 (5%)	81 (53%)	152 (100%)

NOTE: Numbers are number of patients. Numbers in parentheses are percentages.
From McCarthy, P.A., Rubesin, S.E., Levine, M.S., et al.: Colon cancer: Morphology detected with barium enema examination vs. histopathologic stage. Radiology *197*:683, 1995.

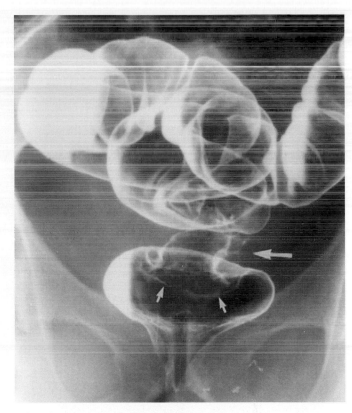

FIGURE 12–22. Annular adenocarcinoma, rectum. Focal circumferential narrowing of the proximal rectum is present. The contour is nodular *(long arrow)*. The distal shelflike margin *(short arrows)* is seen at an angle. No evidence of obstruction is present (either feces impacted proximal to lesion or disproportionate dilatation of colon proximal to lesion).

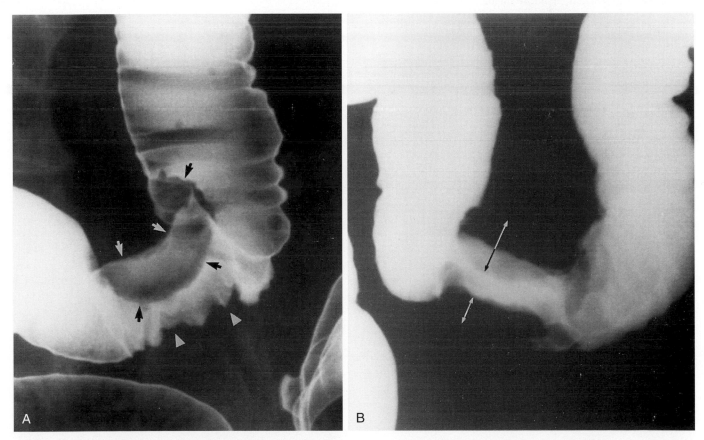

FIGURE 12–23. Semiannular adenocarcinoma (saddle lesion), sigmoid colon. *A,* A polypoid radiolucent mass *(black arrows)* projects into the barium pool. Note that the contour of the polypoid mass *(white arrows)* is indented, so the lesion resembles a saddle. The colonic folds opposite the lesion are tethered *(arrowheads),* indicating the infiltrative nature of the lesion. *B,* When the lesion is studied from a different projection, in single contrast during barium filling, the cancer appears annular. The narrowing is asymmetric, however, thicker at the site of the original polypoid tumor *(double white/black arrow)* than the area of infiltrative spread *(double white arrow)*. This projection is looking at the saddle lesion en face.

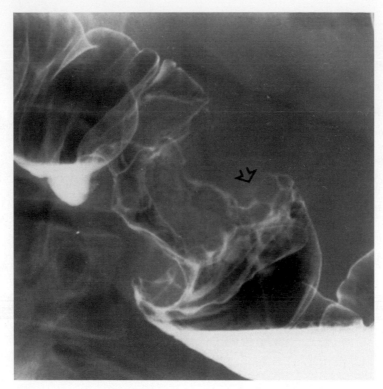

FIGURE 12–24. Annular adenocarcinoma. A 4-cm long annular lesion is seen in the transverse colon. The margins are abrupt, and the mucosa is nodular (representative area identified with *arrow*). (From Rubesin, S.E., et al.: Tumors of the colon. Semin. Colon Rectal Surg. *4*:94–111, 1993, Fig. 13.)

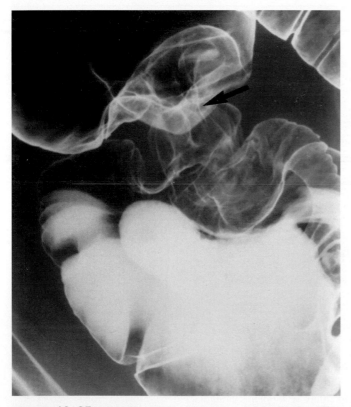

FIGURE 12–25. Annular adenocarcinoma, proximal ascending colon. The distal end of a 3-cm long annular lesion is seen in profile; the proximal end is partly obscured by the ileocecal valve. The narrowed lumen of the cancer is identified. The mucosa is relatively smooth.

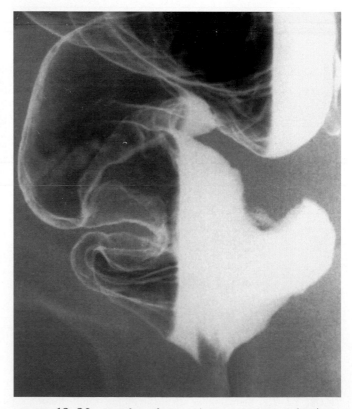

FIGURE 12–26. Annular adenocarcinoma, rectum. A focal circumferential narrowing of the rectum with abrupt margins is seen in the barium pool and etched in white.

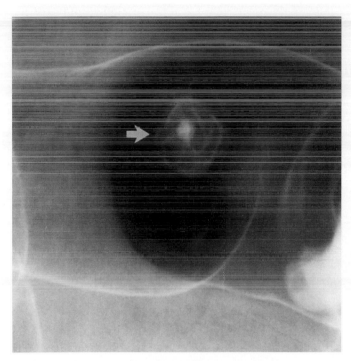

FIGURE 12–27. Polypoid adenocarcinoma. A lobulated polyp *(arrow)* is seen en face. A stalactite hangs off this semipedunculated carcinoma.

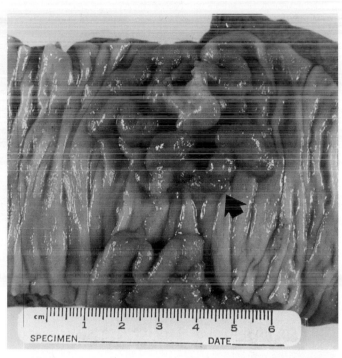

FIGURE 12–28. Polypoid adenocarcinoma. A 5-cm polypoid mass is seen en face. The tumor is composed of cerebriform lobules (representative lobule identified by *arrow*) elevated above the colonic surface. (During opening of the specimen, the tumor was transected.)

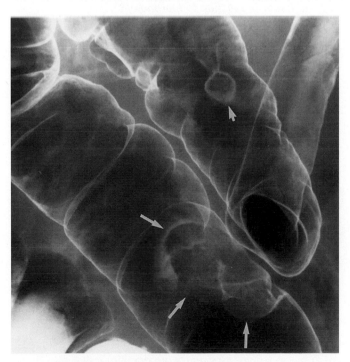

FIGURE 12–29. Polypoid adenocarcinoma, proximal rectum. A large, sessile, polypoid mass *(long arrows)* is etched in white, projecting into the lumen. A pedunculated tubular adenoma *(short arrow)* is seen in the sigmoid colon. (From Rubesin, S.E., et al.: Tumors of the colon. Semin. Colon Rectal Surg. *4*:94–111, 1993, Fig. 11.)

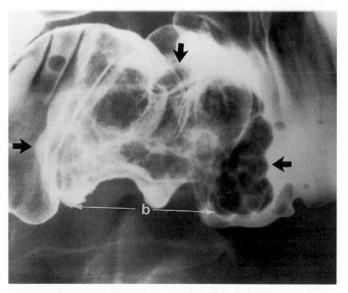

FIGURE 12–30. Polypoid adenocarcinoma, transverse colon. A polypoid mass *(black arrows)* is manifest as a large, lobulated radiolucent filling defect in the barium pool, with barium filling the interstices between tumor lobules. The base of the lesion is broad *(white arrows, b)* but smaller than the transverse diameter, indicating the semipedunculated nature of the lesion.

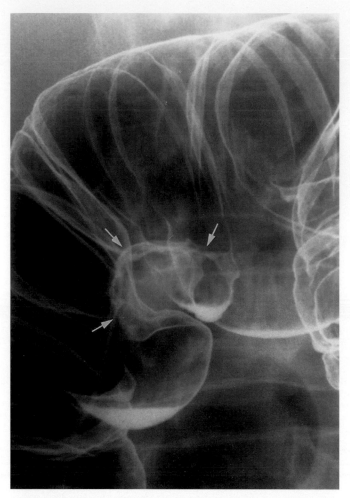

FIGURE 12–31. Polypoid adenocarcinoma, hepatic flexure. The normal contour of the inner margin of the hepatic flexure is missing. Barium-etched lines *(arrows)* project into the lumen, coating the small (2 cm) polypoid cancer.

lignant potential, however, dictates that they must be removed. Carpet lesions should not be confused with cancers infiltrating interhaustral folds or valves of Houston (Fig. 12–32).

Flat Adenomas and Adenocarcinomas

The adenoma-to-carcinoma sequence is found in almost all (96%) early polypoid cancers.[71] Rare, small (5 to 15 mm), flat colonic cancers, however, often have little evidence of prior adenomatous epithelium. These lesions, which are mostly described by Japanese authors,[72] are uncommonly found in the United States. Later reports have shown tiny, flat adenomas which have no carcinoma within them. Therefore it is still not known whether flat, "de novo cancers" truly arise as de novo lesions or in tiny adenomas that are rapidly destroyed by the developing carcinoma.

Small, flat, nonpolypoid adenomas appear as smooth, round, radiolucent lesions, measuring 3 to 5 mm in diameter. They usually have a small central round or irregular barium fleck.[73] Small, flat adenocarcinomas (see Fig.

12–18) average 12 mm in diameter.[71] A few depressed intramucosal cancers may be approximately 5 mm in size, but microscopic invasion does not usually occur until the lesions are 6 to 10 mm in diameter.[74]

Small flat tumors grow more slowly than polypoid lesions. These superficial flat cancers have a doubling time of approximately 52 months.[75] In contrast, the doubling time of large, advanced cancers is approximately 12 months.[75] The slow growth rate of these flat adenomas and flat adenocarcinomas is soothing to the radiologist because these tumors are difficult to detect radiologically. Barium enema will detect only about one half of flat umbilicated tumors less than 5 mm.[74] Barium enema will detect about 85% of flat tumors 6 to 10 mm, however.

We believe that small, flat adenomas and carcinomas may lead to large, plaquelike (Fig. 12–33) or centrally ulcerated tumors (Fig. 12–34). In our series, plaquelike cancers account for approximately 5% of advanced colonic carcinomas.[29]

Size of Tumor in Relation to Symptoms

Patients who are symptomatic and have advanced carcinoma have larger lesions than patients who have advanced carcinoma but are asymptomatic. In our series, symptomatic tumors averaged 5 cm, whereas asymptomatic tumors averaged 3.5 cm.[29] Only 5% of colonic cancers in our nonscreening population were less than 2 cm. In our unscreened population, no colonic cancer less than 2 cm had lymph node or liver metastases.[29]

Stage of Tumor in Relation to Morphology

There are varying classifications of colonic cancer including many variants of the Dukes and TNM classifications.[76–79] In general, the deeper the level of invasion, the worse the prognosis (Table 12–5). In our series of symptomatic or "at-risk" patients, only 4% had lesions confined to the mucosa.[29] Patients who have lesions that have not penetrated the muscularis mucosae have a survival risk equal to an age-matched population.[80,81] Approximately 55% of our patients had lesions confined to the bowel wall (Dukes B), a stage that results in an 80% to 85% 5-year survival. Twenty-eight percent of our "unscreened"

TABLE 12–5. *Modified Dukes Classification of Colonic Carcinoma*

Modified Stage	Depth of Tumor Invasion	5-Year Survival (% of Patients)
Cancer in situ	Above muscularis mucosae	100
A	Invades submucosa	95–100
B_1	Invades muscularis propria	85
B_2	Invades serosa or pericolic fat	80–85
C	Regional lymph node metastasis	50–70
D	Distant metastasis	5–15

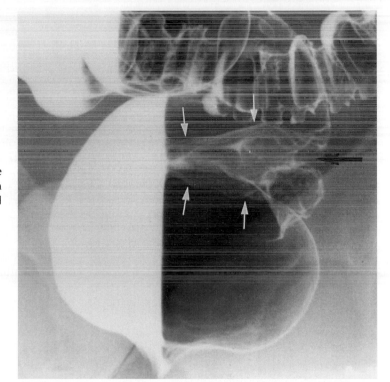

FIGURE 12–32. Adenocarcinoma infiltrating the distal valve of Houston. The lateral wall of the rectum is disrupted by a finely lobulated mass *(black arrow)*, which enlarges the distal valve of Houston *(white arrows)*.

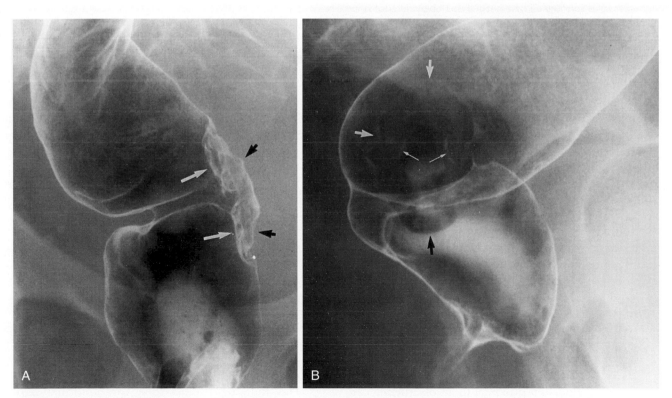

FIGURE 12–33. Plaquelike adenocarcinoma, rectum. *A,* In profile, a 4-cm lesion is etched in white *(white arrows)*. The lesion is much broader than it is elevated. Note the focal irregularity of the contour of the tumor protruding beyond the expected luminal contour *(black arrows)*. This indicates where the plaquelike tumor is centrally ulcerated. *B,* Lateral view of the rectum shows a subtle, large flat lesion as a filling defect in the barium pool distally *(black arrow)* and etched in white proximally *(white arrows)*. The edge of the central ulcer is poorly coated *(thin white arrows)*.

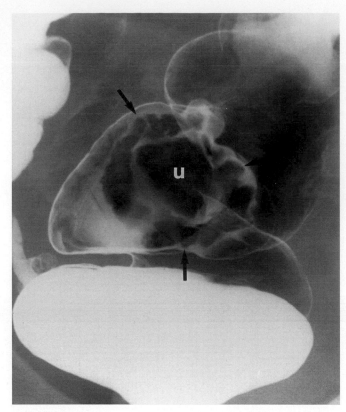

FIGURE **12–34. Flat, ulcerated adenocarcinoma, rectum.** A large central ulcer *(u)* is surrounded by a heaped-up, lobulated edge of tumor *(arrows)*. (From Rubesin, S.E., et al.: Rectum. *In* Gore, R.M., Levine, M.S., and Laufer, I.: Textbook of Gastrointestinal Radiology. Philadelphia, W.B. Saunders Co., 1994, pp. 1261–1309, Fig. 68–24B.)

patients had lymph node metastasis (Dukes C), a 5-year survival rate of approximately 70%. Thirteen percent of our patients had liver metastases or local invasion (Dukes D) documented at the time of initial surgery. Dukes D lesions have an approximate 6% to 14% 5-year survival.[81]

Complications Detected During Barium Enema
Obstruction

Retrograde obstruction to the flow of barium is not equivalent to physiologic obstruction. Obstruction during barium enema may result from a valvelike closure of the lumen when the colon is overdistended distal to the cancer. Physiologic obstruction is best manifested in a symptomatic patient with dilatation of the colon proximal to the tumor. The colon proximal to the cancer will be fecal filled despite a barium enema preparation, if given.

Ischemia

Ischemia of the colon proximal to an obstructing cancer is related to luminal overdistention causing diminished blood flow. The mucosa is the layer of colon most susceptible to decreased blood flow. Barium studies may demonstrate mucosal ischemia as a colonic urticarial pattern (Fig. 12–35). This condition is discussed in Chapter 13.

Intussusception

Colonic cancers are the most common cause of colocolic intussusception in adults. Polypoid adenocarcinomas usually act as the lead point of the intussusceptum (Fig. 12–36). Adenomas and lipomas are the other pedunculated tumors that cause intussusception in adults.

Local Invasion

Local invasion by colonic carcinoma is usually detected during cross-sectional imaging studies. Spread of colonic cancer may be detected if barium enema demonstrates fistula formation, perforation, or invasion of adjacent colonic (Fig. 12–37) or ileal loops. Cancer of the transverse colon may cause a cologastric fistula; cancer of the rectum, a colovaginal fistula; and cancer of the sigmoid colon, a colovesical fistula. Synchronous intraperitoneal metastases may be detected as extrinsic mass effect with spiculation of the luminal contour and tethering of mucosal folds.

Lymphoid Hyperplasia

Hyperplasia of colonic lymph tissue is associated with colonic cancer. The lymphoid hyperplasia can either be diffuse or localized near the region of the tumor (Fig. 12–38).

Technique and Errors

The goals of a radiologist in performing a double contrast barium enema are first to detect lesions, then to give a graded differential diagnosis on the basis of the morphologic characteristics of the lesion. Radiologic detection of precursor adenomas and early colonic cancer is the radiologist's best opportunity to save lives.[82] Technical performance and quality of the barium enema relies heavily on the cleanliness of the patient's preparation and the patient's symptoms, clinical status, and rectal tone. Perceptive errors and a technically poor quality study are the most common reasons that colon cancers are missed radiologically. Most "missed" colonic cancers can be seen in retrospect (Fig. 12–39). Only approximately 10% of "missed" cancers are not visible on good quality films.[83] This fact emphasizes the importance of careful technical performance of barium enemas and careful film review.[83]

The areas of the colon where the radiographic findings of colonic neoplasia may be subtle are the sigmoid colon (Fig. 12–40), the rectosigmoid junction, the anterior wall of the cecum, and the medial wall of the upper ascending (see Fig. 12–39) and descending colon. Most "missed" colonic cancers are hidden in the sigmoid colon in areas of moderate to severe diverticulosis.[84,85]

The radiologist must look for abnormal barium-etched lines where they should not be (Figs. 12–41 and 12–42) or subtle filling defects in the barium pool (see Fig. 12–40). Plaquelike or saddle lesions may be missed[86] if the radiologist does not pay careful attention to the colonic contour. Linitis plastica may mimic Crohn's disease,

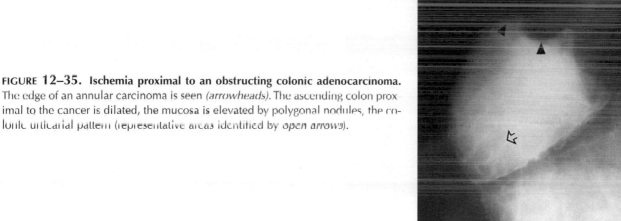

FIGURE 12–35. Ischemia proximal to an obstructing colonic adenocarcinoma. The edge of an annular carcinoma is seen *(arrowheads)*. The ascending colon proximal to the cancer is dilated, the mucosa is elevated by polygonal nodules, the colonic urticarial pattern (representative areas identified by *open arrows*).

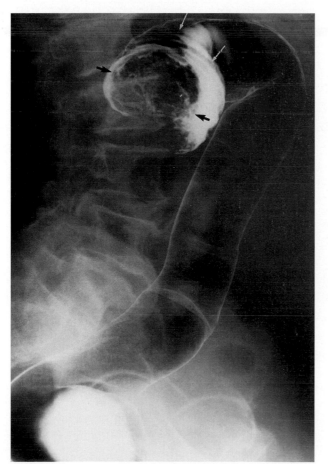

FIGURE 12–36. Colocolic intussusception due to polypoid adenocarcinoma. Barium fills the interstices of a polypoid mass *(black arrows)* in the splenic flexure. This was an adenocarcinoma arising in a villous adenoma. Parallel folds *(white arrows)* just distal to the mass indicate the distal portion of the intussusceptum, which is coated with barium. The remainder of the intussusceptum is not filled. (From Rubesin, S.E., and Laufer, I.: Pictorial glossary of double contrast radiology. *In* Gore, R.M., Levine, M.S., and Laufer, I.: Textbook of Gastrointestinal Radiology. Philadelphia, W.B. Saunders Co., 1994, pp. 50–80, Fig. 5–13A.)

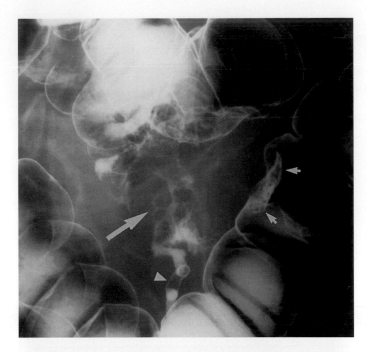

FIGURE 12–37. Carcinoma of cecum invading sigmoid colon. An annular lesion of the cecum *(large arrow)* is seen. The appendix is not dilated *(arrowhead)*. Mass effect and nodularity of the medial wall of the proximal sigmoid colon *(small arrows)* is seen because of direct invasion of the sigmoid colon. An en-bloc resection of cecum and sigmoid colon had to be performed.

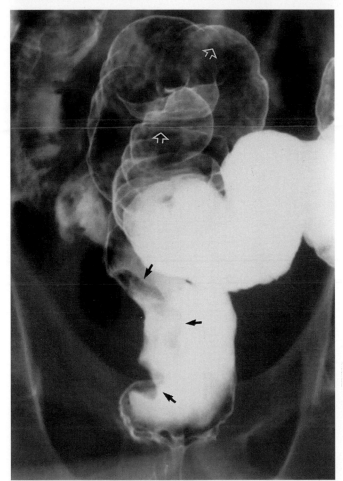

FIGURE 12–38. Lymphoid hyperplasia associated with adenocarcinoma. A subtle, ulcerated mass is seen as a focally abnormal contour of the right lateral wall of the rectum and a heaped-up, nodular margin *(black arrows)*. The mucosa of the sigmoid colon shows many small nodules (representative areas identified with *open arrows*), a marked lymphoid hyperplasia.

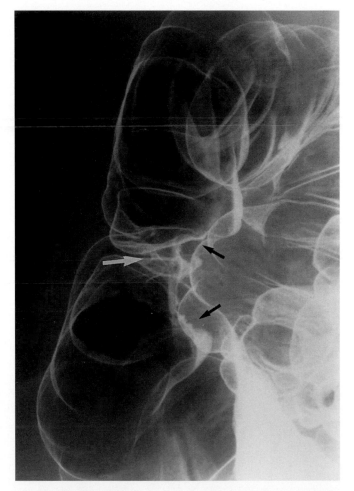

FIGURE 12–39. Colon cancer "missed" during barium enema. Loss of the contour *(black arrows)* and subtle mucosal nodularity are seen focally in the ascending colon. This short lesion spreads circumferentially *(white arrow)*. Missing this lesion is a "perceptive error."

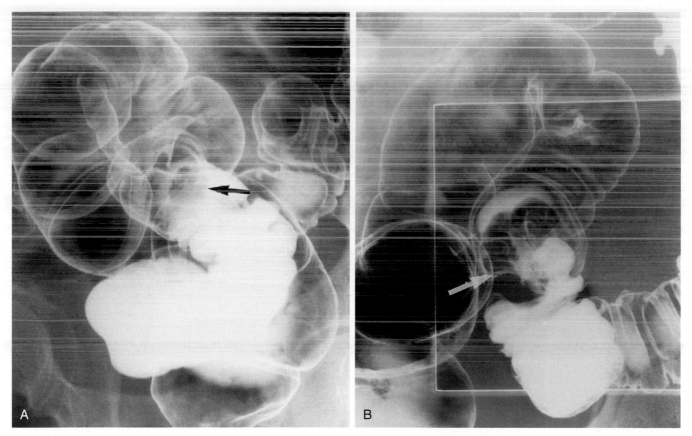

FIGURE 12–40. Missed polypoid tumor progresses to adenocarcinoma. *A,* A 1.5-cm lobulated radiolucent filling defect *(arrow)* is present in the barium pool. This lesion was not reported. *B,* Four years later, a barium enema shows an annular lesion *(arrow)* in the sigmoid colon.

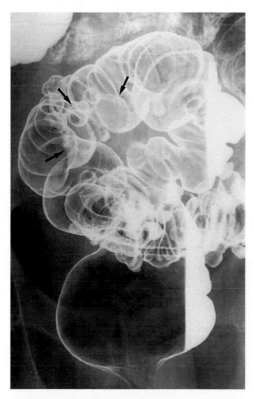

FIGURE 12–41. Polypoid adenocarcinoma, sigmoid colon. Barium etched lines *(arrows)* in an area of diverticulosis are seen on this slightly underexposed left side down decubitus radiograph.

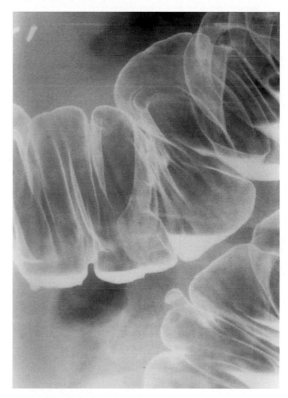

FIGURE 12–42. Tubular adenoma, splenic flexure. Do you see the polyp? Barium etches a 1-cm polyp on a 2.5-cm stalk.

or a perforated carcinoma may mimic an inflammatory process such as diverticulitis.[87,88]

Proper technique is fully discussed in Chapter 11. A quality barium enema requires a clean colon, relatively devoid of fecal particulate debris greater than 2 to 3 mm. The radiologist must use careful fluoroscopy and obtain spot films with the colon well-coated by barium and well-distended by air. The radiologist must be sure that adequate mucosal coating is achieved because with a poor coating, large tumors can be missed.[89] Collapsed colons may hide even sizable lesions. Adequate distention is helped by the use of intravenous glucagon or other hypotonic agent. An adequate number of projections must be taken. A tumor may be seen on only one film.

Special views will help evaluate the areas where colonic cancers are usually missed, the sigmoid colon, the rectosigmoid junction, the anterior wall of the cecum, and the medial wall of the upper ascending and descending colon. The prone angle view is of crucial importance to splay out the rectosigmoid junction, an area that may be obscured on the standard recumbent views. The anterior wall of the cecum may be imaged with the patient in a prone position. Recumbent oblique views of the hepatic and splenic flexure and the ascending and descending colon are complimentary to erect views of the flexures and the ascending and descending colon.

Endoscopy is not infallible either. In fact, even dismissing areas of the colon that were not seen during endoscopy, in our unpublished quality assurance study of 10 years ago, endoscopy missed slightly more cancers than barium studies. Endoscopy may miss flat lesions, lesions on the inner wall of a curve (Fig. 12–43), and even annular lesions. If an endoscope cannot traverse an annular cancer, biopsy may be negative. Even a positive biopsy may underestimate the malignant potential of a colonic tumor (Fig. 12–44).

Postoperative Colon

Barium enemas are frequently performed after surgery for colorectal cancer because of the 5% risk of developing a second cancer and the 2% risk of developing a recurrence at an anastomosis.[90,91] After the immediate postoperative period an anastomosis has a smooth mucosa and is seen as an area of abrupt narrowing, occasionally ringlike (Fig. 12–45). There is frequently a caliber change between the colon on either side of the anastomosis (see Fig. 12–45). An enema performed in the early postoperative period may reveal a smooth or slightly irregular raised polypoid elevation of the mucosa at the anastomosis, which may represent a stitch granuloma. Although a stitch granuloma may be confused with recurrent carcinoma, stitch granulomas are usually seen on early postoperative films and regress with time.[92] In the remote postoperative period, however, if an anastomosis has irregular mucosa (Fig. 12–46), or tethered, radiating folds (Fig. 12–47), or a focal mass (Figs. 12–48 and 12–49), recurrent cancer should be suspected. Biopsy may be negative if the recurrence is submucosal.

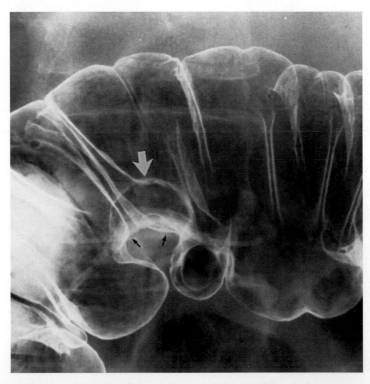

FIGURE 12–43. Polypoid adenocarcinoma missed at endoscopy. Barium enema performed after a "negative" colonoscopy shows a 1.5-cm polypoid lesion in the hepatic flexure. Indentation of the polyp's base *(black arrows)* indicates malignant potential in polyps larger than 1 cm. A repeat endoscopy and surgery confirmed the small carcinoma.

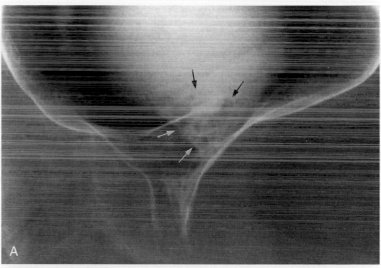

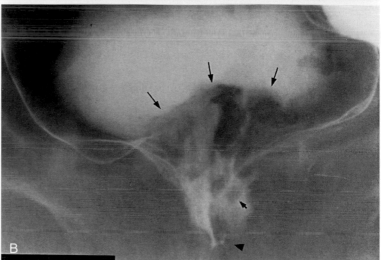

FIGURE 12–44. **Carpet lesion progresses to adenocarcinoma.** *A,* A flat, nodular lesion *(arrows)* is seen in the distal rectum. Barium enema diagnosis was a tubulovillous lesion or worse. Focal endoscopic biopsy revealed tubular adenoma. *B,* Barium enema 1 year later shows nodular folds *(short arrow)* in the distal rectum with mass effect extending both proximally *(long arrows)* and to the anorectal junction *(arrowhead).* Abdominoperineal resection revealed an infiltrating adenocarcinoma. (From Kahn, S., and Rubesin, S.E.: Polypoid lesions at the anorectal junction: Barium enema findings. AJR. Am. J. Roentgenol. *161:*339–342, 1993, Fig. 14*A, B.* © American Roentgen Ray Society.)

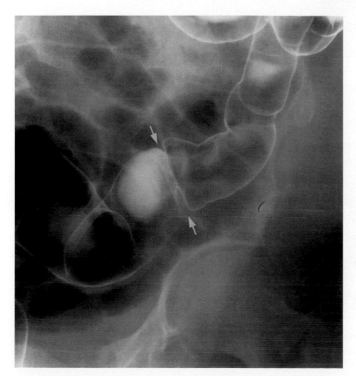

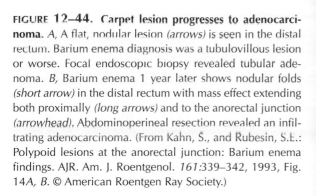

FIGURE 12–45. **Normal colocolic anastomosis.** A smooth, circumferential thin narrowing *(arrows)* is at the junction between colonic loops of differing sizes.

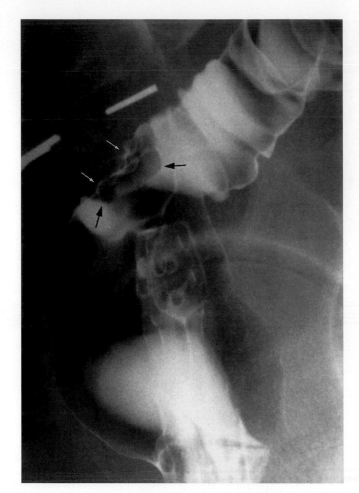

FIGURE 12–46. Recurrent adenocarcinoma at anastomosis. Coarse, lobulated mucosa *(black arrows)* and irregularity and loss of the contour *(white arrows)* are present at the colorectal anastomosis. The radiologic clues that this is an anastomotic region are the caliber change between rectum and distal colon and the loss of the normal rectal size and shape. Surgical clips are present in the presacral space.

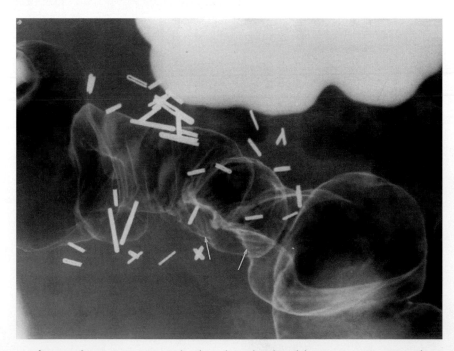

FIGURE 12–47. Recurrent adenocarcinoma at anastomosis. The inferior border of the anastomotic region shows mass effect and tethering of smooth mucosal folds (representative tethered folds identified with *arrows*). The tumor was primarily extrinsic to the bowel wall

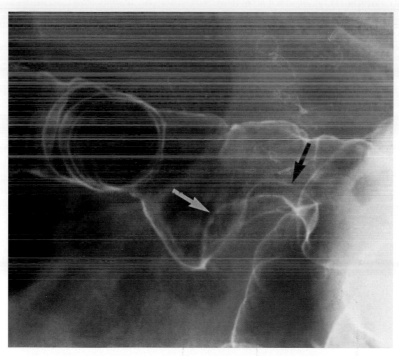

FIGURE **12–48. Recurrent adenocarcinoma near colorectal anastomosis.** A bilobed mass *(arrows)* with an irregular surface is seen.

FIGURE **12–49. Recurrent adenocarcinoma near anastomosis.** A smooth-surfaced mass *(short arrows)* with central ulceration *(long arrow)* is due to submucosal recurrence of tumor.

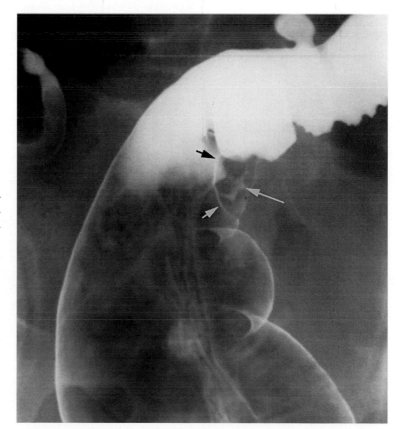

OTHER MUCOSAL POLYPS

Hyperplastic (Metaplastic) Polyps

Hyperplastic (metaplastic) polyps are usually small, less than 0.5 cm, smooth-surfaced sessile polyps, most frequently arising on the crest of mucosal folds (Fig. 12–50).[93] These polyps are common and frequently multiple, occurring in more than 75% of people older than 40.[93] Although most hyperplastic polyps arise in the rectum, these polyps can be found in any part of the colon. Hyperplastic polyps are not precancerous but represent an alteration in the maturation of normal epithelium. Hyperplastic polyps are dome-shaped proliferations composed of elongated crypts lined by a serrated epithelium (see Fig. 12–50B) composed of intermediate cells and a few goblet cells.[94]

If detected radiologically, hyperplastic polyps are usually small, smooth-surfaced sessile polyps (Fig. 12–51), most frequently found in the rectum. Occasionally, hyperplastic polyps are greater than 0.5 cm. These larger hyperplastic polyps may be sessile or pedunculated and have a smooth or slightly lobulated surface.[95] These large hyperplastic polyps are radiographically indistinguishable from tubular adenomas or tubulovillous adenomas.

Juvenile Polyps

Juvenile polyps are nonneoplastic lesions most frequently found in children and adolescents. Juvenile polyps are usually solitary, pedunculated tumors, 1 to 3 cm in diameter. These polyps have a smooth surface lined by normal columnar epithelial cells. In the center of a juvenile polyp are numerous tubules lined by normal epithelium. The tubules are frequently cystically dilated and widely separated by edematous, inflamed stroma (Fig. 12–52). It is unknown whether juvenile polyps are inflammatory or hamartomatous in origin. Previously they were called "retention polyps." Radiographically, juvenile polyps are usually pedunculated, smooth-surfaced polyps (Fig. 12–53), most frequently found in the rectum.[93]

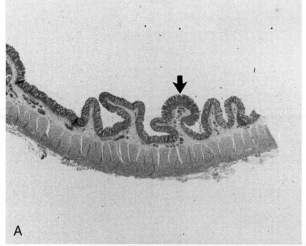

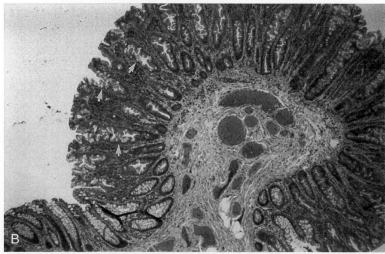

FIGURE 12–50. Hyperplastic polyp. *A*, Low-power photomicrograph of colon shows a hyperplastic polyp *(arrow)* arising on the crest of a mucosal fold. At this magnification, the hyperplastic polyp is seen as an area of increased mucosal thickness. *B*, Medium-power photomicrograph of the same hyperplastic polyp shows the serrated appearance of the epithelium (representative areas identified by *arrows*). The nuclei of goblet and columnar cells are basally located without atypia.

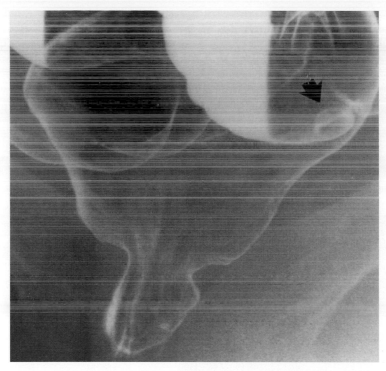

FIGURE 12–51. Hyperplastic polyp. A 5-mm bowler-hat polyp *(arrow)* is seen on the left lateral wall of the rectum. (From Rubesin, S.E., et al.: Rectum. *In* Gore, R.M., Levine, M.S., and Laufer, I. (eds.): Textbook of Gastrointestinal Radiology. Philadelphia, W.B. Saunders, Co., 1994, pp. 1261–1309, Fig. 68–15.)

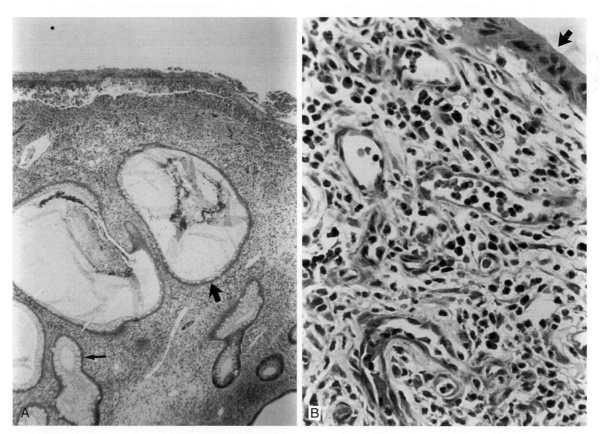

FIGURE 12–52. Juvenile polyp. *A,* Low-power photomicrograph of juvenile polyp shows cystically dilated tubules *(large arrow)* and distorted tubules *(small arrow)* separated by a large volume of edematous and inflamed stroma. The epithelial layer is composed of benign, mucus-secreting cells. *B,* Medium-power photomicrograph shows a marked inflammatory response in the stroma. The inflamed surface epithelium *(arrow)* has lost its mucus but is not dysplastic.

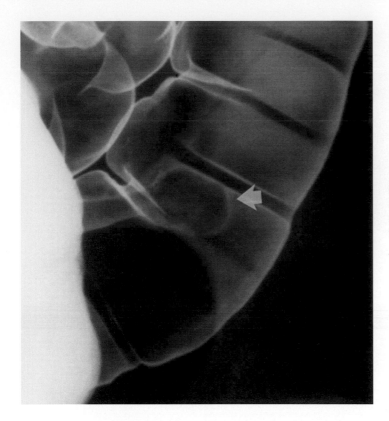

FIGURE **12–53. Juvenile polyp.** A pedunculated polyp *(arrow)* is seen at the junction of the descending and sigmoid colon. Radiographically, this polyp is indistinguishable from an adenomatous polyp.

Fibrovascular Polyps

Fibrovascular polyps, also known as inflammatory fibroid polyps, are rare lesions of the colon or any other portion of the gastrointestinal tract. These growths arise in submucosa and are composed primarily of granulation tissue with a variable eosinophilic infiltrate.[39] Inflammatory fibroid polyps probably are a form of granulation tissue rather than a true tumor.[39] Macroscopically, a fibrovascular polyp may be a pedunculated polyp (Fig. 12–54), sessile submucosal mass, or dumb-bell-shaped lesion.

OTHER BENIGN AND MALIGNANT TUMORS

Vascular Lesions

Hemangioma

Patients with colonic hemangiomas often present at a young age with acute, recurrent, or chronic rectal bleeding, occasionally so severe as to be life-threatening.[96,97] Hemangiomas are associated with a wide variety of syndromes, including Klippel-Trénaunay-Weber syndrome.[98–101] Cavernous hemangiomas are unencapsulated lesions, composed of large multiloculated thin-walled vessels separated by loose connective tissue (Fig. 12–55).[98,102] Cavernous hemangiomas are usually found in the rectum and sigmoid colon, usually arising in the submucosa.

Radiologic diagnosis is important because this tumor may be misdiagnosed as colitis or hemorrhoids at endoscopy.[96] Hemangiomas should be suspected radiologically when plain films demonstrate phleboliths in a young patient with rectal bleeding or a cluster of phleboliths in

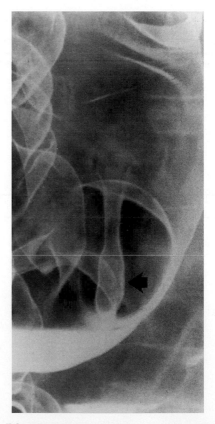

FIGURE **12–54. Fibrovascular polyp.** A 2-cm long, pedunculated polyp is seen in the transverse colon. The elongated nature of the head *(arrow)* suggests that this is a soft lesion such as a lipoma or fibrovascular polyp. Polypectomy is necessary, however, to exclude an adenomatous polyp. (From Rubesin, S.E., et al.: Tumors of the colon. Semin. Colon Rectal Surg. *4:*94–111, 1993, Fig. 7.)

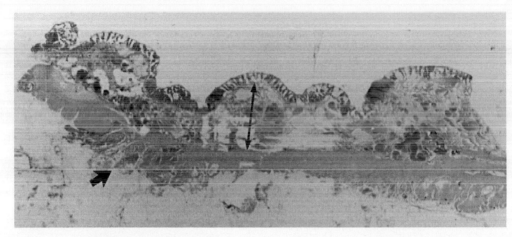

FIGURE 12–55. Hemangioma of the colon. Low-power view of the sigmoid colon shows an undulating colonic surface caused by lobulated widening of the submucosa *(double arrow).* The submucosa is expanded by blood-filled spaces. At a lower power, the cystic spaces were seen to be lined by endothelial cells. Focally, the hemangioma extends through the muscularis propria into the subserosal fat *(arrow).* (From Rubesin, S.E., et al.: Other tumors. *In* Gore, R.M., Levine, M.S., and Laufer, I.: Textbook of Gastrointestinal Radiology. Philadelphia, W.B. Saunders Co., 1994, pp. 1200–1227, Fig. 65–7B.)

the pelvis in a central location or along the expected course of the rectum. Barium enema will usually demonstrate a circumferential lesion with scalloped contours and a nodular mucosal surface (Fig. 12–56).[97] Occasionally, a smooth, sessile, broad-based submucosal mass is seen.[103]

Lymphangioma

Lymphangiomas are extremely rare benign lesions composed of clusters of lymphatic spaces lined by endothelial cells, separated by connective tissue septa. Lymphangiomas are usually solitary, 2 to 4 cm in diameter, often pedunculated polypoid lesions or smooth submucosal masses. These tumors are soft and pliable and change size and shape with compression similar to lipomas. Their radiologic interest is that on CT they are cystic or multicystic masses of water attenuation.[104,105]

Angiodysplasia

Angiodysplasias are extremely common lesions responsible for chronic low gastrointestinal bleeding or massive acute gastrointestinal bleeding in elderly.[106,107] Angiodysplasias are acquired vascular ectasias composed of clusters of dilated, tortuous, thin-walled veins, venules, and capillaries (Fig. 12–57) located in the mucosa or submucosa of the colon.[106] These tumors may be solitary or multiple. They are usually small, less than 5 mm, and are found in the cecum or ascending colon.[106] Because these are flat lesions, angiodysplasias are not detected by barium enema. They must be discovered either at endoscopy or angiography.

Kaposi's Sarcoma

Although Kaposi's sarcoma usually occurs in the colon of patients with AIDS, Kaposi's sarcoma has also been seen in patients with Crohn's disease, ulcerative colitis, and after solid organ transplantation.[100,108,109] On barium enema, Kaposi's sarcoma may be a small polypoid nodule, a plaquelike tumor, or a polypoid or submucosal-appearing mass (Fig. 12–58) with or without central umbilication.[110] Barium enema will not detect the flat, superficial form of Kaposi's sarcoma.

Fatty Lesions
Lipoma

A lipoma of the colon is an encapsulated mass of mature adipose tissue arising in the submucosal layer in 90% of patients and in the appendices epiploicae in 10%.[111,112] About 70% of colonic lipomas are found in the right colon. Lipomas are multiple in approximately 25% of patients.[112] Approximately two thirds of lipomas are pedunculated, arising from a broad-based pedicle covered by normal mucosa. Most lipomas are tumors discovered at autopsy, during endoscopy, or during barium enema performed for symptoms attributed to coexistent lesions.[111] Lipomas causing symptoms are usually larger than 3 cm.

During barium enema, a lipoma is a sessile mass or polypoid lesion (Fig. 12–59).[113] These tumors are round, ovoid, or pear shaped (Fig. 12–60). The submucosal nature of the mass is indicated by its sharply circumscribed nature, by obtuse angles with the colonic wall, or by a broad-based pedicle. Although the surface is smooth (Fig. 12–61), the contour of the tumor may be lobulated. Lipomas are soft, pliable tumors that change size or shape with palpation, varying degrees of colonic distention, during colonic spasm, or after colonic evacuation (see Fig. 12–60).[114,115] Lipomas may cause colocolic intussusception.[116,117]

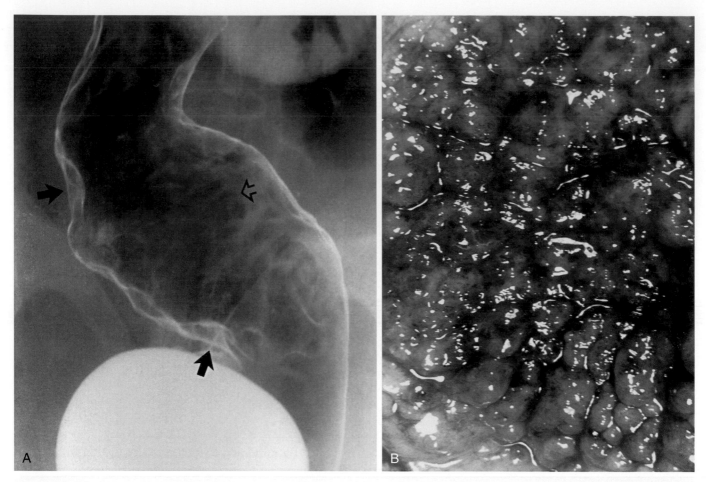

FIGURE 12–56. Hemangioma of the colon. *A,* Prone, angled view of the rectum shows a long lesion manifested by lobulation of the contour *(arrows)* and subtle nodularity of the mucosa *(open arrow)* seen en face. *B,* Close-up photograph of the surgical specimen shows a lobulated/nodular surface with focal areas of hemorrhage. (*A,* From Margulis, A. R.: Case: Cavernous hemangioma of the rectum. Gastrointest. Radiol. *6:*363–364, 1981, Fig. 1*A. B,* From Rubesin, S.E., et al.: Other tumors. *In* Gore, R.M., Levine, M.S., and Laufer, I.: Textbook of Gastrointestinal Radiology. Philadelphia, W.B. Saunders Co., 1994, pp. 1200–1227, Fig. 65–8*B.*)

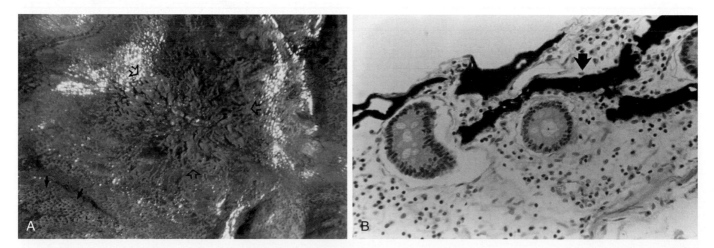

FIGURE 12–57. Angiodysplasia of the ascending colon. *A,* Dissecting photomicrograph shows focal distortion of the normal colonic surface *(open arrows)* by an underlying tangle of vessels. For comparison, an area of normal surface *(arrows)* with its glandular openings is identified. *B,* Medium-power photomicrograph shows thin-walled, endothelium-lined spaces *(arrow)* in the lamina propria. The spaces are filled with a black-staining dye injected into the tumor. (From Rubesin, S.E., et al.: Other tumors. *In* Gore, R.M., Levine, M.S., and Laufer, I.: Textbook of Gastrointestinal Radiology. Philadelphia, W.B. Saunders Co., 1994, pp. 1200–1227, Fig. 65–9.)

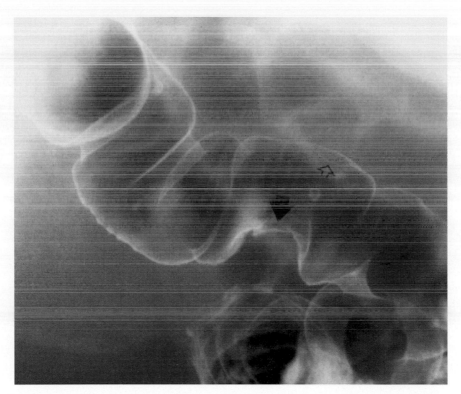

FIGURE 12–58. Kaposi's sarcoma. Spot radiograph of sigmoid colon shows a 1.5-cm submucosal mass *(large arrow)*. A second, more plaquelike tumor *(small arrow)* is faintly visualized as a barium-etched line.

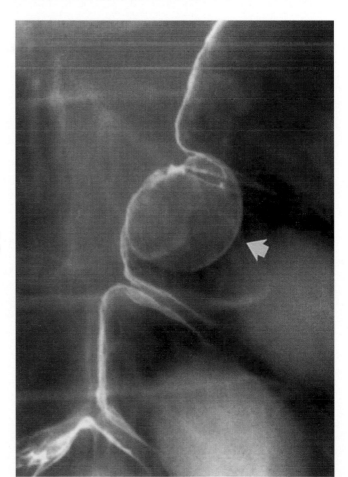

FIGURE 12–59. Colonic lipoma. Spot radiograph of transverse colon shows a smooth-surfaced, round area of increased radiodensity *(arrow)* etched in white.

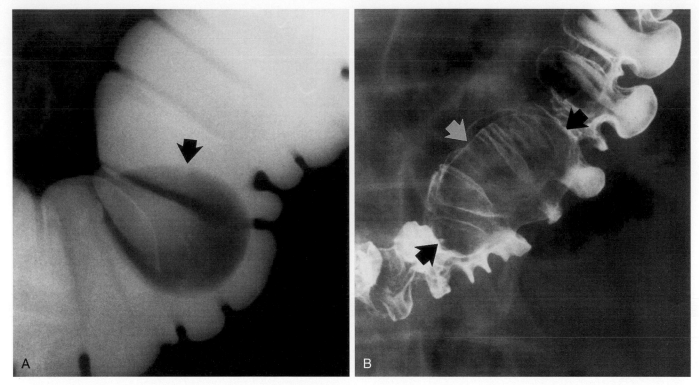

FIGURE 12–60. Colonic lipoma. *A,* Spot radiograph from single contrast barium enema shows a smooth-surfaced, pear-shaped mass *(arrow)* in the mid-transverse colon. *B,* A postevacuation radiograph shows that the lesion *(arrows)* has changed shape with colonic contraction. (From Rubesin, S.E., et al.: Other tumors. *In* Gore, R.M., Levine, M.S., and Laufer, I.: Textbook of Gastrointestinal Radiology. Philadelphia, W.B. Saunders Co., 1994, pp. 1200–1227, Fig. 65–14*A, B.*)

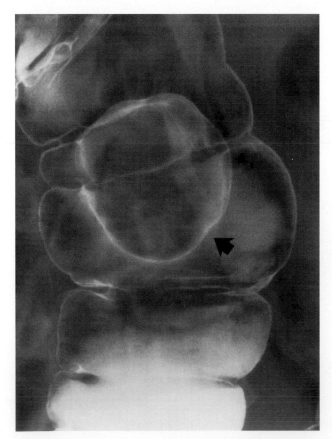

FIGURE 12–61. Colonic lipoma. The contour of this 3-cm lipoma *(arrow)* is slightly lobulated, but the mucosa is smooth. (From Rubesin, S.E., et al.: Other tumors. *In* Gore, R.M., Levine, M.S., and Laufer, I.: Textbook of Gastrointestinal Radiology. Philadelphia, W.B. Saunders Co., 1994, pp. 1200–1227, Fig. 65–13.)

Although barium enema is relatively accurate in the diagnosis of colonic lipoma,[115,116] CT enables a definitive diagnosis.[119,120] On CT, colonic lipoma is usually an intramural or intraluminal mass of uniform, fat density (Fig. 12–62) without large areas of nonfatty tissue.[119-122] Surgery may be avoided in a patient without symptoms or in a patient who is a poor operative risk if CT makes a definitive diagnosis of lipoma. If a colonic lipoma ulcerates and undergoes fat necrosis, CT diagnosis may not be definitive. Furthermore, the radiologist must not mistake mesenteric fat associated with an intussuscepting carcinoma with a lipoma.[123]

Fatty Infiltration of the Ileocecal Valve

Fatty infiltration of the ileocecal valve is distinguished pathologically from a true lipoma of the ileocecal valve by lack of a capsule surrounding the massive accumulation of fat.[93] Fatty infiltration is radiographically manifested as a smooth-surfaced, enlarged ileocecal valve with smooth or lobulated contours. A normal ileocecal valve is less than 4 cm and has stellate folds radiating toward its center.[124,125] Thus the diagnosis of fatty infiltration is suggested when a smooth-surfaced, round or ovoid enlarged ileocecal valve is seen. A discreet, polypoid area arising on the ileocecal valve should not be considered fatty infiltration.

Carcinoid Tumors

There are two relatively distinct subgroups of colonic carcinoid tumors: small, rectal carcinoids and large lesions arising in the right colon. Rectal carcinoids are usually small, submucosal lesions less than 2 cm in diameter, located in the lower third of the rectum (Fig. 12–63). These small polypoid tumors have low malignant potential and are usually cured by complete excision.[126] A rare, large rectal carcinoid appears as an irregular, ulcerated mass and has a poor prognosis.

Colonic carcinoids exclusive of the rectum are advanced tumors with signs, symptoms, and radiographic findings indistinguishable from adenocarcinoma. Colonic carcinoids exclusive of the rectum are usually found in the cecum or ascending colon.[127,128] Radiographically, right colonic carcinoids appear as irregular annular lesions (Fig 12–64) or large, greater than 5 cm fungating sessile masses.[127,129,130]

Lymphoma

Primary lymphoma of the colon is rare, comprising 0.4% of colonic malignancies.[131,132] Colonic involvement by systemic lymphoma is relatively common, but patients with disseminated lymphoma usually do not undergo barium enema.[133] Almost all colonic lymphomas are non-Hodgkin's lymphoma.[134,135]

The signs and symptoms of primary colonic lymphoma are similar to adenocarcinoma, including abdominal pain, weight loss, change in bowel habits, rectal bleeding, diarrhea, and palpable abdominal mass.[135] Patients with long-standing ulcerative colitis, solid organ transplantation, or AIDS are at increased risk for colonic lymphoma.[136-139]

Primary colonic lymphoma usually involves the cecum, ileocecal valve, or rectum, whereas disseminated lymphoma involves long segments of the colon or the entire colon.[140-143] Primary localized lymphoma may appear radiographically as a polypoid mass, a circumferential mural lesion, or a cavitary mass. The most common form of primary colonic lymphoma is a broad-based, sessile, polypoid mass (Fig. 12–65) with a smooth surface with or without central ulceration. The bulky mass may vary from

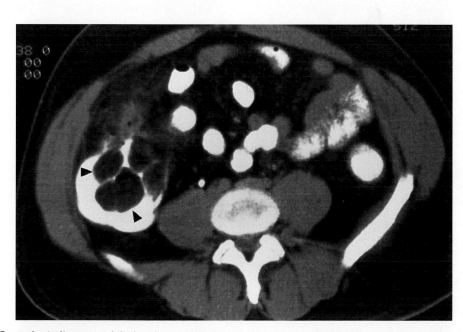

FIGURE 12–62. Colonic lipoma. A lobulated mass of fatty attenuation *(arrowheads)* fills the lumen of the ascending colon.

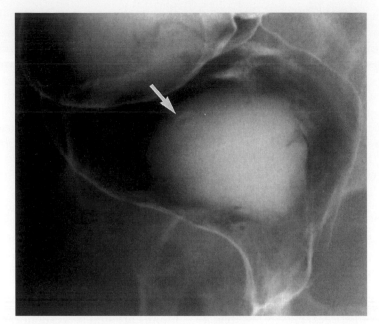

FIGURE 12–63. Carcinoid tumor of rectum. A ring shadow *(arrow)* is faintly seen, partly obscured by the barium pool on the left lateral wall of the rectum.

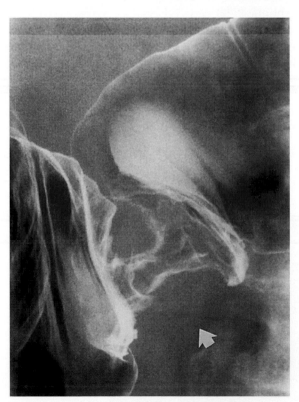

FIGURE 12–64. Carcinoid tumor of hepatic flexure. A short, 2-cm annular lesion *(arrow)* is indistinguishable from an adenocarcinoma. Some primary adenocarcinomas of the colon have extensive neuroendocrine elements, so full pathologic examination is necessary to make the diagnosis of carcinoid tumor. (Courtesy of Seth N. Glick, M.D., Philadelphia, Pennsylvania. From Rubesin, S.E., et al.: Other tumors. *In* Gore, R.M., Levine, M.S., and Laufer, I.: Textbook of Gastrointestinal Radiology. Philadelphia, W.B. Saunders Co., 1994, pp. 1200–1227, Fig. 65–11.)

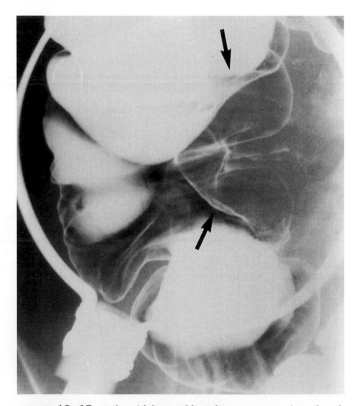

FIGURE 12–65. Polypoid form of lymphoma. A smooth-surfaced, broad-based, sessile, polypoid mass *(arrows)* enlarges the ileocecal valve.

4 to 20 cm and is most frequently located near the ileocecal valve. Ileocecal valve lymphomas frequently invade the adjacent terminal ileum.

The annular, infiltrating form of primary colonic lymphoma (Fig. 12–66) appears radiographically as a concentric narrowing, often with thick interhaustral folds and a coarsely lobulated surface. Although coarsely lobulated, the surface locally is smooth, suggesting a confluence of submucosal nodules (Fig. 12–67). The differential diagnosis of the infiltrating form includes a focal ischemic process versus an unusual colonic carcinoma.[132] Bulky, cavitary masses (Fig. 12–68) have a gross morphology similar to that of gastrointestinal stromal tumors or perforated colonic cancers.

The diffuse form of colonic lymphoma may be associated with disseminated disease from a nodal primary or may be a primary form derived from a subpopulation of mantle cells.[144,145] These tumors, termed mantle cell lymphoma, involve a long segment or the entire colon. Radiographically, mantle cell lymphoma appears as polygonal, smooth, sessile nodules varying from 2 to 25 mm in diameter carpeting the colonic surface (Fig. 12–69),[143,146] hence the term *lymphomatous polyposis*. A conglomerate cecal mass is present in approximately half the patients.[143] The multinodular form of lymphoma must be differentiated from FAPS, lymphoid hyperplasia, or diffuse infections such as pseudomembranous colitis or schistosomiasis. In lymphoid hyperplasia the nodules are round, uniform, 2 to 3 mm, and separated by normal epithelium, whereas the nodules of primary mantle cell lymphoma are usually larger and nonuniform in size.

Differential Diagnosis of Ileocecal Valve Masses

The normal ileocecal valve is usually located on the medial or posterior colonic wall at the junction of the cecum and the ascending colon at the level of the first complete interhaustral fold. The ileocecal valve can be identified by barium filling of the terminal ileum. If an ileocecal valve is mildly enlarged, about 3 to 4 cm in diameter, with a smooth or slightly lobulated contour and a smooth mucosal surface, the most likely diagnosis is fatty infiltration. If the ileocecal valve is greater than 4 cm in diameter and has a gentle, undulating contour with a smooth mucosal surface, an infiltrative process such as lymphoma or Crohn's disease is suggested. In lymphoma the ileocecal valve is moderately enlarged with a lobulated contour. Lymphoma in the ileocecal valve is usually associated with lymphoma in the terminal ileum. In Crohn's disease there is fatty infiltration of the ileocecal valve, usually associated with the typical radiologic changes of Crohn's disease in the terminal ileum and ileocecal fistulas. A focal polypoid projection from the ileocecal valve may represent a tumor such as adenoma or lipoma (Fig. 12–70). Any mucosal surface irregularity of the ileocecal valve suggests a mucosal tumor such as adenoma or carcinoma.

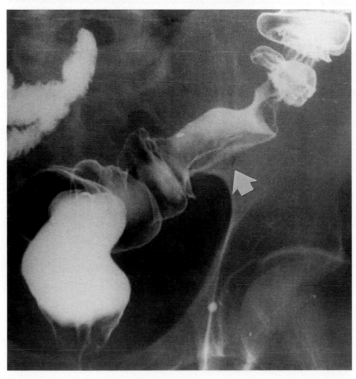

FIGURE 12–66. Annular form of lymphoma. A smooth-surfaced annular lesion *(arrow)* is seen in the sigmoid colon. The proximal margin is tapered, the distal margin is shelflike. The amount of luminal narrowing is mild, given the length of the lesion. (Courtesy of Seth N. Glick, M.D., Philadelphia, Pennsylvania. From Rubesin, S.E., et al.: Other tumors. *In* Gore, R.M., Levine, M.S., and Laufer, I.: Textbook of Gastrointestinal Radiology. Philadelphia, W.B. Saunders Co., 1994, pp. 1200–1227, Fig. 65–3.)

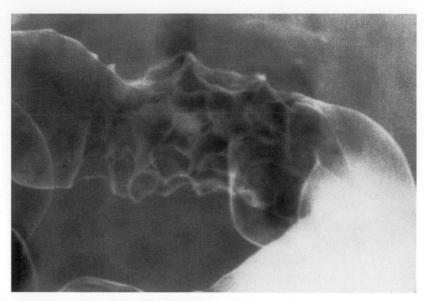

FIGURE 12–67. Lymphoma of sigmoid colon. An annular lesion without much luminal narrowing is seen. The mucosal surface is composed of many small ovoid, smooth nodules. The contour is lobulated, composed of many small "submucosal-appearing" nodules (smooth-surfaced, with right angles to luminal contour). This appearance suggest a lymphoma or hemangioma. (From Rubesin, S.E., et al.: Other tumors. *In* Gore, R.M., Levine, M.S., and Laufer, I.: Textbook of Gastrointestinal Radiology. Philadelphia, W.B. Saunders Co., 1994, pp. 1200–1227, Fig. 65–5.)

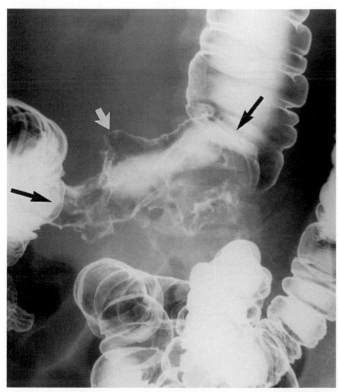

FIGURE 12–68. Cavitary form of lymphoma. A long (>20 cm), circumferential lesion is seen in the transverse colon (limits defined by *black arrows*). Despite the large size, minimal luminal compromise is seen. Protrusion of the luminal contour of the tumor *(white arrow)* beyond the expected lumen of colon indicates cavitation into a bulky mass. (From Rubesin, S.E., et al.: Other tumors. *In* Gore, R.M., Levine, M.S., and Laufer, I.: Textbook of Gastrointestinal Radiology. Philadelphia, W.B. Saunders Co., 1994, pp. 1200–1227, Fig. 65–4A.)

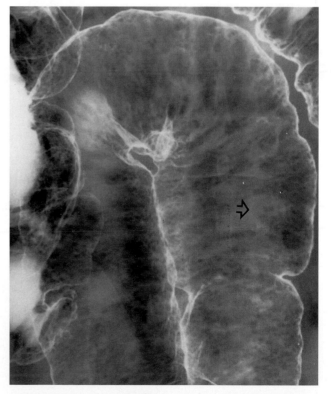

FIGURE 12–69. Disseminated lymphoma involving colon. Numerous 1 to 3 cm, nonuniform nodules (representative area of nodularity identified by *arrow*) disrupt the smooth mucosal surface of the colon. Usually with either disseminated lymphoma or primary mantle cell lymphoma, the nodules are slightly larger and nonuniform. (Courtesy of Seth N. Glick, M.D., Philadelphia, Pennsylvania. From Rubesin, S.E., et al.: Other tumors. *In* Gore, R.M., Levine, M.S., and Laufer, I.: Textbook of Gastrointestinal Radiology. Philadelphia, W.B. Saunders Co., 1994, pp. 1200–1227, Fig. 65–6.)

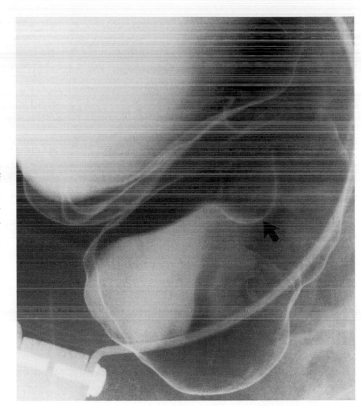

FIGURE 12–70. Lipoma arising on ileocecal valve. A focal, smooth-surfaced polypoid lesion *(arrow)* arises on the inferior lip of the ileocecal valve. The lesion is broad based, with a smooth, abrupt angle with the valve. (From Rubesin, S.E., et al.: Other tumors. *In* Gore, R.M., Levine, M.S., and Laufer, I.: Textbook of Gastrointestinal Radiology. Philadelphia, W.B. Saunders Co., 1994, pp. 1200–1227, Fig. 65–17.)

Gastrointestinal Stromal Tumor

Although radiologists steadfastly call spindle cell and epithelioid tumors of the stomach, small bowel, and colon "leiomyoma" or "leiomyosarcoma," most of these tumors are undifferentiated stromal neoplasms termed gastrointestinal stromal tumors.[147–149] Only a minority of these tumors are shown to be of smooth muscle origin by immunohistochemical or ultrastructural means.

Large colonic stromal tumors are extremely rare, occurring most frequently in the rectum.[150] Radiographically, large gastrointestinal stromal tumors appear as an annular lesion with irregular mucosa, a submucosal mass with or without central ulceration (Fig. 12–71), or a cavitary mass with a large extraluminal component. Gastrointestinal stromal tumors have a high rate of local recurrence and metastasize to the peritoneal surface, liver, and lung.[149,151]

Small, sessile or pedunculated polypoid lesions arising in the muscularis mucosae are extremely rare but are the "true" leiomyomas of the colon. These small tumors have no malignant potential. Radiographically, these small sessile or pedunculated tumors have a smooth or lobulated surface. Small neurofibromas may have a similar appearance.

"Cloacogenic" Carcinoma

The junction of the anal canal and rectum is lined by squamous and columnar epithelium. Many types of tumors arise near the anorectal junction, given the many cell types and structures in this transitional area. Although these tumors have been previously classified as "cloacogenic" carcinomas, their current anatomic classification is based on the tumors' architectural and cellular differentiation. Tumors of the anorectal junction include squamous cell carcinoma, basaloid carcinoma, transitional cell carcinoma, mucoepidermoid carcinoma, and adenoid cystic carcinoma.[100] Many tumors have a mixture of histologic growth patterns. Squamous cell carcinomas have been seen in patients with ulcerative colitis, pelvic irradiation, perianal condylomas (Fig. 12–72) and schistosomiasis.[152] The most common malignancy of the anal canal is adenocarcinoma arising in the rectal mucosa invading inferiorly.

"Cloacogenic" tumors have no distinctive clinical or radiologic features. "Cloacogenic" carcinomas are flat, infiltrative, annular or ulcerative lesions with rolled edges. Radiographically, these tumors appear as infiltrative lesions (Fig. 12–73), a broad-based sessile or polypoid mass (Fig. 12–74), or a submucosal mass with a centrally-ulcerated surface.[153,154]

Metastasis

Symptoms produced by gastrointestinal metastases are often the initial clinical manifestation of a primary tumor. The radiologic features often identify a lesion as a metastasis, identify the mode of dissemination, and indicate possible sites of the primary tumor.[155] Radiologic recognition of metastatic disease alerts the surgeon to perform a wider excision or the need to perform colonic bypass surgery with colostomy.[156]

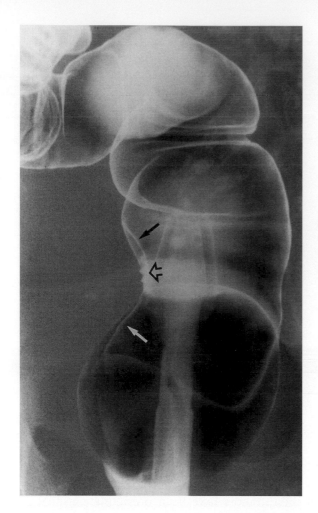

FIGURE 12–71. Gastrointestinal stromal tumor of rectum. A broad-based, smooth surfaced mass *(long arrows)* is seen in the right anterolateral wall of the mid-rectum. Centrally, the mass is focally spiculated *(open arrow)*. (From Rubesin, S.E., et al.: Other tumors. *In* Gore, R.M., Levine, M.S., and Laufer, I.: Textbook of Gastrointestinal Radiology. Philadelphia, W.B. Saunders Co., 1994, pp. 1200–1227, Fig. 65–20A.)

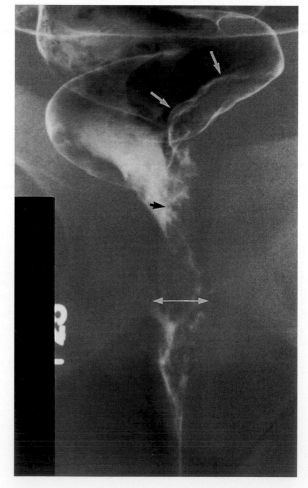

FIGURE 12–72. Squamous cell carcinoma arising in a condyloma acuminatum. This 24-year-old woman had been treated for 5 years for vulvar, cervical, vaginal, and perianal condylomata. An infiltrative lesion extends from the distal rectum through the anal canal. Proximally, the tumor appears polypoid *(white arrows)*. The mucosa of the anorectal junction is nodular *(black arrow)*. The anal canal is expanded and filled with nodular mucosa *(double arrow)*. (From Rubesin, S.E., et al.: Other tumors. *In* Gore, R.M., Levine, M.S., and Laufer, I.: Textbook of Gastrointestinal Radiology. Philadelphia, W.B. Saunders Co., 1994, pp. 1200–1227, Fig. 65–28.)

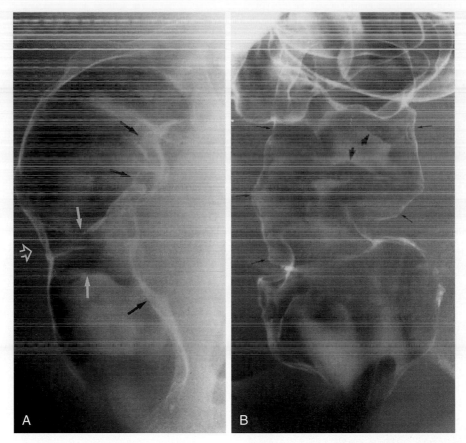

FIGURE 12–73. Infiltrative pattern of "cloacogenic" carcinoma. *A,* Lateral radiograph shows that the anterior wall of the rectum is lobulated *(black arrows).* The tumor expands the distal valve of Houston *(white arrows),* extending circumferentially to flatten the posterior rectal wall *(open arrow). B,* A frontal radiograph shows inbowing and irregularity of the lateral walls of the rectum *(thin arrows)* and thick lobulated folds en face *(thick arrows).* (From Rubesin, S.E., et al.: Other tumors. *In* Gore, R.M., Levine, M.S., and Laufer, I.: Textbook of Gastrointestinal Radiology. Philadelphia, W.B. Saunders Co., 1994, pp. 1200–1227, Fig. 65–30.)

FIGURE 12–74. Cloacogenic carcinoma. A large, sessile, submucosal-appearing polypoid mass *(black arrows)* is seen in the anterior wall of the mid-rectum. Circumferential tumor invasion is manifested by thick folds *(arrowheads)* and narrowing of the rectum *(white arrow)* posteriorly. (From Rubesin, S.E., et al.: Other tumors. *In* Gore, R.M., Levine, M.S., and Laufer, I.: Textbook of Gastrointestinal Radiology. Philadelphia, W.B. Saunders Co., 1994, pp. 1200–1227, Fig. 65–29*A*.)

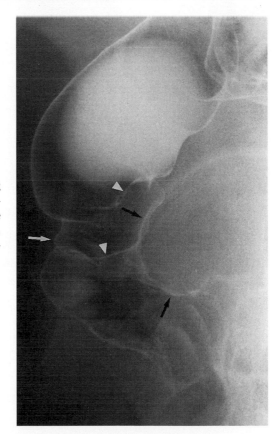

Direct Invasion from Contiguous Primary Tumors

Tumors arising in the ovary, prostate, cervix (Fig. 12–75), uterus, kidney, or gallbladder may directly invade the colon. Prostatic cancer first spreads superiorly into the seminal vesicles, then invades further into the adjacent anterior wall of the rectosigmoid junction (Fig. 12–76). Less frequently, prostatic cancer invades posteriorly through Denonvillier's fascia into the distal rectum (Fig. 12–77).[157] On barium enema, in early cases there is only extrinsic mass effect on the rectosigmoid junction. With colonic invasion, the colonic contour is thrown into spikelike points and the mucosal folds are pleated or tethered (see Figs. 12–76 and 12–77). With advanced metastasis the rectum may be circumferentially narrowed and the presacral space enlarged.[157–160]

Cancers of the left ovary may directly invade the inferior border of the rectosigmoid colon (Fig. 12–78).[161] Barium enema demonstrates angulation of sigmoid loops, with spiculation of the luminal contour, and tethering of mucosal folds.

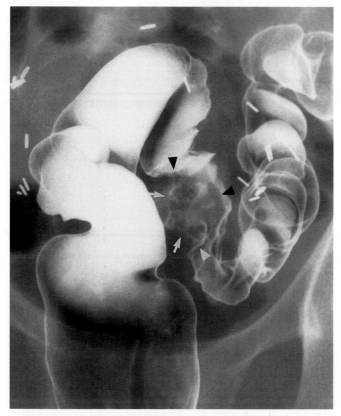

FIGURE 12–75. Direct invasion of the sigmoid colon by recurrent cervical cancer. Close-up from prone view of colon shows extrinsic mass effect manifested as increased radiodensity *(arrowheads)*. Direct invasion is indicated by the spiculated and narrowed inferior contour of the sigmoid colon *(arrows)*. (From Rubesin, S.E., et al.: Other tumors. *In* Gore, R.M., Levine, M.S., and Laufer, I.: Textbook of Gastrointestinal Radiology. Philadelphia, W.B. Saunders Co., 1994, pp. 1200–1227, Fig. 65–21.)

Renal cell carcinoma may invade the colon either at the time of initial diagnosis or at the time of retroperitoneal recurrence of tumor.[162] Right-sided renal cell carcinomas invade the second portion of the duodenum; left-sided renal cell carcinomas invade the distal transverse colon or the proximal descending colon.[162] Radiographically, metastatic renal cell carcinoma invading the colon appears as a bulky, intraluminal mass without signs of obstruction.[162]

Direct Invasion from Noncontiguous Primary Tumors

Cancers may spread to the colon by means of the subperitoneal space or by lymphatic extension.[162] Gastric cancers may spread down the gastrocolic ligament to invade the superior border of the transverse colon.[161] Pancreatic cancers may permeate the transverse mesocolon to spread to the transverse colon (Fig. 12–79). Pancreatic tail cancers may spread along the phrenicocolic ligament to the medial border of the splenic flexure (Fig. 12–80).[155] With direct invasion, there is extrinsic mass effect on the colonic wall that abuts the mesentery, spiculation of the colonic contour, and tethering of mucosal folds.

Intraperitoneal Seeding

Cancers of the ovary, pancreas, stomach, and colon are the most common tumors to seed the intraperitoneal space. Bladder, uterine, and cervical carcinoma and mucinous tumors of the appendix also spread to the peritoneal surface. Lymph node metastases to the retroperitoneum or mesentery, especially from breast carcinoma, may secondarily seed the peritoneal cavity.

The peritoneal reflections direct flow of ascitic fluid to specific locations, which results in characteristic sites of peritoneal implantation.[163] The rectouterine space (pouch of Douglas) and the rectovesicle space are the most common sites of peritoneal metastases in women and men, respectively, as these are the most dependent areas of the peritoneal space.[164] Other common sites of intestinal implantation include the right lower quadrant small bowel loops, the medial border of the cecum, the sigmoid colon (Fig. 12–81), the right pericolic gutter (Fig. 12–82), and the transverse colon (Fig. 12–83).[164] Radiologically, extrinsic mass effect is seen on the side of bowel bathed in peritoneal fluid. The luminal contour is spiculated, and the mucosal folds are tethered toward the implant in a pleated, angulated, or parallel fashion (Fig. 12–84).[165,166] In a woman, endometriosis, tuboovarian abscess, or cervical carcinoma are radiographically indistinguishable from peritoneal metastases to the pouch of Douglas. In a man, prostatic cancer invading the rectum may mimic peritoneal implants. In either sex, spread of an inflammatory process, such as diverticulitis, appendicitis, or Crohn's disease, may mimic intraperitoneal im-

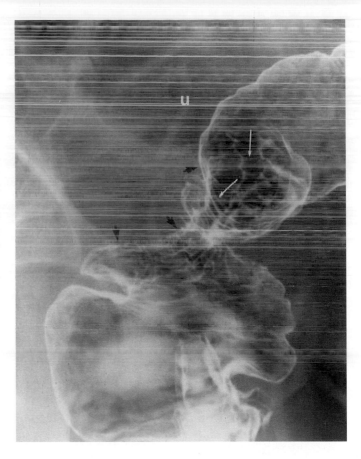

FIGURE 12–76. Direct invasion of rectosigmoid junction by prostatic carcinoma. Slight left oblique view shows extrinsic mass effect *(black arrows)* on the posterolateral wall of the rectosigmoid junction, with mild spiculation of the contour. En face, the mucosal folds are pleated *(white arrows)*. Contrast in the distal right ureter *(u)* from a previous intravenous urogram reflects partial right ureteral obstruction. (From Rubesin, S.E., et al.: Rectal involvement by prostatic carcinoma: Radiographic findings. AJR. Am. J. Roentgenol. *152*:53–57, 1989, Fig. 5*B*. © American Roentgen Ray Society.)

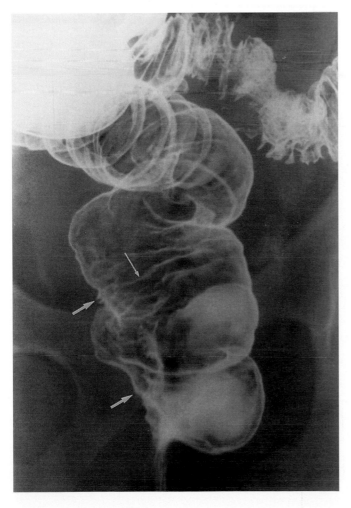

FIGURE 12–77. Direct invasion of lower rectum by prostatic carcinoma. The right lateral wall of the distal rectum is flattened, the contour is spiculated *(thick arrows)*. En face, the mucosa is pleated *(thin arrow)*. (From Rubesin, S.E., et al.: Rectal involvement by prostatic carcinoma: Radiographic findings. AJR. Am. J. Roentgenol. *152*: 53–57, 1989, Fig. 1*A*. © American Roentgen Ray Society.)

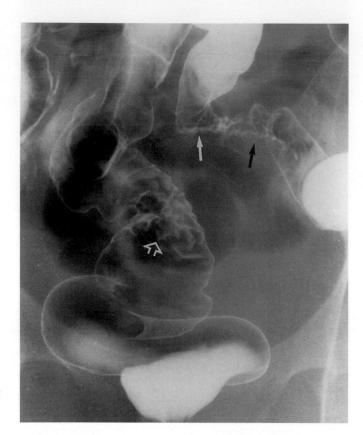

FIGURE **12–78. Direct invasion of rectum and sigmoid colon by left ovarian carcinoma.** Extrinsic mass effect is seen on the inferior border of the sigmoid colon *(arrows)*. The contour of rectum and inferior sigmoid colon is spiculated. En face, the folds of the proximal rectum are pleated *(open arrow)*. (From Rubesin, S.E., et al.: Other tumors. *In* Gore, R.M., Levine, M.S., and Laufer, I.: Textbook of Gastrointestinal Radiology. Philadelphia, W.B. Saunders Co., 1994, pp. 1200–1227, Fig. 65–26.)

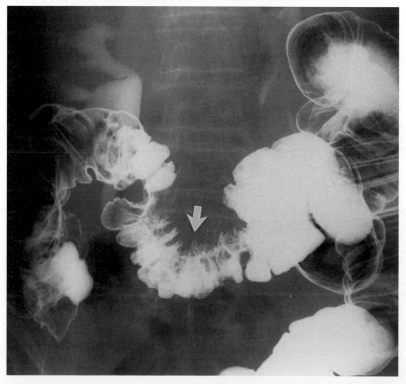

FIGURE **12–79. Pancreatic cancer spreads to transverse colon.** Extrinsic mass effect *(arrow)* and spiculation of the superior border of the transverse colon are seen. (From Rubesin, S.E., et al.: Other tumors. *In* Gore, R.M., Levine, M.S., and Laufer, I.: Textbook of Gastrointestinal Radiology. Philadelphia, W.B. Saunders Co., 1994, pp. 1200–1227, Fig. 65–28.)

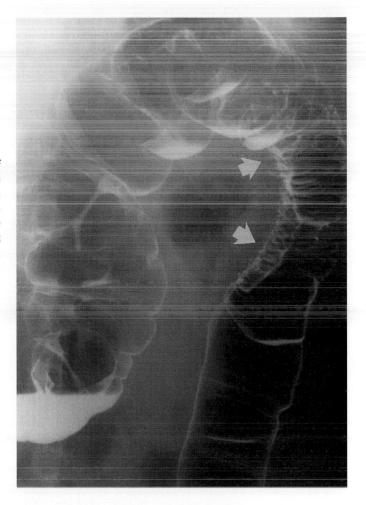

FIGURE 12–80. Pancreatic cancer spreading to splenic flexure of the colon. A cancer in the tail of the pancreas has spread along the phrenicocolic ligament to invade the medial border of the splenic flexure. Extrinsic mass effect upon the medial wall of the splenic flexure *(arrows)* with spiculation of its contour and tethering of folds are typical of serosal disease involving the colon. (From Rubesin, S.E., et al.: Tumors of the colon. Semin. Colon Rectal Surg. *4:*94–111, 1993, Fig. 19.)

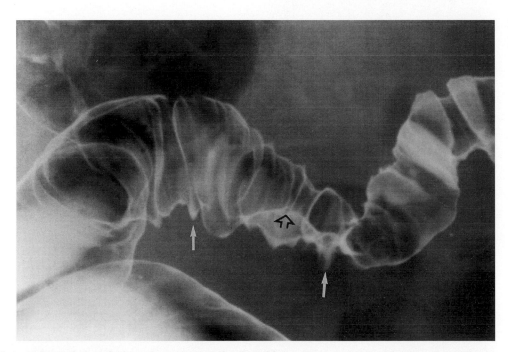

FIGURE 12–81. Intraperitoneal spread of ovarian cancer to the sigmoid mesentery and sigmoid colon. The inferior border of the sigmoid colon is pulled into numerous spikelike points *(white arrows)*. Flattening of the contour and focal asymmetric mass effect *(black arrow)* is seen.

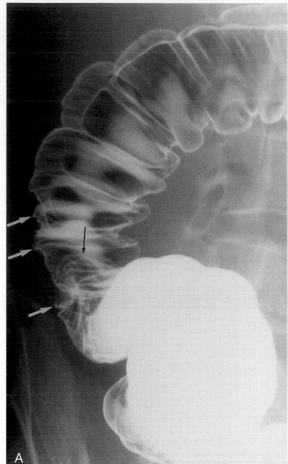

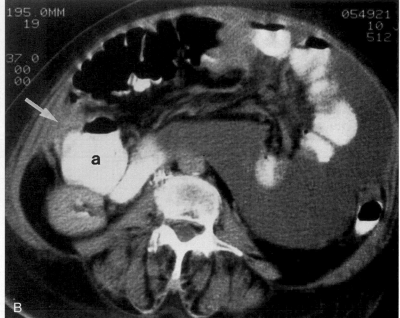

FIGURE 12–82. Intraperitoneal spread of ovarian cancer to right paracolic gutter. *A,* The right lateral wall of the ascending colon is flattened, with spiculation of its contour *(white arrows)* and pleating of mucosal folds *(black arrow).* *B,* CT demonstrates a soft tissue mass *(arrow)* indenting the lateral wall of the ascending colon. The leaves of the small bowel mesentery are thickened because of intraperitoneal implants. Ascites is present. (From Rubesin, S.E., et al.: Tumors of the colon. Semin. Colon Rectal Surg. *4:*94–111, 1993, Fig. 22.)

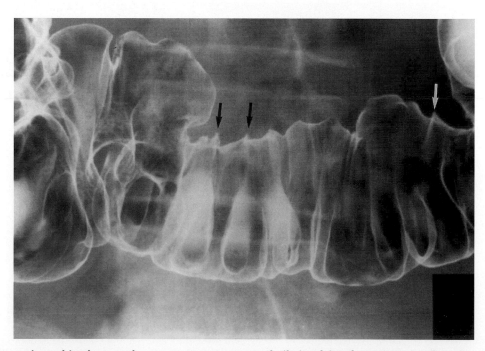

FIGURE 12–83. Intraperitoneal implants to the greater omentum secondarily involving the transverse colon. The superior border of the transverse colon is spiculated *(arrows).*

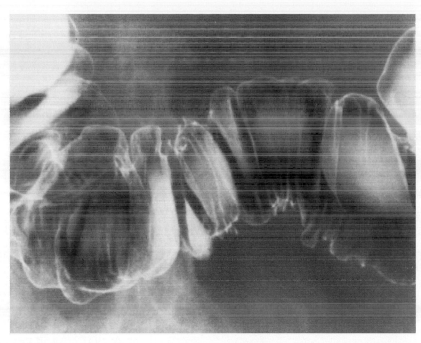

FIGURE 12–84. **Intraperitoneal implants from ovarian cancer spread to greater omentum causing "striping" of colon.** The contour of the transverse colon is spiculated. The mucosa is thrown into parallel folds. (From Rubesin, S.E., et al.: Other tumors. *In* Gore, R.M., Levine, M.S., and Laufer, I.: Textbook of Gastrointestinal Radiology. Philadelphia, W.B. Saunders Co., 1994, pp. 1200–1227, Fig. 65–37A.)

plantation. Consideration of the age of the patient and clinical history will let the radiologist make a graded differential diagnosis.

Peritoneal metastases involving the greater omentum, the so-called omental cakes, may abut or primarily invade the transverse colon.[165] Mass effect, spiculation of the luminal contour, and pleated folds are seen in the transverse colon (Fig. 12–85). The radiologic differential diagnosis at this site includes gastric or pancreatic cancer invading the transverse colon or inflammatory processes from cholecystitis, pancreatitis, or diverticulitis extending into the greater omentum.[165,167]

Hematogenous Metastases

Metastatic melanoma, breast carcinoma, and lung carcinoma are the tumors that most commonly spread to the colon by means of a hematogenous route. Breast metastases are usually small. Patients with metastatic breast cancer are usually asymptomatic, and barium enemas are rarely performed. Metastatic breast carcinoma to the colon appears as mucosal nodules, eccentric strictures, or long circumferential narrowings (linitis plastica) (Fig. 12–86).[155] Metastatic melanoma usually appears as an umbilicated submucosal mass (a target lesion) or as a bulky, polypoid intraluminal mass. Linear fissures radiating around a central ulcer may give metastatic melanoma a "spoke-wheel" appearance. The radiologic differential diagnosis of a colonic target lesion includes gastrointestinal stromal tumor, Kaposi's sarcoma, or lymphoma.

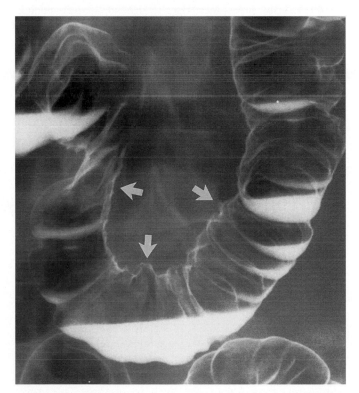

FIGURE 12–85. **"Omental cake" from ovarian cancer spreading to greater omentum.** Flattening of the superior border of the transverse colon *(arrows)* is due to mass effect by greater omental metastases. The superior border is also spiculated. The uninvolved inferior border of the colon is sacculated. (From Rubesin, S.E., et al.: Omental cakes: Colonic involvement by omental metastases. Radiology *154*:593–596, 1985, Fig. 3.)

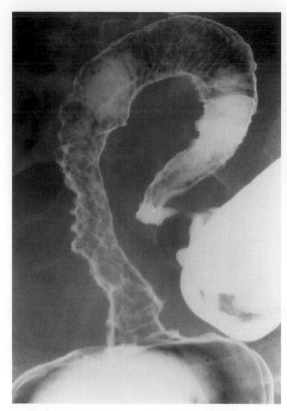

FIGURE 12–86. Breast metastases to sigmoid colon resulting in linitis plastica. The distal sigmoid colon is diffusely narrowed. The contour is focally spiculated. The mucosa is focally nodular. The differential diagnosis includes primary adenocarcinoma of the colon and Crohn's disease, as well as metastatic breast cancer.

PRACTICAL APPROACH TO THE DIAGNOSIS OF TUMORS OF THE COLON

Polyps

A polyp is a polyp (Fig. 12–87). The term *polyp* is not histologically specific. Most colonic polyps, whether sessile or pedunculated, are adenomatous or hyperplastic polyps. The radiologist and clinician assume a worse-case scenario. A polyp detected on barium enema or endoscopy is assumed to be an adenomatous polyp with potential for in situ carcinoma and further development of invasive carcinoma. The most important radiographic criterion for determining the malignant potential of the polyp is the size of the lesion. Approximately 1% of 6- to 10-mm adenomas are malignant.[38] Approximately 10% of 1- to 2-cm adenomas are malignant. Approximately 45% of adenomas larger than 2 cm harbor malignancy. Adenomas less than 5 mm are rarely malignant. Therefore, assuming any polyp is an adenoma, the radiologist and clinician can be reassured that unless there are very strong signs of malignancy in a polyp less than 1 cm, it is doubtful that this lesion will be a carcinoma. On the other hand, polyps greater than 1 cm have more than a 10% chance of being malignant and, therefore, should be excised.

Analysis of a polyp's contour and surface pattern rarely changes clinical decision making. Smooth-surfaced sessile polyps less than 1 cm are almost always benign.[60] Abnormal contour at a polyp's base suggests malignancy in polyps greater than 10 mm but not in small polyps (see Fig. 12–20).[60] A granular or a villous surface pattern may indicate tubulovillous change[45,46,48,168] and greater malignant potential. Centrally umbilicated flat polyps larger than 5 mm (see Fig. 12–18) may be malignant and must be biopsied, if not excised.

If a sessile polyp is small and has a smooth surface, it is hard to distinguish a submucosal from a mucosal lesion. Small, sessile rectal polyps are frequently hyperplastic polyps or occasionally carcinoid tumors.

Once a polyp can be described as a polypoid mass, about 2 cm, it is relatively easy to distinguish a submucosal tumor (Fig. 12–88) from a mucosal mass. This dramatically alters the differential diagnosis. Nodularity or an irregular mucosal surface suggests the possibility of adenocarcinoma in any tumor greater than 1 cm. A smooth-surfaced, bulky polypoid lesion may be a lipoma, lymphoma, or hemangioma. If a perfectly smooth polypoid mass changes size and shape, the diagnosis of lipoma or lymphangioma is made. CT can confirm the diagnosis of lipoma as a tumor of fatty attenuation or a lymphangioma as a cystic or multicystic tumor of water density.[121]

Polypoid masses at the anorectal junction have a wide range of histologic diagnoses (Fig. 12–89) because this is the transition zone between the columnar mucosa of the rectum, nonkeratinizing squamous epithelium of the anal canal, and true skin of the perianal region. Furthermore, the anal sphincter region is a zone of high pressure and frequent trauma. Internal hemorrhoids, solitary rectal ulcer syndrome, and lesions of the distal rectum are discussed in Chapter 15.

Carpet Lesions

Focal disruption of the smooth mucosal surface by a nonneoplastic disorder can be confused with an adenomatous carpet lesion (Fig. 12–90). One macroscopic form of the solitary rectal ulcer syndrome is an irregular surface pattern either focally or diffusely involving the rectum (see Fig. 12–90*A*). This lesion is frequently confused with a flat adenomatous lesion (see Fig. 12–90*B*), both endoscopically and radiologically. Focal trauma or trauma due to biopsy may resemble a carpet lesion (Fig. 12–90*C*). The colonic urticarial pattern, if focal, resembles the reticular pattern of a carpet lesion. When the colonic urticarial pattern is diffuse (Fig. 12–90*D*), there is little difficulty in diagnosis.

Polyposis Syndromes

When numerous polyps disrupt the smooth mucosal surface, pneumatosis coli must first be excluded. Then, inflammatory or postinflammatory polyps or plaques arising in ulcerative colitis, schistosomiasis, or *Clostridium difficile* colitis must be considered (see Chapter 13). Finally,

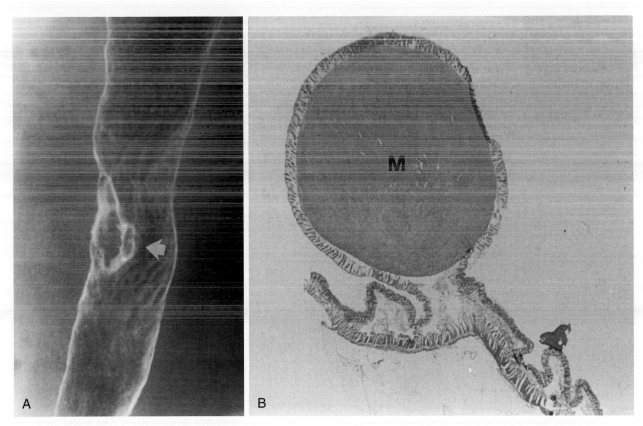

FIGURE 12–87. **A polyp is a polyp.** *A,* A coarsely lobulated polyp *(arrow)* is seen in the descending colon. The background mucosa is finely nodular in this patient with a long-standing history of ulcerative colitis. The pathologic diagnosis was an inflammatory polyp. *B,* A pedunculated polyp is seen in cross section at this low-power view. Rather than being the typical pedunculated adenoma, this polyp is covered by normal colonic epithelium. The lamina propria is expanded by a mass *(M)* of spindle cells, which at a higher power and with immunohistochemistry, proved to be smooth muscle cells. This is a rare true leiomyoma of the colon, presumptively arising in the muscularis mucosae; the final diagnosis is only determined by pathology

FIGURE 12–88. A 3-cm, broad-based, smooth-surfaced polypoid mass *(arrow)* is present in the cecum. The perfectly smooth mucosa in a lesion >2 cm is typical for a submucosal mass. The pathologic diagnosis was a lipoma.

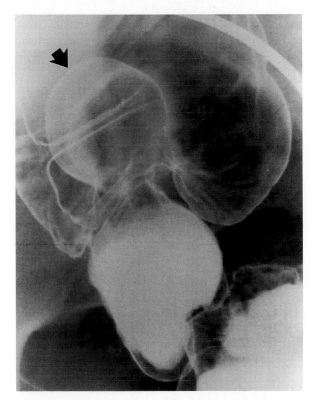

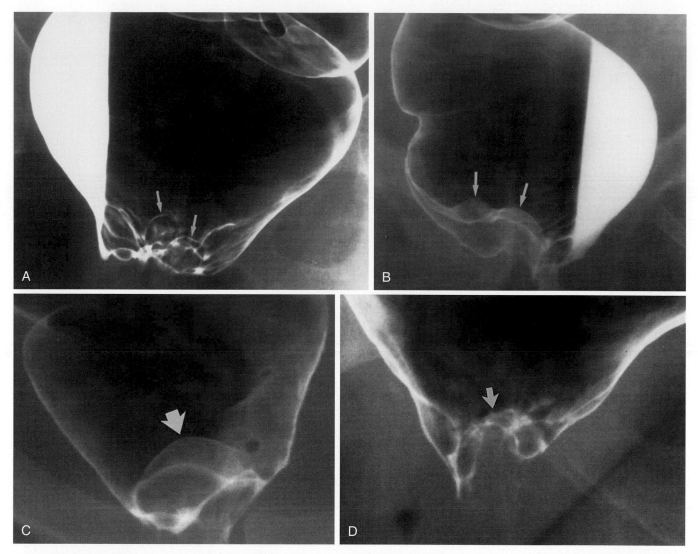

FIGURE 12–89. Polypoid anorectal junction masses. *A,* Four polypoid lesions *(two identified by arrows)* are present just proximal to the anorectal junction. These were internal hemorrhoids. (From Rubesin, S.E., et al.: Rectum. *In* Gore, R.M., Levine, M.S., and Laufer, I.: Textbook of Gastrointestinal Radiology. Philadelphia, W.B. Saunders Co., 1994, pp. 1261–1309, Fig. 65–13*F.) B,* Bilobed, smooth-surfaced polypoid mass *(arrows)* in the distal rectum. Pathologic diagnosis was colitis cystica profunda, part of the spectrum of the chronic mucosal prolapse syndrome. *C,* Smooth-surfaced, polypoid mass in the distal rectum *(arrow).* Pathologic diagnosis was an anal papilloma. *D,* A 2-cm mass *(arrow)* with a nodular surface and enlargement of the columns of Morgagni. Adenocarcinoma arising in distal rectum with invasion of anal canal. (*B* and *D* from Kahn, S., and Rubesin, S.E.: Polypoid lesions at the anorectal junction: Barium enema findings. AJR. Am. J. Roentgenol. *161*:339–342, 1993, Figs. 7 and 11. © American Roentgen Ray Society.)

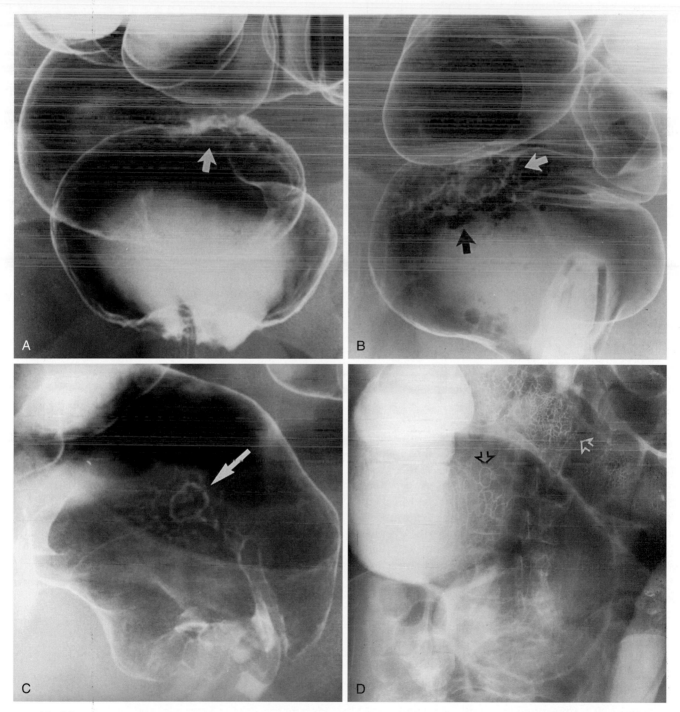

FIGURE 12–90. Carpet lesions of the colon. *A,* A 3-cm focal area of mucosal nodularity *(arrow)* is seen in the mid-rectum. Pathologic diagnosis was solitary rectal ulcer syndrome. *B,* A 3-cm area of confluent mucosal nodularity *(arrows)* is present on the right lateral wall of the mid-rectum. This was a tubular adenoma with a focus of high-grade dysplasia. (From Rubesin, S.E., et al.: Carpet lesions of the colon. Radio-Graphics *5:*537–552, 1985, Fig. 7A.) *C,* A nodular surface pattern radiates from a central ring shadow *(arrow).* Shallow ulcer or carpet lesion? This was a biopsy site. (Courtesy of H. DeGryse, M.D., Antwerp, Belgium. From Rubesin, S.E., et al.: Carpet lesions of the colon. RadioGraphics *5:*537–552, 1985, Fig. 16.) *D,* A reticular, mosaic pattern is seen in the transverse *(white arrow)* and ascending colon *(black arrow).* This colonic urticarial pattern was due to acute adynamic ileus. (From Rubesin, S.E., et al.: Carpet lesions of the colon. RadioGraphics *5:*537–552, 1985, Fig. 19A.) If focal, a colonic urticarial pattern can mimic a carpet lesion.

a diagnosis of a polyposis syndrome (Fig. 12–91) is considered. The age of the patient, family history, and clinical history will greatly narrow the radiologic differential diagnosis before endoscopy and biopsy.

In familial adenomatous polyposis syndrome (FAPS), a positive family history is present in 80% of patients with this autosomal dominant disorder.[169] Adenomas do not develop until the late second decade.[36,169] Colonic symptoms of rectal bleeding, diarrhea, or mucous discharge appear in the fourth decade.[169,170] If a radiologist performs a barium enema on a patient with known FAPS, the purpose of the study is to detect colonic cancers. In asymptomatic patients with positive family history, the purpose of the study is to detect FAPS. In symptomatic patients without family history, barium enema will show numerous (>100) small, sessile polyps (see Fig. 12–91A and B) and frequently one or more coexisting carcinomas. Some patients with FAPS may present with symptoms from a malignant central nervous system tumor, previously classified as Turcot's syndrome.[171] Young patients, especially women, may present with symptoms from a papillary carcinoma of the thyroid gland,[172] part of the previously classified Gardner's syndrome.[173] Other common manifestations of FAPS diagnosed by the abdominal radiologist are fundic gland polyps of the gastric body and fundus,[174,175] duodenal adenomas and carcinomas arising particularly in or near the papilla of Vater,[176,177] intraabdominal mesenteric fibromatosis,[178] and desmoid tumors of the anterior abdominal wall.

A greater percentage of patients with Peutz-Jegher's syndrome are spontaneous mutants than those patients with FAPS. Only 50% to 60% of patients with Peutz-Jegher's syndrome have a family history of this autosomally dominant disorder.[179] The bulk of patients with Peutz-Jegher's syndrome only have a few large, pedunculated hamartomas in the colon and should not be confused with patients who have FAP. In patients with Peutz-Jegher's syndrome there is a greater risk of duodenal cancer (1% to 3%) than of colonic cancer.[180] The abdominal radiologist's main role in Peutz-Jegher's syndrome is the detection of small bowel hamartomas (see Chapter 10).

The small polyps of the multiple hamartoma syndrome (MHS, Cowden's disease) usually do not cause symptoms. Barium studies in patients with family history of this autosomal dominant disease are performed to screen for the presence of the disease, particularly when skin lesions are present. The small (<5 mm), sessile hamartomas are most frequently found in the rectosigmoid colon and stomach but are present in all parts of the gastrointestinal tract.[179] About 50% of patients with known MHS have thyroid abnormalities, including follicular adenocarcinoma of the thyroid that is detected in 10% of patients.[181,182] Screening mammography is essential, as breast carcinoma develops in 30% of women with MHS at an early age, in their fourth decade.[181,182]

Patients with Cronkhite-Canada syndrome have a markedly different clinical history than patients with other polyposis syndromes. Patients with Cronkhite-Canada syndrome present at an elderly age with diarrhea, abdominal pain, and weight loss.[183] The fluid, electrolyte, protein, and blood loss is so severe that electrolyte disturbances, anemia, and hypoproteinemia ensue. The cutaneous hyperpigmentation, alopecia, and nail dystrophy of this sporadic syndrome usually follow the diarrhea.[179] The cutaneous findings precede gastrointestinal symptoms in only 10% of patients. Numerous 0.5- to 1.5-cm sessile polyps are seen in the colon.[184] The stomach is carpeted by tiny polyps.[184]

The two major forms of multiple juvenile polyposis syndromes should not be confused with FAPS. Isolated juvenile polyps have been previously discussed. In the rare form of juvenile polyposis, patients present in the first 2 years of life with a severe mucoid or bloody diarrhea.[179] In the second form, many juvenile polyps are evident throughout the gastrointestinal tract by the second decade.[185] In about one fourth of these patients the disease is transmitted as an autosomal dominant disorder.[179] Patients complain of rectal prolapse, rectal bleeding, and symptoms of small bowel intussusception. Numerous small (2 to 3 mm) polyps are found in the small bowel and colon (Fig. 12–91C). An increased incidence of pancreatic and colonic cancer is present.[185]

Extrinsic Masses

Inflammatory disorders involving the colon (Fig. 12–92) have a similar radiologic appearance to intraperitoneal metastasis, invasion of the colon by a contiguous tumor, or spread of tumor along a fatty mesentery (Table 12–6). Extrinsic masses at the rectosigmoid junction include intraperitoneal metastasis, direct invasion by local cancer (see Figs. 12–76 and 12–78), endometriosis (see Fig. 12–92A), or pelvic abscess (see Fig. 12–92B). Pancreatitis can spread to the transverse colon (see Fig. 12–92C). Inflammation related to appendicitis can spread to the medial base of the cecum (see Fig. 12–92D) and terminal ileum (see Fig. 12–92E), the right pericolic gutter (see Fig. 12–92F), or the pelvis. Some extrinsic masses invad-

TABLE 12–6. *Common Disorders Extrinsically Involving Colon*

Intraperitoneal Metastasis
Ovary, stomach, pancreas, colon: most frequent sites of origin

Direct Invasion by Tumor or Contiguous Spread via Mesentery
Rectum: cancer of cervix or prostate
Sigmoid: ovarian cancer
Splenic flexure: pancreatic cancer, renal cell cancer of left kidney
Transverse colon: gastric cancer
Hepatic flexure: renal cell cancer of right kidney

Inflammatory Disorders
Abscess from appendicitis, diverticulitis, Crohn's disease, tuboovarian abscess
Peritonitis from tuberculosis, peritoneal dialysis
Pancreatitis
Postoperative

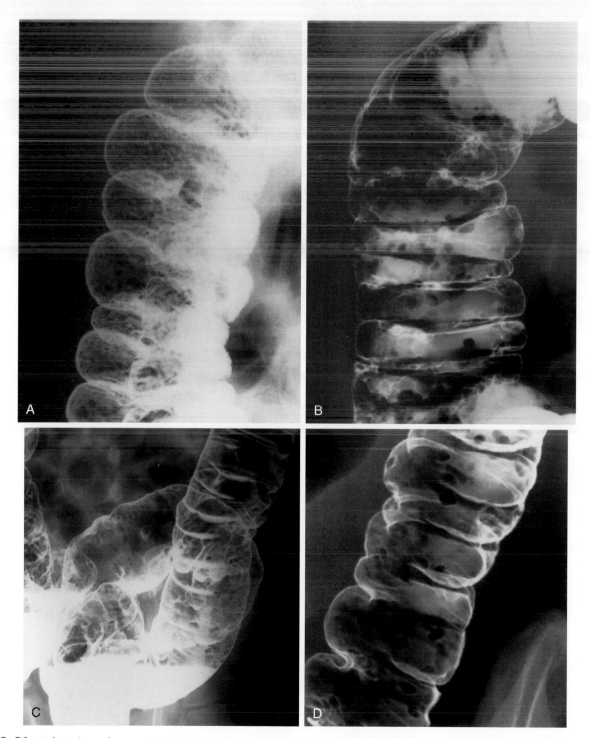

FIGURE 12–91. **Polyposis syndromes.** *A,* Numerous 2- to 3-mm nodules carpet the hepatic flexure. These nodules are more numerous and slightly less uniform than lymphoid hyperplasia. This patient had FAPS. *B,* Numerous 2- to 5-mm in diameter polyps carpet the ascending colon. This patient had FAPS. *C,* Numerous polyps are seen in the descending and sigmoid colon. This seven-year-old had juvenile polyposis. *D,* Numerous polyps are seen in the descending colon. These were neurofibromas in a patient with known neurofibromatosis.

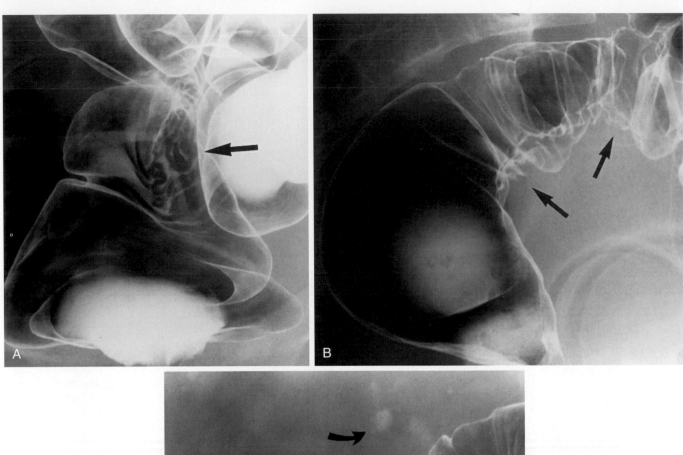

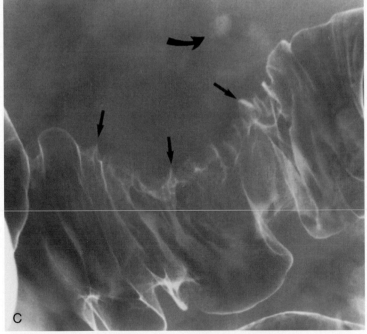

FIGURE 12–92. **Extrinsic abnormalities involving the colon.** *A,* Prone, angle overhead view shows that the colonic mucosa has been pulled into smooth, sinuous folds *(arrow)* by a desmoplastic process in the serosal and muscular layers. Endometriosis involving the rectosigmoid junction. (From Rubesin, S.E., and Laufer, I.: Pictorial glossary of double contrast radiology. *In* Gore, R.M., Levine, M.S., and Laufer, I.: Textbook of Gastrointestinal Radiology. Philadelphia, W.B. Saunders Co., 1994, pp. 50–80, Fig. 38.) *B,* In this patient with fever and a palpable pelvic mass, the anterior wall of the rectosigmoid junction shows extrinsic mass effect and spiculation of the contour *(arrows).* Tubo-ovarian abscess involving the rectosigmoid junction. (From Rubesin, S.E., et al.: Rectum. *In* Gore, R.M., Levine, M.S., and Laufer, I.: Textbook of Gastrointestinal Radiology. Philadelphia, W.B. Saunders Co., 1994, pp. 1261–1309, Fig. 65–37.) *C,* Spiculation *(arrows)* and extrinsic mass effect is seen on the superior border of the transverse colon. Subtle pancreatic calcifications *(curved arrow)* are the radiologic clue to the diagnosis of pancreatitis involving the transverse colon.

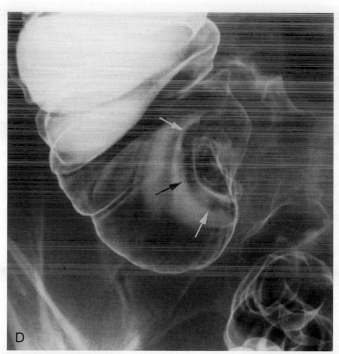

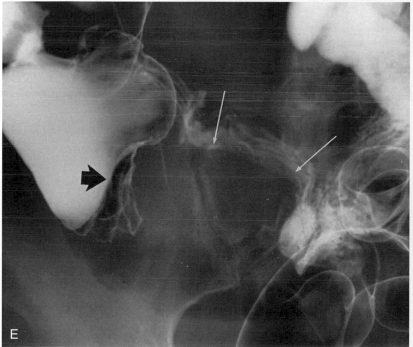

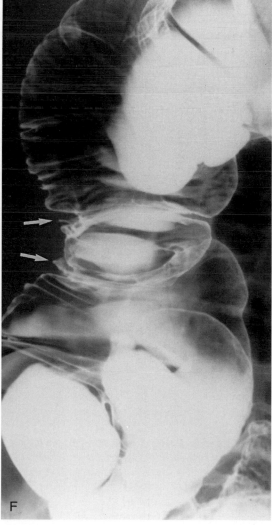

FIGURE **12–92** *Continued* D, Extrinsic mass effect causes concentric ring shadows *(arrows)* on the medial border of the base of the cecum. This patient with chronic right lower quadrant pain had appendicitis. E, Extrinsic mass effect on the medial border of the base of the cecum *(black arrow)* and the lateral border of the terminal ileum *(white arrows)* is seen. This patient with chronic abdominal pain had colonoscopy showing erythema near the orifice of the appendix. At pathologic examination, actinomycosis growing in an appendiceal abscess was detected. F, Spiculation *(arrows)* and mild extrinsic mass effect is seen along the lateral border of the ascending colon. Appendicitis with spread of inflammation up the right paracolic gutter caused this radiographic appearance mimicking intraperitoneal metastases.

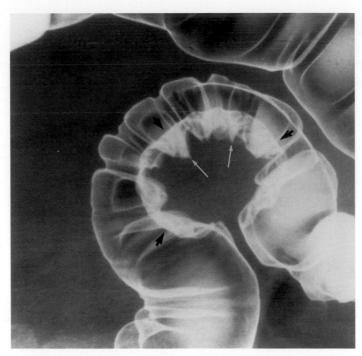

FIGURE 12–93. Endometrioma of sigmoid colon. The contour of the sigmoid colon is focally spiculated *(white arrows).* Part of the mesenteric wall of the sigmoid colon shows deep, smooth-surfaced indentation *(black arrows),* indicating muscular hypertrophy.

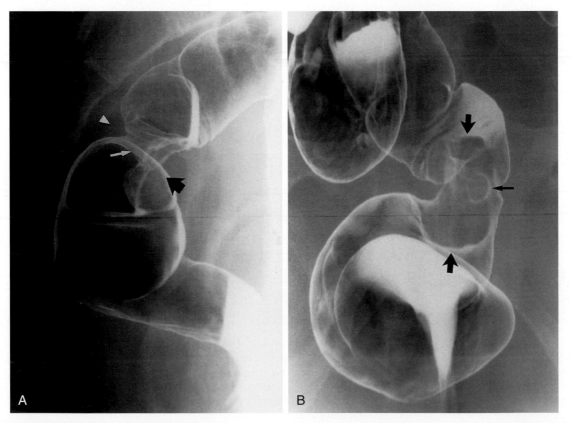

FIGURE 12–94. Endometrioma of rectosigmoid junction. *A,* Prone, cross-table lateral view of rectum shows a polypoid mass *(black arrow)* on the anterior wall of the rectosigmoid junction. The mass has abrupt angles and a focal polypoid projection centrally *(white arrow).* The desmoplastic effect of the lesion has caused focal, smooth, circumferential narrowing of the rectum *(arrowhead). B,* Prone, angled view of rectosigmoid junction shows that the polypoid mass *(large arrows)* has a smooth surface and is very sharply circumscribed. A ring shadow *(small arrow)* is seen centrally, the site of polypoid projection in *A.* (From Rubesin, S.E., et al.: Rectum. *In* Gore, R.M., Levine, M.S., and Lauter, I.: Textbook of Gastrointestinal Radiology. Philadelphia, W.B. Saunders Co., 1994, pp. 1261–1309, Fig. 65–65.)

ing the colon have a large submucosal component. Endometriosis incites smooth muscle hypertrophy, resulting in a prominent submucosal mass (Figs. 12–93 and 12–94). The age and clinical history will narrow the radiologic differential diagnosis in many patients.

REFERENCES

1. Parker, S.H., Torry, T., Bolden, S., et al.: Cancer statistics. Canc. J. Clin. *65*:5, 1996.
2. Bowland, C.R.: Malignant tumors of the colon. *In* Yamada, T. (ed). Textbook of Gastroenterology, ed. 2. New York, JB Lippincott, 1995, p. 1967.
3. Silverberg, E., and Lubera, J.A.: Cancer statistics. Cancer *38*:5, 1988.
4. Kinzler, K.W., Nilbert, M.C., Su, L.K., et al.: Identification of FAP locus genes from chromosome 5q21. Science *253*:661, 1991.
5. Petersen, G.M., Slack, J., and Nakamura, Y.: Screening guidelines and premorbid diagnosis of familial adenomatous polyposis using linkage. Gastroenterology *100*:1658, 1991.
6. Mecklin, J.P.: Frequency of hereditary colorectal carcinoma. Gastroenterology *93*:1021, 1987.
7. Lynch, H.T., Smyrk, T., Lanspa, S.J., et al.: Flat adenomas in a colon cancer–prone kindred. J. Natl. Cancer Inst. *80*:278, 1988.
8. Lynch, H.T., Smyrk, T.C., Watson, P., et al.: Genetics, natural history, tumor spectrum, and pathology of hereditary nonpolyposis colorectal cancer: An updated review. Gastroenterology *104*:1535, 1993.
9. Burt, R.W., Bishop, D.T., Cannon-Albright, L., et al.: Population genetics of colonic cancer. Cancer *70*:1719, 1993.
10. Pollack, E.S., Nomura, A.M.Y., Heilbrun, L.K., et al.: Prospective study of alcohol consumption and cancer. N. Engl. J. Med. *310*:617, 1984.
11. Sandler, R.S., Lyles, C.M., McAuliffe, C., et al.: Cigarette smoking, alcohol, and the risk of colorectal adenomas. Gastroenterology *104*:1445, 1993.
12. Cummings, J.H., Wiggins, H.S., Jenkins, D.J.A., et al.: Influence of diets high and low in animal fat on bowel habit, gastrointestinal transit, fecal microflora, bile acid and fat excretion. J. Clin. Invest. *61*:953, 1978.
13. Willett, W.C., Stamper, M.J., Colditz, G.A., et al.: Relation of meat, fat, and fiber intake to the risk of colon cancer in a prospective study among women. N. Engl. J. Med. *323*:1664, 1990.
14. Cheever, A.W.: Schistosomiasis and colon cancer. Lancet *1*:1369, 1981.
15. Greenstein, A.J., Sachar, D.B., Smith, H., et al.: Cancer in universal and left-sided ulcerative colitis: Factors determining risk. Gastroenterology *77*:290, 1979.
16. Sandler, R.S., and Sandler, D.P.: Radiation-induced cancers of the colon and rectum: Assessing the risk. Gastroenterology *84*:51, 1983.
17. Morson, B.C., and Bussey, H.J.R.: Magnitude of risk for cancer in patients with colorectal adenomas. Br. J. Surg. *72*:S23, 1985.
18. Clark, J.C., Collan, Y., Eide, T.J., et al.: Prevalence of polyps in an autopsy series from areas with varying incidence of large bowel cancer. Int. J. Cancer *36*:179, 1985.
19. Lotfi, A.M., Spencer, R.J., Ilstrup, D.M., et al.: Colorectal polyps and the risk of subsequent carcinoma. Mayo Clin. Proc. *61*:337, 1986.
20. Hastings, J.B.: Mass screening for colorectal cancer. Am. J. Surg. *127*:228, 1974.
21. Miller, M.P., and Stanley, T.V.: Results of a mass screening program for colorectal cancer. Arch. Surg. *123*:63, 1988.
22. Newcomb, P.A., Norfleet, R.G., Storer, B.E., et al.: Screening sigmoidoscopy and colorectal cancer mortality. J. Natl. Cancer Inst. *84*:1572, 1992.
23. Scheitel, S.M., Ahlquist, D.A., Wollan, P.C., et al.: Colorectal cancer screening: A case control community study. J. Gen. Intern. Med. *10*:5103, 1995.
24. Mandel, J.S., Bond, J.H., Church, T.R., et al.: Reducing mortality from colorectal cancer by screening for fecal occult blood. N. Engl. J. Med. *328*:1365, 1993.
25. Simon, J.B.: Occult blood screening for colorectal carcinoma: A critical review. Gastroenterology *88*:820, 1985.
26. Ahlquist, D.A., Wieand, H.S., Moertel, C.G., et al.: Accuracy of fecal occult blood screening for colorectal neoplasia: A prospective study using Hemoccult and HemoQuant Tests. JAMA *269*:1262, 1993.
27. Muller, A.D., Sonnenberg, A.: Protection by endoscopy against death from colorectal cancer. A case-control study among veterans. Arch. Intern. Med. *155*:1741, 1995.
28. Selby, J.V., Friedman, G.D., Quesenberry, C.P., et al.: A case-control study of screening sigmoidoscopy and mortality from colorectal cancer. N. Engl. J. Med. *326*:653, 1992.
29. McCarthy, P.A., Rubesin, S.E., Levine, M.S., et al.: Colon cancer: Morphology detected with barium enema examination versus histopathologic stage. Radiology *197*:683, 1995.
30. Lemmel, G.T., Hageman, J.H., Rex, D.K., et al.: Neoplasia distal to the splenic flexure in patients with proximal colon cancer. Gastrointest. Endosc. *44*:109, 1996.
31. Chodash, H.B., and Ahlquist, D.A.: Are rectosigmoid polyps a sensitive marker for proximal colon cancers? Gastrointest. Endosc. *36*:213, 1990.
32. Eddy, D.M., Nugent, F.W., Eddy, J.F., et al.: Screening for colorectal cancer in a high-risk population. Results of a mathematical model. Gastroenterology *92*:682, 1987.
33. Eddy, D.M.: Screening for colorectal cancer. Ann. Intern. Med. *113*:373, 1990.
34. Winawer, S.J., Zauber, A.G., Ho, M.N., et al.: Prevention of colorectal cancer by colonoscopic polypectomy. N. Engl. J. Med. *329*:1977, 1993.
35. Anderson, M.L., Heigh, R.I., McCoy, G.A., et al.: Accuracy of assessment of the extent of examination by experienced colonoscopists. Gastrointest. Endosc. *38*:560, 1992.
36. Bussey, H.J.R.: Familial Polyposis Coli: Family Studies, Histopathology. Differential Diagnosis and Results of Treatment. Baltimore, Johns Hopkins University Press, 1975, p. 47.
37. Winawer, S.J., Fletcher, R.H., Miller, L., et al.: Colorectal cancer screening: Clinical guidelines and rationale. Gastroenterology *112*:594, 1997.
38. Muto, T., Bussey, H.J.R., and Morson, B.C.: The evolution of cancer of the colon and rectum. Cancer *36*:2251, 1975.
39. Fenoglio-Preiser, C.M., Pascal, R.R., and Perzin, K.H.: Tumors of the Intestines. Atlas of Tumor Pathology, Second Series, Fascicle 27. Washington, DC, Armed Forces Institute of Pathology, 1990.
40. Fung, C.H., and Goldman, H.: The incidence and significance of villous change in adenomatous polyps. Am. J. Clin. Pathol. *53*:21, 1970.
41. Fenoglio-Preiser, C.M., and Hutter, R.V.: Colorectal polyps: Pathologic diagnosis and clinical significance. CA. Cancer J. Clin. *3*:322, 1985.
42. Silverberg, S.G.: Focally malignant adenomatous polyps of the colon and rectum. Surg. Gynecol. Obstet. *131*:103, 1970.
43. Winawer, S.J., Zauber, A.G., O'Brien, M.J., et al.: The National Polyp Study: Designs, methods and characteristics of patients with newly diagnosed polyps. Cancer *70*:1236, 1992.
44. Jacob, H., Schlondorff, D., St. Onge, G., et al.: Villous adenoma depletion syndrome: Evidence for a cyclic nucleotide-mediated diarrhea. Dig. Dis. Sci. *30*:637, 1985.
45. Thompson, J.J., and Enterline, H.T.: The macroscopic appearance of colorectal polyps. Cancer *48*:151, 1981.
46. Wolf, B.S.: Roentgen diagnosis of villous tumors of the colon. AJR. Am. J. Roentgenol. *84*:1093, 1960.
47. Rubesin, S.E., Saul, S.H., Laufer, I., et al.: Carpet lesions of the colon. RadioGraphics *5*:537, 1985.
48. Iida, M., Iwashita, A., Yao, T., et al.: Villous tumor of the colon: Correlation of histologic, macroscopic, and radiographic features. Radiology *167*:673, 1988.
49. Delamarre, J., Descombes, P., Marti, R., et al.: Villous tumors of the colon and rectum: Double-contrast study of 47 cases. Gastrointest. Radiol. *5*:69, 1980.
50. Youker, J.E., Welin, S.: Differentiation of the true polypoid lesions of the colon from extraneous material, a new roentgen sign. Radiology *84*:610, 1965.
51. Miller, W.T., Levine, M.S., Rubesin, S.E., et al.: Bowler-hat sign: A simple principle for differentiating polyps from diverticula. Radiology *173*:615, 1989.
52. Spratt, J.S., and Ackerman, L.V.: Small primary adenocarcinomas of the colon and rectum. JAMA *179*:337, 1962.

53. Gabrielsson, N., Granqvist, S., Ohlsen, H., et al.: Malignancy of colonic polyps: Diagnosis and management. Acta Radiol. *19:*479, 1978.

54. Skucas, J., Spataro, R.F., and Cannucciara, D.P.: The radiographic features of small colon cancers. Radiology *143:*335, 1982.

55. Welin, S., Youker, J., and Spratt, J.S., Jr.: The rates and patterns of growth of 375 tumors of the large intestine and rectum observed serially by double contrast enema study (Malmo technique). AJR. Am. J. Roentgenol. *90:*673, 1963.

56. Smith, T.R.: Pedunculated malignant colonic polyps with superficial invasion of the stalk. Radiology *115:*593, 1975.

57. Maruyama, M.: Radiologic Diagnosis of Polyps and Carcinoma of the Large Bowel. Tokyo, Igaku-Shoin, 1978.

58. Haggitt, R.C., Glotzbach, R.E., Soffer, E.E., et al.: Prognostic factors in colorectal carcinomas arising in adenomas: Implications for lesion removal by endoscopic polypectomy. Gastroenterology *89:*328, 1985.

59. Ament, A.E., Alfidi, R.J., and Rao, P.S.: Basal indentation of sessile polypoid lesions: A function of geometry rather than a sign of malignancy. Radiology *143:*341, 1982.

60. Ott, D.J., Gelfand, D.W., Wu, W.C., et al.: Colon polyp morphology on double-contrast barium enema: Its pathologic predictive value. AJR. Am. J. Roentgenol. *141:*965, 1983.

61. Gohel, V.K., Kressel, H.Y., and Laufer, I.: Double contrast artifacts. Gastrointest. Radiol. *3:*139, 1978.

62. Press, H.C., and Davis, T.W.: Ingested foreign bodies simulating polyposis: Report of six cases. AJR. Am. J. Roentgenol. *127:*1040, 1976.

63. Heald, R.J., and Bussey, H.J.R.: Clinical experiences at St. Mark's Hospital with multiple synchronous cancers of the colon and rectum. Dis. Colon Rectum *18:*6, 1975.

64. Brahme, F., Ekelund, G.R., Norden, J.G., et al.: Metachronous colorectal polyps: Comparison of development of colorectal polyps and carcinomas with and without history of polyps. Dis. Colon Rectum *17:*166, 1974.

65. Kelvin, F.M., Maglinte, D.D.T., and Stephens, B.A.: Colorectal carcinoma detected initially with barium enema examination: Site distribution and implications. Radiology *169:*649, 1988.

66. Maglinte, D.D.T., Keller, K.J., Miller, R.E., et al.: Colon and rectal carcinoma: Spatial distribution and detection. Radiology *147:*669, 1983.

67. Morgenstern, L., and Lee, S.E.: Spatial distribution of colonic carcinoma. Arch. Surg. *113:*1142, 1978.

68. Snyder, D.N., Heston, J.F., Meigs, J.W., et al.: Changes in site distribution of colorectal carcinoma in Connecticut, 1940–1973. Dig. Dis. Sci. *22:*791, 1977.

69. Johnson, H., Jr., and Carstens, R.: Anatomical distribution of colonic carcinomas: Interracial differences in a community hospital population. Cancer *58:*997, 1986.

70. Ishikawa, T., et al: Four cases of colorectal tumors presenting a flat sessile elevated lesion composed of multiple aggregated granules: With particular emphasis on retrospective radiographic study. Stom. Intest. *21:*1379, 1986.

71. Shimoda, T., Ikegami, M., Fujisaki, J., et al.: Early colorectal carcinoma with special reference to its development de novo. Cancer *64:*1138, 1989.

72. Matsui, T., Yao, T., Yao, K., et al.: Natural history of superficial depressed colorectal cancer: Retrospective radiographic and histologic analysis. Radiology *201:*226, 1996.

73. Matsumoto, T., Iida, M., Kohrogi, N., et al.: Minute nonpolypoid adenomas of the colon depicted with barium enema examination. Radiology *187:*377, 1993.

74. Fujiya, M., and Maruyama, M.: Small depressed neoplasms of the large bowel: Radiographic visualization and clinical significance. Abdom. Imaging *22:*325, 1997.

75. Ushio, K., Shima, Y., Goto, Y., et al.: Growth and progression of colorectal cancer: Retrospective study based on roentgenologic findings. Stom. Intest. *20:*843, 1985.

76. Dukes, C.: The classification of cancer of the rectum. J. Pathol. Bacteriol. *35:*323, 1932.

77. Astler, V.B., and Coller, F.A.: The prognostic significance of direct extension of carcinoma of the colon and rectum. Ann. Surg. *139:*846, 1954.

78. Turnbull, R.B., Kyle, K., Watson, F.B., et al.: Cancer of the colon: The influence of the no-touch isolation technique on survival rates. Ann. Surg. *166:*400, 1966.

79. Zinkin, L.D.: A critical review of the classification and staging of colorectal cancer. Dis. Colon Rectum *26:*37, 1983.

80. Boring, C.C., Squires, T.S., and Tong, T.: Cancer statistics. Cancer *42:*19, 1954.

81. McCarty, R.L.: Colorectal cancer: The case for barium enema. Mayo Clin. Proc. *67:*253, 1992.

82. Rice, R.P.: Lowering death rates from colorectal cancer: Challenge for the 1990's. Radiology *176:*297, 1990.

83. Kelvin, F.M., Gardiner, R., Vas, W., et al.: Colorectal carcinoma missed on double contrast barium enema study: A problem in perception. AJR. Am. J. Roentgenol. *137:*307, 1981.

84. Ott, D.J., Gelfand, D.W., and Ramquist, N.A.: Causes of error in gastrointestinal radiology. Gastrointest. Radiol. *5:*99, 1980.

85. Baker, S.R., and Alterman, D.D.: False-negative barium enema in patients with sigmoid cancer and coexistent diverticula. Gastrointest. Radiol. *10:*171, 1985.

86. Dreyfuss, J.R., and Benacerraf, B.: Saddle cancers of the colon and their progression to annular carcinomas. Radiology *129:*289, 1978.

87. Laufer, I., and Joffe, N.: Roentgenologic aspects of chronic perforating carcinoma of the colon: Report of five cases. Dis. Colon Rectum *16:*127, 1973.

88. Raskin, M.M., Viamonte, M., and Viamonte, M., Jr.: Primary linitis plastica carcinoma of the colon. Radiology *113:*17, 1974.

89. Hartzell, H.V.: To err with air. JAMA *187:*455, 1964.

90. Daly, B.D., and Crowley, B.M.: Radiological appearances of colonic ring staple anastomoses. Br. J. Radiol. *62:*256, 1989.

91. Welch, J.P., and Donaldson, G.A.: Detection and treatment of recurrent cancer of the colon and rectum. Am. J. Surg. *135:*505, 1978.

92. Shauffer, I.A., and Sequeira, J.: Suture granuloma simulating recurrent carcinoma. AJR. Am. J. Roentgenol. *128:*856, 1977.

93. Morson, B.C., and Dawson, I.M.P.: Gastrointestinal Pathology, ed. 2. Oxford, Blackwell Scientific Publications, 1979.

94. Fenoglio-Preiser, C.M., Noffsinger, A.E., Franzim, G., et al.: Other tumors of the large intestine. *In* Whitehead, R. (ed.). Gastrointestinal and Oesphageal Pathology. Edinburgh, Churchill Livingstone, 1995, p. 863.

95. Levine, M.S., Barnes, M.J., and Bronner, M.P.: Atypical hyperplastic polyps at double contrast barium enema examination. Radiology *175:*691, 1990.

96. Harned, R.K., Doby, C.A., and Farley, G.E.: Cavernous hemangioma of the rectum and appendix. Dis. Colon Rectum *17:*759, 1974.

97. Dachman, A.H., Ros, P.R., Shekitka, K.M., et al.: Colorectal hemangioma: Radiologic findings. Radiology *167:*31, 1988.

98. Ghahremani, G.G., Kangarloo, H., Volberg, F., et al.: Diffuse cavernous hemangioma of the colon in the Klippel-Trénaunay syndrome. Radiology *118:*673, 1976.

99. Gandolfi, L., Rossi, A., Stasi, G., et al.: The Klippel-Trénaunay syndrome. Gastrointest. Endosc. *33:*442, 1987.

100. Goboes, K.: Rare and secondary (metastatic) tumors. *In* Whitehead, R. (ed.). Gastrointestinal and Oesphageal Pathology. Edinburgh, Churchill Livingstone, 1995, p. 910.

101. Reinhart, W.H., Staubli, M., Mordasini, C., et al.: Abnormalities of the gut vessels in Turner's syndrome. Postgrad. Med. J. *59:*122, 1983.

102. Lyon, D.T., and Mantea, A.G.: Large-bowel hemangiomas. Dis. Colon Rectum *27:*404, 1984.

103. Margulis, A.R.: Selected cases from the film interpretation session of the Society of Gastrointestinal Radiologists. Case 1: Hemangioma of the rectum. Gastrointest. Radiol. *6:*363, 1981.

104. Agha, F.P., Francis, I.R., and Simms, S.M.: Cystic lymphangioma of the colon. AJR. Am. J. Roentgenol. *141:*709, 1983.

105. Young, T.-H., Ho, A.-S., Tang, H.-S., et al.: Cystic lymphangioma of the transverse colon: Report of a case and review of the literature. Abdom. Imaging *21:*415, 1996.

106. Boley, S.J., Sammartano, R., Adams, A., et al.: On the nature and etiology of vascular ectasias of the colon: Degenerative lesions of aging. Gastroenterology *72:*650, 1977.

107. Baum, S., Athanasoulis, C., Waltman, A., et al.: Angiodysplasia of the right colon: A cause of gastrointestinal bleeding. AJR. Am. J. Roentgenol. *129*:789, 1977.

108. Thompson, G.B., Pemberton, J.H., Morris, S., et al.: Kaposi's sarcoma of the colon in a young HIV-negative man with chronic ulcerative colitis. Dis. Colon Rectum *32*:73, 1989.

109. Puy-Montbrun, T., Pigot, F., et al.: Kaposi's sarcoma of the colon in a young HIV-negative woman with Crohn's disease. Dig. Dis. Sci. *36*:528, 1991.

110. Wall, S.D., Friedman, S.L., and Margulis, A.R.: Gastrointestinal Kaposi's sarcoma in AIDS: Radiographic manifestations. J. Clin. Gastroenterol. *6*:165, 1984.

111. Haller, J.D., and Roberts, T.W.: Lipomas of the colon: A clinicopathologic study of 40 cases. Surgery *55*:773, 1964.

112. Castro, D.B., and Stearns, M.W.: Lipomas of the large intestine. Dis. Colon Rectum *15*:441, 1972.

113. Kawamoto, K., Motooka, M., Hirata, N., et al.: Colonic submucosal tumors: New classification based on radiologic characteristics. AJR. Am. J. Roentgenol. *160*:315, 1993.

114. Hurwitz, M.H., Redleaf, P.D., Williams, H.J., et al.: Lipomas of the gastrointestinal tract. AJR. Am. J. Roentgenol. *99*:84, 1967.

115. Margulis, A.R., and Jovanovich, A.: The roentgen diagnosis of submucous lipomas of the colon. AJR. Am. J. Roentgenol. *84*:1114, 1960.

116. Wulff, C., and Jespersen, N.: Colo-colic intussusception caused by lipoma: Case report. Acta Radiol. *36*:478, 1995.

117. Kabaalioglu, A., Gelen, T., Akta, S., et al.: Acute colonic obstruction caused by intussusception and extrusion of a sigmoid lipoma through the anus after barium enema. Abdom. Imaging *22*:389, 1997.

118. Deeths, T.M., and Dodds, W.J.: Lipoma of the colon. Am. J. Gastroenterol. *58*:326, 1972.

119. Heiken, J.P., Forde, K.A., and Gold, R.P.: Computed tomography as a definitive method for diagnosing gastrointestinal lipomas. Radiology *142*:409, 1982.

120. Megibow, A.J., Redmond, P.E., Bosniak, M.A., et al.: Diagnosis of gastrointestinal lipomas by CT. AJR. Am. J. Roentgenol. *133*:743, 1979.

121. Kawamoto, K., Ueyama, T., Iwashita, I., et al.: Colonic submucosal tumors: Comparison of endoscopic US and target air-enema CT with barium enema study and colonoscopy. Radiology *192*:697, 1994.

122. Liesi, G., Pavanello, M., Cesari, S., et al.: Large lipomas of the colon. CT and MR findings in three symptomatic cases. Abdom. Imaging *21*:152, 1996.

123. Buetow, P.C., Buck, J.L., Carr, N.J., et al.: Intussuscepted colonic lipomas: Loss of fat attenuation on CT with pathologic correlation in 10 cases. Abdom. Imaging *21*:153, 1996.

124. Hinkel, C.L.: Roentgenological examination and evaluation of the ileocecal valve. AJR. Am. J. Roentgenol. *68*:171, 1952.

125. Lasser, E.C., and Rigler, L.C.: Ileocecal valve syndrome. Gastroenterology *28*:1, 1955.

126. Sato, T., Sakai, Y., Sonoyama, A., et al.: Radiologic spectrum of rectal carcinoid tumors. Gastrointest. Radiol. *9*:23, 1984.

127. Balthazar, E.J.: Carcinoid tumors of the alimentary tract. Gastrointest. Radiol. *3*:47, 1978.

128. Berardi, R.S.: Carcinoid tumors of the colon (exclusive of the rectum). Review of the literature. Dis. Colon Rectum *15*:383, 1972.

129. Shulman, H., and Giustra, P.: Invasive carcinoids of the colon. Radiology *98*:139, 1971.

130. Crittenden, J.J., Byllesby, J., and Dodds, W.: Carcinoid tumor presenting as an annular lesion in the ascending colon. Radiology *97*:85, 1970.

131. Dragosics, B., Bauer, P., and Radaszkiewicz, T.: Primary gastrointestinal non-Hodgkin's lymphomas: A retrospective clinicopathologic study of 150 cases. Cancer *55*:1060, 1985.

132. Messinger, N.H., Bobroff, L.M., and Beneventano, T.C.: Lymphosarcoma of the colon. AJR. Am. J. Roentgenol. *117*:281, 1973.

133. Herrman, R., Panahon, A.M., Barcos, M.P., et al.: Gastrointestinal involvement in non-Hodgkin's lymphoma. Cancer *46*:215, 1980.

134. Lewin, K.J., Ranchod, M., and Dorfman, R.F.: Lymphomas of the gastrointestinal tract. A study of 117 cases presenting with gastrointestinal disease. Cancer *42*:693, 1978.

135. Wychulis, A.R., Beahrs, O.H., and Woolner, L.B.: Malignant lymphoma of the colon. Arch. Surg. *93*:215, 1966.

136. Renton, P., and Blackshaw, A.J.: Colonic lymphoma complicating ulcerative colitis. Br. J. Surg. *63*:542, 1976.

137. Sataline, L.R., Mobley, E.M., and Kirkham, W.: Ulcerative colitis complicated by colonic lymphoma. Gastroenterology *44*:342, 1963.

138. Hill, D.H., Mill, M., and Maxwell, R.J.: Metachronous colonic lymphomas complicating ulcerative colitis. Abdom. Imaging *18*:369, 1993.

139. Horton, K.M., and Fishman, E.K.: Multifocal primary colonic lymphoma in a patient with posttransplant lymphoproliferative disease: CT findings. AJR. Am. J. Roentgenol. *170*:1672, 1998.

140. Zornoza, J., and Dodd, G.D.: Lymphoma of the gastrointestinal tract. Semin. Roentgenol. *15*:272, 1980.

141. Bragg, D.G., Colby, T.V., and Ward, J.H.: New concepts in the non-Hodgkin lymphomas: Radiologic implications. Radiology *159*:289, 1986.

142. Pochaczevsky, R., and Sherman, R.S.: Diffuse lymphomatous disease of the colon: Its roentgen appearance. AJR. Am. J. Roentgenol. *87*:670, 1962.

143. Williams, S.M., Berk, R.N., and Harned, R.K.: Radiologic features of multinodular lymphoma of the colon. AJR. Am. J. Roentgenol. *143*:87, 1984.

144. Banks, P.M., Chan, J., Cleary, M.L., et al.: Mantle cell lymphoma. A proposal for unification of morphologic, immunologic, and molecular data. Am. J. Surg. Pathol. *16*:637, 1992.

145. Isaacson, P.G., and Wright, D.H.: Gut-associated lymphoid tumors. *In* Whitehead, R. (ed.). Gastrointestinal and Oesphageal Pathology. Edinburgh, Churchill Livingstone, 1995, p. 755.

146. O'Connell, D.J., and Thompson, A.J.: Lymphoma of the colon. The spectrum of radiologic changes. Gastrointest. Radiol. *2*:377, 1978.

147. Appelman, H.D.: Smooth muscle tumors of the gastrointestinal tract. What we know now that Stout didn't know. Am. J. Surg. Pathol. *10*:83, 1986.

148. Saul, S.H., Rast, M.L., and Brooks, J.J.: The immunohistochemistry of gastrointestinal stromal tumors. Evidence supporting an origin from smooth muscle. Am. J. Surg. Pathol. *11*:464, 1987.

149. Kempson, R.L., and Henrickson, W.R.: Gastrointestinal stromal (smooth muscle) tumors. *In* Whitehead, R. (ed.). Gastrointestinal and Oesphageal Pathology. Edinburgh, Churchill-Livingstone, 1995, p. 272.

150. Akwari, O.E., Dozois, R.R., Weiland, L.H., et al.: Leiomyosarcoma of the small and large bowel. Cancer *42*:1375, 1978.

151. Walsh, T.H., and Mann, C.V.: Smooth muscle neoplasms of the rectum and anal canal. Br. J. Surg. *71*:597, 1984.

152. Heenan, P.J.: Other tumors of the anal canal. *In* Whitehead, R. (ed.). Gastrointestinal and Oesphageal Pathology. Edinburgh, Churchill Livingstone, 1995.

153. Kyaw, M.M., Gallagher, T., and Haines, J.O.: Cloacogenic carcinoma. AJR. Am. J. Roentgenol. *115*:384, 1972.

154. Glickman, M.G., and Margulis, A.R.: Cloacogenic carcinoma. AJR. Am. J. Roentgenol. *107*:175, 1969.

155. Meyers, M.A.: Dynamic Radiology of the Abdomen: Normal and Pathologic Anatomy, ed. 3. New York, Springer-Verlag, 1988.

156. Gedgaudas, R.K., Kelvin, F.M., Thompson, W.M., et al.: The value of the preoperative barium enema in the assessment of pelvic masses. Radiology *146*:609, 1983.

157. Becker, J.A.: Prostatic carcinoma involving the rectum and sigmoid colon. AJR. Am. J. Roentgenol. *94*:421, 1965.

158. Gengler, L., Baer, J., and Finby, N.: Rectal and sigmoid involvement secondary to carcinoma of the prostate. AJR. Am. J. Roentgenol. *125*:910, 1975.

159. Winter, C.C.: The problem of rectal involvement by prostatic cancer. Surg. Gynecol. Obstet. *105*:136, 1957.

160. Rubesin, S.E., Levine, M.S., Bezzi, M., et al.: Rectal involvement by prostatic carcinoma: Radiographic findings. AJR. Am. J. Roentgenol. *152*:53, 1989.

161. Meyers, M.A.: Intraperitoneal spread of malignancies and its effect on the bowel. Clin. Radiol. *32*:129, 1981.

162. Meyers, M.A., and McSweeney, J.: Secondary neoplasms of the bowel. Radiology *105*:1, 1972.

163. Meyers, M.A.: The spread and localization of intraperitoneal effusions. Radiology 95:547, 1970.

164. Meyers, M.A.: Distribution of intra-abdominal malignant seeding: Dependency on dynamics of flow of ascitic fluid. AJR. Am. J. Roentgenol. 119:198, 1973.

165. Rubesin, S.E., and Levine, M.S.: Omental cakes: Colonic involvement by omental metastases. Radiology 154:593, 1985.

166. Ginaldi, S., Lindell, M.M., and Zornoza, J.: The striped colon: A new radiographic observation in metastatic serosal implants. AJR. Am. J. Roentgenol. 134:453, 1980.

167. Krestin, G.P., Beyer, D., and Lorenz, R.: Secondary involvement of the transverse colon by tumors of the pelvis: Spread of malignancies along the greater omentum. Gastrointest. Radiol. 10:283, 1985.

168. Rubesin, S.E., Levine, M.S., Laufer, I., et al.: Villous adenomas: The scientific and the practical. Radiology 167:869, 1988.

169. Bartram, C.I., and Laufer, I. Polyposis syndromes. In Laufer, I., Levine, M.S. (eds.): Double Contrast Gastrointestinal Radiology, ed. 2. Philadelphia, W.B . Saunders Co., 1992, pp. 533–554.

170. Watne, A.L.: The syndromes of intestinal polyposis. Curr. Probl. Surg. 24:269, 1987.

171. Turcot, J., Despres, J.P., and Pierre, F.: Malignant tumors of the central nervous system associated with familial polyposis of the colon. Dis. Colon Rectum 2:465, 1959.

172. Plail, R.O., Bussey, J.H., Glazer, G., et al.: Adenomatous polyposis: An association with carcinoma of the thyroid. Br. J. Surg. 74:377, 1987.

173. Gardner, E.J., and Richards, R.C.: Multiple cutaneous and subcutaneous lesions occurring simultaneously with hereditary polyposis and osteomatosis. Am. J. Hum. Genet. 5:139, 1953.

174. Watanabe, J., Enjoji, M., Yao, T., et al.: Gastric lesions in familial adenomatosis coli. Hum. Pathol. 9:269, 1978.

175. Itai, M., Kogure, T., Okuyama, Y., et al.: Radiographic features of the gastric polyps in familial adenomatous coli. AJR. Am. J. Roentgenol. 128:73, 1977.

176. Jagelman, D.G., DeCosse, J.J., and Bussey, H.J.R.: Upper gastrointestinal cancer in familial adenomatous polyposis. Lancet 21:1149, 1988.

177. Bulow, S., Lauritsen, K.B., Johansen, A., et al.: Gastroduodenal polyps in familial polyposis coli. Dis. Colon Rectum 28:90, 1985.

178. Burke, A., Sobin, L.H., Shekitka, K.M, et al.: Intra-abdominal fibromatosis: A pathologic analysis of 130 tumors with comparison of clinical subgroups. Am. J. Surg. Pathol. 14:335, 1990.

179. Harned, R.K., and Buck, J.L.: Polyposis syndromes. In Gore, R.M., Levine, M.S., Laufer, I.: Textbook of Gastrointestinal Radiology. Philadelphia, W.B. Saunders Co., 1994, pp. 1228–1246.

180. Dodds, W.J.: Clinical and roentgen features of the intestinal polyposis syndromes. Gastrointest. Radiol. 1:127, 1976.

181. Starink, T.M., van Der Veen, J.W., De Waal, L.P., et al.: The Cowden syndrome: A clinical and genetic study in 21 patients. Clin. Genet. 29:222, 1986.

182. Salem, O.S., and Steck, W.D.: Cowden's disease (multiple hamartoma and neoplasia syndrome). A case report and review of the literature. J. Am. Acad. Dermatol. 8:686, 1983.

183. Cronkhite, L.W., and Canada, W.J.: Generalized gastrointestinal polyposis: An unusual syndrome of polyposis, pigmentation, alopecia and onychatrophia. N. Engl. J. Med. 252:1011, 1955.

184. Dachman, A.H., Buck, J.L., Burke, A.P., et al.: Cronkhite-Canada syndrome: Radiologic features. Gastrointest. Radiol. 14:285, 1989.

185. Jass, J.R., Williams, C.B., Bussey H.J.R., et al.: Juvenile polyposis: A precancerous condition. Histopathology 13:619, 1988.

Inflammatory Bowel Disease

STEPHEN E. RUBESIN
CLIVE I. BARTRAM
IGOR LAUFER

ULCERATIVE COLITIS

Ulcerative colitis is an inflammatory disease of the colon that is primarily confined to the mucosa and submucosa.[1] Despite a vast amount of research, the etiology of ulcerative colitis is unknown. Similar diseases may be induced in animals by carageenin, bacterial endotoxins, or manipulation of the immune or vascular systems.[2,3]

Clinical Correlation

Ulcerative colitis most frequently occurs in patients between the second and fifth decade, with a peak between ages 15 and 25.[1,4,5] Ulcerative colitis is more commonly found in patients in the United States, Northern Europe, and Israel.[1] The clinical course of ulcerative colitis is variable. Most patients have acute episodes separated by long periods of relative quiescence.[4] In contrast, Crohn's disease has a greater amount of chronic symptoms. Diarrhea is the most common symptom in ulcerative colitis, with nonbloody diarrhea progressing to bloody diarrhea. Frequency, urgency, tenesmus, and weight loss are other symptoms. The acute episodes of bloody diarrhea usually resolve spontaneously or after

therapy. Severe attacks are characterized by fever, leukocytosis, and frequent small amounts of bloody diarrhea. Approximately 5% to 10% of patients require surgery during their first severe attack.[4]

There are numerous extraintestinal manifestations including liver, skeletal, and skin problems. Steatosis of the liver and pericholangitis are found in 50% and 35% to 50% of patients, respectively.[6,7] Sclerosing cholangitis occurs in 1% to 4% of patients.[8] Seronegative migratory polyarthritis and ankylosing spondylitis may be present. Nephrolithiasis is detected in 5% of patients.[9] The incidence of adenocarcinoma of the colon is increased. There is also an increased incidence of carcinoma of the gallbladder and bile ducts, colonic lymphoma, and tumors of the central nervous system and connective tissue.[6,10,11]

Radiographic Findings

Barium studies are complementary to endoscopy in the assessment of ulcerative colitis. Barium studies help confirm or refute the diagnosis of ulcerative colitis, especially in differentiating ulcerative colitis from Crohn's disease. Barium studies help assess the extent of disease, detect complications, and follow the course in response to treatment. Although barium studies correlate beautifully with the gross pathology,[12] they underestimate the extent of histologic involvement.[13]

The macroscopic appearance of ulcerative colitis varies with the severity and duration of disease and the effects of therapy.[1] Ulcerative colitis begins in the rectum and extends retrogradely in a continuous fashion (Fig. 13–1). The rectum is almost always involved, although it may be less severely inflamed than more proximal segments (Fig. 13–2). The mucosal changes of ulcerative colitis are diffuse, symmetrically involving the entire circumference of bowel.

Mucosal Granularity

The earliest radiographic finding in ulcerative colitis is replacement of the normally smooth colonic mucosa by finely granular mucosa (see Fig. 13–1) (Fig. 13–3).[14] Numerous indistinct dots of barium cover the colonic mucosa. In profile, the normally sharp colonic contour is replaced by an indistinct line with punctate dots.[13] Granularity correlates with pathologic changes of mild edema and hyperemia[13,14] and alteration of colonic mucus.[15]

With progression of disease, superficial erosions occur, depicted radiographically as larger dots of barium superimposed on the background of mucosal granularity (Fig. 13–4). The large dots of barium are termed *stippling.* Barium adherence to superficial erosions accounts for the stippling.[15]

With partial healing, the mucosa may appear "coarsely granular," with multiple tiny radiolucent nodules separated by barium coating indistinct colonic depressions (Fig.

13–5). Coarse granularity is usually associated with the chronic changes of ulcerative colitis described below.[13,14]

Acute edema and inflammation also result in widening and blunting of the interhaustral folds and of the valves of Houston. Normally, the valves of Houston and interhaustral folds are approximately 2 to 4 mm in width and are sharply edged. With active inflammation, the folds of the colon widen and appear rounded.

Inflammation is detected in the terminal ileum in approximately 10% to 25% of patients with ulcerative pancolitis.[16] This ileitis is manifested as granular mucosa in the terminal ileum, termed *backwash ileitis* (Fig. 13–6). The distant most 10 to 25 cm of terminal ileum is also dilated and hypoperistaltic. The plicae circulares are absent. The ileocecal valve is patulous. Discrete ulcers are not superimposed on the granular mucosa.[4] The pathogenesis of terminal ileal inflammation is not understood, but this inflammation reverts to normal once the colon is removed.[15] Backwash ileitis is of no clinical significance, and the terminal ileum may be used for ileostomy.[4]

Ulceration

Ulceration implies a severe attack of ulcerative colitis. Shallow ulcers burrow through the mucosa into the submucosa. The ulcers extend laterally in the submucosal fat, undermining the relatively resistant mucosa, resulting in "collar button" ulcers.[17] Radiographically, 2 to 5 mm collections of barium are seen en face on a background of granular mucosa (Fig. 13–7). In profile the mucosal line is clearly disrupted,[13] with barium collections spreading laterally in the submucosa, beneath preserved mucosal

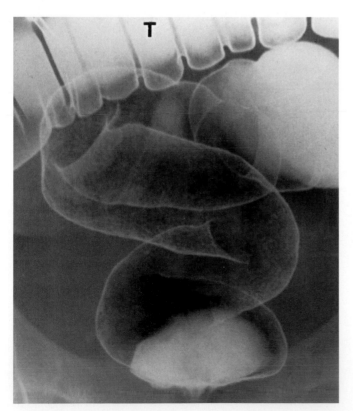

FIGURE 13–1. Ulcerative proctosigmoiditis. Spot radiograph of rectum and sigmoid colon shows a diffusely tubular rectosigmoid with loss of the valves of Houston and diffusely granular mucosa. The overlying transverse colon, *T,* is normal. (From Rubesin, S.E., et al.: Radiologic investigation of inflammatory bowel disease. *In* MacDermott, R.P., and Stenson, W.F.: Inflammatory Bowel Disease. New York, Elsevier Science Publishing Co., 1992.)

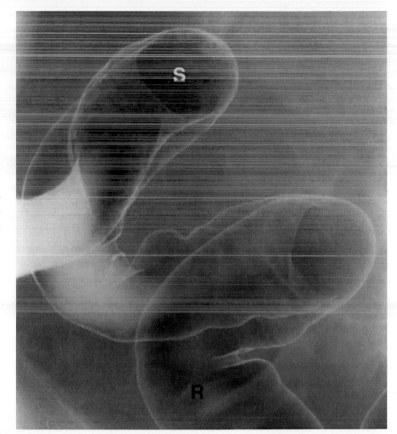

FIGURE **13–2. Rectal sparing after treatment for ulcerative proctosigmoiditis.** After steroid enemas, the rectum, *R,* is relatively normal, but granular mucosa remains at the rectosigmoid junction, *S.*

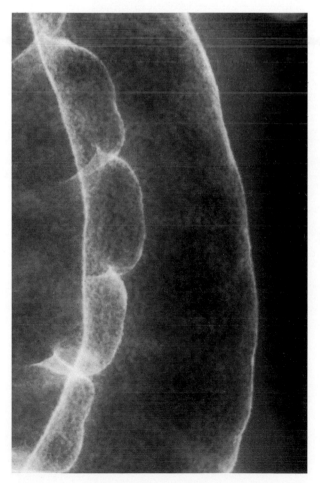

FIGURE **13–3. Granular mucosa in ulcerative colitis.** Tiny punctate dots of barium cover the entire mucosa of the descending colon. (From Laufer, I., et al.: Correlation of endoscopy and double contrast radiography in the early stages of ulcerative and granulomatous colitis. Radiology *118:*1–6, 1976, with permission.)

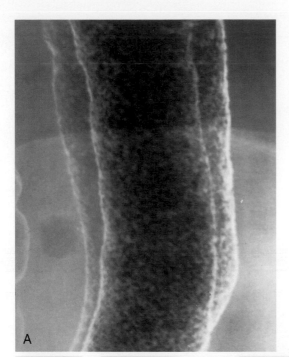

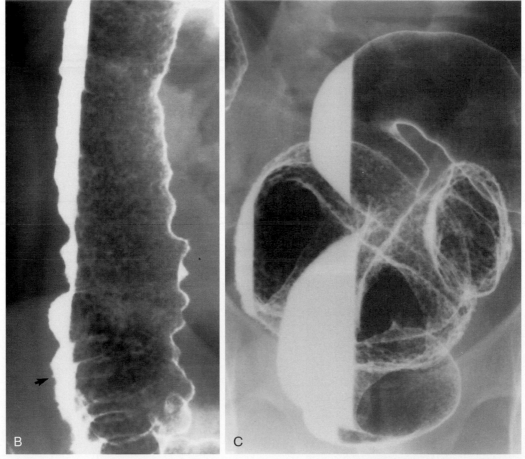

FIGURE 13–4. Stippling in ulcerative colitis. *A,* Spot radiograph of descending colon shows larger, 2- to 3-mm punctate collections of barium superimposed on background granularity. *B,* Right decubitus view of ascending colon shows large dots of barium superimposed on finer granules. Tiny ulcers are seen in profile along the colonic contour *(arrow). C,* Tiny ulcers are superimposed on mucosal granularity in the proximal rectum and sigmoid colon. The distal rectum only has granular mucosa.

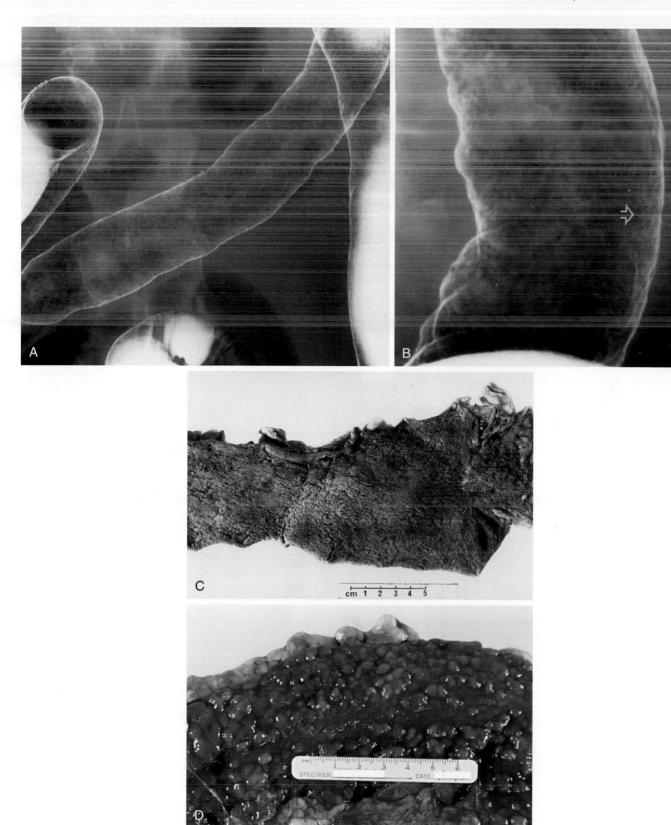

FIGURE 13–5. Coarse granularity in chronic ulcerative colitis. *A,* The transverse colon has a tubular contour and is without interhaustral folds. Coarse granularity is manifested as tiny radiolucent nodules surrounded by shallow barium-filled grooves. (From Rubesin, S.E., et al.: Radiologic investigation of inflammatory bowel disease. *In* MacDermott, R.P., and Stenson, W.F.: Inflammatory Bowel Disease. New York, Elsevier Science Publishing Co., 1992.) *B,* Close-up of descending colon in another patient shows tiny radiolucent nodules in some areas surrounded by barium-filled grooves (representative region identified with *arrow*). *C,* Colectomy specimen in a third patient shows small nodules surrounded by grooves. *D,* Gross photograph of colectomy specimen in a fourth patient shows small mucosal nodules.

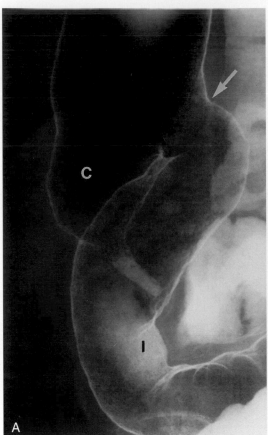

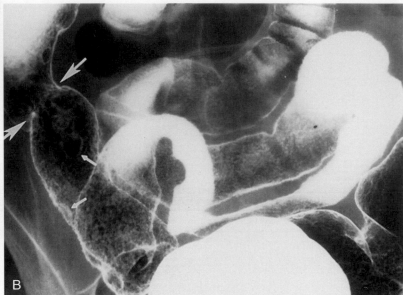

FIGURE 13–6. Backwash ileitis. *A*, Spot film of right lower quadrant shows a cone-shaped cecum *(C)*, a patulous ileocecal valve *(arrow)* and diffusely granular mucosa in the dilated terminal ileum *(I)*. The plicae circulares are absent. *B*, Marked backwash ileitis. The mucosa of the terminal and distal ileum is diffusely granular. The ileocecal valve is patulous *(large arrows)*. Several inflammatory polyps are seen in the terminal ileum *(small arrows)*.

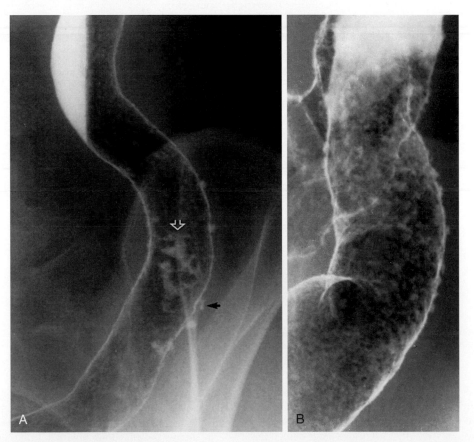

FIGURE 13–7. Ulcers on background of mucosal granularity. *A*, Large, irregular barium collections are seen en face *(open arrow)* and in profile *(arrow)* in a short segment of descending colon. The background mucosa is granular. *B*, Numerous ulcers are superimposed on granular mucosa in the descending colon of a different patient.

tissue (Fig. 13–8). As the ulcers enlarge, broad, round, ovoid, or linear ulcers are formed. Long, linear ulcers follow the course of the taeniae coli.[18] When ulcers interconnect, residual islands of mucosa remain elevated above the sea of ulceration. These remnant mucosal islands rising above the denuded surface appear falsely elevated and are termed *inflammatory pseudopolyps* (Fig. 13–9).

Chronic Changes

Normal interhaustral folds are relatively fixed structures in the right and proximal transverse colon, but they are transient structures in the distal transverse and left colon. Normal interhaustral folds in the left colon are created by contraction of the taeniae coli. The left colon can be normally devoid of interhaustral folds.[4] In long-standing chronic ulcerative colitis the involved portions of colon are shortened and narrowed, with loss of interhaustral folds. The colon becomes tubular in configuration (Fig. 13–10). The flexures are lost (Fig. 13–11), and the sigmoid colon is straightened and shortened. In ulcerative colitis, loss of interhaustral folds may be attributed to both alteration in muscle tone[19] and destruction of the mucosal surface. Loss of the rectal valves of Houston may leave the rectum appearing tubular.[20] With healing, both the valves of Houston and the interhaustral folds may reappear.

Colonic narrowing and shortening is probably due to a combination of altered colonic contractility, chronic inflammation, and loss of mucosal surface area. Pathologically, a narrowed segment of colon shows marked thickening of the muscularis mucosae and widening of the submucosal fat.[19,21] Apparent bowel wall thickening is readily demonstrated pathologically and during CT.[22,23] The narrowed rectum is associated with widening of the retrorectal space greater than 1 cm at the level of S4.[24] The perirectal fat is prominent. Apparent thickening of both muscularis mucosae and submucosa is probably related to change in colonic size rather than true increase of colonic wall volume. It has been shown pathologically that colonic wall thickness varies dramatically, at minimum, from 10 to 40 times, depending on whether the colon is in a stretched or contractile state.[25] A contracted colon shows a much thicker muscularis mucosae and submucosa than the same stretched colon.[25]

Strictures

Strictures develop in approximately 10% of patients with ulcerative colitis of more than 5 years' duration.[26,27] Strictures may be single or multiple and are most frequently found in the sigmoid colon. Strictures are probably due to thickening and contraction of the muscularis mucosae rather than true fibrosis.[26] Obstructive symptoms are unusual, as the loose diarrheal stool easily passes through areas of luminal narrowing. Radiographically, strictures have smooth, symmetrically tapered margins (Fig. 13–12).[28] Strictures are covered by mucosa similar to the adjacent colon. Any irregularity or asymmetry of the contour or nodularity of the mucosa requires biopsy to rule out malignancy.[29] In fact, endoscopy with biopsy is required in smooth strictures as well because some scirrhous cancers may appear as a relatively smooth, tapered stricture. Furthermore, those patients with strictures have long-standing colitis and are at risk for dysplasia and adenocarcinoma.

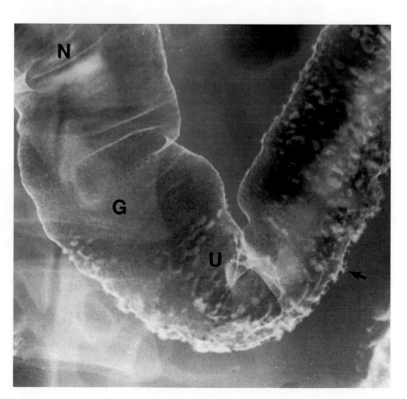

FIGURE 13–8. Collar button ulcers in the transverse colon. Inflammation spreads laterally in the submucosal fat to form collar button ulcers (*arrow* identifies profile view of representative ulcer). Note the transition from relatively normal mucosa (*N*) to granular mucosa (*G*) to ulcers on a background of mucosal granularity (*U*). (From Rubesin, S.E., et al.: Radiologic investigation of inflammatory bowel disease. *In* MacDermott, R.P., and Stenson, W.F.: Inflammatory Bowel Disease. New York, Elsevier Science Publishing Co., 1992.)

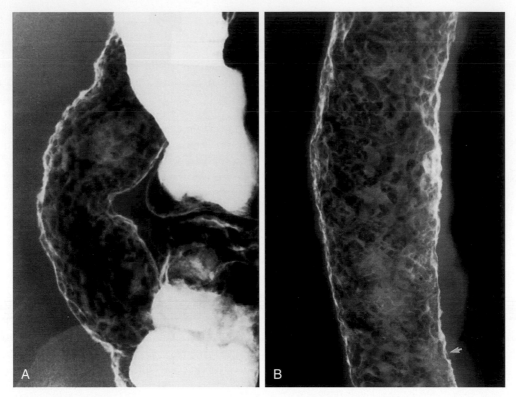

FIGURE 13–9. Inflammatory pseudopolyps. *A,* Spot radiograph of sigmoid colon shows numerous 3- to 5-mm radiolucent islands clearly surrounded by barium-filled grooves. *B,* Barium-coated specimen radiograph from a different patient shows numerous round to ovoid radiolucencies in shallow barium pool or etched in white by barium. Inflamed mucosal remnants create these inflammatory pseudopolyps. When seen in profile, the large nodules are barely elevated above the luminal contour *(arrow).*

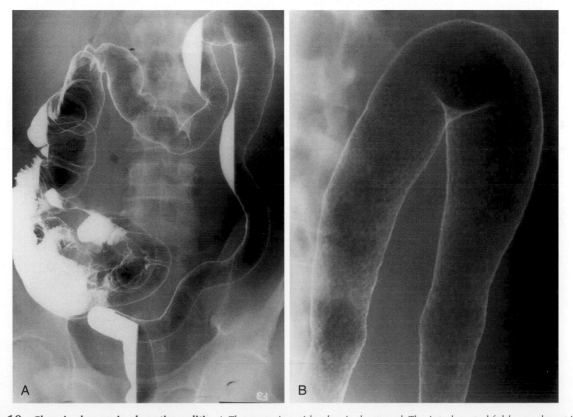

FIGURE 13–10. Chronic changes in ulcerative colitis. *A,* The rectosigmoid colon is shortened. The interhaustral folds are absent in the transverse, descending, and sigmoid colon. The valves of Houston have disappeared. *B,* Close-up of splenic flexure in the same patient shows coarsely granular mucosa.

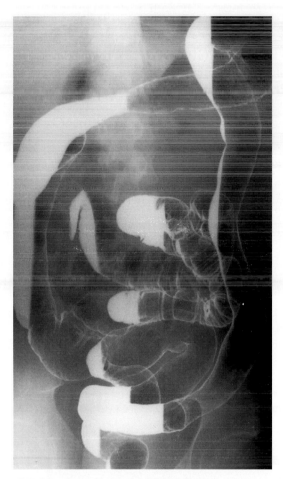

FIGURE 13–11. Chronic changes in ulcerative colitis. The colon is ahaustral. The hepatic flexure is short. The mucosa is diffusely granular. The ileocecal valve is gaping.

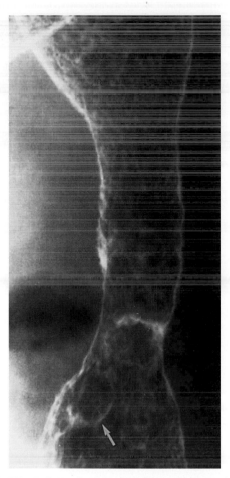

FIGURE 13–12. Stricture in ulcerative colitis. There is a 10 cm long, tapered narrowing in the descending colon that is covered by coarsely granular mucosa. An inflammatory polyp is seen inferiorly *(arrow).*

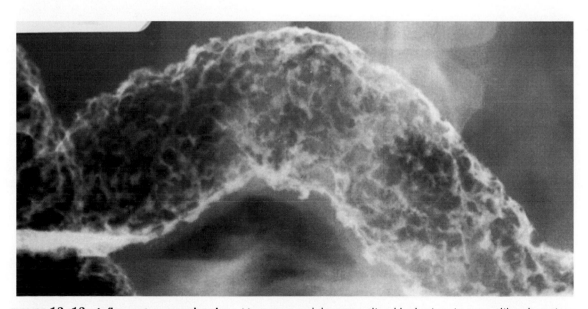

FIGURE 13–13. Inflammatory pseudopolyps. Numerous nodules are outlined by barium in groovelike ulcerations.

Polypoid Lesions

Polypoid lesions are seen in regions of extensive ulceration or after ulcerative colitis has healed. Mucosal remnants between areas of extensive ulceration may appear "elevated" above the denuded surface and are termed *inflammatory pseudopolyps* (Fig. 13–13).[30,31] "Inflammatory polyps" are polypoid masses of granulation tissue and hyperplastic mucosa protruding above inflamed mucosa.[32] These polyps are usually seen on a background of mucosal granularity or ulceration (Fig. 13–14). Inflammatory polyps may be single or multiple, sessile or pedunculated.

Polyps occurring in a colon devoid of inflammatory changes are termed *postinflammatory polyps* and are found in 10% to 20% of patients with chronic ulcerative colitis.[27] Postinflammatory polyps may be single or multiple, arising in a focal segment (Fig. 13–15) or diffusely (Fig. 13–16) throughout the colon. Postinflammatory polyps may be sessile or frondlike. Postinflammatory polyps may also appear as long, tubular elevations with or without clubbed heads, termed *filiform polyps* (see Fig. 13–16).[33] Filiform polyps may be created when ulceration undermines mucosa creating a flap of residual tissue.[33,34] When mucosal repair occurs, tags of residual or hyperplastic mucosa project intraluminally.

Mucosal bridges are long, tubular arches of tissue connected to mucosa at both ends (Fig. 13–17). Mucosal bridges may represent either the adhesion of two filiform polyps[35] or the undermining of mucosa by adjacent ulcers. Filiform polyps and mucosal bridges are not specific for ulcerative colitis, as they are also found in Crohn's disease and other chronic inflammatory conditions.[36,37] Filiform polyps may be present in patients with active colitis (Fig. 13–18), as well as in clinically quiescent states. Filiform polyps are not premalignant.

Colitic Cancer

Patients with ulcerative colitis are at increased risk for colonic adenocarcinoma. Cancers usually develop in patients with long-standing, minimally active colitis. Patients with diffuse colitis and long duration of disease are at the greatest risk for the development of adenocarcinoma.[38–40] Approximately 10 years after the initial diagnosis of ulcerative colitis, the risk of adenocarcinoma developing is approximately 10% per decade.[27,41–43] Patients with ulcerative proctitis do not have an increased risk of adenocarcinoma.[44]

Development of adenocarcinoma follows the dysplasia-to-carcinoma sequence except that early dysplasia usually arises in areas of flat mucosa rather than in typical "ade-

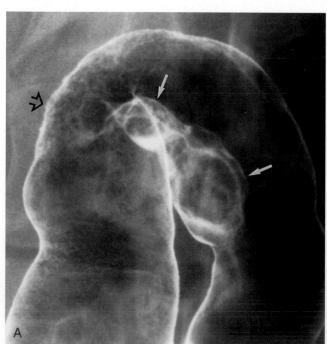
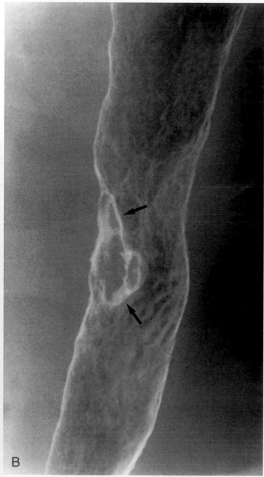

FIGURE 13–14. Inflammatory polyps in ulcerative colitis. *A,* Large pedunculated polyp *(white arrows)* flops down the descending limb of the splenic flexure. Active colitis is manifested by granular mucosa *(black arrow). B,* In another patient an elongated inflammatory polyp *(arrows)* lies on a background of granular mucosa.

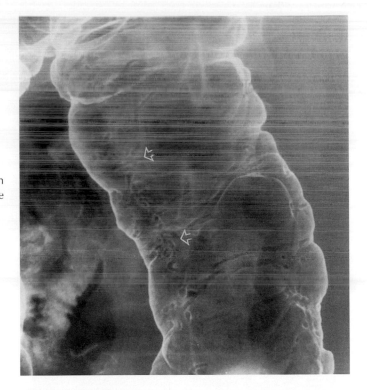

FIGURE 13–15. Focal filiform polyps. A segment of transverse colon has filiform polyps lying along the outer contours (representative polyps identified by *arrows*).

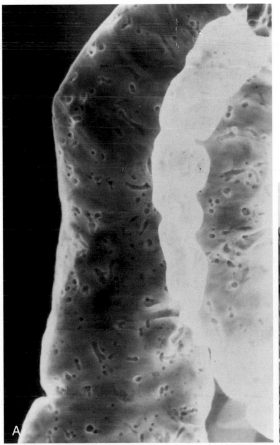

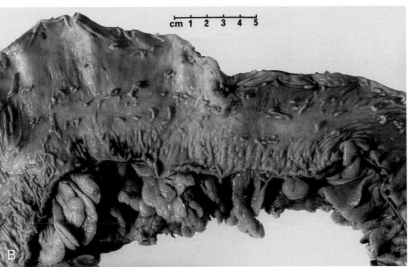

FIGURE 13–16. Diffuse filiform polyps. *A,* Numerous filiform polyps are manifested as radiolucent tubular structures, some with rounded, branching, or clubbed heads. The background mucosa is normal, indicating no active colitis is present. *B,* Surgical specimen in a different patient shows numerous filiform polyps on normal mucosa.

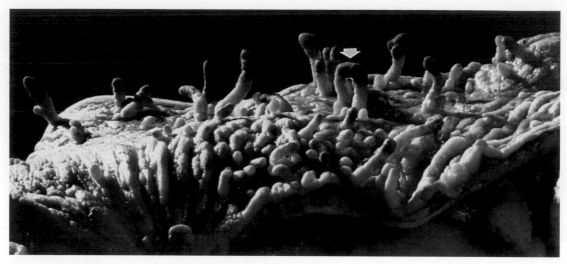

FIGURE 13–17. Mucosal bridges and filiform polyps in ulcerative colitis. Numerous filiform polyps protrude from flat mucosa. Two fronds have joined together *(arrow)* forming a mucosal bridge. (From Morson, B.C.: The Pathogenesis of Colorectal Cancer. Philadelphia, W.B. Saunders Co., 1978, with permission.)

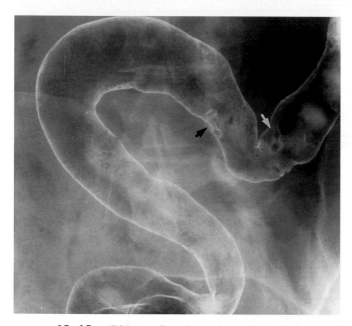

FIGURE 13–18. Filiform polyps in active colitis. The sigmoid colon shows diffusely granular mucosa. Filiform polyps *(arrows)* are seen near the junction of the descending and sigmoid colon.

nomatous polyps." Dysplasia arising in flat mucosa cannot be detected radiographically.[45] However, two thirds of cases of dysplasia arising in ulcerative colitis are detected radiographically.[46] Most frequently, a focal area of "velvety" mucosa resembling a carpet lesion is demonstrated (Fig. 13–19). Barium fills the interstices between round and polygonal islands of dysplastic epithelium (see Fig. 13–19).[47–49] Dysplasia can also be seen as a focal, plaquelike elevation (Fig. 13–20) or as a polypoid lesion.[50,51]

Most polypoid lesions in ulcerative colitis are usually postinflammatory or inflammatory polyps. Polypoid ade-

nomas and polypoid adenocarcinomas are uncommon in ulcerative colitis.[4] Neither radiologist nor endoscopist, however, can determine whether a polypoid lesion is inflammatory or neoplastic. Excision with histologic evaluation is necessary, whether a polyp is sessile or pedunculated or has a smooth or lobulated surface. Filiform polyps are benign lesions, however, and need not be removed. The radiologist must remember that the role of barium studies is determination of the extent of colitis; the configuration of the colon, including detection of strictures; and to suggest areas suspected of having dysplasia or carcinoma.[26]

Most cancers arising in ulcerative colitis are either annular (Fig. 13–21) or plaquelike lesions. Long scirrhous cancers occur but are uncommon (Fig. 13–22).[52,53] Polypoid cancers are uncommon (Fig. 13–23). Synchronous cancers are found in one third of patients with ulcerative colitis.[54] Pathologically, colitic cancers are often infiltrating, mucinous lesions. The radiologist must be vigilant at detecting subtle mucosal nodularity, plaquelike areas, or subtle circumferential narrowings that may indicate dysplasia or infiltrating cancer.

Fulminant Colitis

Although this text focuses on double contrast radiology, the plain film is important in the workup of severely ill patients with ulcerative colitis. Colitis so severe as to be predisposed to transmural disintegration and perforation, termed *fulminant colitis,* is found in 1% to 13% of patients.[55,56] Because the colon is often dilated, this condition has also been described as "toxic megacolon" or "toxic dilatation." Pathologically, the colon is extremely thin, with transmural inflammation, extensive necrosis (Fig. 13–24), and disintegration of tissue cohesiveness.[57,58] The adjacent serosa, mesenteric fat, and omental fat are edematous and inflamed.

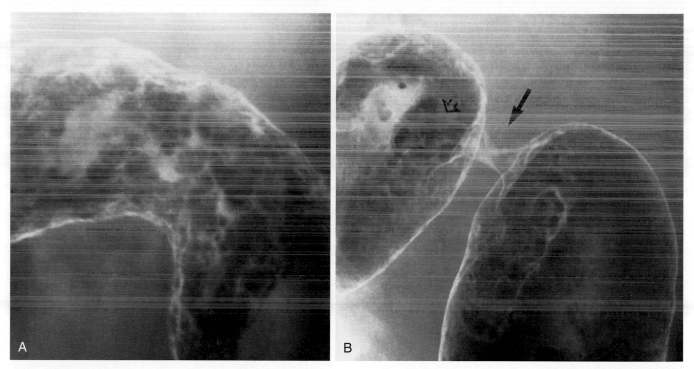

FIGURE 13–19. Dysplasia in ulcerative colitis progressing to adenocarcinoma. *A,* A focal area of "velvety" mucosa is present in the splenic flexure. Numerous round/ovoid 3- to 6-mm nodules carpet the mucosa. *B,* Later, a short annular cancer with abrupt, but smooth margins has developed *(large arrow).* Note the residual dysplastic epithelium lateral to the adenocarcinoma *(small arrow).* (Courtesy of Giles Stevenson, M.D., Hamilton, Ontario, Canada.)

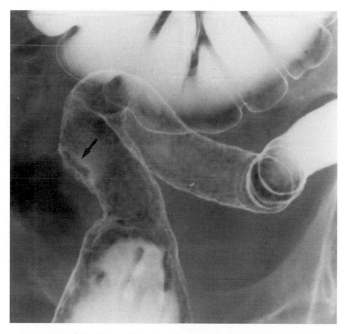

FIGURE 13–20. Plaquelike dysplasia arising in left-sided ulcerative colitis. A 2-cm, slightly raised plaque is etched by barium *(arrow).* The rectosigmoid colon is tubular, covered with coarsely nodular mucosa. The transverse colon is normal. (From Rubesin, S.E., et al.: Radiologic investigation of inflammatory bowel disease. *In* MacDermott, R.P., and Stenson, W.F.: Inflammatory Bowel Disease. New York, Elsevier Science Publishing Co., 1992.)

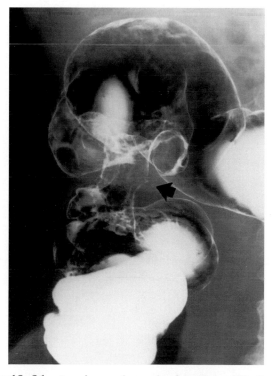

FIGURE 13–21. Annular carcinoma in ulcerative colitis. Spot film shows a 5-cm long annular mass *(arrow)* with abrupt margins and irregular mucosa. The adjacent colonic epithelium is not granular. Colitis is relatively quiescent.

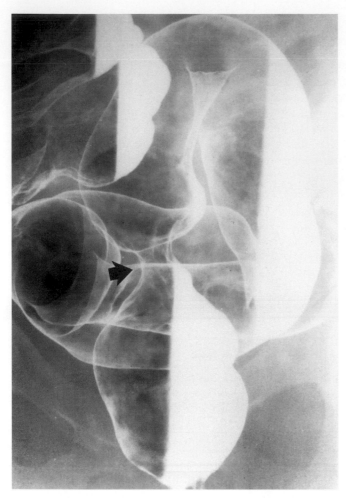

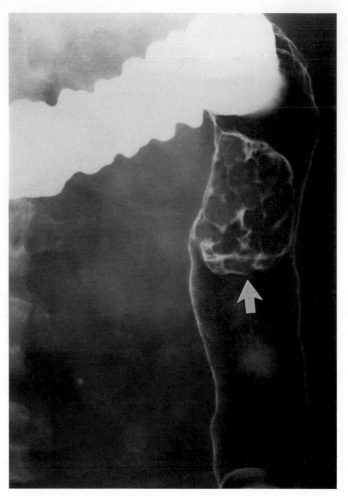

FIGURE 13–22. Scirrhous carcinoma in ulcerative colitis. Despite the smooth mucosa and tapered distal margin, this was an adenocarcinoma *(arrow)* of the proximal rectum.

FIGURE 13–23. Polypoid carcinoma in ulcerative colitis. A coarsely lobulated mass *(arrow)* is seen in the splenic flexure.

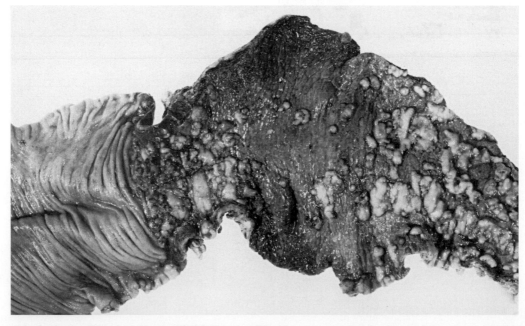

FIGURE 13–24. Colectomy specimen in patient with fulminant colitis. The mucosa is partly sloughed, leaving residual islands of inflamed mucosa.

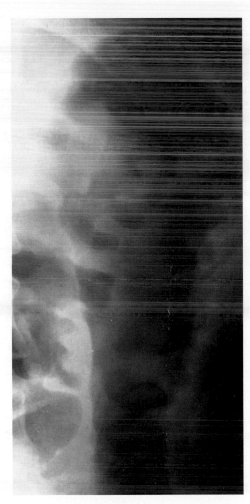

FIGURE 13–25. **Fulminant colitis.** Close-up of splenic flexure from overhead of colon shows a lobulated contour and thick lobulated folds en face.

In these severely ill patients, plain films are used to look for evidence of severe inflammation or perforation. We believe that in the future, CT will ultimately be the examination of choice in assessing patients with fulminant colitis.

The radiologist's threshold for the suggestion of "toxic dilatation" is approximately 5 cm.[59–61] In most patients with fulminant colitis, however, the luminal diameter is greater than 8 cm.[27] The interhaustral folds and haustral sacculations are not identified. The luminal contour has a coarsely lobulated edge, and residual islands of nonsloughed mucosa appear as soft tissue nodules (Fig. 13–25).

CROHN'S DISEASE

Crohn's disease is a chronic inflammatory disease that involves any portion of the gastrointestinal tract. Although described as early as 1913[62] and named after the first author of a 1932 paper,[63] Crohn's disease of the colon was not clinically, pathologically, or radiologically distin-guished from ulcerative colitis until 1959 and the early 1960s.[64–68] Crohn's disease is not a distinct histopathologic entity. The etiology and pathogenesis are unknown.[69] Diagnosis requires consideration of the clinical, radiologic, endoscopic, biopsy, and stool specimen findings. Barium studies are crucial in diagnosis. Barium studies may confirm or refute the clinical and endoscopic diagnosis, especially when biopsy results are equivocal. The distribution and severity of disease and the gross morphology are superbly demonstrated by barium studies.

Clinical Correlation

Crohn's disease is most commonly found in young adults ages 15 to 30,[70] but is discovered at any age from childhood to the elderly. Crohn's disease is more common in patients in Northern Europe and North America. Patients typically have smoldering, chronic symptoms of diarrhea and abdominal pain. Children may present with growth failure,[70] adults with diverticulitis. Severe acute hemorrhage is uncommon, found in approximately 1% of patients.[71]

There are numerous extraintestinal manifestations of Crohn's disease (see Chapter 10). Cholelithiasis is found in 13% to 34% of patients.[72,73] Amyloidosis as a complication of the long-standing chronic inflammation of Crohn's disease is uncommon, seen in 0.5% to 1% of patients.[72] The incidence of adenocarcinoma of the small bowel and colon is slightly increased and is seen in patients who have earlier onset and long-standing duration of the disease. Carcinomas also have a predilection for arising in bypassed segments, strictures, or fistulae.

Distribution and Pathology

The patchy, chronic, inflammatory process may involve any part of the gastrointestinal tract. Crohn's disease is most frequently found in the right lower quadrant, involving terminal ileum and colon in 55% of patients. The terminal ileum is involved alone in 14% of patients, the terminal ileum with proximal extension of disease in 13% of patients, and the colon alone in 15% of patients.[74,75] Proximal small bowel involvement with sparing of the terminal ileum is seen in only 3% of patients.[74] The distribution of disease remains relatively fixed in extent over time. Crohn's disease typically recurs in small bowel adjacent to an anastomosis.[4]

Crohn's disease is typified by granuloma formation, aphthoid ulcers, discontinuous focal inflammation, skip lesions, and fissuring transmural inflammation.[69,70,76] Crohn's disease is typified by asymmetry and discontinuity.[77] Ulceration is discontinuous with inflammatory changes separated by grossly normal mucosa.

Although granulomas are one hallmark of Crohn's disease, they are found in only 25% to 70% of patients.[78–80] Granulomas vary from loosely aggregated collections of histiocytes to densely cellular histiocytic aggregates to large tuberculoid-like granulomas with multinucleated giant cells (Fig. 13–26).[79] Granulomas are most frequently

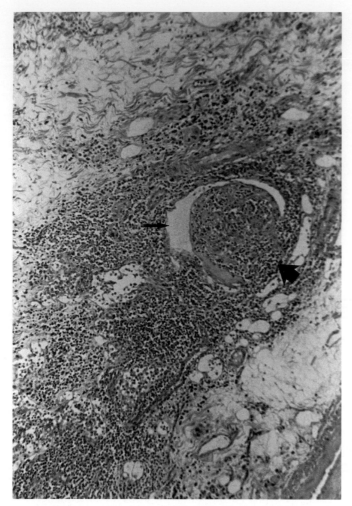

FIGURE 13–26. Granuloma in Crohn's disease. In the submucosa a granuloma *(large arrow)* pushes into a dilated lymphatic *(small arrow)*. The granuloma is composed of histiocytes, lymphocytes, and multinucleated giant cells. (From Rubesin, S.E., and Bronner, M.: Radiologic-pathologic concepts in Crohn's disease. Adv. Gastrointest. Radiol. *1:27,* 1991, with permission.)

found in the submucosa adjacent to lymphatic vessels. Granulomas also form in the mucosa, muscularis mucosae, subserosa, and mesenteric lymph nodes.[80]

Radiographic Findings
Aphthoid Ulcers

The earliest radiographic findings of Crohn's disease are lymphoid hyperplasia (Fig. 13–27) and aphthoid ulcers. Aphthoid ulcers are superficial ulcers overlying aggregates of lymph tissue at the junction of the mucosa and submucosa or at the base of a gland.[14,81–85] Aphthoid ulcers are radiographically manifest as small, 1- to 2-mm round or stellate collections of barium surrounded by thin radiolucent halos (Fig. 13–28). Barium adherent to the sloughed ulcer base forms the punctate collection.[4] The radiolucent halo results from lack of barium adherence to the edematous, inflamed rim of the aphthoid ul-

cer (Fig. 13–29).[4] In profile, aphthoid ulcers appear as shallow barium collections minimally projecting beyond the luminal contour (Fig. 13–30).[4]

Aphthoid ulcers are discrete, separated from other lesions by normal mucosa.[14,84,85] In contrast, in ulcerative colitis, small ulcers are found on a background of granular mucosa.[13] Aphthoid ulcers may be asymmetrically distributed along one side of the colon (Fig. 13–31). When aphthoid ulcers enlarge, they burrow into the submucosa, undermining the mucosa, forming collar-button ulcers or deep ulcers. Folds may radiate toward their margin, similar to folds radiating toward a gastric ulcer (Fig. 13–32).[86]

Aphthoid ulcers may be the only evidence of Crohn's disease or are seen in patients with more advanced disease. Aphthoid ulcers are frequently found at the edges of more severely inflamed segments, in the transition zone from abnormal to normal. Aphthoid ulcers may be isolated, grouped in clusters, or seen throughout the colon. Aphthoid ulcers are not specific for Crohn's disease, and they are also seen in *Yersinia* enterocolitis, salmonellosis, shigellosis, herpetic or cytomegalovirus colitis, amebiasis, tuberculosis, or Behçet's disease.[58,87,88]

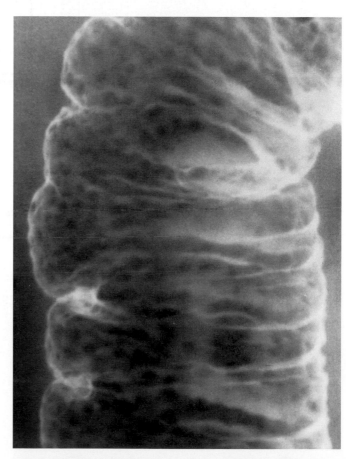

FIGURE 13–27. Lymphoid hyperplasia in Crohn's disease. Spot film of the mid-transverse colon shows numerous 1- to 2-mm, round or ovoid radiolucencies, some in the shallow barium pool, others etched in white.

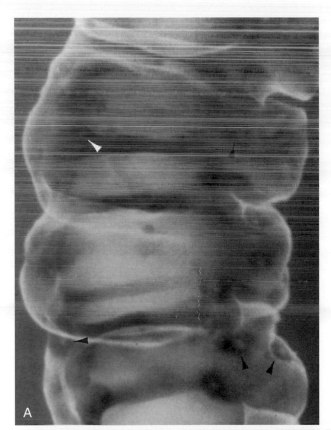

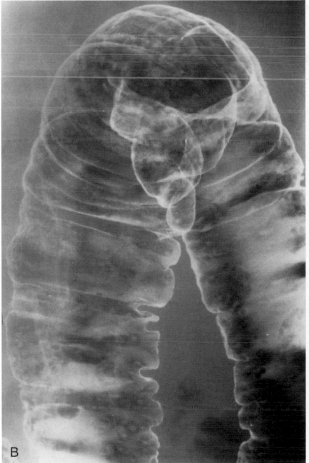

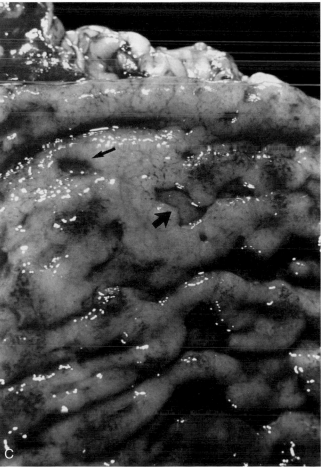

FIGURE 13–28. Aphthoid ulcers in Crohn's disease. *A,* Spot film of descending colon shows punctate collections of barium surrounded by radiolucent halos, some halos etched in white, some less distinct in the shallow barium pool. *B,* Numerous aphthoid ulcers are seen in the splenic flexure. *C,* Close-up specimen photograph of colon shows small aphthoid ulcers *(small arrow)* and larger ulcer with undermined edges *(large arrow).* (From Rubesin, S.E., and Bronner, M.: Radiologic-pathologic concepts in Crohn's disease. Adv. Gastrointest. Radiol. *1*:27, 1991, with permission.)

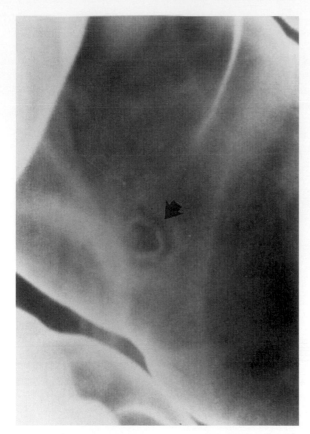

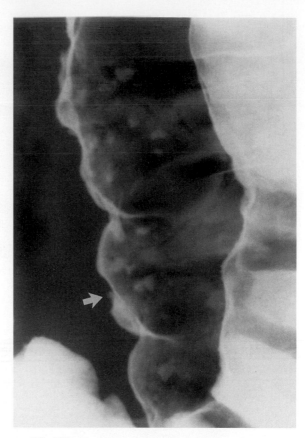

FIGURE 13–29. Aphthoid ulcer as ring shadow. Spot film of sigmoid colon shows a ring of barium surrounded by a radiolucent halo *(arrow)*. Centrally, where the barium has spilled out, the ulcer is devoid of barium.

FIGURE 13–30. Spot film of the splenic flexure shows numerous aphthoid ulcers. In profile a small mound projects slightly into the lumen, with a small central barium collection *(arrow)*.

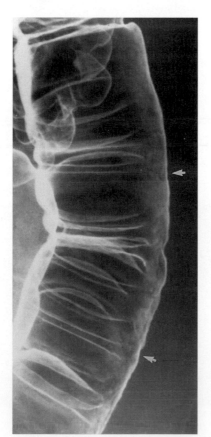

FIGURE 13–31. Asymmetric distribution of aphthoid ulcers. Numerous aphthoid ulcers lie along the lateral border of the descending colon *(arrows)*.

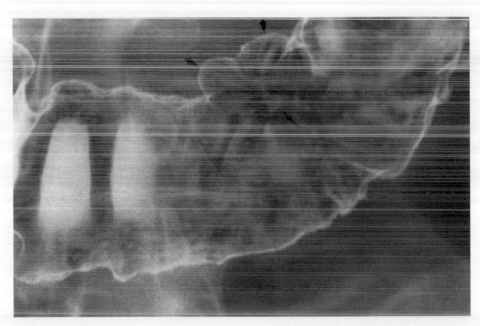

FIGURE 13–32. Numerous aphthoid ulcers are present in the transverse colon. A larger ulcer *(long arrow)* has folds radiating toward its edge. Sacculation of the contour *(small arrows)* results from the folds radiating toward the ulcer. (From Rubesin, S.E., and Bronner, M.: Radiologic-pathologic concepts in Crohn's disease. Adv. Gastrointest. Radiol. *1:27*, 1991, with permission.)

Large Ulcers

Large ulcers (Fig. 13–33) indicate more advanced disease. Long, shallow ulcers may occur in the colon (Fig. 13–34) or small bowel, especially on the mesenteric border of the distal ileum (Fig. 13–35).[86,89] A radiolucent ulcer collar parallels the long barium collection (Fig. 13–36), similar to the halo in an aphthoid ulcer.[86] Smooth, mucosal folds may radiate toward the linear ulcer. The relatively uninvolved wall opposite the linear ulcer may be pulled into sacculations that do not protrude beyond the expected luminal contour (Fig. 13–37). Large, round undermined ulcers are also seen (Fig. 13–38), separated by normal intervening mucosa.

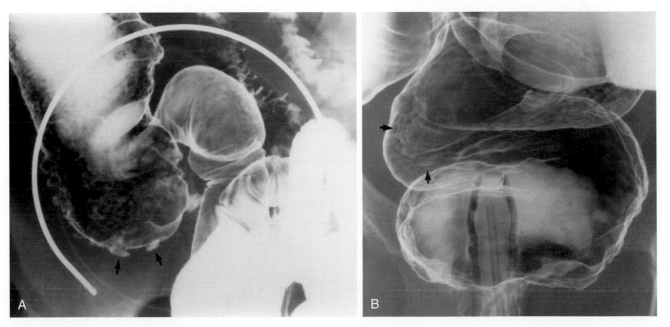

FIGURE 13–33. Large ulcers in Crohn's disease. *A,* Large ulcers *(arrows)* protrude deeply from the inferior border of the cecum. The terminal ileum faintly shows a few aphthoid ulcers. *B,* Shallow ulcers *(arrows)* are seen in the rectum of a different patient, as subtle barium collections surrounded by radiolucent halos. The rectal mucosa appears "boggy."

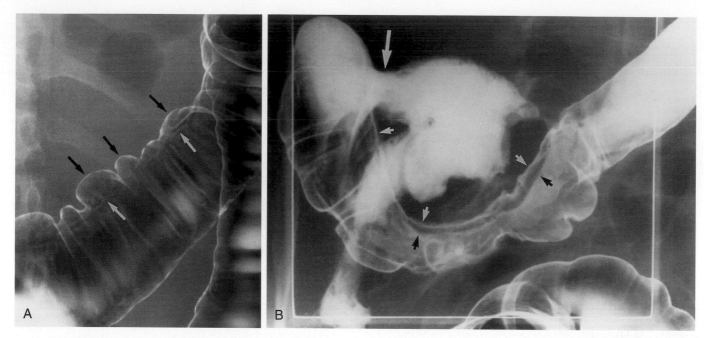

FIGURE 13–34. Longitudinal ulcers in Crohn's disease. *A,* Long, thin ulcers are seen near the superior border of the transverse colon, as barium lines surrounded by a radiolucent halo *(white arrows).* Sacculation *(black arrows)* of the superior border of the transverse colon is present. (From Rubesin, S.E., and Bronner, M.: Radiologic-pathologic concepts in Crohn's disease. Adv. Gastrointest. Radiol. *1:27,* 1991, with permission.) *B,* A long linear ulcer *(short white arrows)* surrounded by a radiolucent halo *(black arrows)* is seen in the transverse colon just distal to the ileocolic anastomosis *(long white arrow).* Recurrent Crohn's disease is also present in the neoterminal ileum.

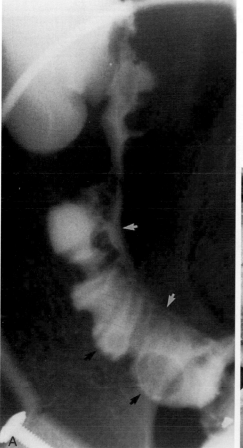

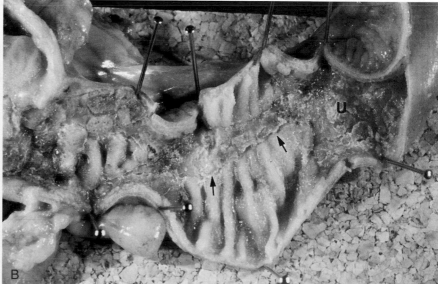

FIGURE 13–35. Mesenteric border ulcer in terminal ileum. *A,* Compression spot radiograph shows a long linear collection of barium *(white arrows)* on the mesenteric border of the terminal ileum. Sacculation *(black arrows)* of the wall opposite the ulcer is seen. *B,* Photograph of the surgical specimen from the same patient shows a 5-mm wide ulcer *(arrows)* faintly coated with barium from a previous specimen radiograph. More extensive ulceration is seen proximally *(U)* and distally. (From Herlinger, H., Rubesin, S.E., and Furth, E.E.: Mesenteric border ulcers in Crohn's disease: Historical, radiologic and pathologic perspectives. Abd. Imaging *23:*122, 1998, with permission.)

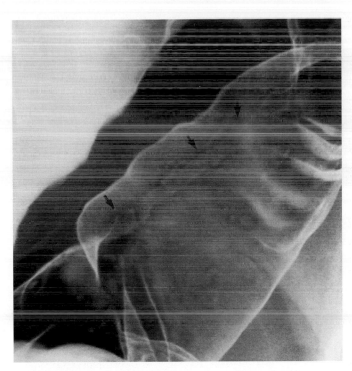

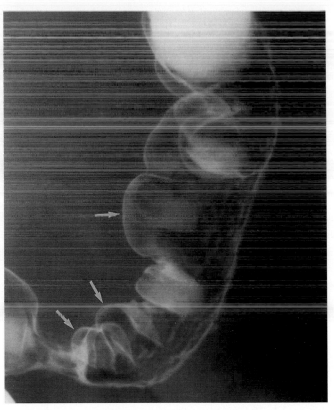

FIGURE 13–36. Spot radiograph of descending colon shows numerous aphthoid ulcers and a long, shallow ulcer. A radiolucent halo *(black arrows)* helps identify the shallow barium collection as an ulcer.

FIGURE 13–37. Sacculation opposite ulceration in Crohn's disease. Numerous shallow ulcers are seen on the lateral wall of the descending colon. The relatively uninvolved medial wall is thrown into sacculations *(arrows).*

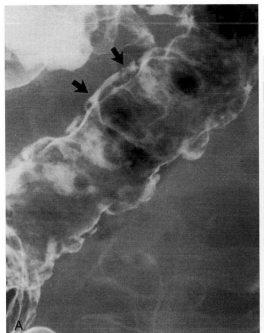

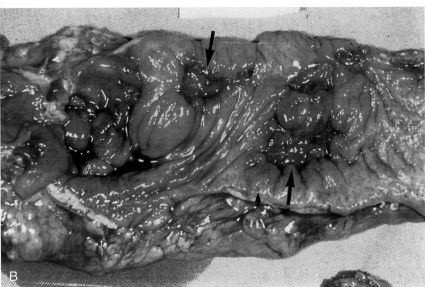

FIGURE 13–38. Deep ulcers in Crohn's disease. *A,* Numerous deep ulcers are present. Two ulcers are joining, forming an intramural track *(arrows). B,* Specimen photograph from a different patient shows deep ulcers *(large arrows)* with undermined edges and folds radiating to their margins. Numerous aphthoid ulcers are also present (representative aphthoid ulcer identified with *small arrow).* (From Rubesin, S.E., and Bronner, M.: Radiologic-pathologic concepts in Crohn's disease. Adv. Gastrointest. Radiol. *1:*27, 1991, with permission.)

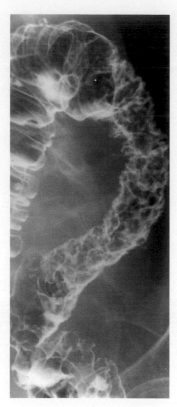

FIGURE 13–39. Cobblestoning in descending colon. Numerous polygonal, radiolucent islands of nondenuded mucosa are surrounded by barium-filled grooves.

Pathologically, Crohn's disease is characterized by knifelike clefts penetrating deep into the submucosa or muscularis propria.[80] When transversely and longitudinally oriented, knifelike clefts communicate, the islands of less inflamed tissue lying between the clefts result in cobblestoning (Figs. 13–39 and 13–40), also called the

"ulceronodular" pattern. Radiographically, barium fills the reticular network of clefts, which are separated by polygonal, radiolucent islands of mucosa (Fig. 13–41). The deeply penetrating ulcers form the basis for fissures and fistulae. Despite deep penetration of large ulcers and fissures, free perforation is uncommon in Crohn's disease.[15,90]

Mural Thickening

Crohn's disease is also characterized by transmural inflammation and fibrosis. The Crohn's inflammatory process spreads downward along the knifelike clefts and lymphatics. The submucosa is widened by edema and a perilymphatic inflammatory infiltrate (Fig. 13–42).[80,86] The inflammatory process may burrow deeply through the muscularis propria into the subserosa. The submucosa may also be thickened by fat.[91]

On barium studies, the submucosal inflammatory process is manifested by fold thickening and mucosal nodularity. Luminal narrowing seen during barium studies may be due to reversible edema, inflammation, or spasm, or by relatively irreversible fibrosis. Therefore a "string sign" or narrowing may be a reversible or fixed process (Figs. 13–43 and 13–44). Luminal narrowing seen on barium studies correlates with wall thickening seen on CT. On CT the wall thickening may be of soft tissue attenuation (Fig. 13–45) due to inflammation or fibrosis or of low attenuation due to submucosal edema or fat.[91] The ileocecal valve is often enlarged, even when Crohn's disease only involves the ileum. Inflammation or fistulous tracks from the terminal ileum through the ileocecal valve region enlarge the ileocecal valve (Fig. 13–46). The radiologist should recommend CT as the first study to be performed in symptomatic patients with Crohn's disease. CT is superior in the demonstration of abscesses (Fig. 13–47) and the causes of separation of bowel loops (Fig. 13–48).

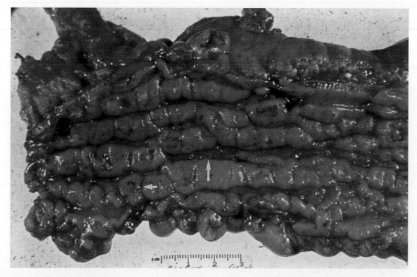

FIGURE 13–40. Cobblestoning in Crohn's colitis. Specimen photograph shows deep longitudinal ulcers (representative longitudinal ulcer— *long white arrow*) and shallow transverse clefts *(short arrow)*. (From Rubesin, S.E., and Bronner, M.: Radiologic-pathologic concepts in Crohn's disease. Adv. Gastrointest. Radiol. *1:27,* 1991, with permission.)

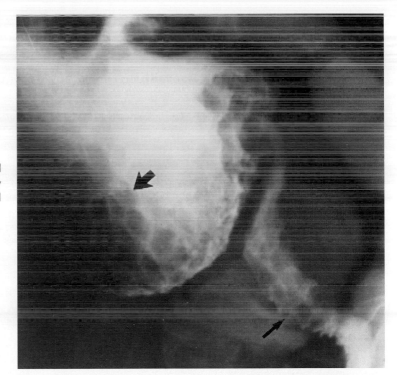

FIGURE 13–41. Cobblestoning in cecum and terminal ileum. Shallow polygonal islands of mucosa are separated by barium-filled clefts in the cecum *(large arrow)* and terminal ileum *(small arrow).*

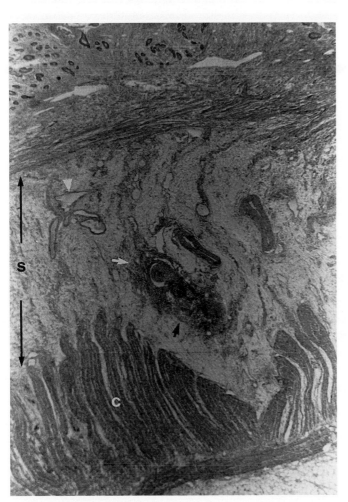

FIGURE 13–42. Wall thickening in Crohn's disease. The submucosa *(s)* of the ileum is widened because of edema and inflammation. There is an extensive perilymphatic inflammatory infiltrate *(short arrows).* Lymphangiectasia *(representative dilated lymphatic—arrowhead)* is also extensive (c—circular muscle layer of muscularis propria). (From Rubesin, S.E., and Bronner, M.: Radiologic-pathologic concepts in Crohn's disease. Adv. Gastrointest. Radiol. *1*:27, 1991, with permission.)

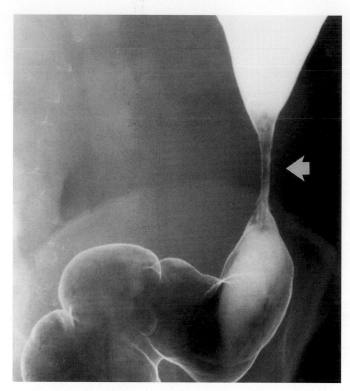

FIGURE 13–43. "String" sign in descending colon. A 5-cm long, tubular segment *(arrow)* with tapered edges is at the junction of the descending and sigmoid colon.

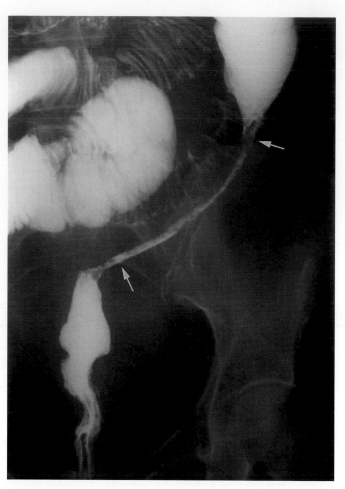

FIGURE 13–44. "String" sign in recurrent Crohn's disease. The segment of small bowel *(arrows)* proximal to the ileocolic anastomosis is diffusely narrowed and has a finely nodular mucosa. (From Rubesin, S.E., and Laufer, I.: Pictorial glossary of double contrast radiology. *In* Gore, R.M., Levine, M.S., and Laufer, I. (eds.): Textbook of Gastrointestinal Radiology. Philadelphia, W.B. Saunders Co., 1994, pp. 50–80, with permission.)

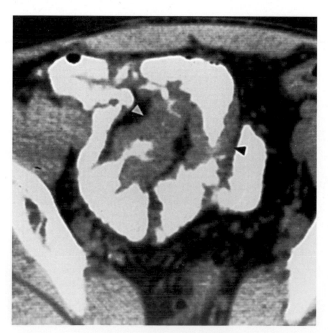

FIGURE 13–45. Wall thickening in Crohn's disease. The distal ileum has moderate thickening *(arrowheads)* of its walls of soft tissue attenuation. (From Rubesin, S.E., and Bronner, M.: Radiologic-pathologic concepts in Crohn's disease. Adv. Gastrointest. Radiol. *1:27,* 1991, with permission.)

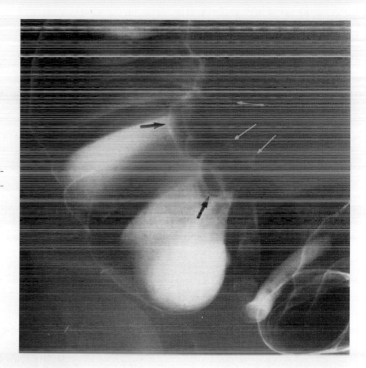

FIGURE 13–46. **Enlarged ileocecal valve in Crohn's disease.** Numerous fistulae *(white arrows)* from unopacified terminal ileum radiate toward an enlarged ileocecal valve region *(black arrows).*

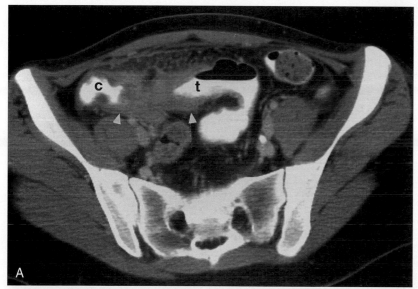

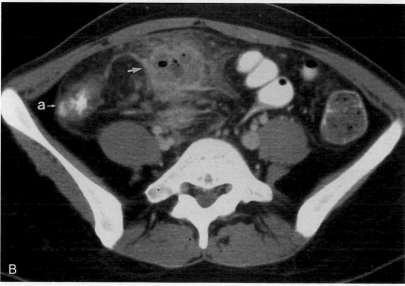

FIGURE **13–47. When in doubt, start with CT.** *A,* Patient with known Crohn's disease and right lower quadrant pain. Marked wall thickening *(arrowheads)* is seen in the terminal ileum *(t)* and cecum *(c).* Moderate stranding of mesenteric fat is seen. *B,* An image more craniad than in *A* through ascending colon *(a)* shows an abscess as soft tissue mass *(arrow)* infiltrating the mesenteric fat. Numerous tiny air pockets are seen.

441

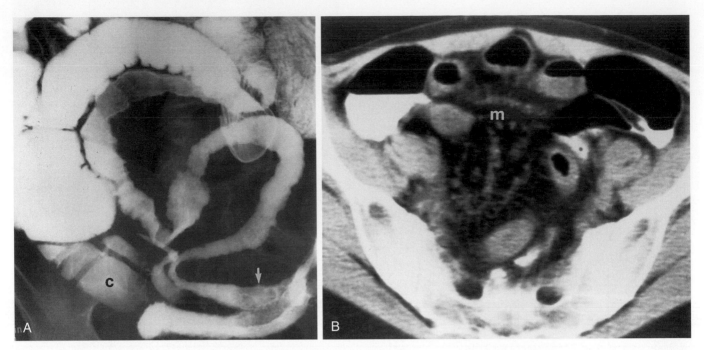

FIGURE 13–48. CT demonstrates the cause for separation of bowel loops. *A,* Ileal loops are separated. Cobblestoning is seen in two pelvic ileal loops *(arrow).* (Cecum—*c*). *B,* CT through pelvis shows "fibrofatty proliferation" of the small bowel mesentery *(m)* with moderate stranding of the fat. (From Rubesin, S.E., and Bronner, M.: Radiologic-pathologic concepts in Crohn's disease. Adv. Gastrointest. Radiol. *1:27,* 1991, with permission.)

Asymmetric changes, a hallmark of Crohn's disease, not only occur opposite longitudinal ulceration but also during healing and fibrosis. Asymmetric scarring results in sacculation of the wall opposite the scar (Fig. 13–49), similar to the sacculation opposite a mesenteric border ulcer. Fibrosis also results in longitudinal shortening and luminal narrowing.[92,93]

Strictures in Crohn's disease are usually long and have tapered margins (see Fig. 13–49) in contrast to colonic cancers, which are short and have abrupt margins. Occasionally, however, Crohn's strictures are short (Fig. 13–50) or have abrupt margins. Therefore a short, abrupt stricture without identifiable ulceration can represent scarring or carcinoma. Cancer arising in Crohn's disease is not only difficult for the radiologist but also for the endoscopist, surgeon, or pathologist. The diagnosis of cancer arising in Crohn's disease is often first made during microscopic evaluation of the surgical pathology specimens.[94]

Fissures, Fistulae, and Abscesses

When knifelike clefts elongate, intramural tracks are formed. Penetration into the serosa results in pericolic fissures (Fig. 13–51) and fistulae. Tracking that parallels the bowel wall frequently occurs, often when Crohn's disease complicates diverticulosis.[95] Tracks paralleling bowel are not specific for Crohn's disease and may occur in either diverticulitis or Crohn's disease (Fig. 13–52).[95–97]

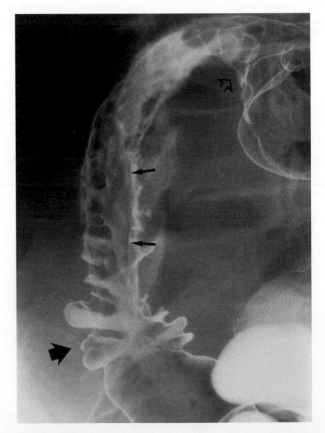

FIGURE 13–49. A long stricture in Crohn's disease has a tapered proximal margin *(open arrow),* a sacculated distal margin *(thick arrow),* and centrally, seen en face, a longitudinal ulcer *(thin arrows).*

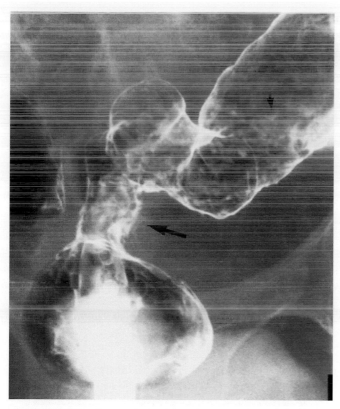

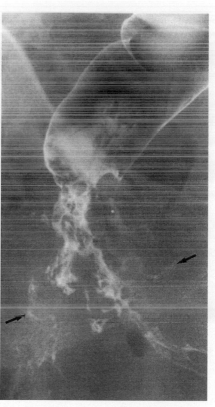

FIGURE 13–50. Short stricture in Crohn's disease. A short stricture *(long arrow)* is present at the rectosigmoid junction. Aphthoid ulcers are seen in the shortened sigmoid colon *(short arrow)*.

FIGURE 13–51. Perirectal fissures in Crohn's disease. The distal rectum is diffusely narrowed. Numerous sinus tracks (representative sinus tracks identified by *arrows*) extend beyond the expected luminal contour. (From Rubesin, S.E., and Bronner, M.: Radiologic-pathologic concepts in Crohn's disease. Adv. Gastrointest. Radiol. 1:27, 1991, with permission.)

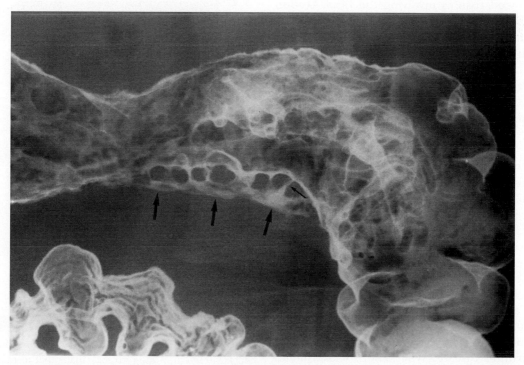

FIGURE 13–52. Pericolic tracking in Crohn's disease. Numerous intramural tracks perpendicular to the longitudinal axis of the colon (representative intramural track identified by *thin arrow*) join a long pericolic track *(thick arrows)* parallel to the wall of the splenic flexure.

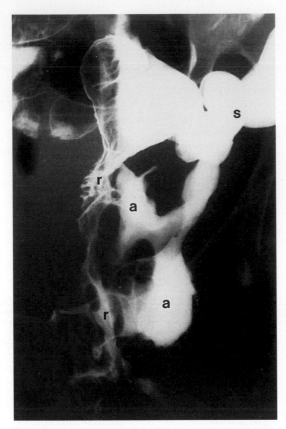

FIGURE 13–53. Perirectal sinus tracks and abscesses in Crohn's disease. The rectosigmoid colon is diffusely narrowed. Numerous fissures emanate from the rectum *(r)* and sigmoid *(s)*, forming abscesses *(a)* in the perirectal fat.

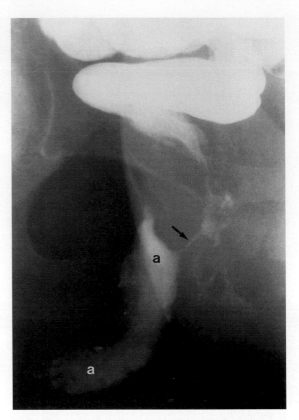

FIGURE 13–54. Perianal abscess caused by Crohn's disease. A sinus track *(arrow)* extends from the anal canal to a long tubular perianal abscess *(a)*. (From Rubesin, S.E., et al.: Radiologic investigation of inflammatory bowel disease. *In* MacDermott, R.P., and Stenson, W.F.: Inflammatory Bowel Disease. New York, Elsevier Science Publishing Co., 1992.)

Deep clefts and fissures involving the distal rectum and anal canal (Fig. 13–53) are hallmarks of Crohn's disease. Approximately two thirds to three quarters of patients with Crohn's disease involving only the colon will have anal involvement.[98,99] Anal disease may be the first clinical manifestation of Crohn's disease. Radiographically, sinus tracks extend deep into perirectal and perianal subcutaneous tissue (see Fig. 13–53)(Fig. 13–54). Distal rectovaginal or anovaginal fistulae may form (Fig. 13–55).

A fistula is defined as a track that communicates with another structure. Ileocolic (Fig. 13–56) and enterovesical (Fig. 13–57) fistulae are the most common types of fistulae in Crohn's disease.[100,101] Of ileocolic fistulae, ileocecal and ileosigmoid are the most frequent types. Enterocutaneous, colocolic (Fig. 13–58), and enterovaginal fistulae are less commonly seen. Crohn's fistulas can extend up the gastrocolic portion of the greater omentum to involve the stomach (Fig. 13–59). Ileosigmoid fistulae are usually related to Crohn's disease of the ileum, tracking inferiorly to involve normal sigmoid colon (Fig. 13–60).[102] The sigmoid mucosa is not involved with Crohn's disease. When the diseased ileum and fistula are resected, the sigmoid colon returns to its normal state.[102]

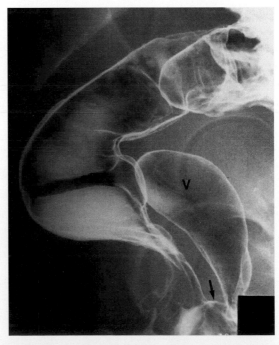

FIGURE 13–55. Anovaginal fistula in Crohn's disease. A barium track *(arrow)* from the proximal anal canal to the distal vagina is seen. The vagina *(V)* is distended with air during the air contrast study. Numerous aphthoid ulcers are seen in the proximal rectum.

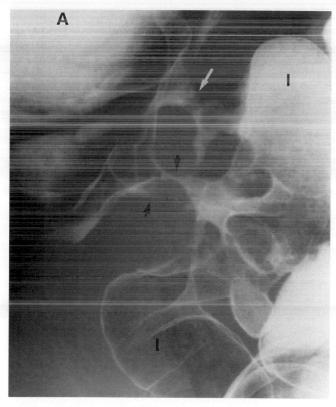

FIGURE **13–56. Ileocolic fistulae in Crohn's disease.** Two fistulae *(black arrows)* and a distorted ileocecal valve *(white arrow)* bridge the distorted terminal ileum *(I)* to the cecum. *A* = ascending colon. (From Rubesin, S.E., et al.: Radiologic investigation of inflammatory bowel disease. *In* MacDermott, R.P., and Stenson, W.F.: Inflammatory Bowel Disease. New York, Elsevier Science Publishing Co., 1992.)

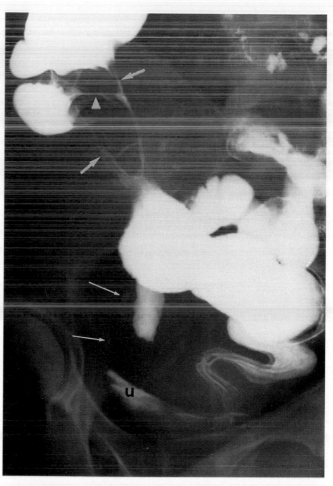

FIGURE **13–57. Enterovesical fistula.** The urinary bladder *(u)* is filled with barium from a faintly opacified fistula *(thin arrows)* from the ileum. Two ileocecal fistulae *(thick arrows)* are seen. The ileocecal valve is identified *(arrowhead)*. (From Rubesin, S.E., and Bronner, M.: Radiologic-pathologic concepts in Crohn's disease. Adv. Gastrointest. Radiol. *1:27,* 1991, with permission.)

FIGURE **13–58. Colocolic fistula.** A fistula *(arrows)* parallels the inferior wall of the sigmoid colon. The sigmoid colon is narrowed with nodular mucosa.

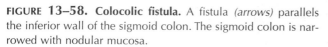
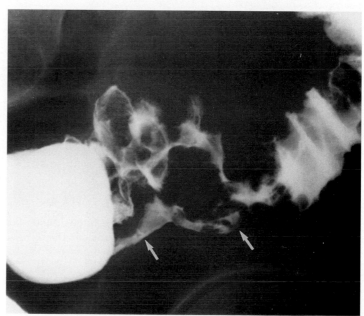

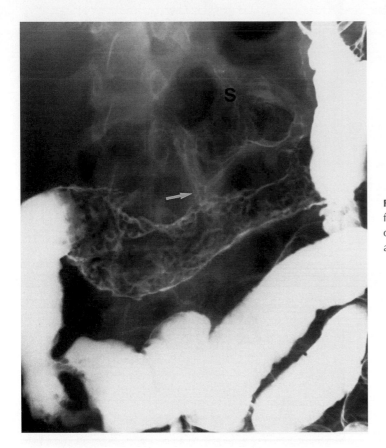

FIGURE 13–59. Gastrocolic fistula. The transverse colon is diffusely narrowed with numerous postinflammatory polyps. A track of barium *(arrow)* heads superiorly. Barium faintly coats the antrum of the stomach.

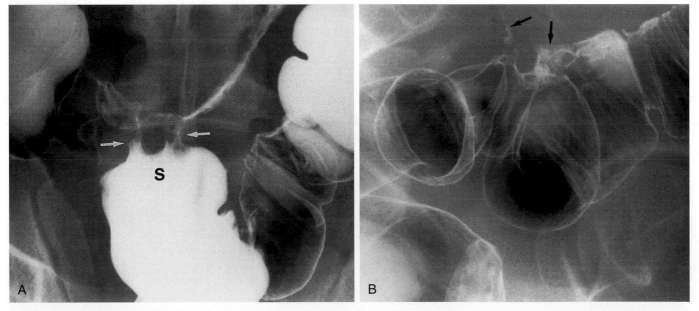

FIGURE 13–60. Ileosigmoid fistulae. *A,* Two tracks *(arrows)* course from the diffusely narrowed ileum to the sigmoid colon *(S). B,* The sigmoid colon is relatively uninvolved. The mucosa is smooth. During resection of the fistulae *(arrows),* the sigmoid colon was found to be free of primary Crohn's disease. (From Rubesin, S.E., and Bronner, M.: Radiologic-pathologic concepts in Crohn's disease. Adv. Gastrointest. Radiol. *1:*27, 1991, with permission.)

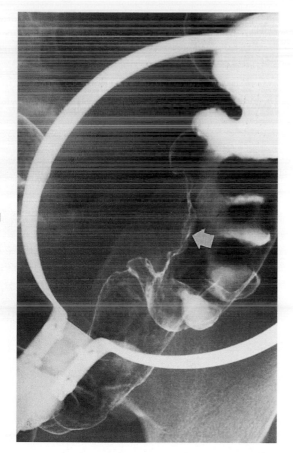

FIGURE 13–61. Inflammatory mass in Crohn's colitis. A long, sessile polypoid mass *(arrow)* protrudes into the medial wall of the descending colon.

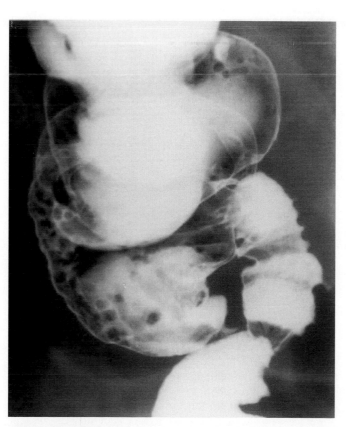

FIGURE 13–62. Numerous round, postinflammatory polyps are seen on the lateral wall of the cecum.

Polypoid Lesions

Almost all polyps arising in Crohn's disease are related to inflammation. Islands of mucosa between areas of extensive ulceration are termed *inflammatory pseudopolyps.*[4] Inflammatory polypoid masses may occur (Fig. 13–61).[4] After inflammation has healed, reparative or hyperplastic tissue may form polyps of varying sizes and shapes. Postinflammatory polyps may be round (Fig. 13–62), sessile, pedunculated, or filiform in shape (Fig. 13–63).[33,103] When the tips of filiform polyps fuse, mucosal bridges are formed (Fig. 13–64).[104]

Uncommon Findings

Reversibility is less common in Crohn's disease than in ulcerative colitis, occurring in 7% of patients.[105] When Crohn's disease heals, it usually results in scarring, unlike ulcerative colitis, which usually heals without scarring.[4] Crohn's disease involving the entire colon is unusual but, when present, may be difficult to distinguish from ulcerative colitis.

Other Sites

Details of Crohn's disease involving the upper gastrointestinal tract and small bowel are discussed in Chapters 7 and 10 and in references 106 to 116. Aphthoid ulcers are the most common gastroduodenal manifestation of Crohn's disease, seen in 40% to 75% of patients (Fig.

FIGURE 13–63. Filiform polyps in Crohn's disease. *A,* A focal group of filiform polyps *(arrow)* are seen in a stricture of the sigmoid colon. *B,* In a different patient, numerous filiform polyps are seen in the descending colon.

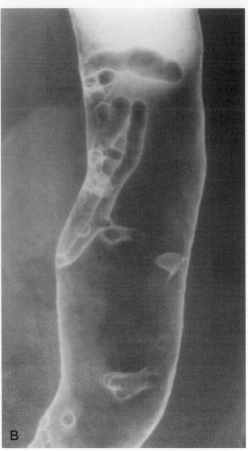

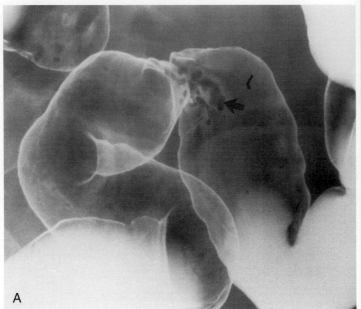

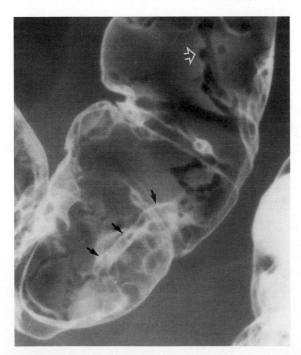

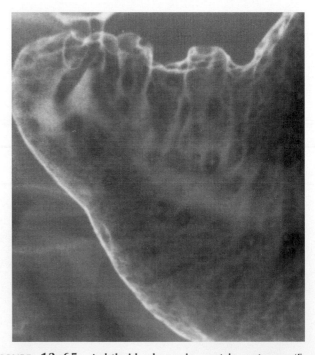

FIGURE 13–64. Mucosal bridges and filiform polyps in Crohn's disease. A mucosal bridge is etched in white *(black arrows)*. Some of the filiform polyps are branching; others have clubbed heads *(white arrow).* (From Rubesin, S.E., and Bronner, M.: Radiologic-pathologic concepts in Crohn's disease. Adv. Gastrointest. Radiol. *1:*27, 1991, with permission.)

FIGURE 13–65. Aphthoid ulcers in gastric antrum. (From Rubesin, S.E., et al.: Radiologic investigation of inflammatory bowel disease. *In* MacDermott, R.P., and Stenson, W.F.: Inflammatory Bowel Disease. New York, Elsevier Science Publishing Co., 1992.)

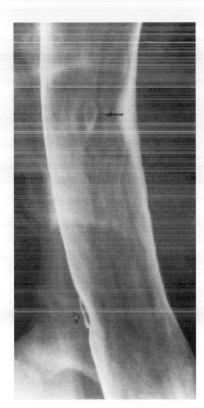

FIGURE 13–66. Aphthoid ulcers in esophagus seen en face *(arrow)* and in profile *(open arrow)*. (From Gohel, V.J., et al.: Aphthous ulcers in the esophagus with Crohn disease. AJR Am. J. Roentgenol. *137*:872, 1981. © American Roentgen Ray Society.)

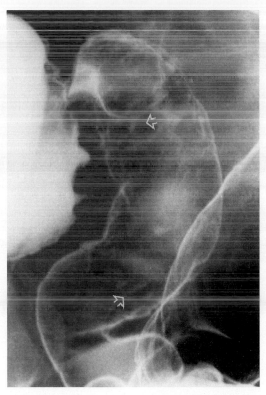

FIGURE 13–67. **Aphthoid ulcers in the terminal ileum** in Crohn's disease. Representative aphthoid ulcers are identified by arrows. (From Rubesin, S.E., and Bronner, M.: Radiologic-pathologic concepts in Crohn's disease. Adv. Gastrointest. Radiol. *1*:27, 1991, with permission.)

13–65). Aphthoid ulcers in Crohn's disease are radiographically indistinguishable from other causes of erosions. Esophageal involvement (Fig. 13–66) is uncommon.[115,116] Terminal ileal changes are similar to colonic changes, including aphthoid ulcers (Fig. 13–67), thickening of folds or mucosal nodularity (Fig. 13–68), mesenteric border ulceration (see Fig. 13–35), cobblestoning, strictures, and fistulae.[117] Granular mucosa, rare in the colon, is not uncommon in the small bowel (Fig. 13–69). Wide and blunted, edematous, and inflamed villi radio-

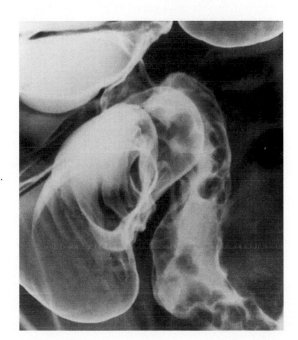

FIGURE 13–68. **Nodular mucosa in terminal ileum** of patient with Crohn's disease.

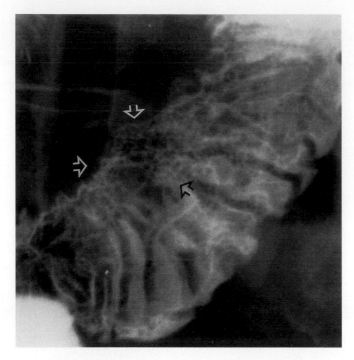

FIGURE 13–69. Granular mucosa in Crohn's disease. Spot film of distal ileum shows numerous 0.5 to 1 mm fine nodules *(arrows)* surrounded by a reticular network of barium. The tiny nodules represent villi enlarged by edema and inflammatory cells.

graphically appear as 0.5 to 2 mm round or angulated nodules surrounded by barium in the interstices between villi. The enlarged villi result in the "granular" or finely nodular pattern.[86,118–120]

DISTINCTION BETWEEN ULCERATIVE COLITIS AND CROHN'S DISEASE

Distinguishing ulcerative colitis and Crohn's disease is important because the two diseases have different medical treatment strategies and surgical approaches and different prognoses for either recurrent disease or cancer risk. Barium enemas can distinguish colonic Crohn's disease from ulcerative colitis in more than 95% of patients (Table 13–1).[121] Barium enema distinction between Crohn's disease and ulcerative colitis is relatively simple

compared with distinguishing the mimics of ulcerative colitis from ulcerative colitis and the mimics of Crohn's disease from Crohn's disease (Table 13–2).

Ulcerative colitis extends retrogradely from the anorectal junction in a continuous, symmetric fashion. Ulcerative colitis extends circumferentially around a bowel loop. In contrast, Crohn's disease is patchy and discontinuous, involving bowel segments asymmetrically. Only rarely does Crohn's disease form a pancolitis (Fig. 13–70). Small ulcers in ulcerative colitis are seen on a

TABLE 13–1. *Ulcerative Colitis versus Crohn's Disease*

Ulcerative Colitis	Crohn's Disease
Mucosal granularity	Aphthoid ulcers
Ulcers on background of granular mucosa	Ulcers on background of normal mucosa
Continuous	Discontinuous
Symmetric	Asymmetric
Begins in rectum, spreads retrogradely in continuous fashion	Any segment of gastrointestinal tract
Fulminant colitis	Severe anal and perianal disease
	Sinus tracks and fistulae
Colon cancer in large percentage of patients	Abscesses

TABLE 13–2. *Mimics of Ulcerative Colitis versus Mimics of Crohn's Disease*

Mimics of Ulcerative Colitis	Mimics of Crohn's Disease
Pancolitis	**Colonic**
Campylobacter	Amebiasis
Shigellosis	Tuberculosis
Salmonellosis	Ischemic colitis
E. coli infection	LGV
C. difficile infection	
	Ileocecal
Amebiasis	Carcinoma/lymphoma
	Tuberculosis
Proctosigmoiditis	
Chlamydia	**Small Intestinal**
Radiation colitis	*Yersinia* (early Crohn's disease)
	Salmonella (early Crohn's disease)
	Eosinophilic enteritis
	Radiation change
	Carcinoid
	Tuberculosis

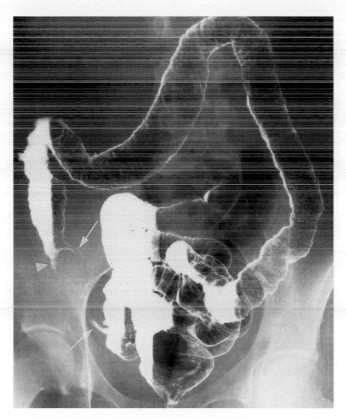

FIGURE 13–70. Pancolitis in Crohn's disease. Numerous aphthoid ulcers carpet the colon. The rectum is relatively spared. The background mucosa is smooth. The terminal ileum *(long arrows)* is diffusely narrowed. The cecum *(arrowhead)* is contracted.

background of granular mucosa. In contrast, in the early phase of Crohn's disease, aphthoid ulcers are separated by normal intervening mucosa. Anal and perianal fissures are typically seen in Crohn's disease, as well as sinus tracks and fistulae. Ulcerative colitis does not result in sinus tracks or fistulae. Crohn's disease is a chronic, debilitating condition complicated by abscess formation and fistulae. Ulcerative colitis has frequent flares of bloody diarrhea separated by relatively long periods of clinical quiescence. Cancer complicates long-standing ulcerative colitis much more frequently than long-standing Crohn's disease.

ISCHEMIA

Ischemia is the most common cause of colitis in patients older than 50.[122,123] Ischemic colitis has a broad clinical spectrum, from transient colitis to acute fulminant necrosis.[124,125] Patients complain of colicky, lower abdominal pain, rectal bleeding, or bloody diarrhea.

Ischemic colitis is often multifactorial, but the most common causes of ischemia are low flow states due to diminished cardiac output or depletion of intravascular volume (Table 13–3).[126] Common low-flow conditions leading to ischemic colitis include congestive heart failure, shock, or arrhythmia. Small vessel disease such as vasculitis and diabetes frequently results in ischemia. Large ves-

sel occlusion of the superior mesenteric artery or inferior mesenteric artery because of atherosclerosis, embolism, or other causes less frequently results in ischemic colitis because the collateral circulation is rich, which prevents ischemic change. Medium-sized arterial occlusion in combination with deficiency of the collateral arcs, however, may result in ischemia. Venous occlusion related to portal venous thrombosis, pancreatitis, or hypercoagulable states such as sickle cell disease may result in ischemia. Acute colonic dilatation due to acute adynamic ileus or obstructing lesions such as carcinoma or volvulus may also result in ischemia. Fecal impaction causes rectal ischemia by overdistention and pressure necrosis, resulting in stercoral ulcers. Stercoral ulcers typically occur in elderly patients with constipation.

The spectrum of ischemic change depends on the cause, rate, duration, and extent of vascular injury. The mucosa is the colonic layer most susceptible to ischemia.

TABLE 13–3. *Common Causes of Ischemic Colitis*

Low Flow States
Carcinogenic shock: Drugs, dehydration, sepsis
Congestive heart failure
Arrhythmia
Myocardial infarction

Small Vessel Disease
Vasculitis
   Collagen vascular: Systemic lupus erythematosus, rheumatoid arthritis
   Hypersensitivity: Henoch-Schönlein purpura, cryoglobulinemia
   Behçet's disease
Amyloidosis
Irradiation
Organ transplantation
Disseminated intravascular coagulation

Arterial Occlusion
Atherosclerosis
Embolism
Thrombosis
Takayasu's disease
Giant cell arteritis

Venous Occlusion
Thrombosis
Portal vein thrombosis
Pancreatitis
Hypercoaguable states: Idiopathic thrombocytopenic purpura, sickle cell disease

Vascular Compression
Carcinoid
Lymphoma

Colonic Obstruction
Carcinoma
Volvulus
Fecal impaction
Diverticulitis

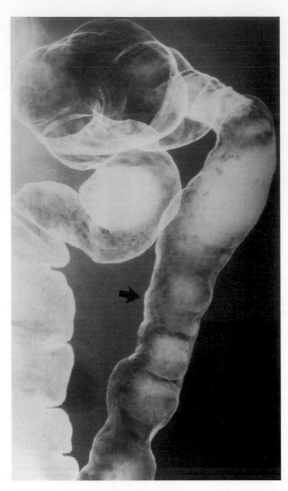

FIGURE 13–71. Ischemia in watershed area. Diffuse narrowing of the splenic flexure is seen. The mucosa has numerous tiny nodules on its surface (representative nodular mucosa identified by *arrow*).

Mild ischemia results in edema, hemorrhage, or superficial ulceration in the mucosa and submucosa.[127] This form of ischemia is usually reversible, healing within 1 to 2 weeks.[125] Moderately severe ischemia affects deeper colonic layers as well, resulting in deep ulceration and fibrosis. Massive ischemia leads to fulminant necrosis, pneumatosis, perforation, and toxic megacolon.

Any portion of the colon can become ischemic. The splenic flexure and descending colon are the most frequent sites of ischemia (Fig. 13–71), especially in the presence of deficiency of the marginal artery between the superior mesenteric and inferior mesenteric artery distribution. Approximately two thirds of cases of colonic ischemia occur in the watershed area of the transverse and descending colon.[126,128] Ischemia is not uncommon, however, in the cecum or sigmoid colon. Ischemia may even occur in the rectum,[129] especially in patients with stercoral ulceration. Short, focal areas of ischemia usually are due to vasculitis or cholesterol emboli.[130]

In young adults, transient ischemia of the right colon has been described in a wide variety of clinical settings, including hypotension related to trauma[131] and use of drugs such as cocaine[132] and amphetamines.[133,134] Transient right-sided colitis has also been associated with hypersensitivity vasculitis due to penicillin derivatives[135] and to the use of oral contraceptives.[136]

Barium enemas are contraindicated in patients with suspected perforation. Because CT is often performed in severely ill patients with bloody diarrhea or acute abdominal pain, CT is often the first study to suggest colonic ischemia. On CT, ischemia usually appears as symmetric bowel wall thickening (Fig. 13–72).[137] Submucosal edema may result in low attenuation "target" or "double halo" signs.[138] CT is superb at demonstrating pneumatosis coli

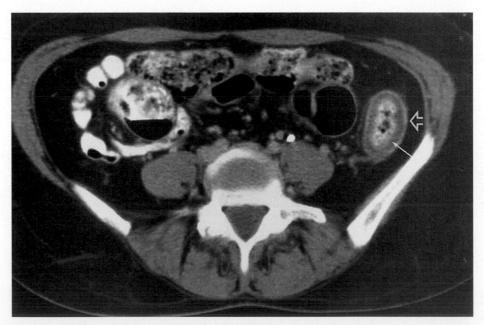

FIGURE 13–72. Ischemia in descending colon in patient with acute left lower, quadrant pain. The descending colon wall is thickened. The submucosa *(thin arrow)* is widened and of low attenuation. The muscular wall enhances with intravenous contrast material *(open arrow)*.

(Fig. 13–73), free intraperitoneal gas, or other signs of perforation (Fig. 13–74).

Despite the primacy of CT in acutely ill patients, if a barium study is performed, it is relatively accurate, detecting ischemic colitis in 80% to 90% of patients.[139-141] Barium enema findings depend on the severity of ischemia and the duration of symptoms. Ischemic findings change with follow-up examinations.

Early mucosal and submucosal hemorrhage and edema lead to thick colonic folds and thumbprinting (Fig. 13–75). The thick folds often form "transverse ridges" perpendicular to the longitudinal axis of bowel. Thumbprints are smooth, round elevations protruding into the lumen (Fig. 13–76).[139,140] Thumbprints are usu-

ally multiple. Spasm may be prominent because of anoxic change in smooth muscle. Early and mild changes may be effaced with colonic overdistention.[142]

Mucosal ischemia may occur in areas of colonic distention proximal to an obstructing lesion or in markedly dilated colon as a result of acute adynamic ileus. Mucosal ischemia is radiographically manifest as relatively flat and polygonal nodules outlined by barium within grooves between nodules. These flat nodules were originally described in patients with urticaria, hence the name "colonic urticarial pattern" (Fig. 13–77).[143] Colonic urticaria is not specific for urticaria and is seen in a wide variety of conditions, including viral infections, Crohn's disease, and colonic obstruction.

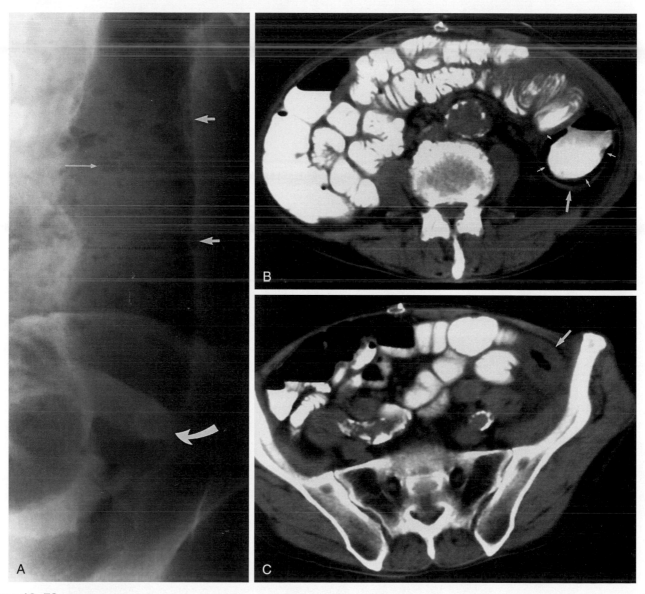

FIGURE 13–73. Pneumatosis coli in ischemic colitis. *A,* Plain film of descending colon shows small collections of air in the wall of the bowel en face (representative lucency of air—*long arrow*) and in profile *(short arrows).* Folds at the descending/sigmoid junction are thick *(curved arrow). B,* CT from same patient shows a curvilinear collection of air *(small arrows)* in the wall *(large arrow)* of descending colon. *C,* CT from same patient at level of descending/sigmoid junction shows diffuse thickening of the wall of the colon *(arrow)* corresponding to the thick folds seen inferiorly on the plain film.

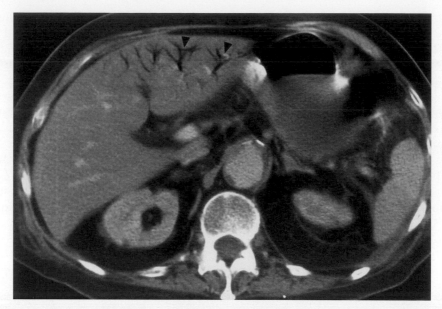

FIGURE 13–74. Air in portal venous vessels in liver. In another patient with ischemic colitis, numerous gas-attenuation, "seagull"-shaped densities *(arrowheads)* are seen in the nondependent portion of the left lobe of the liver.

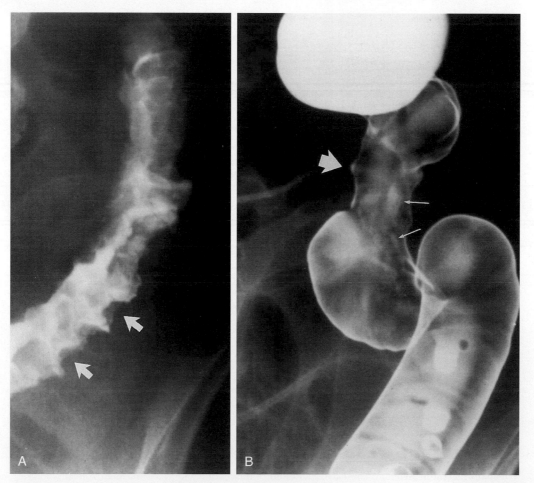

FIGURE 13–75. Thumbprinting and mucosal nodularity in ischemia. *A,* The folds at the junction of the descending and sigmoid colon are thick, the mucosa is nodular, and "thumbprints" *(arrows)* are present as hemispheric indentations of the colonic wall. *B,* Several weeks later, most of the descending colon has healed. A focal narrowing *(large arrow)* has developed. Superficial ulcers within this early stricture are manifest as focal barium collections (representative ulcers identified by *thin arrows*).

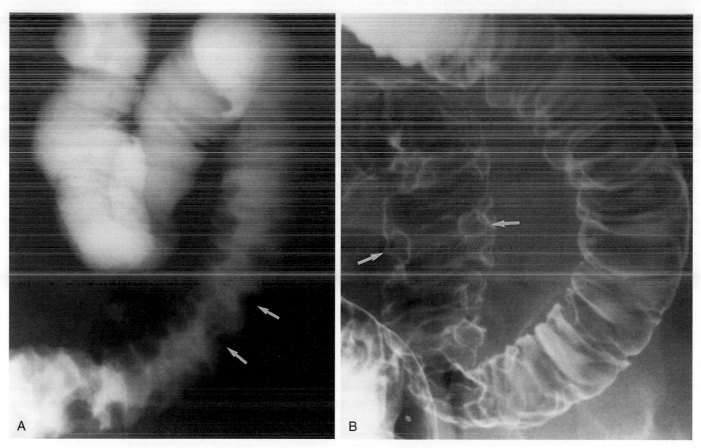

FIGURE 13–76.   Thumbprinting in ischemic colitis. *A,* Single contrast phase of barium enema shows numerous "thumbprints" *(arrows)* in sigmoid colon. *B,* Air contrast phase from the same barium enema shows thumbprints as round, barium-etched nodules *(arrows).*

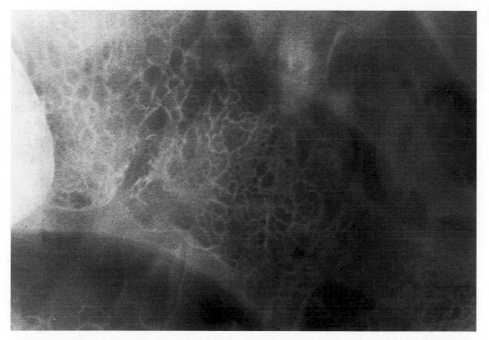

FIGURE 13–77.   Colonic urticarial pattern. Close-up of dilated transverse colon shows numerous polygonal islands surrounded by barium etched grooves. (From Rubesin, S.E., et al.: Carpet lesions of the colon. RadioGraphics, *5:*537–552, 1985.)

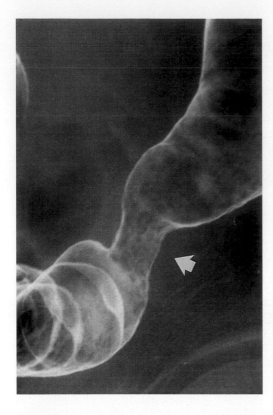

FIGURE 13–78. Stricture in ischemic colitis. A focal narrowing *(arrow)* with tapered margins is covered by mildly nodular mucosa.

After the initial ischemic insult, the colon may heal completely or form chronic ulcers or strictures. Within 1 to 3 weeks after the initial ischemic event, sloughing of the necrotic layer results in ulceration in approximately 40% to 60% of patients.[141,144] Ulcers may be small or large (see Fig. 13–75*B*), punctate, or longitudinally oriented. Strictures develop in a minority of patients as early as 3 weeks after the initial insult.[141] Strictures usually appear smooth or tapered (Fig. 13–78) (see Fig. 13–75*B*) but occasionally are eccentric and sacculated.

RADIATION THERAPY

Acute radiation colitis is usually self-limited, occurring in the first weeks after radiation therapy because of direct toxic damage to the colonic epithelium. Patients complain of diarrhea, tenesmus, abdominal cramping, and rectal bleeding. Barium enemas are rarely performed during the acute phase of radiation colitis.

Chronic radiation colitis is usually caused by destruction of the microvasculature of the colon. A progressive obliterative endarteritis leads to ulceration and fissuring of the mucosa, hypertrophy of the muscularis mucosae, fibrosis, and with time, mucosal atrophy.[145] Severe radiation change is complicated by deep ulceration, stricture formation, colitis cystica profunda, and rectovaginal fistula formation.[145–147]

In patients with a history of pelvic irradiation, barium enemas are performed to exclude other lesions causing bloody discharge, diarrhea, or lower abdominal pain. Radiographically, the rectosigmoid colon is smooth, featureless, and narrow (Fig. 13–79).[148] The valves of Houston are diminished in number or are absent. In some patients the mucosa is granular (Fig. 13–80), similar in appearance to ulcerative colitis. Strictures may be long or short but show tapered margins. Fistulas to the bladder or vagina may be seen.

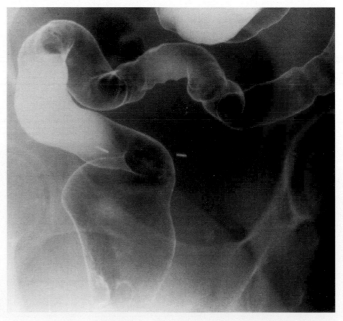

FIGURE 13–79. Radiation colitis. The rectosigmoid colon is tubular: diffusely narrowed, with loss of the valves of Houston and the sigmoid folds. Clips in the pelvis are from a total abdominal hysterectomy for cervical cancer.

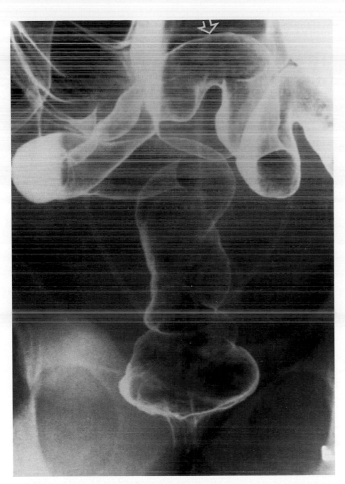

FIGURE 13–80. Radiation colitis with granular mucosa. The rectosigmoid colon has a tubular configuration. Mucosal granularity is best seen in the sigmoid colon *(arrow)*. Bilateral ureteral stents are in place.

INFECTIOUS COLITIS

A huge variety of pathogens infect the colon.[149] Patients with infectious colitis usually present with acute lower abdominal pain, tenesmus, and relatively low-volume diarrhea with passage of bloody stools or blood-tinged mucus. Diagnosis is usually made by considering the clinical history, the microscopic examination of stool for ova and parasites, stool cultures and blood titers, and sigmoidoscopy. Barium studies are not usually performed in patients with acute diarrhea (Fig. 13–81). Barium enemas may be performed in those patients in whom symptoms persist (Fig. 13–82) or are intermittent, if diarrhea relapses, or in patients with minimal symptoms (Fig. 13–83). Barium enemas may be performed if cultures are falsely negative. Some cultures, such as those for *Yersinia enterocolitica* or *Mycobacterium tuberculosis,* take up to 6 weeks for diagnosis.

Shigellosis

Various species of *Shigella* cause acute dysentery. In some patients a subacute form develops that is confused

clinically, endoscopically, and radiologically with ulcerative colitis (Fig. 13–84).[149,150] The gram-negative bacilli multiply in the epithelial cells, then enter the lamina propria, resulting in acute ulceration and mucosal necrosis covered by a pyogenic exudate. Radiologically, the rectosigmoid colon will appear ulcerated with pseudomembrane formation.[151,152]

Clostridium difficile Colitis

A broad spectrum of severity of colitis occurs with infection by *C. difficile,* a gram-positive bacillus.[153] *C. difficile* colonizes colons whose endogenous flora is altered by antibiotic therapy, endogenous pathogens such as *Salmonella* or *Shigella,* chemotherapeutic agents, or coexisting diseases such as ulcerative colitis. *C. difficile* produces several endotoxins that incite both secretion of fluid into the colonic lumen and necrosis and inflammation of the colonic epithelium.

The most typical symptoms are watery, nonbloody diarrhea, crampy abdominal pain, fever, and leukocytosis. When the diagnosis of *C. difficile* colitis is suspected, diagnosis is confirmed by stool analysis for cytotoxin and flex-

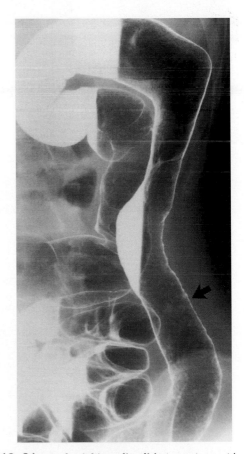

FIGURE 13–81. *Escherichia coli* colitis in patient with persistent colitis 2 weeks after return from Mexico. The left colon is tubular, with mucosal granularity and small ulcers in the distal descending colon (representative inflamed area identified with *arrow*). Acute loss of interhaustral folds is indicative of their "motor" nature.

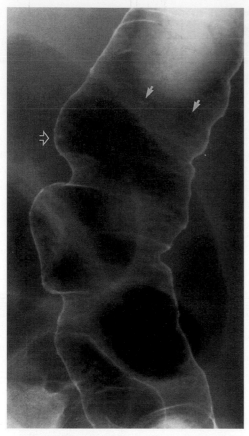

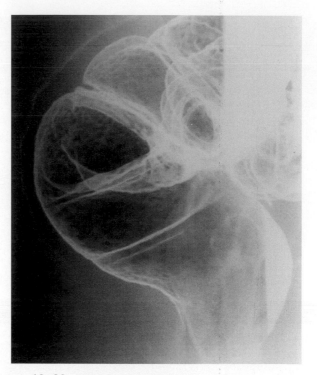

FIGURE 13–83. Follicular proctitis. Patient with increased passage of mucus per rectum. A diffuse lymphoid follicular pattern is seen in the rectum. No cultures were obtained. No recurrent diarrheal episodes occurred. This is a presumed response to an unknown pathogen, either infectious or immunologic in nature.

FIGURE 13–82. *Salmonella* colitis in patient with 2 months of persistent low-grade diarrhea. Tiny linear barium collections are identified *(arrows)*. The barium collections are slightly larger than the normal innominate pits of the colon. The interhaustral folds *(open arrow)* are enlarged.

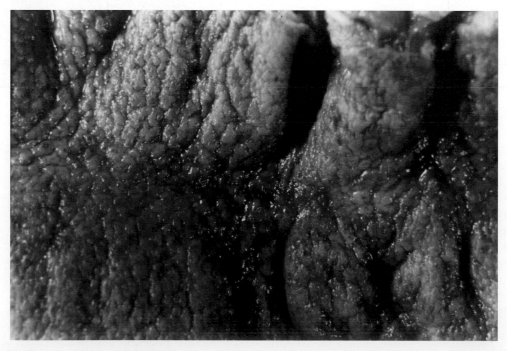

FIGURE 13–84. Shigellosis in patient with leukemia. Photograph of colectomy specimen shows coarsely nodular mucosa similar in dimension to the nodules in chronic ulcerative colitis.

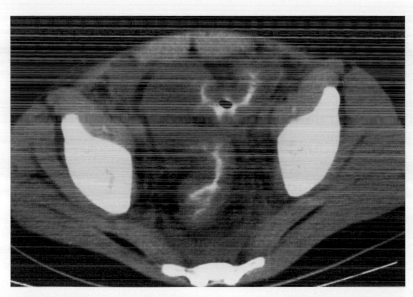

FIGURE 13–85. ***Clostridium difficile* colitis** in postoperative patient with fever. The "wall" of the rectosigmoid colon is diffusely thickened. Ascitic fluid is present unrelated to the colitis.

ible sigmoidoscopy. At flexible sigmoidoscopy, numerous 2 to 5 mm, well-circumscribed, yellow-white plaques are scattered over the mucosal surface giving rise to the term *pseudomembranous colitis.* There is such a broad spectrum of severity of *C. difficile* colitis, however, that the radiologist is often the first physician to suggest the diagnosis in patients with atypical clinical histories or nonspecific endoscopic findings. In postoperative patients with fever and leukocytosis, CT is often performed to rule out an abscess, and a diagnosis of pseudomembranous colitis may be made (Fig. 13–85). CT often shows a thick colonic wall with scalloped, nodular contour.[154–156] Wall thickening may be of low attenuation (Fig. 13–86).

Barium studies may be performed in patients with atypical clinical histories such as blood-tinged mucus or bloody diarrhea. The rectosigmoid colon is spared in 20% to 70% of patients with *C. difficile* colitis.[157–161] Therefore barium studies may be performed in patients in whom flexible sigmoidoscopies are normal or show nonspecific colitis.[162] Barium enema may demonstrate diffuse mucosal granularity, small nodules, or plaques (Fig. 13–87) in a pancolitic, left-sided, or right-sided distribution. The interhaustral folds are thickened and finely lobulated (Fig. 13–88), especially in the transverse and ascending colon.[163] The rectum and sigmoid colon may appear normal or finely granular.[162]

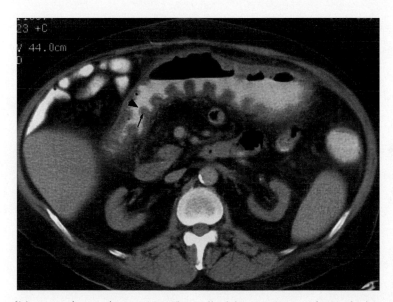

FIGURE 13–86. ***C. difficile* colitis** in renal transplant patient. The wall of the transverse colon is thickened. The pseudomembranes and mucosa *(arrowhead)* are relatively high attenuation. The submucosa *(arrow)* is of low attenuation because of edema. The native kidneys are atrophic.

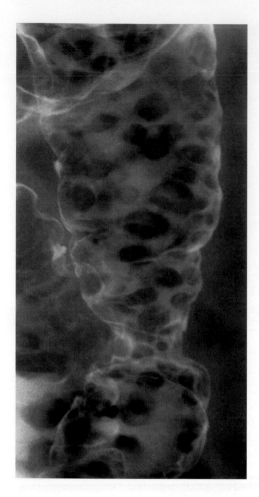

FIGURE 13–87. Plaques in *C. difficile* colitis. Numerous radiolucent plaques cover the descending colon. This patient had sparing of the rectosigmoid colon and a negative sigmoidoscopy but positive toxin titers. (From Rubesin, S.E., et al.: Pseudomembranous colitis with rectosigmoid sparing on barium studies. Radiology *170*:811, 1989.)

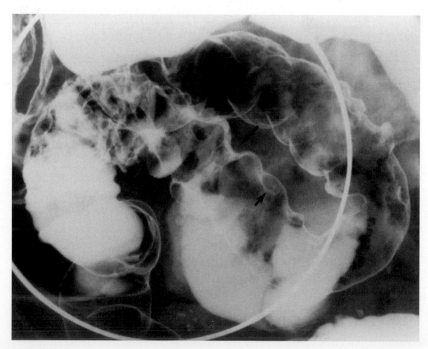

FIGURE 13–88. *C. difficile* colitis. Plaques (representative plaque identified with *short arrow*), coarse mucosal nodularity, and thick folds *(long arrow)* are seen in the rectosigmoid colon.

Neutropenic Colitis

In neutropenic colitis (typhlitis), acute inflammation and necrosis is found in the ascending colon and cecum or rarely the small intestine. Typhlitis occurs in neutropenic patients, typically patients with leukemia, lymphoma, aplastic anemia, organ transplants, or AIDS.[164,165] Patients complain of right lower quadrant pain and diarrhea. A variety of organisms are cultured. CT shows marked low-attenuation wall thickening in the cecum and ascending colon (Fig. 13–89).[166,167] The pericolic fat is stranded, and pericolic fluid may be present. Perforation may be present. The barium radiologist should suggest that a CT be first performed in toxic, neutropenic patients with right lower quadrant pain and diarrhea.

Lymphogranuloma Venereum

Lymphogranuloma venereum (LGV) is a venereally transmitted infection of *Chlamydia trachomatis* characterized by inguinal lymphadenopathy and proctosigmoiditis. Proctitis in men is usually related to anal intercourse. Proctitis in women may be related to spread of infected vaginal discharge into the rectum, anal intercourse, or dissemination from inguinal lymphadenopathy.[148] Rectal involvement by LGV varies from the asymptomatic carrier state to bloody diarrhea with mucopurulent discharge, rectal pain, and tenesmus. Clinical diagnosis requires a careful clinical history and culture by special transport media, immunofluorescent staining of biopsy specimens, or serologic diagnosis. Untreated infections may lead to

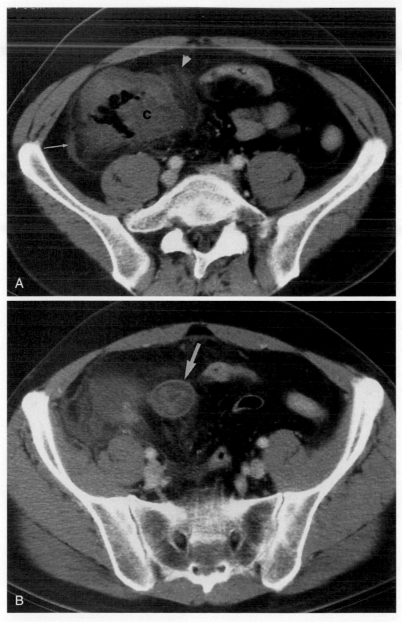

FIGURE 13–89. Neutropenic colitis and ileitis in leukemic patient with right lower quadrant pain. *A,* The cecal wall *(c)* is massively thickened. Stranding of pericecal fat *(arrowhead)* and fluid in the right paracolic gutter *(arrow)* are also seen. *B,* The terminal ileal wall *(arrow)* is also markedly thickened, manifested as a "target sign." (Courtesy of Bernard A. Birnbaum, M.D., Philadelphia, Pennsylvania.)

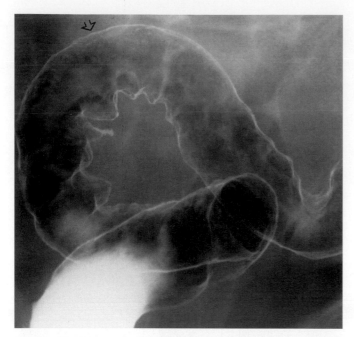

FIGURE 13–90. lymphogranuloma venereum. The rectosigmoid colon is tubular, with numerous punctate collections of barium (representative collections identified with *arrow*). This man complained of 3 months of diarrhea and admitted to anal intercourse. Chlamydial titers were elevated. (From Rubesin, S.E., and Schnall, M.: Rectum. *In* Gore, R.M., Levine, M.S., and Laufer, I. (eds.): Textbook of Gastrointestinal Radiology. Philadelphia, W.B. Saunders Co., 1994, p. 1261.)

rectal strictures due to marked fibrotic thickening of the rectal wall.[168,169]

A barium enema performed in the acute stage shows a nonspecific proctitis with boggy or granular mucosa (Fig. 13–90). A barium enema performed in a chronically infected, untreated patient shows deep ulceration, fissures (Fig. 13–91), diffuse rectosigmoid narrowing with loss of the valves of Houston, perianal fissures, and rectovaginal fistulae.[170] Thus a barium enema performed early in the course of disease mimics either ulcerative colitis (see Fig. 13–90) or nonspecific colitis. A barium enema performed late in the course of disease mimics Crohn's disease (see Fig. 13–91) or radiation proctitis (Fig. 13–92).

Tuberculosis

Tuberculosis involving the intestine is a common problem in tropical developing countries. Although uncommon in the West, tuberculosis is increasing in incidence in patients with AIDS and in immigrants.[171] Tuberculosis usually results from ingestion of infected sputum from pulmonary infections (*M. tuberculosis*) or drinking unpasteurized milk (*Mycobacterium bovis*). Immunocompromised patients can be infected with *Mycobacterium avium-intracellulare* or *Mycobacterium kansasii* as well. Patients have chronic symptoms of fever, abdominal pain, weight loss, diarrhea, and right lower quadrant tenderness.

Tuberculosis is located in areas in the intestine with large amounts of lymph tissue or in areas of the intestine where lymph nodes secondarily abut the bowel. Thus tuberculosis is most frequently localized in the ascending (Fig. 13–93) and proximal transverse colon and in the distal ileum.[169,172] Tuberculosis is characterized by transversely oriented ulcers and stenotic lesions. Unlike Crohn's disease, there is a relative absence of deep fissures and fistulae.[150] Granulomas are found in areas of ulceration or in areas of caseous necrosis, especially within lymph nodes.

Radiographically, deep or superficial, large or aphthoid ulcers are present (Fig. 13–94).[173,174] The ulcers have a predilection for the ascending colon, cecum, or terminal ileum. Fibrosis causes a short ascending colon and a cone-shaped cecum (Fig. 13–95). Focal or diffuse narrowing may be present in the ileum.[175,176] The ileocecal valve is gaping with thick lips, forming a right angle to the ascending colon, termed Fleischner's sign.[169] Loss of demarcation between the distal ileum and ascending

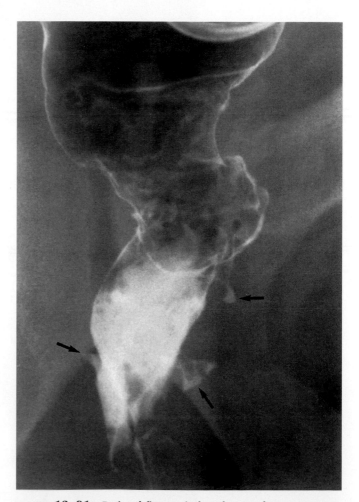

FIGURE 13–91. Perianal fissures in lymphogranuloma venereum. Numerous barium-filled tracks *(arrows)* extend into the perirectal tissue. The rectum is diffusely narrowed with mildly nodular mucosa. This example of chronic LGV mimics Crohn's disease.

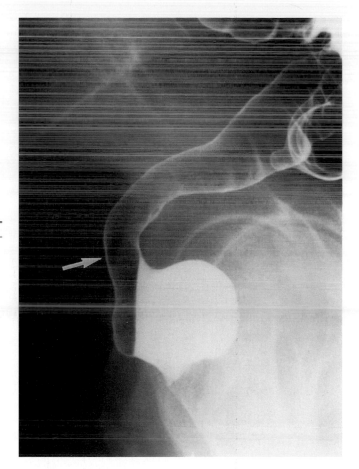

FIGURE 13–92. **Lymphogranuloma venereum mimics radiation colitis.** The rectum is tubular with loss of the valves of Houston. The mid-rectum *(arrow)* is disproportionately narrowed, a mild stricture.

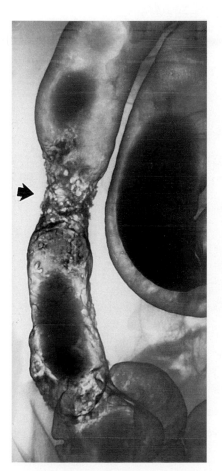

FIGURE 13–93. ***M. tuberculosis* of ascending colon.** The ascending colon has lost its interhaustral folds. Focal narrowing is seen *(arrow)*. Numerous inflammatory polyps are present, particularly near the stricture and the ileocecal valve. The terminal ileum only shows lymphoid hyperplasia. (Courtesy of M. Maruyama, M.D., Tokyo. From Maruyama, M.: Diagnosis of ileocecal tuberculosis—Clinicopathological study on 12 operated cases [in Japanese]. Stomach Intestine *9*:865, 1974, with permission.)

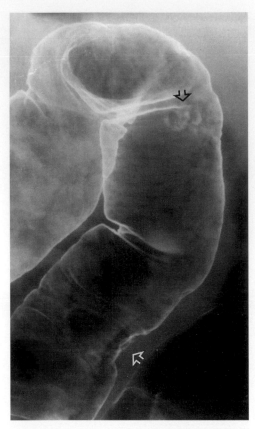

FIGURE 13–94. *M. avium-intracellulare* **in patient with AIDS.** Two large, shallow, barium-etched ulcers *(black arrow)* are present in the splenic flexure. Distally, several plaquelike elevations are seen *(white arrow)*. Mild lymphoid hyperplasia is present.

colon is termed Stierlin's sign.[169] Filiform polyps may be present.[177] On CT, markedly enlarged low attenuation or isoattenuation lymph nodes are detected in the small bowel mesentery.[178]

Amebiasis

Although amebiasis is rare in the United States, up to 20% of the world's population harbors amebae.[179] Amebiasis is more common in the tropics and subtropics and is especially found in areas of poor nutrition.[179] Man ingests water or food contaminated by cysts. Trophozoites excyst in the small intestine, pass into the colon, and invade the colonic mucosa. The clinical spectrum varies from the asymptomatic carrier state to a fulminant colitis. Patients may have recurrent bouts of diarrhea with passage of mucus and blood, alternating with intermittent constipation. Colitis may persist for weeks, months, or even years. Early, there is mild edema, which progresses to erosions or small ulcers. Larger ulcers may develop. With progression, deep, flask-shaped ulcers with undermined edges and overlying pseudomembranes may form (Fig. 13–96). The right colon is more frequently involved. The terminal ileum is spared.

Radiographically, mild colitis may be manifest as mucosal granularity, similar to ulcerative colitis. When small

erosions form, the radiographic findings may mimic the aphthoid ulcers of Crohn's disease (Fig. 13–97). Although typically a right-sided disease, occasionally pancolitis is seen. Amebiasis is also characterized by skip areas. "Amebomas" are usually long strictures with tapered edges, resulting from exuberant granulation tissue causing marked bowel wall thickening. Amebomas have a predilection for the cecum and the hepatic and splenic flexures[180] and are seen in 1% to 10% of patients. Occasionally short, annular amebomas mimic colonic carcinoma.

Viral Colitis

The barium radiologist will rarely encounter viral colitis, except venereal proctitis such as herpetic proctitis (Fig. 13–98) or cytomegalovirus (CMV) colitis (Fig. 13–99) in immunocompromised patients. Although described in immunocompetent patients, CMV colitis is most commonly found in patients with AIDS. CMV primarily attacks mesothelial cells: endothelial cells, fibroblasts, and smooth muscle cells.[181] CMV causes vasculitis resulting in thrombosis and ischemia. In the colon, segmental or diffuse abnormalities are found, including hemorrhagic mucosa, ulceration, and perforation.[182–183] Patients complain of rectal bleeding, diarrhea, or severe symptoms due to

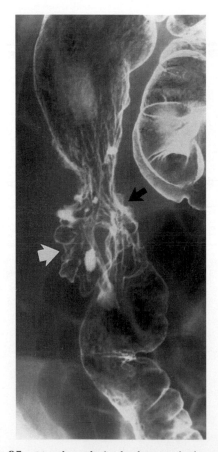

FIGURE 13–95. *M. tuberculosis* **of colon.** Marked contraction and sacculation of the cecum is seen *(white arrow)*. Granular mucosa is present in the ascending colon. The ileocecal valve *(black arrow)* is open. The terminal ileum is relatively spared.

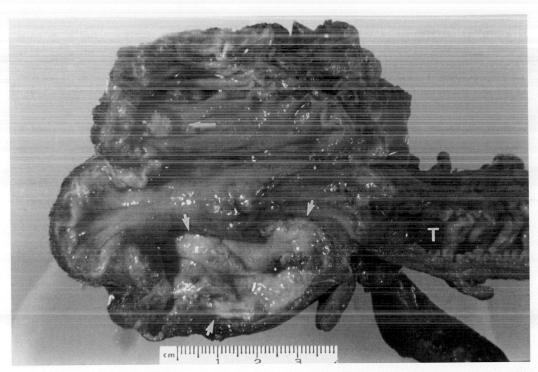

FIGURE 13–96. Amebiasis. Photograph of right hemicolectomy specimen shows numerous deep ulcers (representative ulcer identified with *long arrow*) in the cecum and ascending colon. The mucosa of the inferior cecum is denuded and covered by a white pseudomembrane of inflammatory detritus *(short arrows)*. The terminal ileum *(T)* is normal.

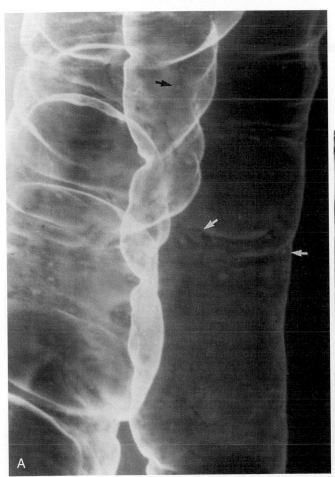

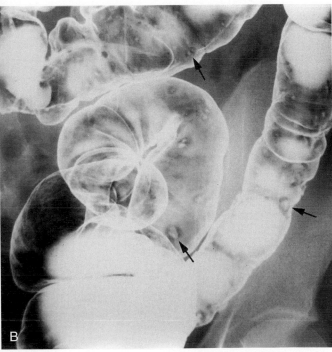

FIGURE 13–97. Amebiasis. *A,* Numerous aphthoid ulcers (representative ulcers identified with *arrows*) are present in the splenic flexure in a homosexual male patient. *B,* Numerous large and small ulcers are seen in the rectum and descending and transverse colon (representative ulcers identified with *arrows*). The radiographic findings in *A* and *B* mimic Crohn's colitis. (*A* and *B* Courtesy of Harvey Goldstein, M.D., San Antonio, Texas.)

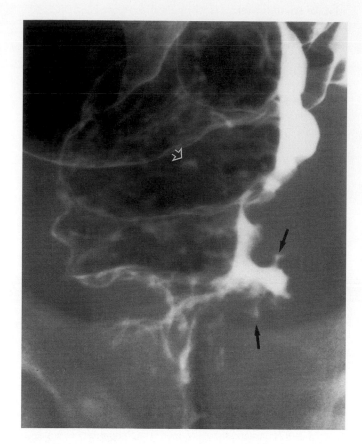

FIGURE 13–98. Herpetic proctitis due to anal intercourse. Numerous small aphthoid ulcers (representative ulcer identified with *open arrow*) are present in the rectum. Some ulcers deeply extend into the rectal wall *(arrows)*. (Courtesy of Francis J. Scholz, M.D., Burlington, MA. From Shah, S.J., and Scholz, F.J.: Anorectal herpes: Radiographic findings. Radiology *147*:81, 1983, with permission.)

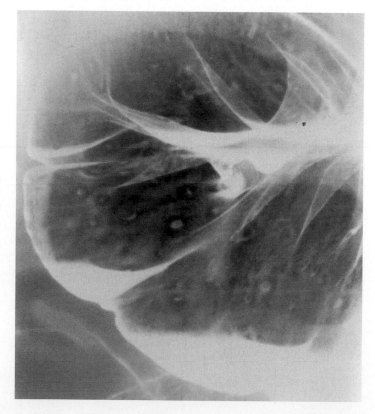

FIGURE 13–99. Cytomegalovirus colitis in patient with AIDS. Close-up view of splenic flexure shows numerous aphthoid ulcers separated by normal mucosa. The radiographic findings are identical to those of Crohn's disease. The clinical history, culture, and biopsy results allow the diagnosis.

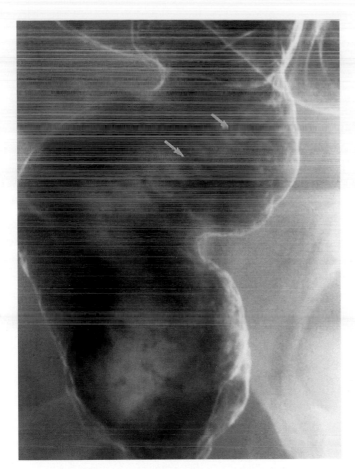

FIGURE 13–100. Nonspecific viral proctosigmoiditis. Shallow aphthoid and large ulcers are seen in the mid-rectum (representative ulcers identified by *arrows*). The valves of Houston are effaced—the rectum has a tubular configuration. Biopsy specimen revealed viral inclusion bodies in the cytoplasm of epithelial cells. (From Rubesin, S.E., and Schnall, M.: Rectum. *In* Gore, R.M., Levine, M.S., and Laufer, I. (eds.): Textbook of Gastrointestinal Radiology. Philadelphia, W.B. Saunders Co., 1994, p. 1261.)

perforation. Radiologically, granular mucosa resembling ulcerative colitis or aphthoid ulcers (Fig. 13–100, see Fig. 13–99) resembling Crohn's disease may be seen. With severe disease, deep ulcers and marked inflammatory change are present. The radiologist must be wary about performing a barium enema on an acutely ill patient with AIDS, given the risk of perforation. On CT, the colonic wall is thickened, and the adjacent fat is inflamed.[184]

DIVERSION COLITIS

Diversion of the fecal stream leads to nutritional deficiency of short chain fatty acids, a source of energy for colonic epithelial cells.[185,186] Thus a colitis, termed *diversion colitis,* may ensue after end-ileostomy or end-colostomy with a rectosigmoid pouch in the treatment of Crohn's disease, diverticulitis, or cancer. Symptoms and histologic changes

resolve after reanastomosis of the rectosigmoid pouch to colon or small bowel.[187] Barium studies of the rectosigmoid pouch may be performed for symptoms or before reanastomosis. In diversion colitis, fine or coarse mucosal nodularity or lymphoid hyperplasia may be seen.[188]

REFERENCES

1. Whitehead, R.: Ulcerative colitis. *In* Whitehead, R. (ed.): Gastrointestinal and Esophageal Pathology, ed. 2. Edinburgh, Churchill-Livingstone, 1995, p. 622.
2. Strober, W.: Animal models of inflammatory bowel disease—An overview. Dig. Dis. Sci. 30(Suppl):3S, 1985.
3. Onderdonk, A.B.: Experimental models for ulcerative colitis. Dig. Dis. Sci. 30(Suppl):40S, 1985.
4. Bartram, C.: Inflammatory bowel disease. *In* Laufer, I., and Levine, M.S. (eds.): Double Contrast Gastrointestinal Radiology, ed. 2. Philadelphia, W.B. Saunders Co., 1992, p. 579.
5. Podolsky, D.K.: Inflammatory bowel disease. Part 1. N. Engl. J. Med. *325:*928, 1991.
6. Schrumpf, E., Fausa, O., Elgjo, K., et al.: Hepatobiliary complications of inflammatory bowel disease. Semin. Liver Dis. *8:*201, 1988.
7. Williams, S.M., and Harned, R.K.: Hepatobiliary complications of inflammatory bowel disease. Radiol. Clin. North Am. *25:*175, 1987.
8. Olsson, R., Danielsson, A., Jarnerot, G.I., et al.: Prevalence of primary sclerosing cholangitis in patients with ulcerative colitis. Gastroenterology *100:*1319, 1991.
9. Fukushima, T., Ishiguro, N., Matsude, Y., et al.: Clinical and urinary characteristics of urolithiasis in ulcerative colitis. Am. J. Gastroenterol. *77:*238, 1982.
10. Ekbom, A., Helmick, C., Zack, M., and Adami, H.O.: Extracolonic malignancies in inflammatory bowel disease. Cancer *67:*2015, 1991.
11. Greenstein, A.J., Mullin, G.E., Strauchen, J.A., et al.: Lymphoma in inflammatory bowel disease. Cancer *69:*1119, 1992.
12. Laufer, I.: Air contrast studies of the colon in inflammatory bowel disease. CRC Crit. Rev. Diagnost. Imaging *9:*421, 1977.
13. Bartram, C.I., and Walmesley, K.: A pathological and radiological correlation of the mucosal changes in ulcerative colitis. Clin. Radiol. *29:*323, 1978.
14. Laufer, I., Mullens, J.E., and Hamilton, J.: Correlation of endoscopy and double-contrast radiography in the early stages of ulcerative and granulomatous colitis. Radiology *118:*1, 1976.
15. Lichtenstein, J.E.: Radiologic-pathologic correlation of inflammatory bowel disease. Radiol. Clin. North Am. *25:*3, 1987.
16. Counsell, B.: Lesions of the ileum associated with ulcerative colitis. Br. J. Surg. *185:*276, 1956.
17. Lichtenstein, J.E., Madewell, J.E., and Feigen, D.S.: The collar button ulcer. Gastrointest. Radiol. *4:*79, 1979.
18. Suekane, H., Iida, M., Matsui, T., et al.: Radiographic demonstration of longitudinal ulcers in patients with ulcerative colitis. Gastrointest. Radiol. *4:*103, 1980.
19. Gore, R.M.: Colonic contour changes in chronic ulcerative colitis: Reappraisal of some old concepts. AJR Am. J. Roentgenol. *158:*59, 1992.
20. Simpkins, K.C., and Stevenson, G.W.: The modified Malmö double contrast barium enema in colitis: An assessment of its accuracy in reflecting sigmoidoscopic findings. Br. J. Radiol. *45:*486, 1972.
21. Goulston, S.J.M., and McGovern, V.J.: The nature of benign strictures in ulcerative colitis. N. Engl. J. Med. *281:*290, 1969.
22. Gore, R.M.: Cross-sectional imaging of inflammatory bowel disease. Radiol. Clin. North Am. *25:*115, 1987.
23. Gore, R.M., Marn, C.S., Kirby, D.F., et al.: CT findings in ulcerative, granulomatous and indeterminate colitis. AJR Am. J. Roentgenol. *143:*279, 1983.
24. Edling, N.P.G., and Eklof, O.: The retrorectal soft tissue space in ulcerative colitis: A roentgen diagnostic study. Radiology *80:*949, 1963.
25. Rubesin, S.E., Furth, E.E., Rose, D., et. al.: Pictorial essay. The effects of distention on colonic morphology: Barium radiography and anatomic correlation. AJR Am. J. Roentgenol. *164:*1387, 1995.

26. Bartram, C.I.: Ulcerative colitis. *In* Bartram, C.I. (ed): Radiology in Inflammatory Bowel Disease. New York, Marcel Dekker, 1983, p. 31.

27. de Dombal, F.T., Watts, J., Watkins, G., et al.: Local complications of ulcerative colitis, strictures, pseudopolyps, and carcinoma of colon and rectum. BMJ *1*:1442, 1966.

28. Marshak, R.H., Boch, C., and Wolf, B.S.: The roentgen findings in strictures of the colon associated with ulcerative and granulomatous colitis. AJR Am. J. Roentgenol. *90*:709, 1963.

29. Simpkins, K.C., and Young, A.C.: The differential diagnosis of large bowel strictures. Clin. Radiol. *22*:449, 1971.

30. Jalan, K.N., Walker, R.J., Sircus, W., et al.: Pseudopolyposis in ulcerative colitis. Lancet *11*:555, 1969.

31. Kelly, J.K., and Gabos, S.: The pathogenesis of inflammatory polyps. Dis. Colon Rectum *30*:251, 1987.

32. Joffe, N.: Localized giant pseudopolyposis secondary to ulcerative or granulomatous colitis. Clin. Radiol. *28*:609, 1977.

33. Zegel, N., and Laufer, I.: Filiform polyposis. Radiology *127*:615, 1978.

34. Bozna, J.P., Fisher, R.L., and Barwick, K.W.: Filiform polyposis: An unusual complication of inflammatory bowel disease. J. Clin. Gastroenterol. *7*:451, 1985.

35. Goldberger, L.E., Neely, H.R., and Stammer, J.L.: Large mucosal bridges. An unusual roentgenographic manifestation of ulcerative colitis. Gastrointest. Radiol. *3*:81, 1978.

36. Hammerman, A.M., Shatz, B.A., and Susman, N.: Radiographic characteristics of colonic "mucosal bridges": Sequelae of inflammatory bowel disease. Radiology *127*:611, 1978.

37. Bray, J.F.: Filiform polyposis of the small bowel in Crohn's disease. Gastrointest. Radiol. *8*:155, 1983.

38. Ekbom, A., Helmick, C., Zack, M., et al.: Ulcerative colitis and colorectal cancer: A population-based study. N. Engl. J. Med. *323*:1228, 1990.

39. MacDougall, I.P.M.: Clinical identification of those cases of ulcerative colitis most likely to develop cancer of the bowel. Dis. Colon Rectum *7*:447, 1964.

40. Hinton, J.M.: Risk of malignant change in ulcerative colitis. Gut *7*:427, 1966.

41. Lennard-Jones, J.F., Misiewicz, J.J., Parish, J.A., et al.: Prospective study of outpatients with extensive colitis. Lancet *1*:1065, 1974.

42. Devroede, G., and Taylor, W.F.: On calculating cancer risk and survival of ulcerative colitis patients with the life table method. Gastroenterology *71*:505, 1976.

43. Lennard-Jones, J.E., Morson, B.C., Ritchie, J.K., et al.: Cancer in colitis: Assessment of the individual risk by clinical and histological criteria. Gastroenterology *73*:1280, 1977.

44. Bröstrom, O., Löfberg, R., Nordenvall, B., et al.: The risk of colorectal cancer in ulcerative colitis. Scand. J. Gastroenterol. *22*:1193, 1987.

45. Hooyman, J.R., MacCarty, R.L., Carpenter, H.A., et al.: Radiographic appearance of mucosal dysplasia associated with ulcerative colitis. AJR Am. J. Roentgenol. *149*:47, 1987.

46. Matsumoto, T., Iida, M., Kuroki, F., et al.: Dysplasia in ulcerative colitis: Is radiography adequate for diagnosis? Radiology *199*:85, 1996.

47. Frank, P.H., Riddell, R.H., Feczko, P.J., et al.: Radiological detection of colonic dysplasia (precarcinoma) in chronic ulcerative colitis. Gastrointest. Radiol. *3*:209, 1978.

48. Kelvin, F.M., Woodward, B.H., McLeod, M., et al.: Prospective diagnosis of dysplasia (pre-cancer) in chronic ulcerative colitis. AJR Am. J. Roentgenol. *138*:347, 1982.

49. Stevenson, G.W., Goodacre, R., and Jackson, M.: Dysplasia to carcinoma transformation in ulcerative colitis. AJR Am. J. Roentgenol. *143*:108, 1984.

50. Blackstone, M.O., Riddell, R.H., Rogers, B.H., and Levin, B.: Dysplasia-associated lesion or mass (DALM) detected by colonoscopy in long-standing ulcerative colitis: An indication for colectomy. Gastroenterology *80*:366, 1981.

51. Butt, J.H., Konishi, F., Morson, B.C., et al.: Macroscopic lesions in dysplasia and carcinoma complicating ulcerative colitis. Dig. Dis. Sci. *28*:18,1983.

52. Edling, N.P.G., Lagercrantz, R., and Rosenquist, H.: Roentgenologic findings in ulcerative colitis with malignant degeneration. Acta Radiol. *52*:123, 1959.

53. Hodgson, J.R., and Sauer, W.G.: The roentgenologic features of carcinoma in chronic ulcerative colitis. AJR Am. J. Roentgenol. *86*:91, 1961.

54. Fennessey, J.J., Sparberg, M.B., and Kirsner, J.B. Radiological findings in carcinoma of the colon complicating chronic ulcerative colitis. Gut *9*:388, 1968.

55. Truelove, S.C., and Marcks, C.G.: Toxic megacolon. Part I. Pathogenesis, diagnosis and treatment. Clin. Gastroenterol. *10*:107, 1981.

56. Grant, C.S., and Dozois, R.R.: Toxic megacolon: Ultimate fate of patients after successful medical management. Am. J. Surg. *147*: 106, 1984.

57. Bucknell, N.A., Williams, G.T., Bartam, C.I., and Lennard-Jones, J.E.: Depth of ulceration in acute colitis. Gastroenterology *79*:19, 1980.

58. Gore, R.M., and Laufer, I.: Ulcerative and granulomatous colitis: Idiopathic inflammatory bowel disease. *In* Gore, R.M., Levine, M.S., and Laufer, I. (eds.): Textbook of Gastrointestinal Radiology. Philadelphia, W.B. Saunders Co., 1994, p. 1098.

59. McConnell, F., Hanelin, J., and Robbins, L.L.: Plain film diagnosis of fulminating ulcerative colitis. Radiology *71*:674, 1958.

60. Simpson, S.A., and Lewis, J.R.: Plain roentgenography in diagnosis of chronic ulcerative colitis and terminal ileitis. Radiology *84*: 306, 1960.

61. Caprilli, R., Vernia, P., Latella, G., et al.: Early recognition of toxic megacolon. J. Clin. Gastroenterol. *9*:160, 1987.

62. Dalziel, T.K.: Chronic interstitial enteritis. BMJ *2*:1068, 1913.

63. Crohn, B.B., Ginzburg, L., and Oppenheimer, G.D.: Regional ileitis: A pathologic and clinical entity. JAMA *99*:1323, 1932.

64. Brooke, B.N.: Granulomatous diseases of the intestine. Lancet *2*:745, 1959.

65. Morson, B.C., and Lockhart-Mummery, H.E.: Crohn's disease of the colon. Gastroenterologica (Basel) *92*:168, 1959.

66. Marshak, R.H., Wolf, B.S., Eliasoph, J.: Segmental colitis. Radiology *73*:707, 1959.

67. Lindner, A.E., Marshak, R.H., Wolf, B.S., et al.: Granulomatous colitis: A clinical study. N. Engl. J. Med. *269*:379, 1963.

68. Lockhart-Mummery, H.E., and Morson, B.C.: Crohn's disease of the large intestine. Gut *5*:493, 1964.

69. Gilmour, H.M.: The small intestine: Crohn's disease. *In* Whitehead, R. (ed.): Gastrointestinal and esophageal pathology, ed. 2. Edinburgh, Churchill-Livingstone, 1995, p. 547.

70. Gilmour, H.M.: The large intestine: Crohn's disease. *In* Whitehead, R. (ed.): Gastrointestinal and esophageal pathology, ed. 2. Edinburgh, Churchill-Livingstone, 1995, p. 604.

71. Robert, J.R., Sachar, D.B., and Greenstein, A.J.: Severe gastrointestinal haemorrhage in Crohn's disease. Ann. Surg. *213*:207, 1991.

72. Greenstein, A.J., Janowitz, H.D., and Sachar, D.B.: The extraintestinal complications of Crohn's disease and ulcerative colitis: A study of 700 patients. Medicine *55*:401, 1976.

73. Whorwell, P.J., Hawkins, R., Dewbury, K., and Wright, R.: Ultrasound survey of gallstones and other hepatobiliary disorders in patients with Crohn's disease. Dig. Dis. Sci. *29*:930, 1984.

74. Goldberg, H.I., Carruthers, S.B., Jr., Nelson, J.A., et al.: Radiographic findings of the National Cooperative Crohn's Disease Study. Gastroenterology *77*:925, 1979.

75. Dyer, N.H., Rutherford, C., Visick, J.H., et al.: The incidence and reliability of individual radiographic signs in the small intestine in Crohn's disease. Br. J. Radiol. *43*:401, 1980.

76. Whitehead, R.: Pathology of Crohn's disease. *In* Kirsner, J.B., and Shorter, R.G. (eds.): Inflammatory Bowel Disease. Philadelphia, Lea & Febiger, 1980, p. 296.

77. Laufer, I., and Hamilton, J.: The radiological differentiation between ulcerative and granulomatous colitis by double contrast radiology. Am. J. Gastroenterol. *66*:259, 1976.

78. Chambers, T.J., and Morson, B.C.: The granuloma in Crohn's disease. Gut *20*:269, 1979.

79. McGovern, V.J., and Goulston, S.J.M.: Crohn's disease of the colon. Gut *9*:164, 1968.

80. Morson, B.C., and Dawson, I.M.P.: Large intestine: Inflammatory disorders. *In* Morson, B.C., and Dawson, I.M.P. (eds.): Gastrointestinal Pathology. Boston, Blackwell Scientific, 1979, p. 512.

81. Whitehead, R.: Mucosal biopsy of the gastrointestinal tract. Philadelphia, W.B. Saunders Co., 1985, p. 227.

82. Marshak, R.H.: Granulomatous disease of the intestinal tract (Crohn's disease). Radiology *114*:3, 1975.

83. Ni, X.Y., and Goldberg, H.I.: Aphthoid ulcers in Crohn's disease: Radiographic course and relationship to bowel appearance. Radiology 158:589, 1986.

84. Laufer, I., and Costopoulos, L.: Early lesions of Crohn's disease. AJR Am. J. Roentgenol. 130:307, 1978.

85. Simpkins, K.C.: Aphthoid ulcers in Crohn's colitis. Clin. Radiol. 28:601, 1978.

86. Rubesin, S.E., and Bronner, M.: Radiologic-pathologic concepts in Crohn's disease. In Herlinger, H. (ed.): Advances in Gastrointestinal Radiology. Vol. 1. Chicago, Mosby–Year Book, 1992, p. 27.

87. Max, R.J., and Kelvin, F.M.: Nonspecificity of discrete colonic ulceration on double-contrast barium enema study. AJR Am. J. Roentgenol. 134:1265, 1980.

88. Kelly, R.J., and Sutherland, L.R.: The chronological sequence in the pathology of Crohn's disease. J. Clin. Gastroenterol. 10:28, 1988.

89. Herlinger, H., Rubesin, S.E., and Furth, E.E.: Mesenteric border ulcers in Crohn's disease: Historical, radiologic and pathologic perspectives. Abd. Imaging 23:122, 1998.

90. Bartram, C.I.: Complications of Crohn's disease. In Bartram, C.I. (ed.): Radiology in Inflammatory Bowel Disease. New York, Marcel Dekker, 1983, p. 169.

91. Jones, B., Fishman, E.K., Hamilton, S.R., et al.: Submucosal accumulation of fat in inflammatory bowel disease: CT/pathologic correlation. J. Comput. Assist. Tomogr. 10:759, 1986.

92. Sommer, S.C.: Ulcerative and granulomatous colitis. AJR Am. J. Roentgenol. 130:817, 1977.

93. Price, A.B., and Morson, B.C.: Inflammatory bowel disease: The surgical pathology of Crohn's disease and ulcerative colitis. Hum. Pathol. 6:7, 1987.

94. Greenstein, A.J., and Janowitz, H.D.: Cancer in Crohn's disease. Am. J. Gastroenterol. 64:122, 1976.

95. Marshak, R.H., Janowitz, H.D., and Present, D.H.: Granulomatous colitis in association with diverticula. N. Engl. J. Med. 283:1080, 1970.

96. Ferrucci, J.T., Jr., Ragsdale, B.D., Bartrett, P.J., et al.: Double tracking in the sigmoid colon. Radiology 120:307, 1976.

97. Meyers, M.A., Alonso, D.R., Morson, B.C., et al.: Pathogenesis of diverticulitis complicating granulomatous colitis. Gastroenterology 74:23, 1978.

98. Rankin, B.G., Watts, H.D., Melnyk, C.J., et al.: National Cooperative Crohn's Disease Study: Extraintestinal manifestations and perianal complications. Gastroenterology 77:914, 1979.

99. Yousem, D.M., Fishman, E.K., and Jones, B.: Crohn's disease: Perirectal and perianal findings at CT. Radiology 167:331, 1988.

100. Glass, R.E.: The management of internal fistulae in Crohn's disease. Br. J. Surg. 72(Suppl):S93, 1985.

101. Kelly, J.K., and Preshaw, R.M.: Origin of fistulas in Crohn's disease. J. Clin. Gastroenterol. 11:193, 1989.

102. Herlinger, H., O'Riordan, D., Saul, S., et al.: Nonspecific involvement of bowel adjoining Crohn's disease. Radiology 159:47, 1986.

103. Munyer, T.P., Montgomery, C.K., Thoeni, R.F., et al.: Postinflammatory polyposis (PIP) of the colon: The radiologic-pathologic spectrum. Radiology 145:607, 1982.

104. Hammerman, A.M., Shatz, B.A., and Sussman, N.: Radiographic characteristics of colonic "mucosal bridges": Sequelae of inflammatory bowel disease. Radiology 127:611, 1978.

105. Brahme, F.: Granulomatous colitis: Roentgenologic appearance and course of the lesion. AJR Am. J. Roentgenol. 97:35, 1967.

106. Wilder, W.M., and Davis, W.D.: Duodenal enteritis. South. Med. J. 59:884, 1966.

107. Legge, D.A., Carlson, H.C., and Judd, E.S.: Roentgenologic features of regional enteritis of the upper gastrointestinal tract. AJR Am. J. Roentgenol. 110:355, 1970.

108. Laufer, I., Trueman, T., and deSa, D.: Multiple superficial gastric erosions due to Crohn's disease of the stomach: Radiologic and endoscopic diagnosis. Br. J. Radiol. 49:726, 1976.

109. Laufer, I., Hamilton, J., and Mullens, J.E.,: Demonstration of superficial gastric erosions by double contrast radiology. Gastroenterology 68:387, 1975

110. Ariyama, J., Wehlin, L., Lindstrom, C.G., et al.: Gastroduodenal erosions in Crohn's disease. Gastrointest. Radiol. 5:121, 1980.

111. Gore, R.M., and Ghahremani, G.G.: Crohn's disease of the upper gastrointestinal tract. CRC Crit. Rev. Diagn. Imaging 25:305, 1986.

112. Tanaka, M., Kimura, K., Sakai, H., et al.: Long-term follow-up for minute gastroduodenal lesions in Crohn's disease. Gastrointest. Endosc. 32:206, 1986.

113. Levine, M.S.: Crohn's disease of the upper gastrointestinal tract. Radiol. Clin. North Am. 25:79, 1987.

114. Nugent, F.W., and Roy, M.A.: Duodenal Crohn's disease: An analysis of 89 cases. Am. J. Gastroenterol. 84:249, 1989.

115. Gohel, V., Long, B.W., and Richter, G.: Aphthous ulcers in the esophagus with Crohn colitis. AJR Am. J. Roentgenol. 137:872, 1981.

116. Ghahremani, G.G., Gore, R.M., Breuer, R.I., et al.: Esophageal manifestations of Crohn's disease. Gastrointest. Radiol. 7:199, 1982.

117. Rubesin, S.E., Laufer, I., and Dinsmore, B.: Radiologic investigation of inflammatory bowel disease. In MacDermott, R.P., and Stenson, W.F. (eds.): Inflammatory Bowel Disease. New York, Elsevier Science Publishing Company, 1992, p. 453.

118. Glick, S.N., and Teplick, S.K.: Crohn's disease of the small intestine. Diffuse mucosal granularity. Radiology 154:313, 1985.

119. Glick, S.N.: Crohn's disease of the small intestine. Radiol. Clin. North Am. 25:25, 1987.

120. Jones, B., Hamilton, S.R., Rubesin, S.E., et al.: Granular small bowel mucosa: A reflection of villous abnormality. Gastrointest. Radiol. 12:219, 1987.

121. Williams, H.J., Stephens, D.H., and Carlson, H.C.: Double contrast radiography: Colonic inflammatory disease. AJR Am. J. Roentgenol. 137:315, 1981.

122. Eisenberg, R.L., Montgomery, C.K., and Margulis, A.R.: Colitis in the elderly: Ischaemic colitis mimicking ulcerative and granulomatous colitis. AJR Am. J. Roentgenol. 133:1113, 1979.

123. Brandt, L.J., Boley, S.J., Goldberg, L., et. al.: Colitis in the elderly: A reappraisal. Am. J. Gastroenterol. 76:239, 1981.

124. Boley, S.J.: Colonic ischemia—25 years later. Am. J. Gastroenterol. 85:931, 1990.

125. Marston, A., Pheils, M.T., Thomas, M.L., and Morson, B.C.: Ischaemic colitis. Gut 7:1, 1966.

126. Reeders, J.W.A.J., Tytgat, G.N.J., Rosenbusch, G., et al.: Ischaemic Colitis. Boston, Martinus Nijhoff, 1984.

127. Whitehead, R., and Gratama, S.: The large intestine. Ischaemic colitis. In Whitehead, R. (ed.): Gastrointestinal and Esophageal Pathology, ed. 2. Edinburgh, Churchill-Livingstone, 1995, p. 687.

128. Griffiths, J.D.: Surgical anatomy of the distal colon. Ann. R. Coll. Surg. Engl. 19:241, 1956.

129. Kilpatrick, Z.M., Farman, J., Yesner, R., et al.: Ischemic proctitis. JAMA 205:74, 1968.

130. Whitehead, R.: The pathology of ischaemia of the intestines. Pathol. Ann. 11:1, 1976.

131. Reickert, R.R., Johnson, R.G., and Wignarajan, K.R.: Ischaemic colitis in a young adult patient: Report of a case. Dis. Colon Rectum 17:112, 1974.

132. Turnbull, A.R., and Isaacson, P.: Ischaemic colitis and drug abuse. BMJ 2:1000, 1977.

133. Yang, R.D., Han, M.W., and McCarthy, J.H.: Ischemic colitis in a crack abuser. Dig. Dis. Sci. 36:238, 1991.

134. Johnson, T.D., and Berenson, M.M.: Methamphetamine-induced ischemic colitis. J. Clin. Gastroenterol. 13:687, 1991.

135. Toffler, R.B., Pingoud, E.G., and Burell, M.L.: Acute colitis related to penicillin and penicillin derivatives. Lancet 2:707, 1978.

136. Kilpatrick, Z.M., Silverman, J.F., Betancourt, E., Farman, J., and Lawson, J.P.: Vascular occlusion of the colon and oral contraceptives. Possible relation. N. Engl. J. Med. 278:438, 1968.

137. Fisher, J.K.: Abnormal colonic bowel wall thickening on computed tomography. J. Comput. Assist. Tomogr. 7:90, 1983.

138. Jones, B., Fishman, E.K., and Siegelman, S.S.: Ischemic colitis demonstrated by computed tomography. J. Comput. Assist. Tomogr. 6:1120, 1982.

139. Wittenberg, J., Athanasoulis, C.A., Williams, L.F., et al.: Ischemic colitis. Radiology and pathophysiology. AJR Am. J. Roentgenol. 123:287, 1975.

140. Gore, R.M., Calenoff, L., and Rogers, L.F.: Roentgenographic manifestations of ischemic colitis. JAMA 241:1171, 1979.

141. Iida, M., Matsui, T., Fuchigami, T., et al.: Ischemic colitis: Serial changes in double contrast barium enema examinations. Radiology 159:337, 1986.

142. Bartram, C.I.: Obliteration of thumbprinting with double contrast enemas in acute ischemic colitis. Gastrointest. Radiol. 4:85, 1979.

143. Greenberg, H.M., Goldberg, H.I., and Axel, L.: Colonic "urticaria" pattern due to early ischemia. Gastrointest. Radiol. *6:*145, 1981.

144. Boley, S.J., Schwartz, S., Lash, J., et al.: Reversible vascular occlusion of the colon. Surg. Gynecol. Obstet. *116:*53, 1963.

145. Fajardo, L.F.: Radiation-induced pathology of the alimentary tract. *In* Whitehead, R. (ed.): Gastrointestinal and esophageal pathology, ed. 2. Edinburgh, Churchill-Livingstone, 1995, p. 962.

146. Gardiner, G.W., McAuliffe, N., and Murray, D.: Colitis cystica profunda occurring in a radiation-induced colonic stricture. Hum. Pathol. *15:*295, 1984.

147. Baratz, M., Werbin, N., Wiznitzer, T., et al.: Irradiation-induced colonic stricture and colitis cystica profunda. Report of case. Dis. Colon Rectum *21:*75, 1978.

148. Kelvin, F.M., and Gardiner, R.: Clinical Imaging of the Colon and Rectum. New York, Raven Press, 1987, p. 422.

149. Lamont, J.T.: Bacterial infections of the colon. *In* Yamada, T. (ed.): Textbook of Gastroenterology, ed. 2. Philadelphia, J.B. Lippincott, 1995, p. 1891.

150. Mathan, M.M.: Specific infections of the large intestine. *In* Whitehead, R. (ed.): Gastrointestinal and Esophageal Pathology, ed. 2. Edinburgh, Churchill-Livingstone, 1995, p. 589.

151. Speelman, P., Kabir, I., and Islam, M.: Distribution and spread of colonic lesions in shigellosis: A colonoscopic study. J. Infect. Dis. *150:*899, 1984.

152. Dammin, G. J.: Acute diarrhea and dysenteries. *In* Binford, C.H., and Connor, D.H.: Pathology of Tropical and Extraordinary Diseases. Washington, DC, Armed Forces Institute of Pathology, 1976, p. 135.

153. Barlett, J.G., Moon, N., Chang, T.W., et al.: Role of *Clostridium difficile* in antibiotic-associated pseudomembranous colitis. Gastroenterology *75:*778, 1978.

154. Megibow, A.J., Streiter, M.L., Balthazar, E.J., et al.: Pseudomembranous colitis: Diagnosis by computed tomography. J. Compt. Assist. Tomogr. *8:*281, 1984.

155. Brunner, D., Feifarek, C., McNeely, D., et al.: CT of pseudomembranous colitis. Gastrointest. Radiol. *9:*73, 1984.

156. Letourneau, J.G., Day, D.L., Steely, J.W., et al.: CT appearance of antibiotic-induced colitis. Gastrointest. Radiol. *12:*257, 1987.

157. Tedesco, F.J.: Antibiotic associated pseudomembranous colitis with negative proctosigmoidoscopy exam. Gastroenterology *77:*295, 1979.

158. Tedesco, F.J., Corless, J.K., and Brownstein, R.E.: Rectal sparing in antibiotic pseudomembranous colitis: A prospective study. Gastroenterology *83:*1259, 1982.

159. Burbige, E.J., and Radigan, J.J.: Antibiotic-associated colitis with normal appearing rectum. Dis. Col. Rectum *24:*198, 1981.

160. Seppala, K., Kjelt, L., and Sipponen, P.: Colonoscopy in the diagnosis of antibiotic-associated colitis. Scand. J. Gastroenterol. *16:*465, 1981.

161. Gerding, D.N., Olson, M.M., Peterson, L.R., et al.: *Clostridium difficile*-associated diarrhea and colitis in adults: A prospective case-controlled epidemiologic study. Arch. Intern. Med. *146:*95, 1986.

162. Rubesin, S.E., Levine, M.S., Glick, S.N., et al.: Pseudomembranous colitis with rectosigmoid sparing on barium studies. Radiology *170:*811, 1989.

163. Strada, M., Meregaglia, D., and Donzelli, R.: Double-contrast enema in antibiotic-related pseudomembranous colitis. Gastrointest. Radiol. *8:*67, 1983.

164. Mulholland, M.W., and Delaney, J.P.: Neutropenic colitis and aplastic anemia: A new association. Ann. Surg. *197:*84, 1983.

165. Wagner, M.L., Rosenberg, H.S., Fernbach, D.J., et al.: Typhlitis: A complication of leukemia in childhood. AJR Am. J. Roentgenol. *109:*341, 1970.

166. Frick, M.P., Maile, C.W., Crass, J.R., et al.: Computed tomography of neutropenic colitis. AJR Am. J. Roentgenol. *143:*763, 1984.

167. Merine, D.S., Fishman, E.K., Jones, B., et al.: Right lower quadrant pain in the immunocompromised patient. CT findings in 10 cases. AJR Am. J. Roentgenol. *149:*1177, 1987.

168. Strano, A.J.: Lymphogranuloma venereum. *In* Binford, C.H., and Connor, D.H.: Pathology of Tropical and Extraordinary Diseases. Washington, DC, Armed Forces Institute of Pathology, 1976, p. 82.

169. Glick, S.N.: Other inflammatory conditions. *In* Gore, R.M., Levine, M.S., and Laufer, I. (eds.): Textbook of Gastrointestinal Radiology. Philadelphia, W.B. Saunders Co., 1994, p. 1142.

170. Levine, J.S., Smith, P.D., and Brugge, W.R.: Chronic proctitis in male homosexuals due to lymphogranuloma venereum. Gastroenterology *79:*563, 1980.

171. Palmer, K.R., Patil, D.H., Basran, G.S., et. al.: Abdominal tuberculosis in urban Britain—A common disease. Gut *26:*1296, 1985.

172. Vaidya, M.G., and Sodhi, J.S.: Gastrointestinal tract tuberculosis: A study of 102 cases including 55 hemicolectomies. Clin. Radiol. *29:*189, 1978.

173. Carr-Locke, D.L., and Finlay, D.B.L.: Radiological demonstration of colonic aphthoid ulcers in a patient with intestinal tuberculosis. Gut *24:*453, 1983.

174. Downey, D.B., and Nakielny, R.A.: Aphthoid ulcers in colonic tuberculosis. Br. J. Radiol. *58:*561, 1985.

175. Balthazar, E.J., and Bryk, D.: Segmental tuberculosis of the distal colon: Radiographic features in 7 cases. Gastrointest. Radiol. *5:*75, 1980.

176. Werbeloff, L., Novis, B.H., Banks, S., et al.: The radiology of tuberculosis of the gastrointestinal tract. Br. J. Radiol. *46:*329, 1973.

177. Peh, W.C.: Filiform polyposis in tuberculosis of the colon. Clin. Radiol. *39:*534, 1988.

178. Balthazar, E.J., Gordon, R., and Hulnick, D.: Ileocecal tuberculosis: CT and radiologic evaluation. AJR Am. J. Roentgenol. *154:*499, 1990.

179. Connor, D.H., Neafie, R.C., and Meyers, W.M.: Amebiasis. *In* Binford, C.H., and Connor, D.H.: Pathology of Tropical and Extraordinary Diseases. Washington, DC, Armed Forces Institute of Pathology, 1976, pp 308–316.

180. Cardosa, J.M., Kimura, K., Stoopen, M., et al.: Radiology of invasive amebiasis of the colon. AJR Am. J. Roentgenol. *128:*935, 1977.

181. Dieterich, D.T., and Rahmin, M.: Cytomegalovirus colitis in AIDS: Presentation in 44 patients and a review of the literature. J. Acquir. Immune Defic. Syndr. *4:*S29, 1991.

182. Frank, D., and Raicht, R.F.: Intestinal perforation associated with cytomegalovirus infection in patients with acquired immunodeficiency syndrome. Am. J. Gastroenterol. *79:*201, 1984.

183. Tatum, E.T., Sun, P.C.J., and Cohn, D.L.: Cytomegalovirus vasculitis and colon perforation in a patient with acquired immunodeficiency syndrome. Pathology *21:*235, 1989.

184. Balthazar, E.J., Megibow, A.J., Fazzini, E., et. al.: Cytomegalovirus colitis in AIDS: Radiographic findings in 11 patients. Radiology *155:*585, 1985.

185. Glotzer, D.J., Glick, M.E., and Goldman, H.: Proctitis and colitis follow-up diversion of the fecal stream. Gastroenterology *80:*438, 1981.

186. Bosshardt, R.T., and Abel, M.E.: Proctitis following fecal diversion. Dis. Colon Rectum *27:*605, 1984.

187. Korelitz, B.I., Cheskin, L.J., Sohn, N., et al.: Proctitis after fecal diversion in Crohn's disease and its elimination with reanastomosis: Implications for surgical management. Gastroenterology *87:*710, 1984.

188. Scott, R.L., and Pinstein, M.L.: Diversion colitis demonstrated by double-contrast barium enema. AJR Am. J. Roentgenol. *143:*767, 1984.

Diverticular Disease

STEPHEN E. RUBESIN
IGOR LAUFER

PATHOLOGIC FEATURES

CLINICAL CORRELATION

DIVERTICULOSIS

DIVERTICULITIS
Complications Related to Diverticulitis
Pericolic Tracking and Fistula Formation
Obstruction
Perforation

DIVERTICULAR HEMORRHAGE

COEXISTING LESIONS
Inflammatory Bowel Disease
Polyps and Carcinoma

PATHOLOGIC FEATURES

Diverticular disease of the colon is composed of two primary pathologic abnormalities: (1) the presence of multiple diverticula and (2) alteration of the normal structure of the longitudinal and circular muscle layers.[1] Diverticula are acquired herniations of mucosa and submucosa through areas of colonic wall weakness.[2] Because the herniations only contain mucosa and submucosa, these protrusions have been termed "false" diverticula or "pseudodiverticula."[3] The diverticula protrude at sites of penetrating arterioles on the mesenteric side of the antimesenteric teniae.[4] These large diverticula form two rows, each row running between the one mesenteric tenia and one of the two antimesenteric teniae. Small diverticula also protrude near the mesenteric tenia.

A diverticulum ranges from 0.2 to 2 cm in diameter; it is flask shaped, and its narrow neck is surrounded by circular muscle. The protruding mucosa and submucosa are separated from the pericolic fat by a thin layer of longitudinal muscle (Fig. 14–1).[5] An artery and vein are usually seen at the neck of a diverticulum. Lymph follicles are frequently seen at the apex of a diverticulum, a response to chronic inspissation of feces and food.[6]

Diverticula, if present, are most frequently found in the sigmoid colon (90%) (Fig. 14–2), the descending colon (30%), or throughout the colon (16%).[7,8] Right-sided diverticulosis (Fig. 14–3) is the most frequent form of diverticulosis in Japan, although it is relatively uncommon in Western populations.[1,9] Appendiceal diverticula are found in 0.2% to 2% of patients (Fig. 14–4). Rectal diverticula (Fig. 14–5) are extremely rare because the longitudinal muscle layer spreads laterally in the distal colon to encircle the rectum. Thus the rectal wall is thicker, preventing formation of diverticula.

The bulk of the longitudinal muscle layer of the colon is primarily found in three longitudinal bands—the teniae coli. The haustral sacculations are formed between the teniae. In diverticular disease, elastin deposits between normal muscle fibers in the teniae coli. This microscopic finding is associated with macroscopic shortening and thickening of the teniae coli.[10] Shortening of the teniae coli leads to shortening of the colon, with resultant bunching of the circular muscle layer and its overlying mucosa. The corrugated circular muscle layer appears as semilunar ridges between the mesenteric and antimesenteric teniae (Fig. 14–6).[2] Histologically, there is neither increased size of muscle cells (hypertrophy) nor increased number of cells (hyperplasia). Morson, for want of a better term, describes the secondary effect on the circular muscle layer as circular muscle "thickening" or "bunching." This has been termed *myochosis* by radiologists. The colonic wall between the bunched circular muscle layer is sacculated. Diverticula may protrude from the sacculations. The bunched-up mucosa becomes so redundant that it may fill the colonic lumen, adding to the stenosis caused by the circular muscle thickening.

Either the diverticula or the muscle abnormality may be present independently. Approximately 8% of patients display only the muscle change and 20% of patients only the diverticula.[7] The term *diverticulosis* refers to the presence of sacs with or without the muscle abnormality (Fig. 14–7). The term *diverticular disease* implies that the muscle abnormality is present (Fig. 14–8). *Diverticulitis* implies that a diverticulum is inflamed.

471

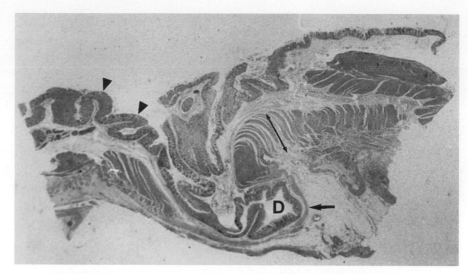

FIGURE 14–1. Diverticulosis of the colon. Low-power photomicrograph of a segment of sigmoid colon shows a thick circular muscle layer *(double arrow)* and redundant folds of mucosa *(arrowheads)*. A diverticulum *(D)* protrudes through the circular muscle layer into the pericolic fat. The diverticulum is surrounded by a thin layer of longitudinal muscle *(arrow)*.

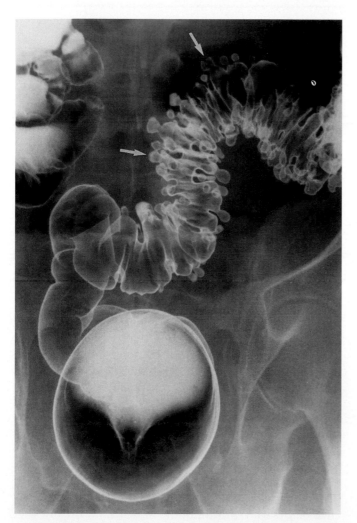

FIGURE 14–2. Diverticulosis of the sigmoid colon. Prone, angled view of the colon shows numerous diverticula in a typical sigmoid distribution *(arrows)*.

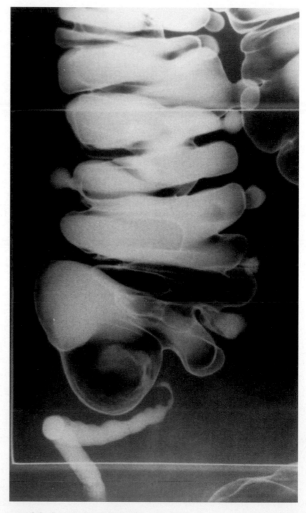

FIGURE 14–3. Right-sided diverticulosis. Scattered diverticula are located in the ascending colon.

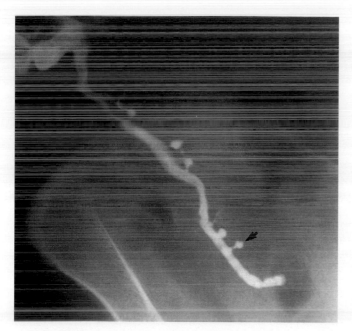

FIGURE 14–4. Appendiceal diverticulosis. Compression-aided view of appendix shows numerous barium-filled diverticula (representative diverticulum identified with *arrow*).

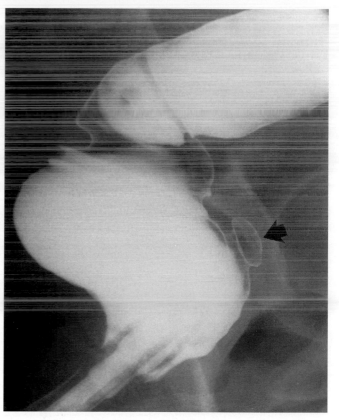

FIGURE 14–5. Rectal diverticulum. Spot film of the rectum shows a 1.5-cm air-filled, contrast-etched diverticulum *(arrow)* arising from the anterior rectal wall. (Reproduced with permission from Rubesin, S.E., and Schnall, M.D.: Rectum. *In* Gore, R.M., Levine, M.S., and Laufer, I. (eds.): Textbook of Gastrointestinal Radiology. Philadelphia, W.B. Saunders Co., 1994, p. 1306, Fig. 60–73.)

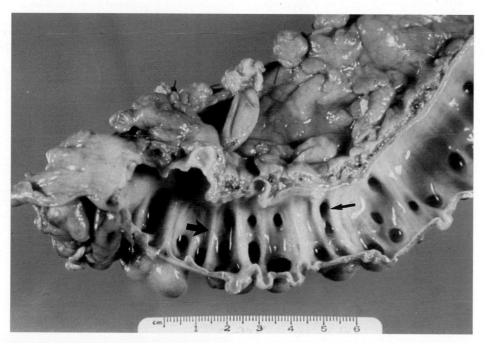

FIGURE 14–6. Diverticulosis. Photograph of a formalin-fixed specimen shows numerous circular muscle folds (representative fold identified with *large arrow*). The orifices of the diverticula are seen en face as black, ovoid-shaped shadows (representative diverticular orifice identified with *small arrow*).

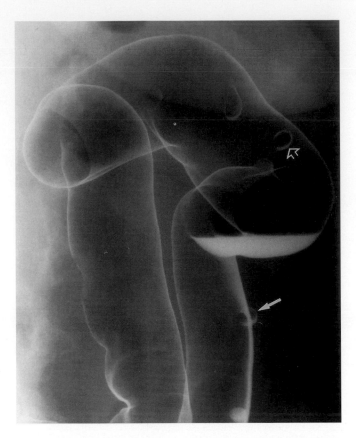

FIGURE 14–7. Diverticulosis. Diverticula in the splenic flexure are seen as ring shadows en face *(open arrow)* and as protrusions from the wall either filled with barium or etched in white by barium *(arrow).* No circular muscle thickening is present.

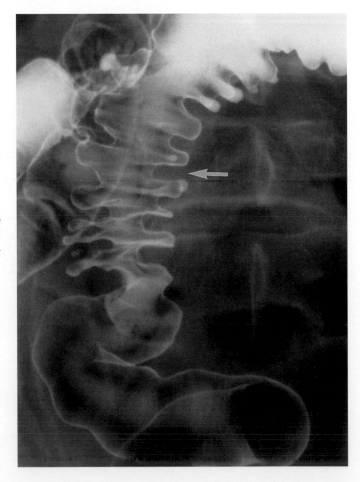

FIGURE 14–8. Circular muscle thickening. Spot radiograph of the sigmoid colon shows thick folds perpendicular to the longitudinal axis of the bowel (representative fold identified with *arrow*). A few diverticula are present.

CLINICAL CORRELATION

The incidence of diverticulosis has dramatically increased in the Western world since the turn of the century.[7,11,12] Before 1900, diverticulosis was a pathologic curiosity. Today, in Western populations, more than 50% of people older than 40 have diverticulosis.[11,13] Most people with diverticulosis are asymptomatic. Of the 10% to 25% of people with diverticulosis who become symptomatic, most present with acute symptoms at an elderly age (50 to 70 years).[14] Only 1 in 200 people with diverticulosis will require an operation. However, if symptoms present at an early age, the disease will be more severe.[15] Patients taking nonsteroidal antiinflammatory agents will have more severe complications.[16]

The cause of the development of diverticulosis is unknown. Clearly, diverticulosis is a disease of developed or developing nations. Diverticulosis is uncommon in underdeveloped areas of Africa and Asia.[17-20] The incidence of diverticulosis increases in specific populations who migrate to developing countries. It is postulated that lack of dietary fiber leads to increased intraluminal pressure, which leads to mucosal herniation through areas of muscular weakness.[21] Diverticulosis has been shown to be of increased incidence and to be present at an earlier age in Marfan syndrome and in Ehlers-Danlos syndrome, presumptively related to increased bowel wall weakness.[22]

DIVERTICULOSIS

Patients with uncomplicated diverticulosis are usually asymptomatic. Some patients may complain of left lower quadrant pain related to muscular spasm.

A radiologist should become thoroughly familiar with diverticulosis, as it is present in most patients undergoing barium enema. During barium enema, diverticula appear as round or flask-shaped protrusions, often with narrow necks. Diverticula may be filled with barium or may be etched in white by barium and distended with air (Fig. 14–9). Diverticula may not always fill with air or barium and may only be filled after colonic spasm or colonic evacuation.

A diverticulum's appearance depends on the amount of barium within its lumen or the angle in which it is viewed.[3] En face, a diverticulum appears as a sharply demarcated collection of barium, or if unfilled, a ring shadow (Fig. 14–10). Barium will frequently fade away from the sharp luminal margin of an incompletely filled diverticulum, forming an irregular "meniscus" on the inside of the diverticulum (Fig. 14–11). Barium-etched diverticula, seen en face, may resemble a bowler hat (Fig. 14–12). The luminal margin of the diverticulum appears as an ovoid ring shadow (the "brim" of the bowler hat). The apex of the diverticulum appears as a hemispheric line (the "dome" of the bowler hat). The apex of the hemispheric line will point toward the extraluminal

space, away from the longitudinal axis of the lumen.[23] In contrast, a polyp that resembles a bowler hat will protrude inward toward the longitudinal axis of the colonic lumen.

When seen en face, small diverticula (Fig. 14–13) may resemble aphthoid ulcers. Tiny diverticula have less of a radiolucent shadow surrounding the barium collection than aphthoid ulcers. In profile, tiny diverticula may be round or conical.[3]

Portions of a diverticulum may bulge into the colonic lumen. The orifice of a diverticulum may invaginate into the colonic lumen, or the apex of a diverticulum may prolapse into the lumen of the diverticulum itself.[24] These prolapsing diverticula have been termed *inverted diverticula*. Inverted diverticula are usually seen proximal to the splenic flexure. Inverted diverticula (Fig. 14–14) may initially be mistaken for a small submucosal mass or polyp.[24,25] The key to the radiologic diagnosis of an inverted diverticulum is recognition of a central barium collection in a small, right-sided "submucosal mass" (see Fig. 14–14) or umbilication of barium beyond the expected luminal contour of the colon. Sometimes, a central barium collection is not seen during early fluoroscopy or on early radiographs. With time, manual compression, insufflation of more air, or postevacuation radiography, portions of inverted diverticula will fill with barium allowing correct diagnosis.

Occasionally, large barium collections resembling giant diverticula are detected, especially in the sigmoid colon (Fig. 14–15).[26,27] Pathologically, these "giant diverticula" are lined by inflammatory and granulation tissue

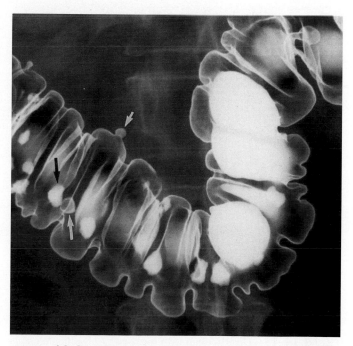

FIGURE 14–9. Diverticulosis. Supine radiograph of transverse colon shows diverticula manifested en face as barium-filled sacs *(black arrow)* or ring shadows *(long white arrow),* and diverticula seen in profile as sacs etched in white *(short white arrow).*

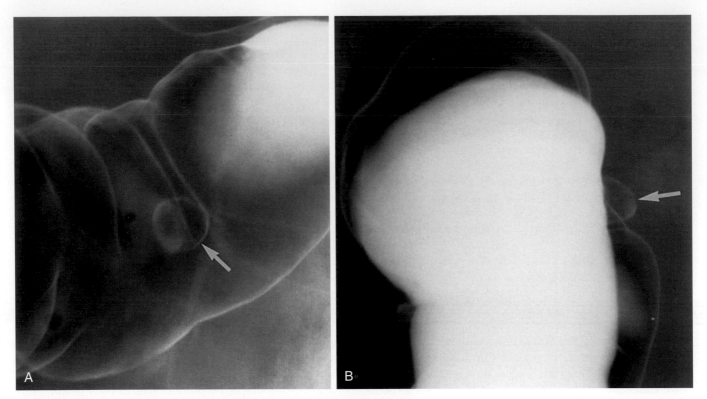

FIGURE 14–10. Diverticulosis. *A,* En face, a diverticulum appears as a ring shadow *(arrow)* containing a small droplet of barium. *B,* In profile the same diverticulum *(arrow)* protrudes from the contour of the colon.

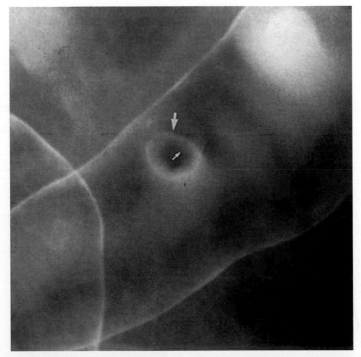

FIGURE 14–11. Diverticulum with meniscus. A diverticulum appears en face as a ring shadow with a relatively sharp outer edge *(large arrow).* A meniscus of barium has a irregular margin on its inner border *(small arrow).*

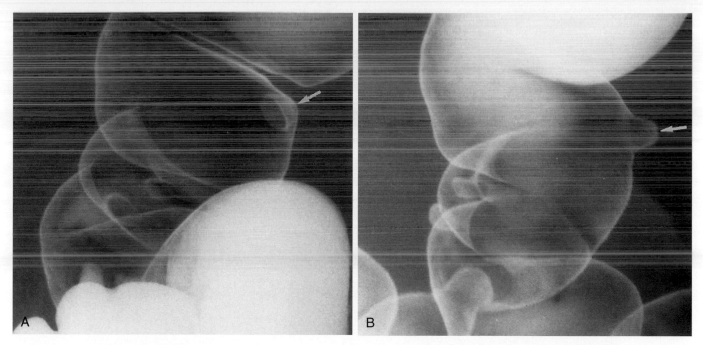

FIGURE 14–12. Bowler hat diverticulum. *A,* A Bowler hat shadow *(arrow)* is seen on the lateral wall of the descending colon. The apex of the Bowler hat points away from the longitudinal axis of the bowel. Several other diverticula are seen. *B,* When the patient is turned, the same diverticulum *(arrow)* is seen protruding outside the luminal contour of the colon. (From Miller, W.T., Jr., Levine, M.S., Rubesin, S.E., and Laufer, I.: Bowler hats: A simple principle for differentiating polyps from diverticula. Radiology 173:615–617, 1989.)

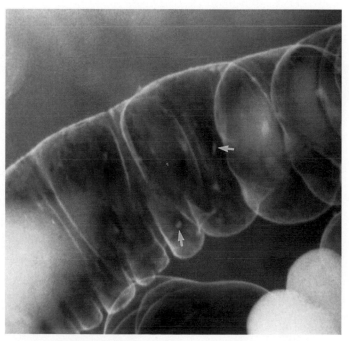

FIGURE 14–13. Tiny diverticula. Spot radiograph of transverse colon shows numerous punctate collections of barium mimicking aphthoid ulcers (representative diverticula identified with *arrows*).

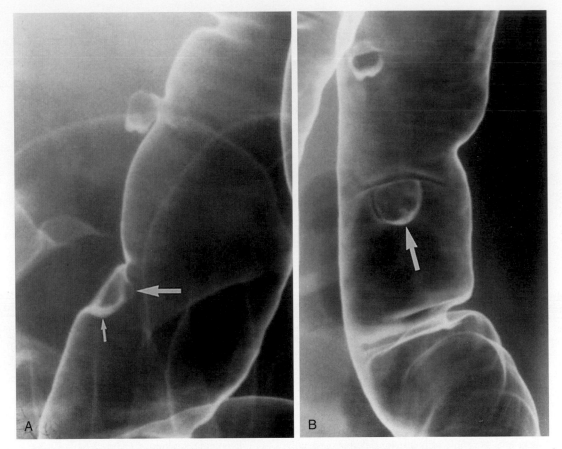

FIGURE 14–14. Inverted diverticulum. *A,* Spot radiograph of descending colon demonstrates an inverted diverticulum as a barium-etched "submucosal-appearing" mass protruding intraluminally *(large arrow).* There is, however, a barium collection *(small arrow)* on the inside of the "polypoid" diverticulum. *B,* En face, a ring shadow is seen, with a barium collection on its dependent wall *(arrow).*

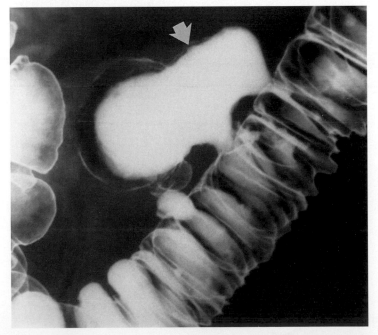

FIGURE 14–15. "Giant sigmoid diverticulum." Spot radiograph of the junction of the descending colon and sigmoid colon shows a 5 × 3 cm barium-filled "giant diverticulum" *(arrow),* the result of a prior diverticular abscess. Pathologic study showed that this space was not lined by mucosa but by granulation tissue and was therefore not a colonic diverticulum.

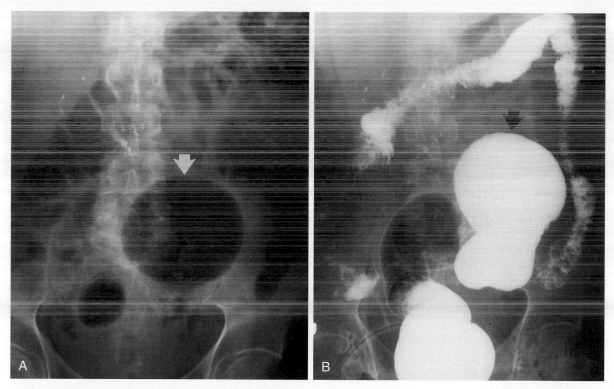

FIGURE 14–16. Giant sigmoid diverticulum retaining air. *A,* Plain film of the abdomen shows a large air-filled sac *(arrow)* in the left lower quadrant. *B,* Overhead radiograph from a barium enema shows that the air-filled sac *(arrow)* is now filled with barium. This was a giant sigmoid diverticulum.

and not epithelium. Thus these "giant diverticula" are probably the sequelae of diverticulitis with abscess formation. After the abscess heals, the cavity of the abscess remains distended with air (Fig. 14–16) or debris. The reason air is trapped in these large "diverticula" remains unknown.

Longitudinal muscle shortening and thickening leads to a shortened sigmoid and descending colon, circular muscle bunching, and redundant mucosa. Radiographi-

cally, the sigmoid colon is shortened and straight (see Fig. 14–8). The barium or air-filled lumen has a zigzag course resembling an accordion or concertina. The bunched folds of circular muscle protrude into the lumen as fingerlike filling defects in the barium column or as parallel folds etched in white. The circular muscle folds may hide polyps or may be mistaken for polyps.[28]

On CT, circular muscle thickening is depicted as mural thickening >4 mm in thickness (Fig. 14–17).[29] Di-

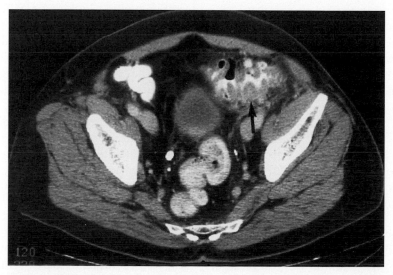

FIGURE 14–17. Circular muscle thickening. A thick, undulating wall *(arrow)* is seen in the sigmoid colon, the CT manifestation of circular muscle thickening.

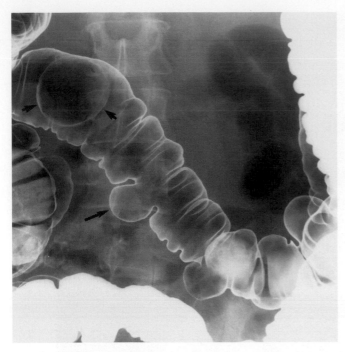

FIGURE **14–18. Sacculations in scleroderma.** Overhead view of the transverse colon shows broad-mouthed sacculations in profile *(large arrow)* and en face *(small arrows).*

verticula on CT will appear as outpouchings containing air, feces, or contrast extending into the pericolonic fat. These diverticula are easily distinguished from pneumatosis coli.

Diverticula of the colon are to be distinguished from sacculations of the colon, which contain all elements of the colonic wall. Sacculations that protrude beyond the expected luminal contour of the colon are usually due to colonic wall weakening. Broad-based sacculations due to weakening are most commonly found in scleroderma (Fig. 14–18).[30,31] The colonic wall may also appear sacculated opposite an inflammatory or scarring disorder. As colonic folds are pulled toward an inflammatory or scarring process, the uninvolved wall becomes sacculated but does not extend beyond the luminal contour. Crohn's disease and healing ischemia show sacculations related to scarring.

DIVERTICULITIS

Feces, food, or foreign material inspissated in a diverticulum may lead to chronic inflammation in the mucosa of the tip of the diverticulum. Lymphoid aggregates will develop in the subserosal fat as a response to the chronic inflammation. When the mucosa is destroyed, the inflammatory process will extend into the pericolic fat, resulting in a continuum from microperforation to focal peritonitis to pericolic abscess formation.[32] The inflammatory process may spread long distances in the pericolic gutters

or into the pelvis. Fistulae most commonly communicate with the urinary bladder,[33] vagina, small bowel, and skin. Longitudinal spread of inflammation may form tracks communicating with other diverticula.[34] With healing, the colon may return to its baseline diverticulosis or may become chronically narrowed.

Patients with moderate to severe sigmoid diverticulitis usually have fever, left lower quadrant pain, and leukocytosis. The initial attack of diverticulitis in young patients may be severe.[35,36] Some patients, however, have minimal symptoms or complain of mild rectal bleeding. Patients with diverticulitis arising in right or transverse colon diverticula may have symptoms in places less commonly associated with diverticulitis. Debilitated or elderly patients or patients taking corticosteroids may have minimal symptoms.[37]

Computed tomography (CT) has become the radiologists' modality of choice for patients with suspected diverticulitis.[38–40] CT is less invasive than contrast enema and has less risk of perforation in ill patients.[41] CT shows the pericolic inflammatory process that contrast enemas can sometimes only infer. CT demonstrates spread of disease long distances from the colon and demonstrates the presence of colovesical fistulae better than barium enema.

On CT, in patients with diverticulitis, the pericolic fat shows increased attenuation and stranding (Fig. 14–19). Small fluid collections or bubbles of air will be seen in the pericolic fat (see Fig. 14–19*B*), especially associated with a heterogeneous soft tissue mass. The root of the sigmoid mesentery will be indurated. Air-fluid levels can be seen in some pericolic abscesses (Fig. 14–20). Abscesses can also be detected in the liver, subphrenic space, groin, or thigh. If free perforation is present, an air-fluid level may be seen in the pelvis.

Contrast enemas are rarely indicated in acutely ill patients with suspected diverticulitis. However, barium enemas may be the first study obtained in patients who have mild symptoms such as left lower quadrant pain or mild rectal bleeding. Contrast enemas may also be the first study obtained in patients with symptoms in an atypical location, such as the right lower quadrant or mid-abdomen in patients with right-sided or transverse colon diverticulitis (Fig. 14–21). Therefore a radiologist must know the barium enema findings of diverticulitis and suspect this disease in middle-aged or elderly patients with mild pain or bleeding.

Contrast enemas are also often obtained after treatment of diverticulitis. Contrast enemas or endoscopy are performed after patient treatment to differentiate cancer from diverticulitis. Contrast enemas are superior to CT in demonstration of diverticula, luminal narrowing, muscular spasm, and circular muscle bunching and in differentiating diverticulitis from colonic carcinoma. Contrast enemas are safe in patients whose symptoms have resolved or are resolving. Free extravasation of barium or air into the intraperitoneal space is uncommon in treated patients and is even uncommon in patients with acute diverticulitis.

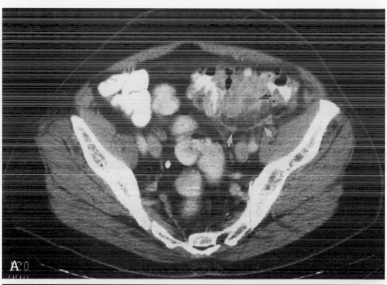

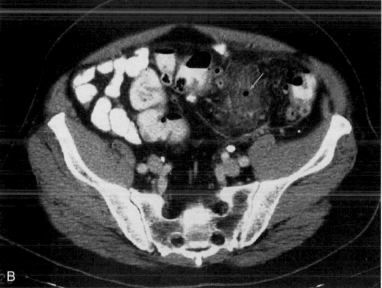

FIGURE **14–19. Diverticulitis.** A, CT scan through the pelvis shows stranding of the fat and induration of the root of the sigmoid mesentery *(white arrows)*. A low attenuation collection *(black arrow)* posterior to the thick, circular muscle folds represents an inflammatory process within the wall of the colon or in the serosal fat tucked between the undulating colonic contour. B, Just superior to the sigmoid loop in A, there is extensive stranding of the pericolic fat and a focal collection of air *(arrow)*, which is well above the expected location of a diverticulum.

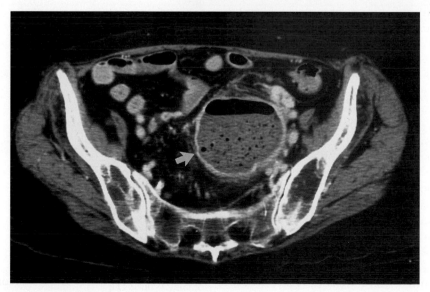

FIGURE **14–20. Abscess due to diverticulitis.** CT through the pelvis shows a large debris and air-filled collection *(arrow)*. Other evidence of diverticulitis was present on images taken more inferiorly through the pelvis.

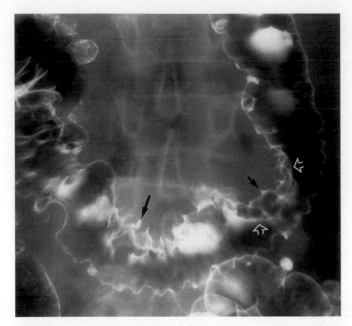

FIGURE 14–21. Diverticulitis of the transverse colon. Overhead view shows spiculation of the superior border of the transverse colon (representative "spicule" identified by *short arrow*), several areas of mass effect *(open arrows),* and a few deformed diverticula *(long arrow).* (Courtesy of Michael Davis, M.D.)

Definitive diagnosis of diverticulitis can be made on barium studies when air or barium is seen outside the expected luminal contour in sinus tracks (Fig. 14–22), fistulae, or abscesses (Fig. 14–23). Otherwise, contrast enema findings only infer the diagnosis of diverticulitis on the basis of secondary effects on the colonic contour adjacent to the pericolic inflammatory process.[41] The pericolic abscess may narrow the colonic contour on one side (Fig. 14–24) or circumferentially (Fig. 14–25). Mucosal folds are pulled toward the inflammatory process forming spikelike points. Diverticula near the pericolic abscess are tethered, flattened, or deformed (Fig. 14–26).[42]

Deformity of the colonic contour and tethering of mucosal folds are not diagnostic of diverticulitis. Tethered mucosal folds may be seen in any desmoplastic inflammatory or neoplastic process involving the serosa or mesentery (Fig. 14–27). The key to the diagnosis of diverticulitis is demonstration of air or barium outside of the expected luminal contour of the colon.

If the inflammatory process is confined to the wall of the colon or extends only minimally into the serosal fat, a diagnosis of "intramural diverticulitis" may be made. On barium enema, intramural diverticulitis is manifested as focal, asymmetric spiculation of the colonic contour associated with a deformed diverticulum (Fig. 14–28) or tiny contrast collection within the expected colonic contour (Fig. 14–29). Only minimal, if any, extrinsic mass is seen.

Although CT is safer than and superior to contrast enema in diagnosing the presence of mild diverticulitis,

contrast enemas are probably superior in differentiating diverticulitis from colon cancer.[38] Some authors believe that after CT diagnosis and treatment for diverticulitis, a contrast enema or endoscopy should be performed to rule out colonic cancer.[41,43] At minimum, barium enema or endoscopic follow-up is probably necessary in patients with marked eccentric or circumferential wall thickening >2 cm as demonstrated by CT scan.

On contrast enema, cancers have abrupt shelflike margins and nodular mucosa, whereas diverticulitis usually has smooth, slightly tapered edges and preserved mucosal folds (Figs. 14–30 and 14–31). Cancers are usually shorter lesions associated with higher grades of obstruction. Barium enema cannot always unequivocally differentiate diverticulitis from cancer (Fig. 14–32). If there is any doubt about distinguishing diverticulitis from cancer, endoscopy must be performed. On the other hand, endoscopy also cannot always distinguish diverticulitis from colonic cancer, especially if the lesion cannot be traversed by the endoscope or biopsy specimens are taken from the edge of an obstructing lesion. If there is any endoscopic doubt, barium enema should be performed.

When large colonic cancers perforate into adjacent pericolic fat, a secondary inflammatory process may ensue. On CT, any inflammatory-appearing process that has a thick colonic wall or a large amount of mass extending into the pericolic fat should be suspected of being a perforated colonic cancer. Endoscopy or barium enema or a combination thereof may be required to make the diagnosis of perforated colonic cancer.

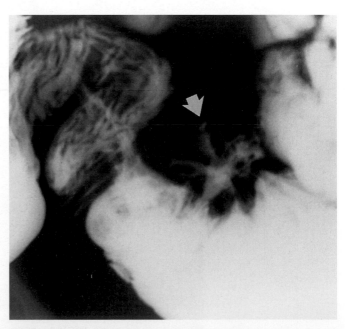

FIGURE 14–22. Pericolic tracks in diverticulitis. Spot radiograph obtained during barium filling shows numerous contrast-filled tracks *(arrow)* arising from the superior border of the sigmoid colon, extending into the pericolic space.

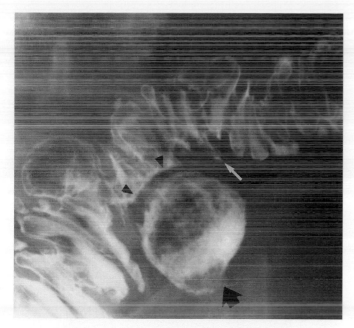

FIGURE 14–23. Barium filling pericolic abscess. Spot radiograph shows barium filling a 3-cm diameter collection *(black arrow)* arising from the inferior border of the sigmoid colon. Extrinsic mass effect on the inferior border of the sigmoid colon *(arrowheads)* and deformed diverticula *(white arrow)* are seen.

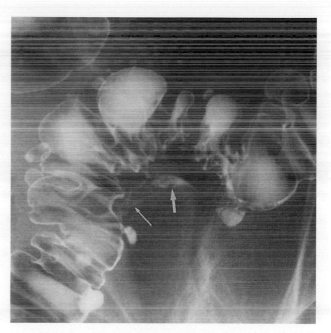

FIGURE 14–24. Diverticulitis of sigmoid colon. Spot radiograph shows a flame-shaped, barium-filled collection *(thick arrow)* communicating with the inferior border of the sigmoid colon via several fistulous tracks *(thin arrow)*. The pericolic abscess results in a mass effect along the inferior border of the sigmoid colon and spiculation of the colonic contour.

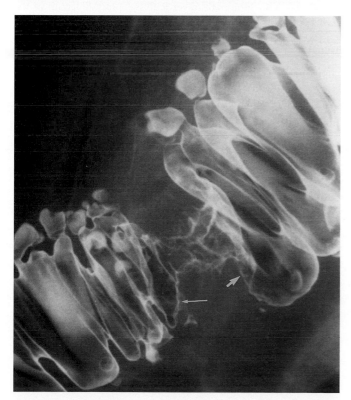

FIGURE 14–25. Circumferential extension of diverticulitis. Spot radiograph of the sigmoid colon shows circumferential narrowing of the colon. The narrowing is mildly tapered distally *(long arrow)* and shelflike proximally *(short arrow)*. The mucosa is preserved. Endoscopy, biopsy, and repeat barium enema showed no evidence of cancer.

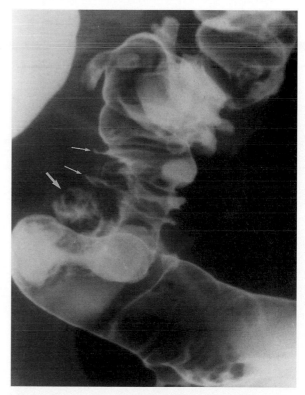

FIGURE 14–26. Deformed diverticula enveloped by sigmoid diverticulitis. Spot radiograph of sigmoid colon shows barium filling a small pericolic abscess *(thick arrow)*. Diverticula adjacent to the collection are deformed *(thin arrows)*.

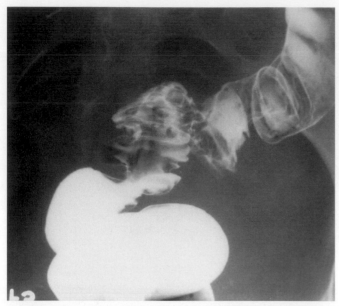

FIGURE 14–27. Ovarian cancer involving sigmoid colon. A segment of sigmoid colon is narrowed and angulated in several places. The mucosal folds are tethered.

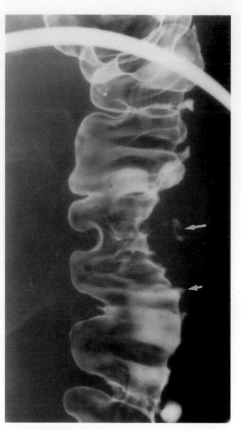

FIGURE 14–28. Intramural diverticulitis. Spot radiograph of the descending colon shows barium extending into a deformed diverticulum *(long arrow)*. Moderate spiculation *(short arrow)* and mild flattening of the colonic contour is seen.

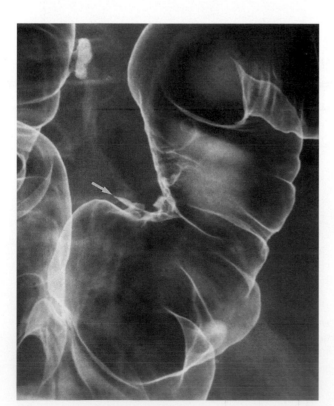

FIGURE 14–29. Intramural diverticulitis, transverse colon. Mild spiculation *(arrow)* and focal contour deformity of the superior contour of the transverse colon is present.

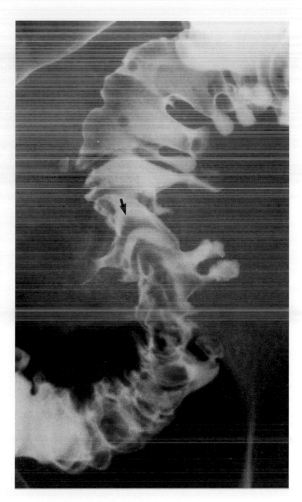

FIGURE 14–30. Preservation of mucosal folds in diverticulitis. Spot radiograph of sigmoid colon demonstrates tapered narrowing and many deformed diverticula. The mucosal folds (representative fold identified by *arrow*) are preserved. No barium is seen outside of the expected luminal contour in a pericolic track or abscess, however.

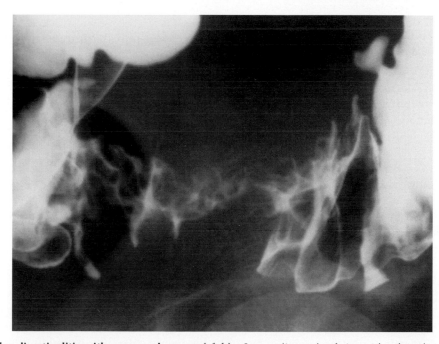

FIGURE 14–31. Annular diverticulitis with preserved mucosal folds. Spot radiograph of sigmoid colon shows an annular narrowing with preserved mucosa. Although the narrowing is abrupt, the edges are not shelflike. The edges are minimally tapered and the mucosa is preserved.

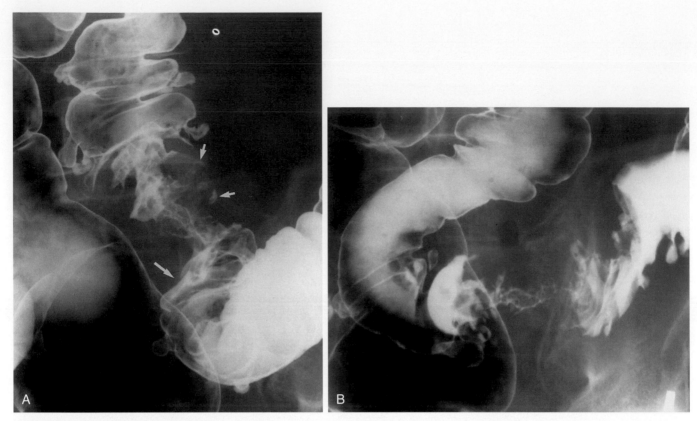

FIGURE 14–32. Diverticulitis versus cancer. *A,* Spot radiograph of the proximal sigmoid colon shows a focal annular lesion. The margins are abrupt, but tapered *(long arrow),* with smooth mucosa. Centrally, the mucosa is thrown into nondiagnostic nodular folds. Deformed diverticula *(short arrows)* are present in what would be the wall of a tumor, if this was a tumor. The presence of deformed diverticula within the walls of the annular narrowing is another sign that this is circumferential diverticulitis. Endoscopy with biopsy should be performed to confirm the radiologic diagnosis of probable diverticulitis. *B,* Spot radiograph of the sigmoid colon obtained during a barium enema performed 3 years after the study in *A* shows persistence of the focal annular area of chronic diverticulitis.

Complications Related to Diverticulitis
Pericolic Tracking and Fistula Formation

Barium may fill longitudinally oriented tracks that join adjacent diverticula in the pericolic space (Figs. 14–33 and 14–34).[34] Pericolic tracks or fistulae may fill slowly (Fig. 14–35) or on postevacuation films (Fig. 14–36).

Obstruction

Adenocarcinoma is the most common cause of colonic obstruction in adults. Diverticulitis, however, is the second most common cause of colonic obstruction in adults. Plain films or barium enema show a transition zone, with disproportionate dilatation of colon proximal to the obstructing lesion (Fig. 14–37). Feces and fluid fill the colon proximal to the obstruction. The inflammatory process of diverticulitis may spread to the small bowel, causing small bowel obstruction or adynamic ileus.

Perforation

Focal, contained perforation into the pericolic fat is the essential radiographic finding in diverticulitis. Free perforation into the intraperitoneal space is rare, however. Barium studies are not usually performed while a patient is acutely ill. Only extremely rarely is barium seen spilling into the peritoneal space (Fig. 14–38).

DIVERTICULAR HEMORRHAGE

Brisk, severe rectal bleeding is often due to diverticulosis, especially in elderly or hypertensive patients. As diverticula herniate at sites of wall weakening adjacent to arterioles, the penetrating arteries suffer eccentric damage.[44] Eccentric rupture of an arteriole into the lumen of a diverticulum leads to massive bleeding. Minor bleeding from granulation tissue is common. Bleeding from a diverticulum more frequently occurs in the right colon.[45] The increased prevalence of right-sided diverticular bleeding is probably related to the larger diverticula in this region. Bleeding from left-sided diverticula does occur, however.

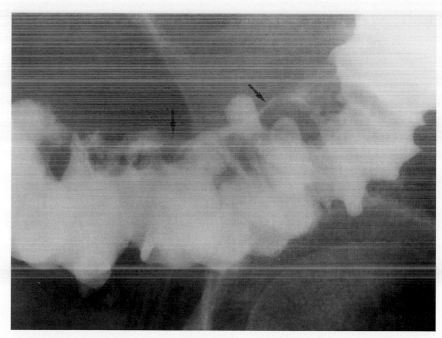

FIGURE 14–33. Pericolic tracking in diverticulitis. Spot radiograph shows a barium-filled track *(arrows)* running parallel to the superior border of the sigmoid colon.

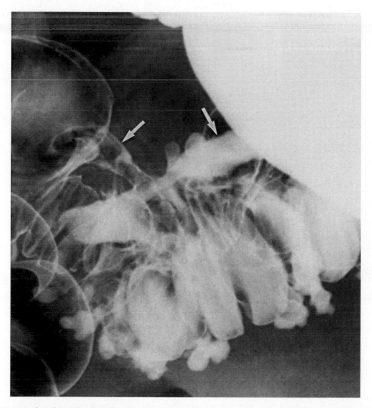

FIGURE 14–34. Pericolic tracking and colocolic fistulae in diverticulitis. Spot radiograph shows several barium-filled tracks *(arrows)* along the superior border of the transverse colon. Because the tracks communicate with each other, colocolic fistula formation is present.

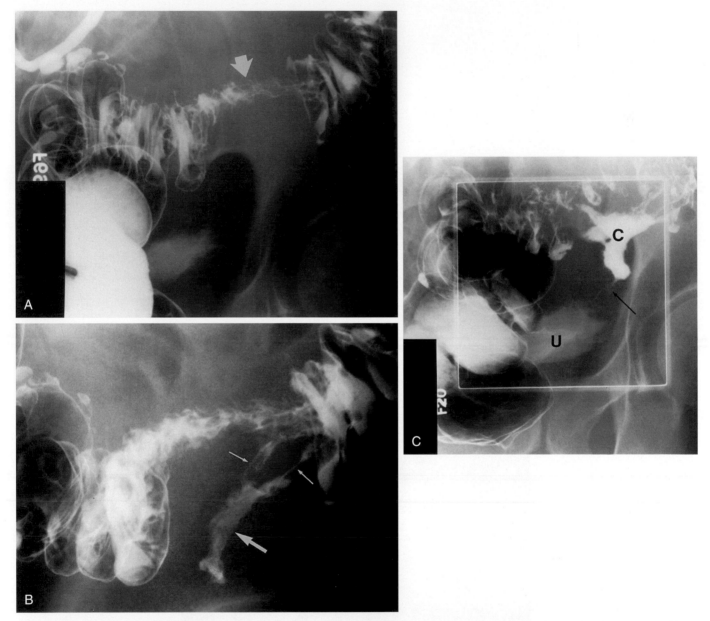

FIGURE 14–35. Sigmoid diverticulitis with delayed filling of fistula. *A,* Early spot radiograph shows circumferential narrowing *(arrow)* with preservation of mucosal folds in the proximal sigmoid colon. *B,* Spot radiograph obtained later during the study shows two fistulous tracks *(thin arrows)* arising from the more proximal end of the area involved by diverticulitis. A pericolic collection *(thick arrow)* is beginning to fill. *C,* Overhead radiograph shows filling of a Y-shaped collection *(C),* with a fistula *(arrow)* extending to the urinary bladder *(U).*

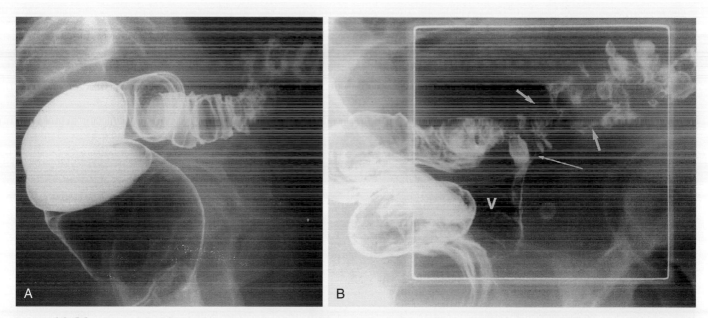

FIGURE 14–36. **Rectovaginal fistula demonstrated only on postevacuation radiograph.** *A,* Lateral spot radiograph of rectum does not show contrast in the vagina. Mild narrowing and diverticulosis is seen in the sigmoid colon. *B,* Spot radiograph obtained after the patient evacuated shows filling of several pericolic tracks *(short arrows).* A fistula *(long arrow)* to the vagina *(V)* is now filled with barium.

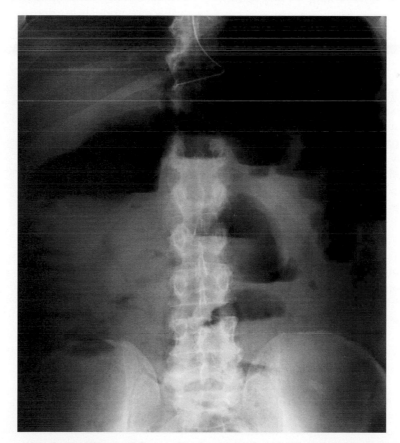

FIGURE 14–37. **Colonic obstruction due to diverticulitis.** Overhead radiograph with the patient in the erect position shows diffusely dilated transverse and descending colon with numerous air-fluid levels. The sigmoid and ascending colon also have air-fluid levels, but their lumens are less distended because these loops are more inferiorly located. A few air-fluid levels are also seen in the distal small intestine.

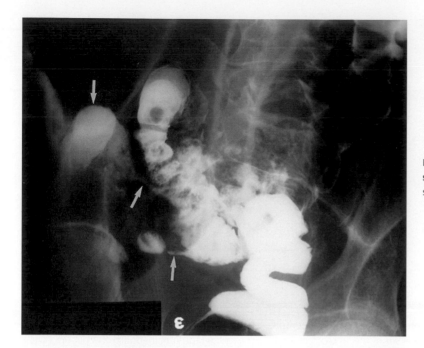

FIGURE **14–38. Free intraperitoneal perforation during single contrast barium enema.** Overhead radiograph shows barium streaming *(arrows)* into the right pelvis.

COEXISTING LESIONS

Diverticulosis is so common in developed countries that it is not infrequent that coexisting lesions or other diseases are present.

Inflammatory Bowel Disease

There are second peak incidences of both ulcerative colitis and Crohn's disease in the elderly. When Crohn's disease and ulcerative colitis occur in the elderly, diverticulosis is frequently a coexistent disorder. Idiopathic colitides are easily differentiated by their typical radiographic findings. For example, a patient with ulcerative colitis and diverticulosis will usually have mucosal granularity or small ulcers superimposed on mucosal granularity and diverticulosis. Patients who have ulcerative colitis in the presence of diverticulosis may have a grave prognosis, however.[46] Patients with Crohn's disease and diverticulosis are at increased risk for diverticulitis.[47] The radiographic findings of Crohn's disease, including aphthoid ulcers, anal fistulae, and mesenteric border ulcers, should be seen. Longitudinal sinus tracks may occur in both Crohn's disease and diverticulitis and are not helpful in distinguishing the two entities.[48–50]

Polyps and Carcinoma

Barium enema diagnosis of polyps would be easy if colons were free of feces and there were no diverticula. Diverticular disease is the most common reason that polyps are missed (Fig. 14–39).[51] Circular muscle bunching may obscure polyps or make diagnosis difficult for both radiologists and endoscopists. Fecaliths projecting out of a diverticulum may mimic a polyp (Fig. 14–40).[52] Usually, however, barium will enter at least part of a fecal-

filled diverticulum to surround the fecalith. En face, the fecal-filled diverticulum will appear as a sharp edge with a jagged barium-etched inner margin surrounding the feces. In contrast, barium surrounding a polyp will result in a sharp or nodular border with barium fading toward the periphery.

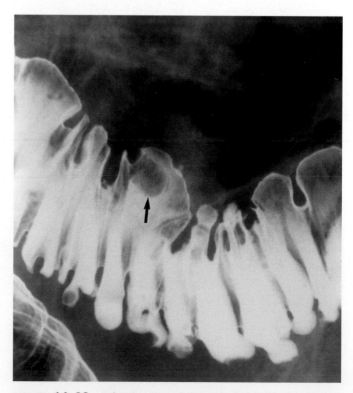

FIGURE **14–39. Polyp in area of sigmoid diverticulosis.** Spot radiograph shows a 0.4 × 0.6 cm ovoid radiolucency *(arrow)* in the barium pool. This was a tubular adenoma.

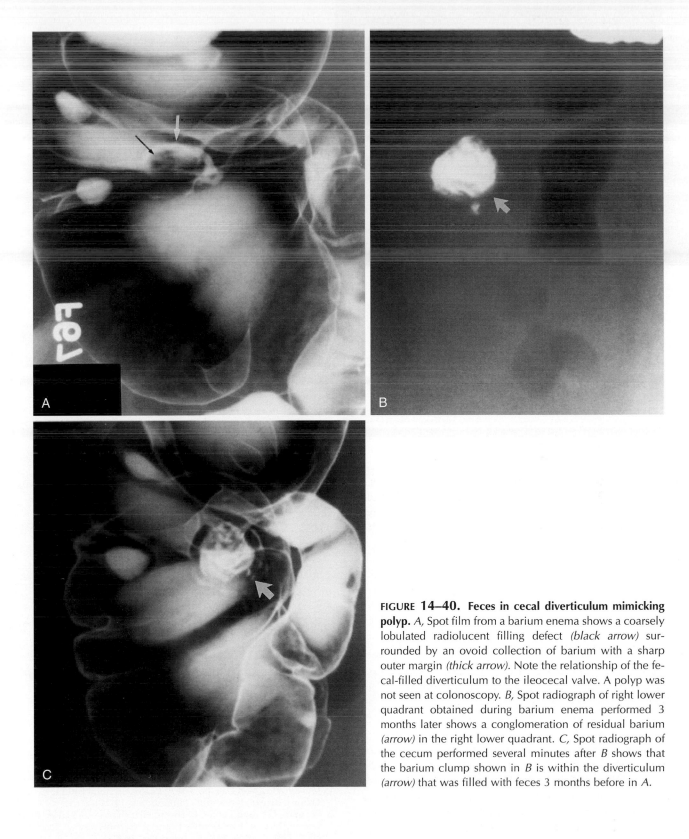

FIGURE **14–40. Feces in cecal diverticulum mimicking polyp.** *A,* Spot film from a barium enema shows a coarsely lobulated radiolucent filling defect *(black arrow)* surrounded by an ovoid collection of barium with a sharp outer margin *(thick arrow)*. Note the relationship of the fecal-filled diverticulum to the ileocecal valve. A polyp was not seen at colonoscopy. *B,* Spot radiograph of right lower quadrant obtained during barium enema performed 3 months later shows a conglomeration of residual barium *(arrow)* in the right lower quadrant. *C,* Spot radiograph of the cecum performed several minutes after *B* shows that the barium clump shown in *B* is within the diverticulum *(arrow)* that was filled with feces 3 months before in *A.*

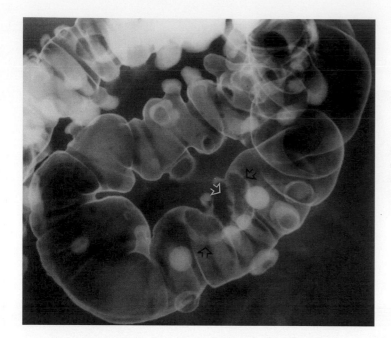

FIGURE 14–41. Polypoid adenocarcinoma arising in area of sigmoid diverticulosis. Barium etches a 3-cm polypoid mass *(black arrows)*. The colonic contour is focally disrupted *(white arrow)*.

FIGURE 14–42. Polypoid adenocarcinoma arising in area of sigmoid diverticulosis. Barium etches a focal polypoid lesion *(arrowheads)*. Barium within the interstices between nodular mucosa *(arrow)* helps identify this area as a tumor hiding in diverticulosis. Compressed, deformed diverticula make the diagnosis even harder.

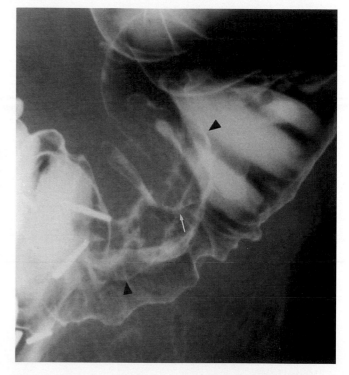

The presence of diverticulosis also makes diagnosis of colonic cancer more difficult. Polypoid cancers may hide in areas of diverticulosis (Fig. 14–41) or may rarely cause diverticulitis. The key to discovering cancer in the presence of diverticulosis is to look for a polypoid filling defect in the barium pool, barium-etched lines where they should not be (see Fig. 14–41), disruption of the luminal contour, and focal mucosal nodularity (Fig. 14–42).

REFERENCES

1. duBoulay, C.E.H.: Diverticular disease of the colon and solitary ulcer syndrome. *In* Whitehead, R. (ed.): Gastrointestinal and Oesophageal Pathology. Edinburgh, Churchill-Livingstone, 1989.
2. Morson, B.C., and Dawson, I.M.P.: Gastrointestinal Pathology, ed. 2. Oxford, Blackwell Scientific Publications, 1979.
3. Bartram, C.I., and Laufer, I.: Diverticular disease. *In* Laufer, I., and Levine, M.S. (eds.): Double Contrast Gastrointestinal Radiology, ed. 2. Philadelphia, W.B. Saunders Co., 1992.
4. Meyers, M.A., Volberg, F., Katzen, B., et al.: The angioarchitecture of colonic diverticula. Radiology *108*:249, 1973.

5. Morson, B.C.: The muscle abnormality in diverticular disease of the sigmoid colon. Br. J. Radiol. *36*:385, 1963.

6. Ming, S.: Diverticular disease of the colon. *In* Ming, S.C., and Goldman, H. (eds.): Pathology of the Gastrointestinal Tract. Philadelphia, W.B. Saunders Co., 1992.

7. Hughes, L.E.: Postmortem survey of diverticular disease of the colon. I. Diverticulosis and diverticulitis. II. The muscular abnormality of the sigmoid colon. Gut *10*:336, 1969.

8. Zollinger, R.W.: The prognosis of diverticulitis of the colon. Arch. Surg. *97*:418, 1968.

9. Sugihara, K., Muto, T., Morioka, Y., et al.: Diverticular disease of the colon in Japan: Review of 615 cases. Dis. Colon Rectum *27*:531, 1984.

10. Whiteway, J., and Morson, B.C.: Elastosis in diverticular disease of the sigmoid colon. Gut *26*:258, 1985.

11. Manousos, O.N., Truelove, S.C., and Lumsden, K.: Prevalence of colonic diverticulosis in the general population of Oxford area. BMJ *3*:762, 1967.

12. Hartwell, J.A., and Cecil, R.L.: Intestinal diverticula: A pathological and clinical study. Am. J. Med. Sci. *140*:174, 1910.

13. Hughes, L.E.: Complications of diverticular disease: Inflammation, obstruction and bleeding. Clin. Gastroenterol. *4*:147, 1975.

14. Parks, T.G.: Natural history of diverticular disease of the colon. Clin. Gastroenterol. *4*:53, 1975.

15. Acosta, J.A., Grebenc, M.L., Doberneck, R.C., et al.: Colonic diverticular disease in patients 40 years old or younger. Am. Surg. *58*:605, 1992.

16. Campbell, K., and Steele, R.J.: Non-steroidal anti-inflammatory drugs in diverticular disease: A case-control study. Br. J. Surg. *78*:190, 1991.

17. Kubo, A., Ishiwata, J., Maeda, Y., et al.: Clinical studies on diverticular disease of the colon. Jpn. J. Med. *22*:185, 1983.

18. Trotman, I.F., and Misiewicz, J.J.: Sigmoid motility in diverticular disease and the irritable bowel syndrome. Gut *29*:218, 1988.

19. Manousos, O., Day, N.E., Tzonou, A., et al.: Diet and other factors in the aetiology of diverticulosis: An epidemiological study in Greece. Gut *26*:544, 1985.

20. Segal, I., Solomon, A., and Hunt, J.A.: Emergence of diverticular disease in the urban South African black. Gastroenterology *72*:215, 1977.

21. Painter, N.S., and Burkitt, D.P.: Diverticular disease of the colon, a 20th century problem. Clin. Gastroenterol. *4*:3, 1975.

22. Mielke, J.E., Becker, K.L., and Gross, J.B.: Diverticulitis of the colon in a young man with Marfan's syndrome. Gastroenterology *48*:379, 1965.

23. Miller, W.T., Levine, M.S., Rubesin, S.E., et al.: Bowler-hat sign: A simple principle for differentiating polyps from diverticula. Radiology *173*:615, 1989.

24. Glick, S.N.: Inverted colonic diverticulum: Air contrast barium enema findings in six cases. AJR Am. J. Roentgenol. *156*:961, 1991.

25. Freeny, P.C., and Walker, J.H.: Inverted diverticula of the gastrointestinal tract. Gastrointest. Radiol. *4*:57, 1979.

26. Kricun, R., Stasik, J.J., Reither, R.D., et al.: Giant colonic diverticulum. AJR Am. J. Roentgenol. *135*:507, 1980.

27. Muhletaler, C.A., Berger, J., and Robinette, C.L.: Pathogenesis of giant colonic diverticula. Gastrointest. Radiol. *6*:217, 1981.

28. Htoo, A.M., and Dartram, C.I.: The radiological diagnosis of polyps in the presence of diverticular disease. Br. J. Radiol. *52*:263, 1979.

29. Balthazar, E.J.: Colon. *In* Megibow, A.J., and Balthazar, E.J. (eds.): Computed Tomography of the Gastrointestinal Tract. St. Louis, Mosby, 1986.

30. Heinz, E.R., Steinberg, A.J., and Sackner, M.A.: Roentgenographic and pathologic aspects of intestinal scleroderma. Ann. Intern. Med. *59*:822, 1963.

31. Cohen, S., Laufer, I., Snape, W.J., et al.: The gastrointestinal manifestations of scleroderma: Pathogenesis and management. Gastroenterology *79*:155, 1980.

32. Fleischner, F.G., and Ming, S.C.: Revised concepts on diverticular disease of the colon. 2. So-called diverticulitis: Diverticular sigmoiditis and perisigmoiditis, diverticular abscess, fistula, frank peritonitis. Radiology *84*:599, 1965.

33. Woods, R.J., Lavery, J.C., Fazio, V.W., et al.: Internal fistulas in diverticular disease. Dis. Colon Rectum *31*:591, 1988.

34. Ferrucci, J.T., Ragsdale, B.D., Barrett, P.J., et al.: Double tracking in the sigmoid colon. Radiology *120*:307, 1976.

35. Freischlag, J., Bennion, R.S., and Thompson, J.E., Jr.: Complications of diverticular disease of the colon in young people. Dis. Colon Rectum *29*:639, 1986.

36. Chodak, G.W., Rangel, D.M., and Passaro, E., Jr.: Colonic diverticulitis in patients under age 40: Need for earlier diagnosis. Am. J. Surg. *141*:699, 1981.

37. Canter, J.W., and Shorb, P.E., Jr.: Acute perforation of colonic diverticula associated with prolonged adrenocorticosteroid therapy. Am. J. Surg. *121*:46, 1971.

38. Cho, K.C., Morehouse, H.T., Alterman, D.D., et al.: Sigmoid diverticulitis: Diagnostic role of CT—comparison with barium enema studies. Radiology *176*:111, 1990.

39. Hulnick, D.H., Megibow, A.J., Balthazar, E.J., et al.: Computed tomography in the evaluation of diverticulitis. Radiology *152*:491, 1984.

40. Feldberg, M.S., Hendriks, M.J., and van Waes, P.F.: Role of CT in diagnosis and management of complications of diverticular disease. Gastrointest. Radiol. *10*:370, 1985.

41. Balthazar, E.J.: Diverticular disease. *In* Gore, R.M., Levine, M.S., and Laufer, I. (eds.). Textbook of Gastrointestinal Radiology. Philadelphia, W.B. Saunders Co., 1994.

42. Marshak, R.H., Lindner, A.E., and Maklansky, D.: Diverticulosis and diverticulitis of the colon. Mt. Sinai J. Med. *46*:261, 1979.

43. Balthazar, E.J., Megibow, A., Schinella, R.A., et al.: Limitations in the CT diagnosis of acute diverticulitis: Comparison of CT, contrast enema, and pathologic findings in 16 patients. AJR Am. J. Roentgenol. *154*:281, 1990.

44. Meyers, M.A., Alonso, D.R., Gray, G.F., et al.: Pathogenesis of bleeding colonic diverticulosis. Gastroenterology *71*:577, 1976.

45. Casarella, W.J., Kantor, I.E., and Seaman, W.B.: Right-sided colonic diverticula as a cause of acute rectal hemorrhage. N. Engl. J. Med. *286*:450, 1972.

46. Bates, T., and Kaminsky, V.: Diverticulitis and ulcerative colitis. Br. J. Surg. *61*:293, 1974.

47. Meyers, M.A., Alonso, D.R., Morson, B.C., et al.: Pathogenesis of diverticulitis complicating granulomatous colitis. Gastroenterology *74*:24, 1978.

48. Marshak, R.H., Linder, A.E., Pochaczevsky, R., et al.: Longitudinal sinus tracts in granulomatous colitis and diverticulitis. Semin. Roentgenol. *11*:101, 1976.

49. Marshak, R.H., Janowitz, H.D., and Present, D.H.: Granulomatous colitis in association with diverticula. N. Engl. J. Med. *283*:1080, 1970.

50. Loeb, P.M., Berk, R.N., and Saltzstein, S.L.: Longitudinal fistula of the colon in diverticulitis. Gastroenterology *67*:720, 1974.

51. Williams, C.B., Hunt, R.D., Loose, H., et al.: Colonoscopy in the management of colon polyps. Br. J. Surg. *61*:673, 1974.

52. Ott, D.J., Kerr, R.M., and Gelfand, D.W.: Colonic diverticula with stool simulating polyps. Gastrointest. Endosc. *33*:252, 1987.

Rectum

MARC S. LEVINE
IGOR LAUFER

Because the rectum is inaccessible to fluoroscopic palpation or compression, the conventional single contrast barium enema has been ineffective in diagnosing inflammatory or neoplastic lesions in this area.[1] As a result, the rectum has traditionally been considered the domain of the endoscopist rather than the radiologist. However, it is now recognized that endoscopy also has limitations in evaluating the rectum and that significant abnormalities may remain undetected.[2-5] This is partly because proctosigmoidoscopy is often done by examiners who are not expert in performing the procedure or in interpreting the findings.[6] Even experienced examiners can miss lesions in endoscopic "blind spots" behind a valve of Houston or on the posterior wall of the distal rectum near the anal verge (see Figs. 15–7 and 15–24).[3,4] Other lesions can be missed because of patient discomfort, anatomic variation, or distortion of the rectosigmoid by underlying disease that prevents complete insertion of the sigmoidoscope. For all these reasons, the rectum should be carefully evaluated during the routine barium enema examination, even in patients who have recently undergone or are about to undergo endoscopy. The major advantage of double contrast technique is that it permits visualization of the rectum in double contrast without an overlying column of barium, so that lesions can be demonstrated both en face and in profile.

TECHNIQUE

A complete study of the rectum is included in the routine double contrast enema (see Chapter 11). A high-quality examination of the rectum requires drainage of excess barium through the enema tip before final air insufflation.[7] This is best accomplished by placing the patient in a prone or left lateral position with the head of the table elevated 20 to 40 degrees and gently depressing the enema tip between the patient's legs to facilitate drainage of barium from the rectum.[8] It should be recognized that the enema tip itself may obscure lesions in the distal rectum (see Fig. 15–19). In patients with adequate sphincter tone, the tip therefore should be removed before obtaining spot films of the rectum. Early removal of the enema tip results not only in greater diagnostic accuracy in evaluating the rectum but also in better patient acceptance of the procedure.[9]

After the enema tip has been removed, spot films of the rectum should be obtained in prone, supine, and lateral projections. Frontal views often provide better mucosal detail because of decreased scatter. However, lateral views permit better delineation of perirectal disease involving the anterior wall of the rectosigmoid due to inflammatory conditions, endometriosis, or metastatic tumor (see later discussion, Extrinsic Abnormalities). Additional spot films may be obtained in appropriate projections when rectal lesions are suspected at fluoroscopy.

Two of the routine overhead radiographs included in the double contrast enema—the prone, angled view of the rectosigmoid and the prone, cross-table lateral view of the rectum—are particularly helpful for evaluating this region.[10,11] Some small lesions near the rectosigmoid junction may be visible only on the prone, angled view, whereas larger lesions that are suspected on other views may be demonstrated conclusively only on the angled view (see Fig. 15–21). The prone, cross-table lateral view is ideal for demonstrating abnormalities involving the anterior or posterior wall of the rectum.

A double contrast enema may be performed on patients with poor or absent sphincter tone by inflating a balloon in the rectum at the beginning of the examination and applying gentle traction on the enema tip to prevent leakage of barium and air. It is safe to use a balloon as long as there is no history of rectal disease or pelvic irradiation. The balloon should be inflated only under fluoroscopic guidance, and no more than 100 cc of gas should be injected into the balloon. When a balloon is used, it is still possible to evaluate the rectum by deflating the balloon at the end of the study and obtaining frontal and lateral spot films of the rectum at that time. Otherwise, proctoscopy is required to rule out rectal disease.

Recently, there has been considerable interest in the use of defecography or excretory proctography to evaluate patients with rectal prolapse, incontinence, or other defecation disorders.[12,13] However, this subject is beyond the scope of this text.

NORMAL APPEARANCES

The normal anatomy of the rectum is well demonstrated on double contrast studies. There are usually three prominent transverse folds, known as the valves of Houston, which are best seen on lateral views of the rectum (Fig. 15–1A).[14] The largest of these folds has been called the fold of Kohlrausch (Fig. 15–1B). When the distal rectum is partially collapsed, the columns of Morgagni may also be recognized as relatively straight, 2- to 4-mm wide folds extending 2 to 3 cm from the anorectal junction (Fig. 15–2). Aside from these normal structures, the rectal mucosa usually has a smooth, featureless appearance. On lateral views the posterior wall of the rectum generally lies 1 cm or less from the curve of the sacrum, but there is considerable variation, particularly in older patients, in whom a presacral space of 1 to 2 cm may be observed as a normal finding.[15] A sharp angulation almost always occurs at the rectosigmoid junction, as the distal rectum heads anteriorly and inferiorly.

FIGURE 15–1. Normal anatomy of rectum. *A,* Lateral view showing valves of Houston *(arrows). B,* Prone, angled view showing prominent valve of Kohlrausch *(arrow).*

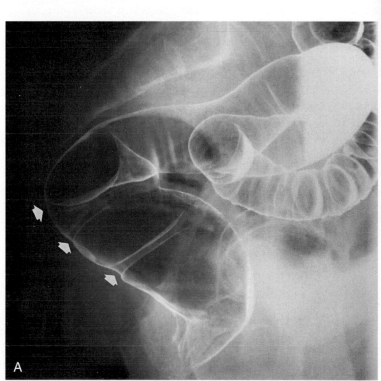

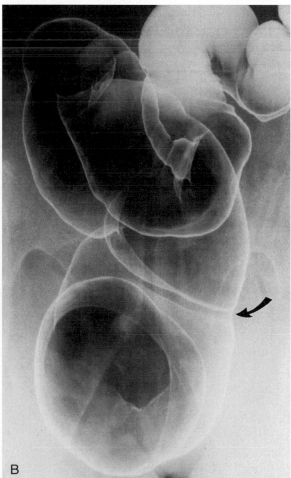

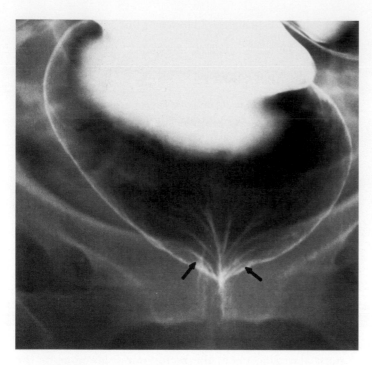

FIGURE 15–2. Rectal columns of Morgagni, appearing as thin, straight folds *(arrows)* near anorectal junction.

INTRINSIC ABNORMALITIES
Hemorrhoids

Hemorrhoids are a common source of rectal bleeding in older patients. They may be classified as internal or external, depending on their location above or below the anorectal junction. Although external hemorrhoids are readily detectable by visual inspection, internal hemorrhoids may be diagnosed by digital examination of the rectum, proctoscopy, or double contrast barium enema. In many cases, the patient is already known to have hemorrhoids, and a barium enema is performed to search for other more proximal sources of rectal bleeding. Nevertheless, it is important to be aware of the radiographic appearance of internal hemorrhoids, so that they can be differentiated from other more serious pathologic lesions.

Internal hemorrhoids are typically manifested on double contrast enemas by lobulated folds extending 3 cm or less from the anorectal junction (Fig. 15–3) or by multiple, small submucosal nodules (usually two to four) in the distal rectum, often resembling a small cluster of grapes (Fig. 15–4).[16,17] Much less frequently, internal hemorrhoids may appear as lobulated folds extending more than 3 cm from the anorectal junction or as solitary nodules or polypoid lesions in the distal rectum (Fig. 15–5).[17] Conversely, rectal carcinomas that infiltrate the submucosa can mimic the appearance of internal hemorrhoids (Fig. 15–6).[17] Occasionally, hypertrophied anal papillae or proctitis may produce similar findings.[17,18] Thus, any lesions that have an atypical appearance for internal hemorrhoids on double contrast enema should be evaluated by proctoscopy to rule out other pathologic conditions.

Neoplastic Lesions
Polyps

Because they are predominantly located in the distal colon, polyps are particularly common in the rectosigmoid region. Rectal polyps are more likely to be missed at endoscopy if they lie just beyond the anal verge or behind a valve of Houston (Fig. 15–7).[3] These polyps are usually hyperplastic or adenomatous. Hyperplastic polyps tend to be smooth, rounded elevations less than 5 mm in size, whereas adenomatous polyps tend to be larger and more lobulated.[19] Occasionally, small villous tumors may be indistinguishable from tubular adenomas (Fig. 15–8). It is important to visualize all surfaces of the rectum in double contrast because polyps can easily be obscured by the barium pool (Fig. 15–9). The radiologic aspects of polyps are discussed in more detail in Chapter 12.

Rectal polyps occasionally may be simulated by a variety of see-through artifacts projected over the rectum, such as calcified uterine fibroids, phleboliths, injection granulomas, and lymphangiographic contrast in pelvic lymph nodes (Fig. 15–10). However, the true nature of these findings is easily recognized by visualizing the rectum in other projections.

Double contrast enemas performed 2 weeks or less from the time of biopsy or resection of rectal polyps occasionally may reveal areas of shallow ulceration or deformity at the biopsy or polypectomy sites (Figs. 15–11 to 15–13).[20-22] The radiographic findings erroneously may suggest Crohn's disease or other inflammatory conditions involving the rectum. However, some postbiopsy or postpolypectomy ulcers may have a ringlike appearance that

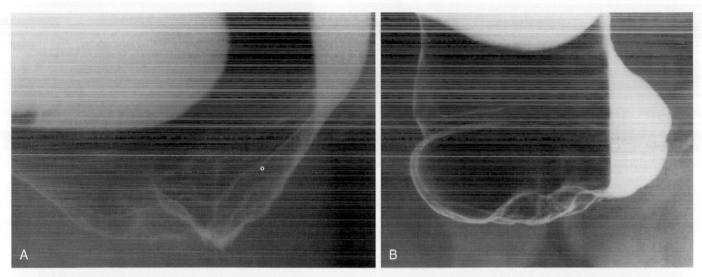

FIGURE 15–3. Two examples (*A* and *B*) of internal hemorrhoids manifested by lobulated folds near anorectal junction.

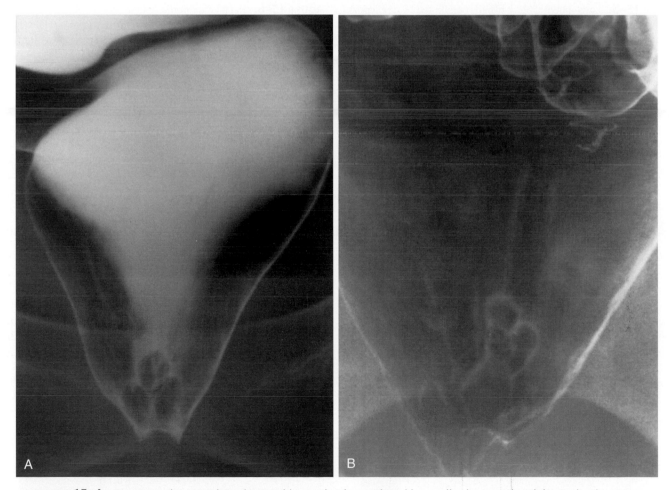

FIGURE 15–4. Two examples (*A* and *B*) of internal hemorrhoids manifested by small submucosal nodules in distal rectum.

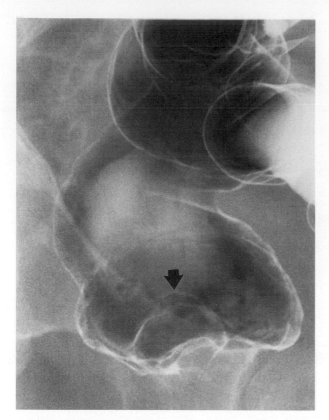

FIGURE 15–5. Large internal hemorrhoids manifested by a polypoid mass *(arrow)* in distal rectum. Proctoscopy is required in this patient because a polypoid carcinoma could produce similar findings.

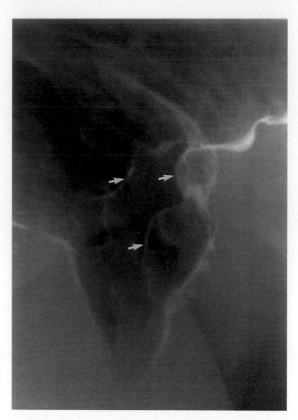

FIGURE 15–6. Rectal carcinoma with irregular, lobulated folds *(arrows)* in distal rectum, raising the possibility of prominent hemorrhoids. However, the folds extend farther proximally from the anorectal junction than expected for most internal hemorrhoids. (From Levine, M.S., et al.: Internal hemorrhoids: Diagnosis with double-contrast barium enema examinations. Radiology *177*:141, 1990, with permission.)

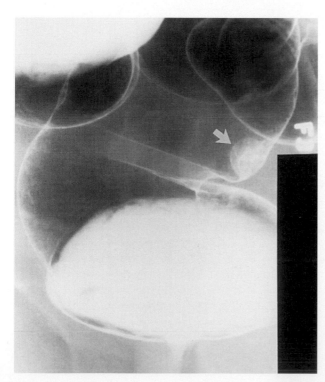

FIGURE 15–7. Rectal polyp *(arrow)* missed at proctoscopy because of its location behind valve of Houston.

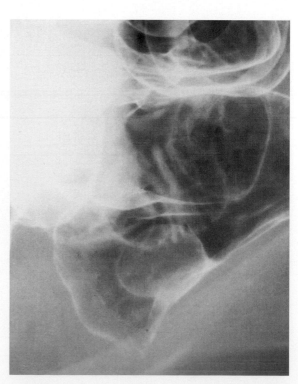

FIGURE 15–8. Villous adenoma in rectum. Note smooth surface of polyp, which has none of the radiologic features of a villous tumor.

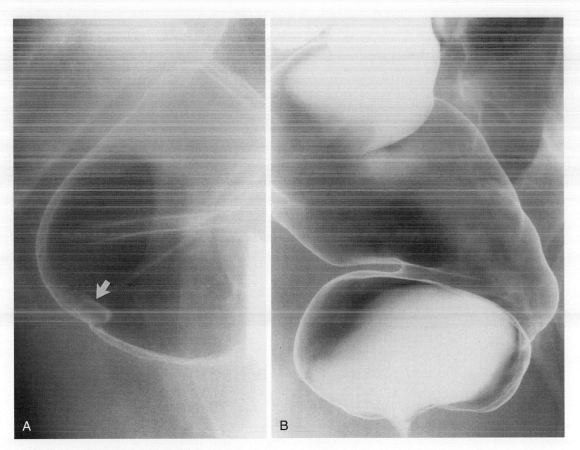

FIGURE 15–9. Importance of projection for demonstrating rectal polyps. *A,* Lateral view shows sessile polyp *(arrow)* on posterior wall of rectum. *B,* Prone view shows no evidence of polyp, which is obscured by barium pool on dependent surface *(the anterior wall).*

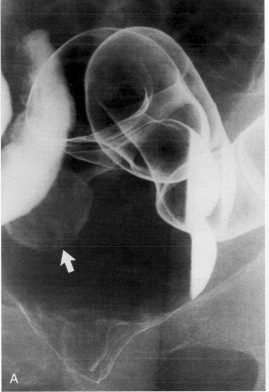

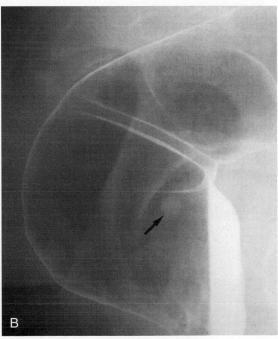

FIGURE 15–10. Pelvic calcifications *(arrows)* mimicking rectal polyps. *A,* Calcified uterine fibroid. *B,* Phlebolith.

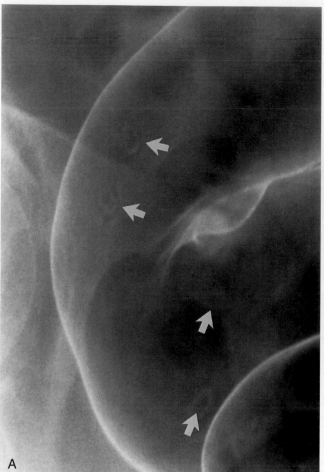

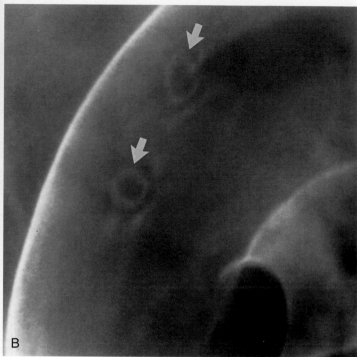

FIGURE 15–11. Multiple rectal ulcers at sites of biopsies taken 4 days earlier. *A,* Note characteristic ringlike appearance of ulcers *(arrows)* with surrounding radiolucent halos. *B,* Close-up view better delineates these ring-like ulcers *(arrows),* which should be differentiated from the aphthous ulcers of Crohn's disease. (*B,* From Lev-Toaff, A.S., et al.: Ringlike rectal ulcers after biopsy or polypectomy. AJR Am. J. Roentgenol. *148:*285, 1987, with permission, © by American Roentgen Ray Society.)

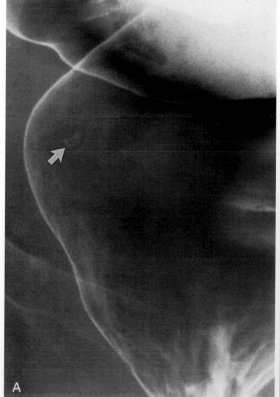

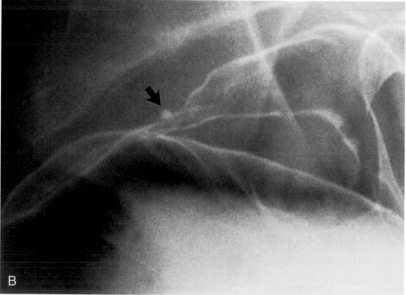

FIGURE 15–12. Rectal ulcer at site of polypectomy done 3 days earlier. *A,* Frontal view shows tiny, ringlike ulcer *(arrow)* with faint halo surrounding ulcer. (From Lev-Toaff, A.S., et al.: Ringlike rectal ulcers after biopsy or polypectomy. AJR Am. J. Roentgenol. *148:*285, 1987, with permission, © by American Roentgen Ray Society.) *B,* Lateral view shows ulcer in profile *(arrow).* Note deformity and puckering of adjacent rectal wall.

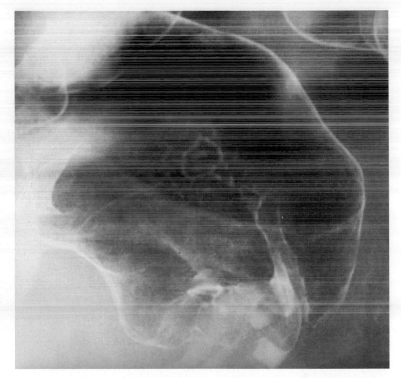

FIGURE 15–13. "Fried-egg" appearance after electrocoagulation biopsy of rectal polyp. Note irregular periphery representing coagulated base of polyp and smooth, domed center at point of separation from resected fragment. (Courtesy of Henry Degryse, M.D., Antwerp, Belgium.)

should distinguish these lesions from the aphthous ulcers of Crohn's disease (Figs. 15–11 and 15–12).[21] A hot (electrocoagulation) biopsy of a polyp may also result in a "fried egg" appearance, with an irregular, peripheral area representing the partially coagulated base of the polyp and a smooth, domed center representing the point of separation from the resected fragment (Fig. 15–13).[22] When these lesions are encountered, it is important to ascertain whether there has been a recent biopsy or polypectomy, so that unnecessary follow-up studies can be avoided.

Carpet Lesions

Carpet lesions of the colon are defined as flat, lobulated lesions that may involve a considerable surface area of the bowel with little or no protrusion into the lumen.[23] For reasons that are unclear, they are found predominantly in the rectum and cecum.[23] Most carpet lesions are benign adenomas with varying degrees of villous change (tubulovillous adenomas).[23] Resection is warranted because of the risk of malignant degeneration.

Carpet lesions of the rectum may be recognized en face by a nodular or reticular surface pattern of the mucosa (Fig. 15–14).[23,24] Some can be relatively extensive lesions, involving the entire circumference of the rectum (Fig. 15–15). Despite their large size, these lesions may cause only minimal alteration in the appearance of the mucosa, so that they can be missed at endoscopy.[5] One or more repeat endoscopic examinations therefore may be required when the double contrast enema arouses suspicion of a carpet lesion of the rectum.

Malignant Tumors

Nearly 50% of all colonic carcinomas missed on single contrast barium enemas are located in the rectum.[25] Double contrast technique is therefore particularly important for detecting lesions in this location. Like malignant tumors elsewhere in the colon, rectal carcinomas may be polypoid (Figs. 15–16 and 15–17), ulcerated (Fig. 15–18), plaquelike (Fig. 15–19), or annular lesions (Fig. 15–20).[4] In general, polypoid lesions on the dependent wall of the rectum appear as filling defects in the barium pool, whereas those on the nondependent wall are etched in white (Fig. 15–17; see Chapter 2). Lesions near the rectosigmoid junction may be seen exclusively or to best advantage on prone, angled views (Fig. 15–21), whereas lesions on the posterior wall may be seen best on prone, cross-table lateral views. In any case, lesions that are visible on one projection may be partially or completely obscured by the barium pool in other projections, so that all the spot films and overhead radiographs must be scrutinized carefully to avoid missing polypoid or plaquelike lesions in the rectum. Finally, lesions in the distal rectum may be hidden by the rectal tip itself (Fig. 15–19*A*), so that it is important to obtain views of the rectum after the tip has been removed (Fig. 15–19*B*).

Because colorectal cancer often results from malignant degeneration of preexisting adenomatous polyps, early rectal cancers are virtually always polypoid lesions, and they may be indistinguishable radiographically from benign-appearing polyps (Fig. 15–22). Not surprisingly, some early lesions may be detected as incidental findings in asymptomatic patients. The patient illustrated in

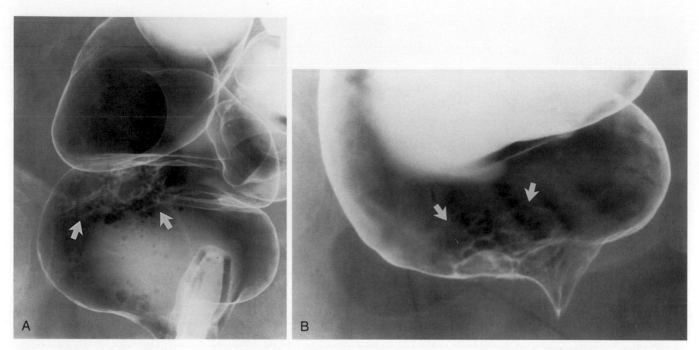

FIGURE 15–14. Two examples (*A* and *B*) of carpet lesions *(arrows)* in rectum manifested by finely nodular or reticular surface pattern of mucosa. Both patients had tubular adenomas with varying degrees of villous change. (*A*, From Rubesin, S.E., et al.: Carpet lesions of the colon. Radiographics *5*:537, 1985, with permission.)

FIGURE 15–15. *A,* Extensive carpet lesion of distal rectum, causing diffuse coarsening and irregularity of mucosa. *B,* Surgical specimen from similar case showing flat, carpetlike growth involving entire circumference of distal rectum. (From Rubesin, S.E., et al.: Carpet lesions of the colon. Radiographics *5*:537, 1985, with permission.)

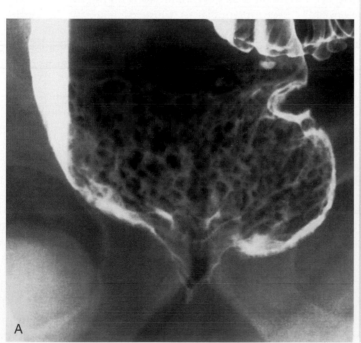

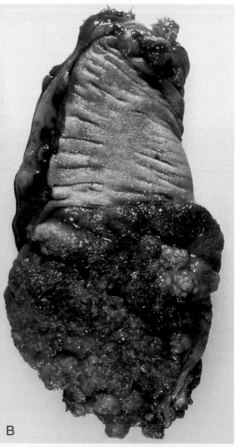

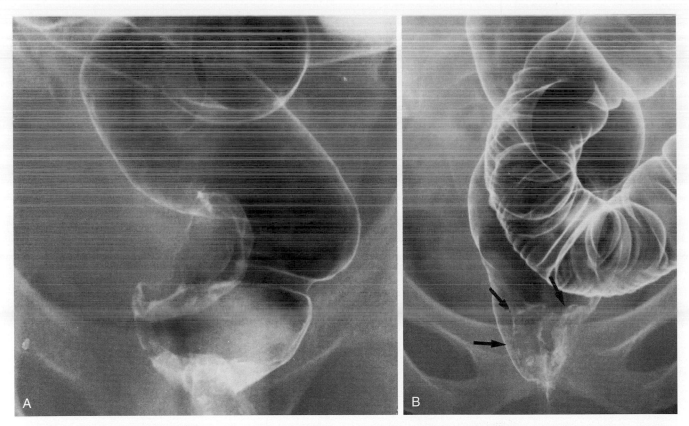

FIGURE 15–16. Two examples (*A* and *B*) of polypoid carcinomas *(arrows in B)* in rectum.

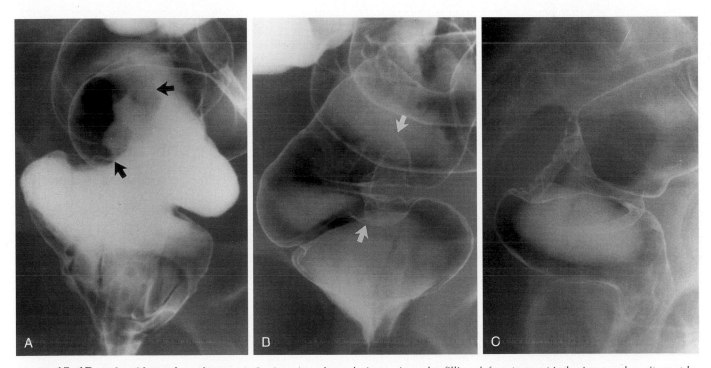

FIGURE 15–17. Polypoid rectal carcinoma. *A,* Supine view shows lesion as irregular filling defect *(arrows)* in barium pool, so it must be located on posterior wall. *B,* Prone view shows lesion etched in white *(arrows)* on nondependent surface. *C,* Lateral view confirms location of mass on posterior wall.

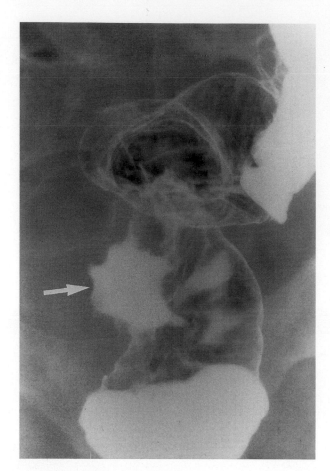

FIGURE 15–18. Rectal carcinoma containing large area of ulceration *(arrow)*.

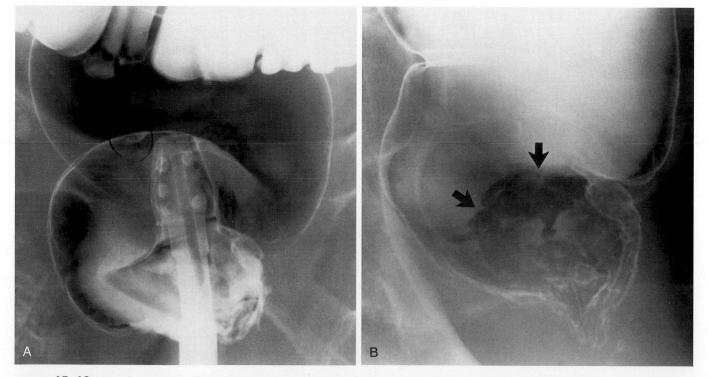

FIGURE 15–19. Rectal carcinoma obscured by enema tip. *A,* Initial view shows small polyp *(circle)* in proximal rectum. However, the enema tip prevents adequate visualization of distal rectum. *B,* Another view after removal of enema tip shows plaquelike cancer *(arrows)* that had been obscured by tip. (From Evers, K., et al.: Double-contrast enema examination for detection of rectal carcinoma. Radiology *140*:635, 1981, with permission.)

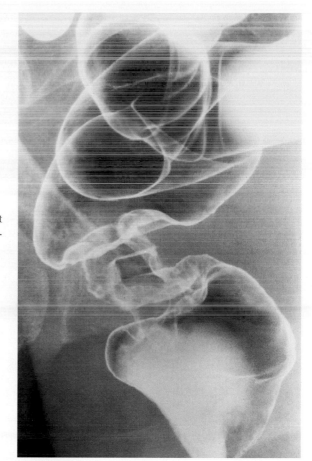

FIGURE **15–20.** Annular carcinoma in proximal rectum, which was missed at sigmoidoscopy. Angulation caused by the tumor apparently prevented the sigmoidoscope from reaching the cancer.

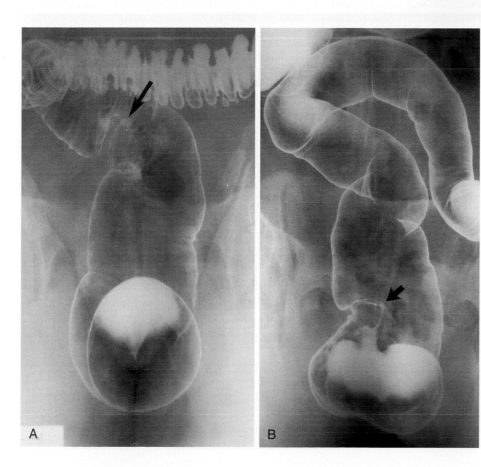

FIGURE **15–21. Polypoid carcinomas *(arrows)* best seen on prone, angled view.** *A,* Carcinoma of rectosigmoid junction. *B,* Carcinoma of rectum.

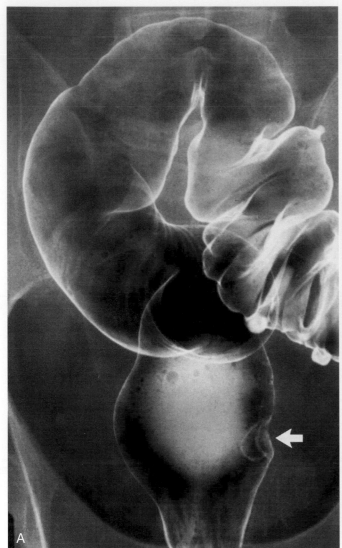

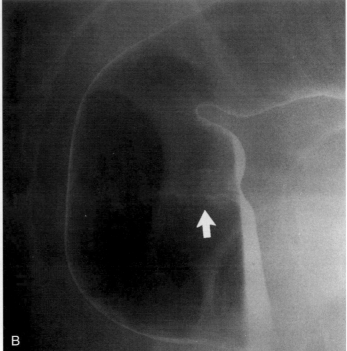

FIGURE 15–22. Early rectal carcinoma. *A,* Frontal view shows small, sessile polyp *(arrow)* in rectum. Note slight retraction of base of polyp. *B,* Polyp *(arrow)* is barely visible on prone, cross-table lateral view.

Figure 15–23 had a double contrast enema because of right lower quadrant pain. The polypoid lesion in the rectum, which proved to be an early cancer, was detected as a fortuitous finding.

Some rectal cancers may be located at endoscopic "blind spots" discussed previously (Fig. 15–24; see previous discussion, Polyps).[4] Others can be missed if the sigmoidoscope is not advanced to its full extent, particularly if angulation or fixation of the bowel by tumor prevents complete insertion of the scope. The patient illustrated in Figure 15–20 had undergone sigmoidoscopy twice in the previous 1½ years without detection of the lesion. In one study, 91% of rectal carcinomas were diagnosed on double contrast enema, whereas 86% were diagnosed on proctoscopy.[4] Thus, the double contrast enema detects most rectal cancers, including some that are missed at proctoscopy.

Primary scirrhous carcinoma of the rectum is a rare type of malignancy characterized by a linitis plastica appearance due to an extensive desmoplastic response in-

cited by the tumor. Some lesions may be associated with narrowing and rigidity of the rectosigmoid with a smooth contour and effaced mucosal folds, whereas others may be associated with an irregular rectal contour and distorted, spiculated folds.[26,27] The latter findings erroneously may suggest that the rectosigmoid colon has been encased by metastatic tumor (see later discussion, Extrinsic Abnormalities). Cloacogenic carcinoma is another unusual malignant tumor arising from the transitional cloacogenic zone of the anorectal junction. These tumors typically appear as plaquelike or polypoid lesions involving the distal rectum near the anal verge (Fig. 15–25).[28,29] However, adenocarcinoma of the distal rectum or even squamous cell carcinoma of the anus invading the rectum may produce similar findings (Figs. 15–26 and 15–27).[30] Other malignant tumors that rarely may involve the rectum are carcinoid, lymphoma, and leiomyosarcoma (Fig. 15–28).[31–33] However, pathologic specimens are required for a definitive diagnosis.

Primary anorectal lymphoma recently has been en-

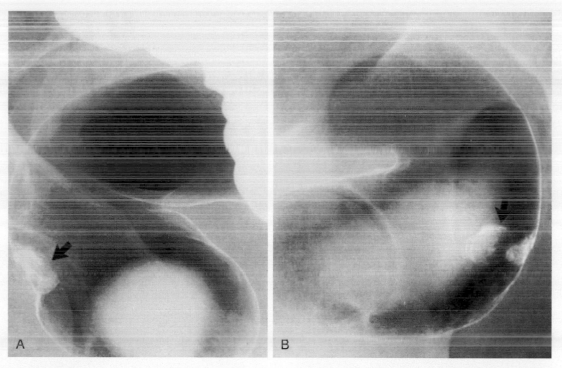

FIGURE 15–23. *A* and *B*, Early, asymptomatic rectal carcinoma appearing as a sessile, polypoid lesion *(arrows)*. This patient presented with right lower quadrant pain. The rectal tumor was an incidental finding.

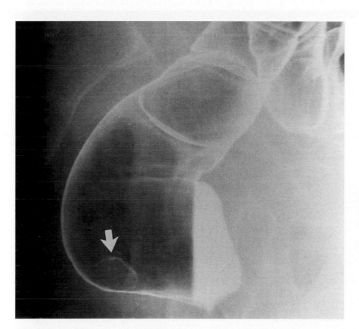

FIGURE 15–24. Small, polypoid rectal carcinoma *(arrow)* missed at sigmoidoscopy. This lesion probably was not detected by the endoscopist because of its location at a potential blind spot on posterior wall of rectum just inside anal verge.

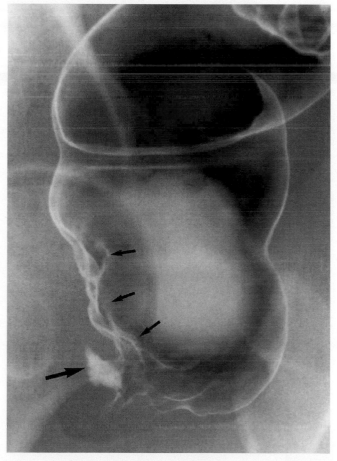

FIGURE 15–25. Cloacogenic carcinoma appearing as plaquelike lesion *(small arrows)* on posterolateral wall of distal rectum with area of ulceration *(large arrow)*. (Courtesy of Seth N. Glick, M.D., Philadelphia, Pennsylvania.)

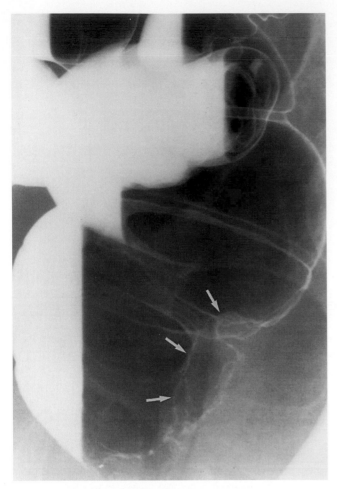

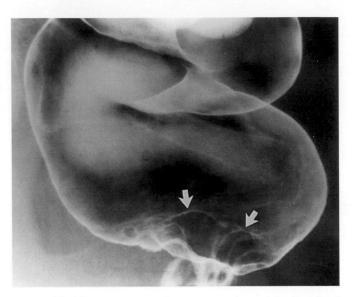

FIGURE 15–27. Squamous cell carcinoma of anus invading distal rectum *(arrows).*

FIGURE 15–26. Plaquelike carcinoma *(arrows)* in distal rectum. Note resemblance to the cloacogenic carcinoma illustrated in Figure 15–25.

FIGURE 15–28. *A* and *B,* Leiomyosarcoma of the rectum, appearing as giant submucosal mass.

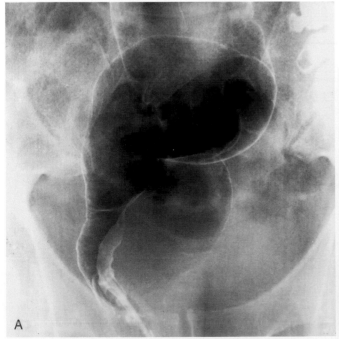

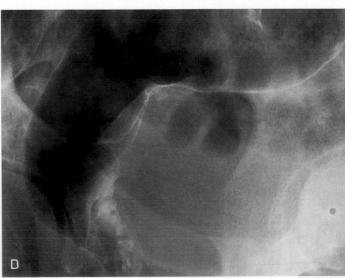

countered with increased frequency in patients with AIDS, especially homosexual men.[34] AIDS-related anorectal lymphoma may be manifested on double contrast studies by a perianal mass with marked rectal narrowing.[35,36] CT in these patients may show dramatic soft-tissue thickening of the rectal wall.

Inflammatory Conditions
Ulcerative Proctitis

Ulcerative proctitis is a mild variant of ulcerative colitis, in which involvement is limited to the rectum. Conventional single contrast barium enemas usually reveal no abnormalities in these patients.[37] With double contrast techniques, however, inflammatory changes can readily be demonstrated in the rectum, even in its most distal portion (Fig. 15–29).[38] As in patients with ulcerative colitis, ulcerative proctitis is initially manifested by a granular-appearing rectum due to mucosal edema and hyperemia (Fig. 15–29A). As the disease progresses, areas of shallow ulceration may be superimposed on a diffusely granular background mucosa (Fig. 15–29B).

Crohn's Disease

The rectum is involved endoscopically in about 50% of patients with granulomatous colitis.[39,40] However, the involvement tends to be patchy and asymmetric rather than the diffuse involvement seen in ulcerative colitis. As in the remainder of the colon, early Crohn's disease in the rectum may be manifested radiographically by discrete "aphthous" ulcers separated by normal mucosa (see Chapter 13).[41] In more advanced disease, relatively deep, collar-button ulcers may be seen in the rectum, as well as perirectal or perianal fistulas (Fig. 15–30).[42] These findings are rarely seen in the rectum in ulcerative colitis.[43] Thus, it usually is possible to differentiate Crohn's disease and ulcerative colitis involving the rectum on double contrast enemas.

Venereal Proctitis

Venereal proctitis has become a relatively common disease in homosexual men. Gonorrhea and herpes simplex are the most common organisms responsible for this condition.[44] Both gonococcal and herpetic proctitis may be manifested by edema, spasm, and ulceration.[45,46] Some patients with anorectal herpes may have discrete aphthous ulcers indistinguishable from those of Crohn's disease involving the rectum (Fig. 15–31A).[47] Lymphogranuloma venereum is another less common cause of venereal proctitis characterized by diffuse rectosigmoid narrowing, deep ulcers, and perirectal fistulae (Fig.

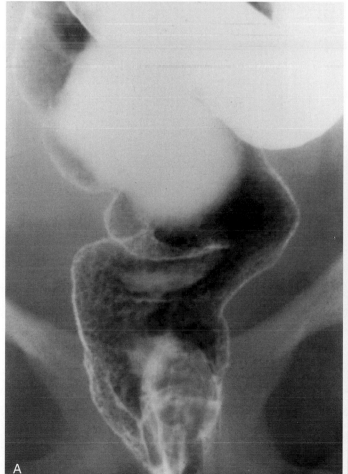
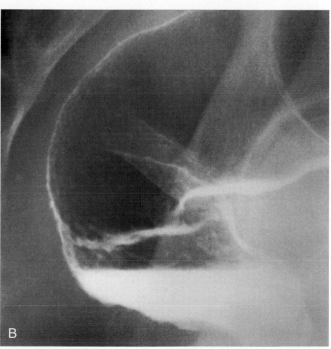

FIGURE **15–29. Ulcerative proctitis.** *A,* Frontal view shows coarse granularity of rectum due to chronic inflammation. *B,* Lateral view in another patient shows stippling of mucosa in distal rectum due to superficial ulceration.

A

B

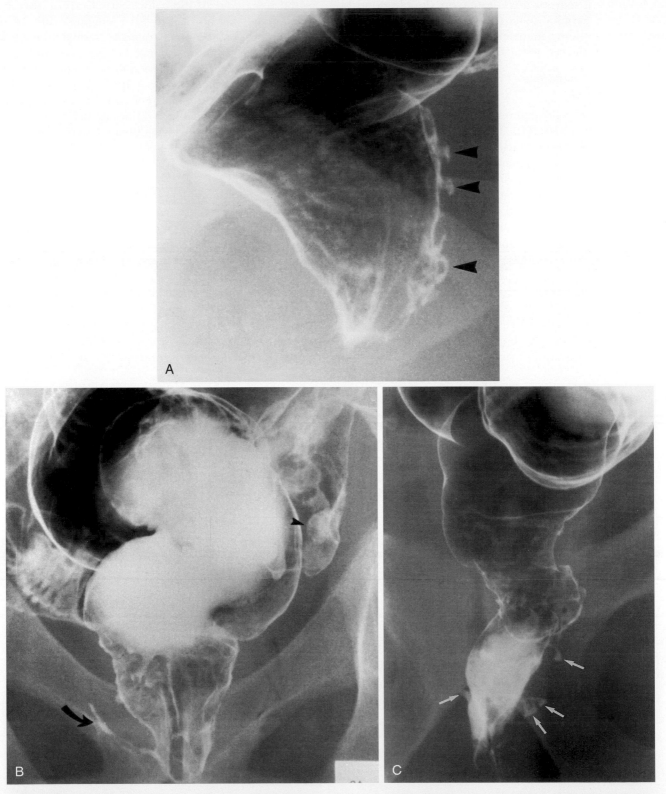

FIGURE 15–30. Rectal involvement by Crohn's disease. *A,* Deep, collar-button ulcers *(arrowheads)* in the rectum. When found in the rectum, these ulcers are characteristic of Crohn's disease rather than ulcerative colitis. *B,* Ulcers and a sinus tract *(arrow)* in rectum. Inflammatory polyps *(arrowhead)* are also present. *C,* More severe disease with narrowing, ulceration, and multiple perirectal fistulas *(arrows).*

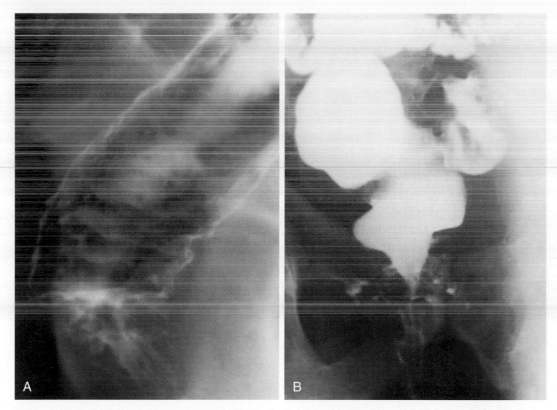

FIGURE 15–31. Venereal proctitis. *A,* Herpetic proctitis with multiple aphthous ulcers in rectum. Rectal involvement by Crohn's disease could produce identical findings. (Courtesy of Francis J. Scholz, M.D., Burlington, Massachusetts. From Shah, S.J., and Scholz, F.J.: Anorectal herpes: Radiographic findings. Radiology *147*:81, 1983, with permission.) *B,* Lymphogranuloma venereum with narrowing of distal rectum and multiple anorectal fistulas.

15–31*B*).[48] Although the possibility of venereal proctitis may be suspected from the clinical history, stool cultures are required for a definitive diagnosis.

Other Forms of Proctitis

Injury to the rectosigmoid colon frequently occurs as the result of pelvic irradiation for cervical carcinoma or other malignant tumors.[49] In the acute phase, the mucosa may have a granular or ulcerated appearance indistinguishable from that of ulcerative proctitis (Fig. 15–32).[50] In the chronic phase, diffuse narrowing and loss of haustration may produce a rigid, tubular structure that has a smooth, featureless appearance (Fig. 15–33).[49] The rectum usually is spared in patients with ischemic colitis. When it is involved, however, the appearance may be similar to that of ulcerative proctitis (Fig. 15–34).[51]

HIV proctitis is another recently described entity thought to be caused by primary infection of rectal mucosa by HIV.[52] As in patients with HIV esophagitis (see Chapter 5), HIV proctitis is a diagnosis of exclusion that can only be suggested when other opportunistic infections have been ruled out by stool cultures or endoscopic biopsy specimens. HIV proctitis may be manifested on double contrast studies by granularity or ulceration of the mucosa (Fig. 15–35*A*) or by the development of a

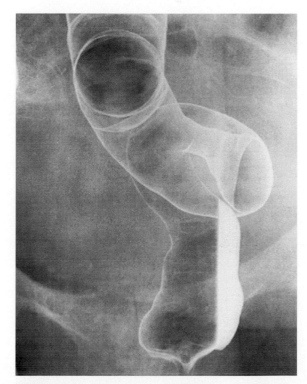

FIGURE 15–32. Acute radiation proctitis with minimal granularity of mucosa.

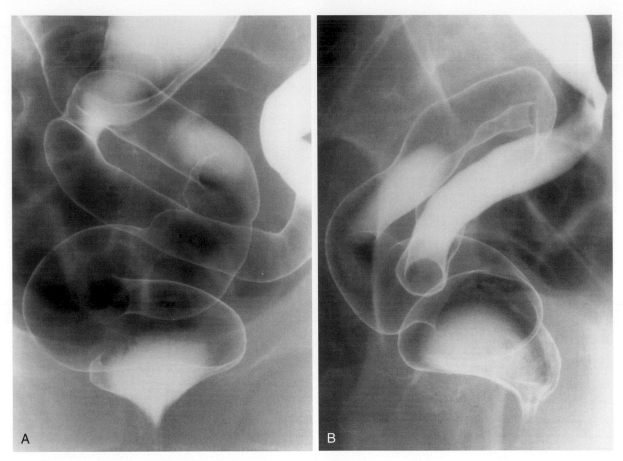

FIGURE 15–33. **Chronic radiation changes in rectosigmoid colon with diffuse narrowing and loss of haustration.** *A,* Frontal view. *B,* Steep oblique view.

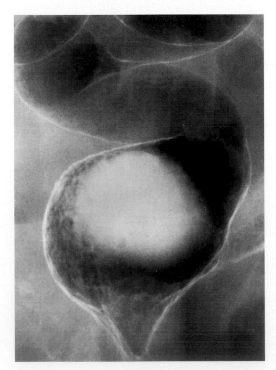

FIGURE 15–34. Ischemic proctitis with coarse granularity of rectal mucosa.

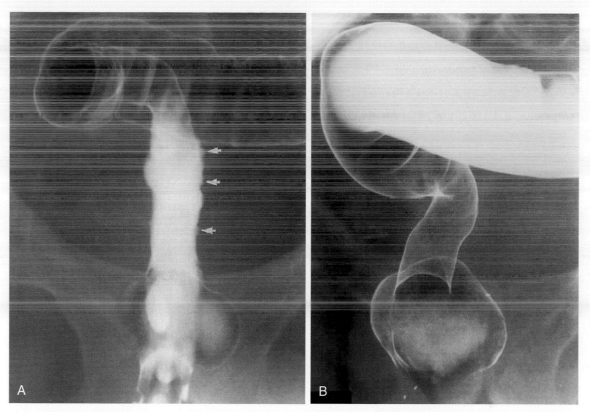

FIGURE 15–35. HIV proctitis. *A,* Rectosigmoid narrowing with multiple tiny ulcers *(arrows)* seen in profile in proximal rectum and distal sigmoid colon. *B,* Follow-up study 9 years later shows tubular narrowing of rectosigmoid colon with obliterated haustral folds and smooth, featureless mucosa. (From Solomon, J.A., Levine, M.S., O'Brien, C., et al.: HIV colitis: Clinical and radiographic findings. AJR Am. J. Roentgenol. *168:*681, 1997, with permission, © by American Roentgen Ray Society.)

smooth, tapered stricture of the rectosigmoid colon due to progressive scarring (Fig. 15–35*B*).[53] The possibility of HIV infection should be considered when an acute proctosigmoiditis is diagnosed on double contrast enema in an HIV-positive patient in whom there is no pathologic evidence of venereal proctitis.

Some patients may have nonspecific proctitis on double contrast enemas with nodular mucosa or thickened, edematous valves of Houston, producing a "boggy" rectum (Fig. 15–36). Other patients with proctitis may have enlarged lymphoid follicles in the rectum, a condition known as "follicular proctitis" (Fig. 15–37).[54] In our experience, mild forms of proctitis may even be caused by the laxatives that the patient takes for the barium enema examination.

Solitary Rectal Ulcer Syndrome and Colitis Cystica Profunda

Solitary rectal ulcer syndrome is a benign clinical entity in which a persistent, nonhealing ulcer is classically found on the anterior wall of the rectum in young patients with rectal bleeding.[55] However, the name of the condition is misleading because some patients may have multiple ulcers and others may have localized proctitis without ulceration.[55] Although the pathogenesis is uncertain, there frequently is a history of rectal straining or prolapse, so that ulceration of the anterior rectal wall may be traumatic or ischemic in origin. The diagnosis may be confirmed by rectal biopsy, which reveals classic histopathologic findings (fibromuscular obliteration of the lamina propria and thickening and fraying of the muscularis mucosae).[55]

The diagnosis of solitary rectal ulcer syndrome may be suggested radiographically by the presence of a discrete, benign-appearing ulcer on the anterior rectal wall near the first valve of Houston (Fig. 15–38). In the majority of patients, however, double contrast enemas demonstrate thickened, edematous valves of Houston or nodular mucosa without ulcers (Fig. 15–39).[56,57] The latter findings therefore should raise the possibility of solitary rectal ulcer syndrome, particularly in young patients with rectal bleeding. Proctoscopy and biopsy can then be performed for a definitive diagnosis.

Colitis cystica profunda is an unusual condition characterized by the presence of mucus-filled, epithelial-lined cysts in the submucosa. Some investigators have reported an association between a localized form of colitis cystica profunda involving the rectum and solitary rectal ulcer syndrome, possibly due to extension of regenerating surface epithelium into the submucosa.[55,58] The lesions of colitis cystica profunda may appear radiographically as one

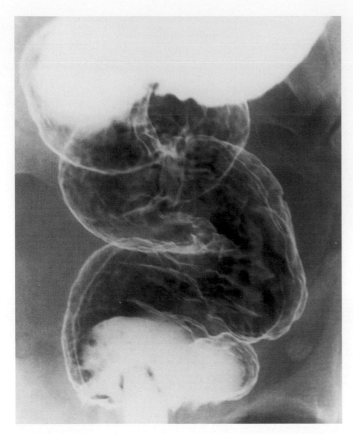

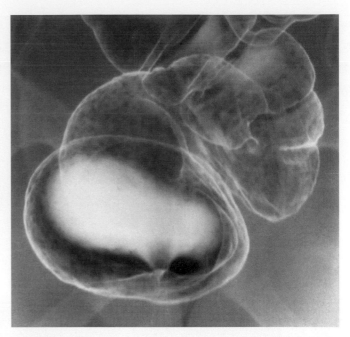

FIGURE 15–37. Follicular proctitis with enlarged lymphoid follicles appearing as multiple small nodules in rectum.

FIGURE 15–36. Nonspecific proctitis with nodular mucosa and thickened folds in rectum, producing "boggy" appearance. (From Rubesin, S.E., et al.: Carpet lesions of the colon. Radiographics *5*:537, 1985, with permission.)

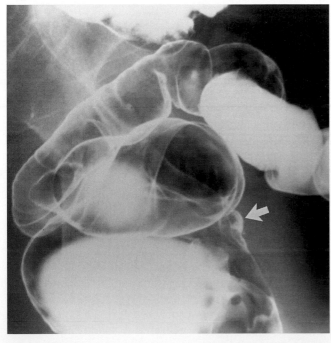

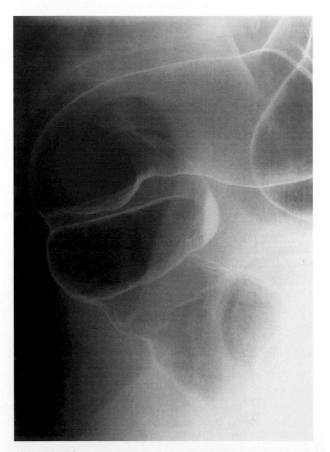

FIGURE 15–38. Solitary rectal ulcer syndrome with single, discrete ulcer *(arrow)* on anterior wall of rectum. (Courtesy of Harvey N. Goldstein, M.D., San Antonio, Texas.)

FIGURE 15–39. Solitary rectal ulcer syndrome with thickened, edematous valves of Houston but no ulcers. (From Levine, M.S., et al.: Solitary rectal ulcer syndrome: A radiologic diagnosis? Gastrointest. Radiol. *11*:187, 1986, with permission.)

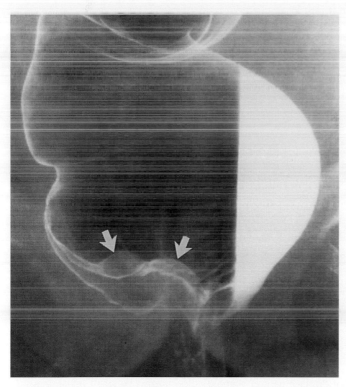

FIGURE 15–40. Solitary rectal ulcer syndrome with localized colitis cystica profunda. Note slightly lobulated submucosal-appearing mass *(arrows)* in distal rectum near anal verge due to mucus-filled, epithelium-lined cysts in submucosa. (From Levine, M.S., et al.: Solitary rectal ulcer syndrome: A radiologic diagnosis? Gastrointest. Radiol. *11:*187, 1986, with permission.)

or more lobulated submucosal masses in the rectum (Fig. 15–40).[58,59] Although it is a benign condition, pathologists occasionally have mistaken these mucus filled cysts for invasive mucinous adenocarcinoma. Thus, it is important to be aware of the association between solitary rectal ulcer syndrome and colitis cystica profunda, so that unnecessary radical surgery can be avoided in these patients.

EXTRINSIC ABNORMALITIES

Various types of perirectal disease are well demonstrated on double contrast studies. Extrinsic compression of the rectosigmoid colon may be caused by soft tissue masses (uterine or ovarian tumors; Figs. 15–41 and 15–42), fluid collections (ascites, hematomas, lymphoceles, and others), or even accumulation of fat in the pelvis (pelvic lipomatosis; Fig. 15–43).[60,61] A pelvic mass may be manifested by a smooth, gently sloping indentation on the anterior border of the rectosigmoid that usually is most obvious on lateral projections (Fig. 15–41). In some patients, the findings may be quite subtle (Fig. 15–42A) and may be easiest to recognize on prone, cross-table lateral views (Fig. 15–42B). Less frequently, extrinsic compression of the lateral borders of the rectosigmoid colon may be seen best on frontal projections (Fig. 15–43A). Regardless of the location of the mass, the absence of irregularity, spiculation, tethering, or ulceration generally indicates that it is compressing the bowel and not invading it.[62]

FIGURE 15–41. Extrinsic compression of rectosigmoid by uterine fibroids. *A,* Lateral view shows smooth, gently sloping indentation on anterior border of rectosigmoid. Also note impression on bladder *(arrows).* *B,* Frontal view shows area of mass effect en face *(arrows),* but findings are more subtle in this projection.

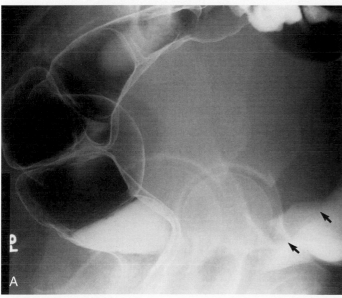

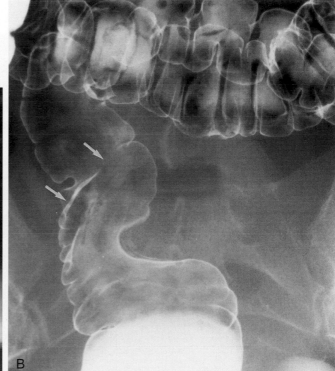

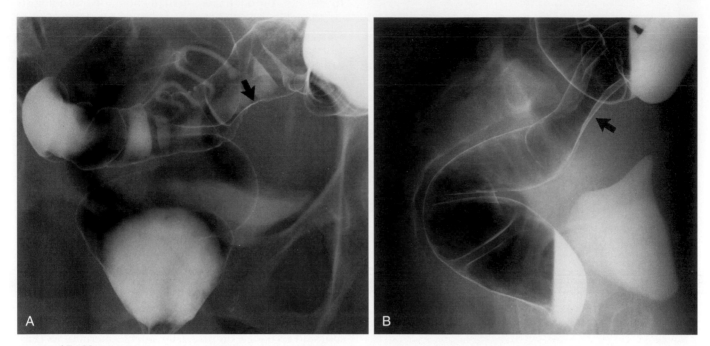

FIGURE 15–42. Subtle areas of mass effect on rectosigmoid. *A,* Slight displacement of sigmoid colon *(arrow)* by small pelvic mass. *B,* Cross-table lateral view showing minimal compression of rectosigmoid *(arrow)* by pelvic mass.

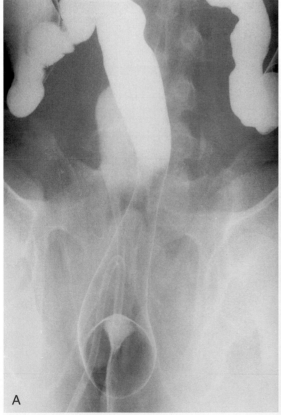

FIGURE 15–43. Extrinsic compression of rectosigmoid by fat in pelvis. *A,* Prone, angled view shows smooth, symmetric compression of lateral walls of rectosigmoid colon. *B,* CT scan shows marked amount of adipose tissue surrounding rectum *(arrow)* in this patient with pelvic lipomatosis.

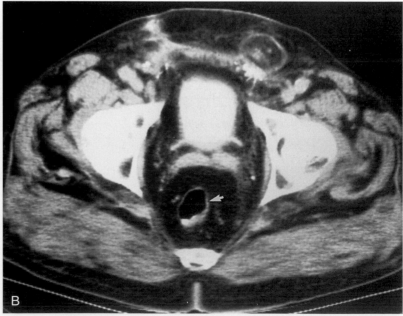

Because the rectosigmoid colon directly abuts the most dependent portion of the peritoneal cavity, it is the most common site of involvement by intraperitoneal seeding of metastatic tumor from ovarian, gastric, colonic, or pancreatic carcinoma.[63,64] These metastatic deposits in the rectovesical space (the pouch of Douglas in a woman) may incite a marked desmoplastic response in the wall of the bowel, causing mass effect, irregularity, spiculation, or tethering of the anterior border of the rectosigmoid (Fig. 15–44). Although these changes may be recognized en face (Fig. 15–44B), they are best seen in profile on lateral views of the rectum (Fig. 15–44A). Involvement of the rectovesical space by inflammatory conditions such as appendicitis, diverticulitis, Crohn's disease, and tuboovarian abscess may produce similar radiographic findings (Fig. 15–45).[60] In the latter patients, spread of inflammation to the serosa of the bowel may result in thickened, spiculated folds (Fig. 15–46). The rectosigmoid is also a common site of colonic involvement by endometriosis.[65] These hormonally stimulated endometriosis implants may cause mass effect, crenulation, and tethering of the anterior border of the rectosigmoid due to bleeding and subsequent fibrosis in the wall of the bowel (Figs. 15–47 and 15–48A).[66] Additional implants may be found in the sigmoid and cecum (Fig. 15–48B). Thus, intraperitoneal metastases, inflammatory diseases, and endometriosis may produce similar changes in the rectosigmoid colon, so that the clinical history is essential for differentiating these conditions.

Pelvic malignancies such as cervical, uterine, and bladder cancer may directly invade the rectum, causing mass effect and tethered, spiculated folds on its anterior or lateral walls or, in advanced cases, circumferential narrowing of the bowel (Fig. 15–49). However, these tumors tend to involve the distal portion of the rectum below the level of the peritoneal reflection, whereas intraperitoneal metastases to the rectosigmoid rarely extend below this level. Although prostatic carcinoma may also invade the distal rectum (Fig. 15–50), this malignancy tends to spread superiorly to the seminal vesicles before invading the rectum.[67] As a result, the majority of patients have localized rectosigmoid involvement with sparing of the distal rectum (Fig. 15–51). Invasion of the bowel wall may be manifested by mass effect and spiculated, tethered folds on the anterior border of the rectosigmoid, mimicking the appearance of intraperitoneal metastases.[67] However, prostatic carcinoma often spreads posteriorly around the bowel, causing circumferential narrowing and widening of the presacral space (Fig. 15–51),[67] whereas intraperitoneal seeding of the rectosigmoid almost always produces abnormalities that are confined to the anterior border of the bowel. Thus, it is often possible to suggest the nature and origin of malignant spread to the rectosigmoid colon on the basis of the radiographic findings.

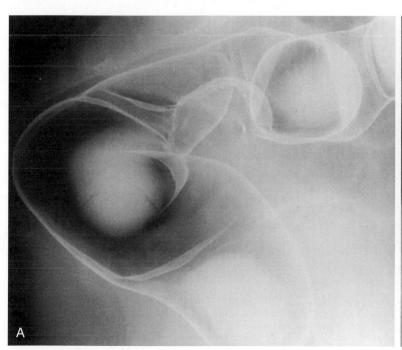
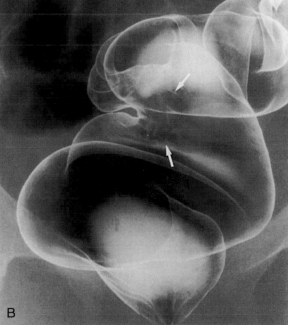

FIGURE 15–44. Intraperitoneal-seeded metastasis to rectosigmoid colon. *A,* Lateral view shows area of mass effect, spiculation, and irregularity on anterior border of rectosigmoid due to metastatic seeding. *B,* This metastatic deposit can also be recognized en face by pleated, tethered appearance of mucosa *(arrows)* on frontal view.

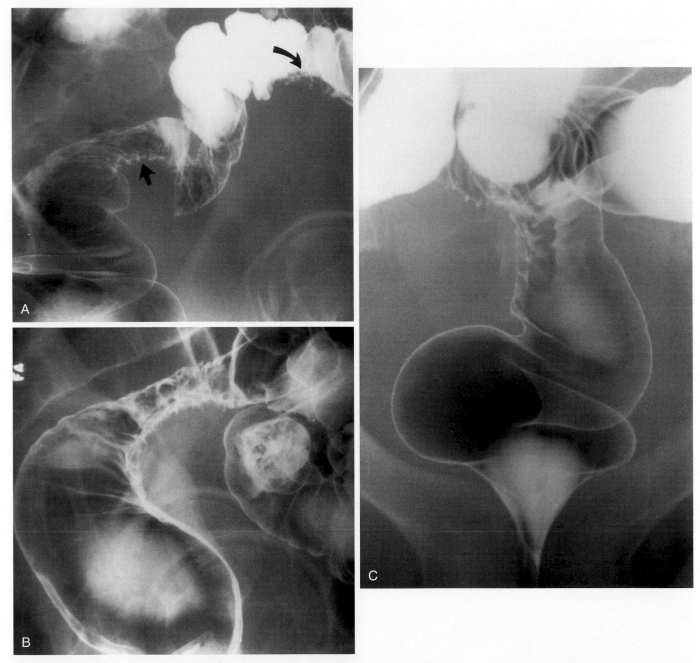

FIGURE 15–45. Rectosigmoid involvement by inflammatory conditions in rectovesical space. *A,* Sigmoid diverticulitis *(curved arrow)* with extension of inflammatory process to rectosigmoid *(straight arrow)*. *B,* Crohn's disease with findings indistinguishable from those of metastatic disease or endometriosis involving rectosigmoid colon. *C,* Tuboovarian abscess with mucosal pleating seen en face on frontal view of rectum.

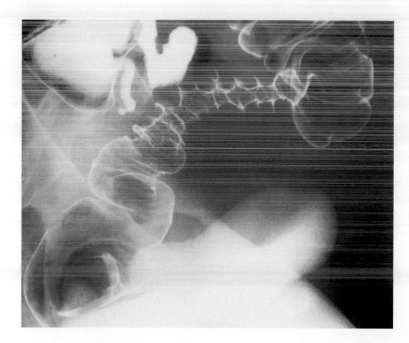

FIGURE 15–46. Tuberculous tuboovarian abscess involving sigmoid colon. Note thickened, spiculated folds.

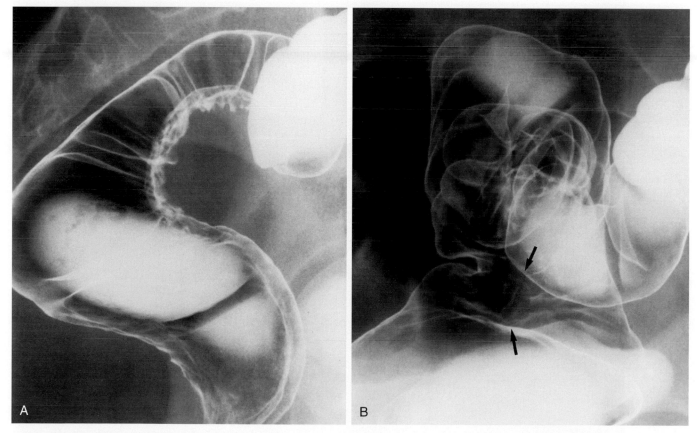

FIGURE 15–47. Rectosigmoid involvement by endometriosis. *A,* Lateral view shows mass effect on anterior border of rectosigmoid colon with spiculated, tethered mucosal folds. *B,* Frontal view shows mucosal pleating en face *(arrows).* Intraperitoneal metastases or inflammatory processes in rectovesical space may produce identical findings, so the clinical history is essential for differentiating these conditions.

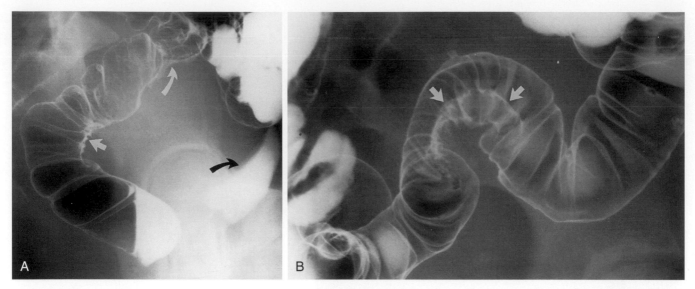

FIGURE 15–48. Colonic involvement by endometriosis. *A,* Lateral view shows spiculation and tethering of anterior border of rectosigmoid *(straight white arrow).* Also note pelvic mass compressing sigmoid colon *(curved white arrow)* and bladder *(curved black arrow).* *B,* Endometriosis implant in sigmoid colon *(arrows)* in another patient. Note mucosal pleating in this region.

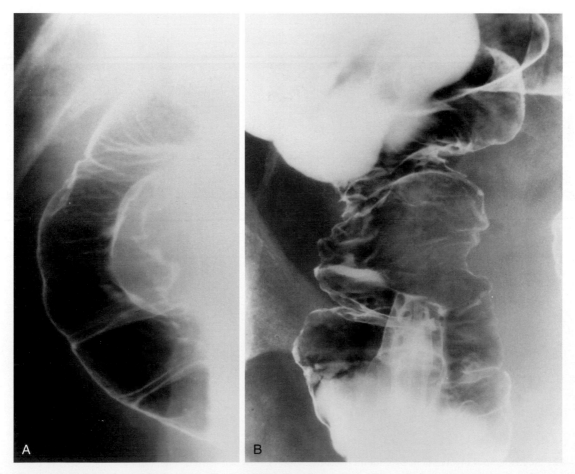

FIGURE 15–49. Rectal invasion by cervical carcinoma. *A,* Lateral view shows mass effect and irregular mucosa on anterior border of rectum. *B,* Frontal view also shows area of mass effect and pleated mucosal folds in rectum. Unlike in patients with intraperitoneal metastases to rectosigmoid, note how rectum is involved below level of peritoneal reflection.

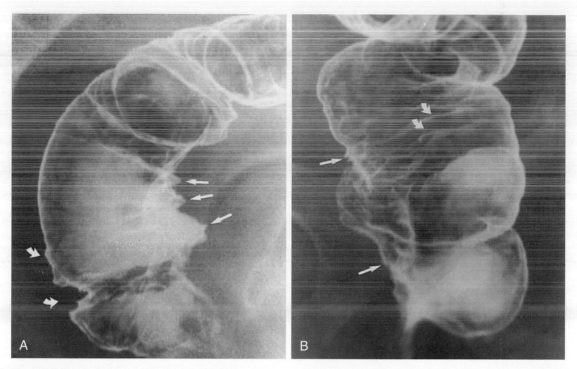

FIGURE 15–50. Rectal invasion by prostatic carcinoma. *A,* Lateral view shows flattening and spiculation of anterior border of rectum *(straight arrows).* Mild circumferential extension is seen distally *(curved arrows). B,* Frontal view shows mass effect and spiculation along right lateral wall of rectum *(straight arrows)* and mucosal pleating en face *(curved arrows).* (From Rubesin S.E., et al.: Rectal involvement by prostatic carcinoma: Barium enema findings. AJR Am. J. Roentgenol. *152:*53, 1989, with permission, © by American Roentgen Ray Society.)

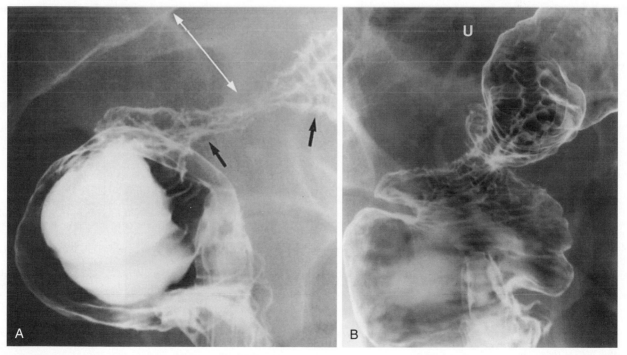

FIGURE 15–51. Rectosigmoid invasion by prostatic carcinoma. *A,* Lateral view shows mass effect and spiculated contour along anterior border of rectosigmoid *(black arrows)* with widening of presacral space *(double white arrow).* Note sparing of distal rectum. *B,* Oblique view shows narrowing of rectosigmoid and mucosal pleating en face. Although intraperitoneal metastases could produce similar findings, circumferential narrowing of rectosigmoid colon and widening of presacral space should suggest the correct diagnosis. (*U,* Opacified ureter from intravenous urography.) (From Rubesin, S.E., et al.: Rectal involvement by prostatic carcinoma: Barium enema findings. AJR Am. J. Roentgenol. *152:*53, 1989, with permission, © by American Roentgen Ray Society.)

REFERENCES

1. Cooley, R.N.: The diagnostic accuracy of radiologic studies of the biliary tract, small intestine and colon. Am. J. Med. Sci. 246:610, 1963.
2. Simpkins, K.C., and Young, A.C.: The radiology of colonic and rectal polyps. Br. J. Surg. 55:731, 1968.
3. Laufer, I., Smith, N.C.W., and Mullens, J.E.: The radiologic demonstration of colorectal polyps undetected by endoscopy. Gastroenterology 70:167, 1976.
4. Evers, K., Laufer, I., Gordon, R.L., et al.: Double-contrast enema examination for detection of rectal carcinoma. Radiology 140:635, 1981.
5. Glick, S.N., Teplick, S.K., Balfe, D.M., et al.: Large colonic neoplasms missed by endoscopy. AJR Am. J. Roentgenol. 152:513, 1989.
6. Kirsner, J.B.: Problems in the differentiation of ulcerative colitis and Crohn's disease of the colon: The need for repeated diagnostic evaluation. Gastroenterology 68:187, 1975.
7. Miller, R.E.: Barium enema examination with large bore tubing and drainage. Radiology 82:905, 1964.
8. Miller, R.E., and Peterson, G.H.: Drainage of the rectum: A simple maneuver to improve the accuracy of colon examinations. Radiology 128:506, 1978.
9. Maglinte, D.D.T., Miller, R.E., and Chernish, S.M.: Early rectal tube removal for improved patient tolerance during double-contrast barium enema examination. Radiology 155:525, 1985.
10. Dysart, D.N., and Stewart H.R.: Special angled roentgenography for lesions of the rectosigmoid. AJR Am. J. Roentgenol. 96:285, 1966.
11. Niizuma, S., and Kobayashi, S.: Rectosigmoid double contrast examination in the prone position with a horizontal beam. AJR Am. J. Roentgenol. 128:519, 1977.
12. Goei, R.: Anorectal function in patients with defecation disorders and asymptomatic subjects: Evaluation with defecography. Radiology 174:121, 1990.
13. Goei, R., and Baeten, C.: Rectal intussusception and rectal prolapse: Detection and postoperative evaluation with defecography. Radiology 174:124, 1990.
14. Cohen, W.N.: Roentgenographic evaluation of the rectal valves of Houston in the normal and ulcerative colitis. AJR Am. J. Roentgenol. 104:580, 1968.
15. Kattan, K.R., and King, A.Y.: Presacral space revisited. AJR Am. J. Roentgenol. 132:437, 1979.
16. Thoeni, R.F., and Venbrux, A.C.: The anal canal: Distinction of internal hemorrhoids from small cancers by double-contrast barium enema examination. Radiology 145:17, 1982.
17. Levine, M.S., Kam, L.W., Rubesin, S.E., et al.: Internal hemorrhoids: Diagnosis with double-contrast barium enema examinations. Radiology 177:141, 1990.
18. Heiken, J.P., Zuckerman, G.R., and Balfe, D.M.: The hypertrophied anal papilla: Recognition on air-contrast barium enema examinations. Radiology 151:315, 1984.
19. Ott, D.J., and Gelfand, D.W.: Colorectal tumors: Pathology and detection. AJR Am. J. Roentgenol. 131:691, 1978.
20. Millward, S.F., Chapman, A., Somers, S., et al.: Rectal biopsy as a cause of rectal ulceration. Radiology 156:42, 1985.
21. Lev-Toaff, A.S., Levine, M.S., Laufer, I., et al.: Ringlike rectal ulcers after biopsy or polypectomy. AJR Am. J. Roentgenol. 148:285, 1987.
22. Bartram, C.I., and Hall-Craggs, M.A.: Interventional colorectal endoscopic procedures: Residual lesions on follow-up double-contrast barium enema study. Radiology 162:835, 1987.
23. Rubesin, S.E., Saul, S.H., Laufer, I., et al.: Carpet lesions of the colon. RadioGraphics 5:537, 1985.
24. Herman, T.E., Koehler, R.E., and Lee, J.K.T.: Focal irregularity of the rectal mucosa. AJR Am. J. Roentgenol. 133:677, 1979.
25. Cooley, R.N., Agnew, C.H., and Rios, G.: Diagnostic accuracy of the barium enema study in carcinoma of the colon and rectum. AJR Am. J. Roentgenol. 84:316, 1960.
26. Balthazar, E.J., Rosenberg, H.D., and Davidian, M.M.: Primary and metastatic scirrhous carcinoma of the rectum. AJR Am. J. Roentgenol. 132:711, 1979.
27. Oliver, T.W., Somogyi, J., and Gaffney, E.F.: Primary linitis plastica of the rectum. AJR Am. J. Roentgenol. 140:79, 1983.
28. Kyaw, M.M., Gallagher, T., and Haines, J.O.: Cloacogenic carcinoma of the anorectal junction: Roentgenologic diagnosis. AJR Am. J. Roentgenol. 115:384, 1972.
29. Hertz, I., Train, J., and Keller, R.: Cloacogenic carcinoma. J. Clin. Gastroenterol. 3:367, 1981.
30. McConnell, F.M.: Squamous carcinoma of the anus: A review of 96 cases. Br. J. Surg. 57:89, 1970.
31. Sato, T., Sakai, Y., Sonoyama, A., et al.: Radiologic spectrum of rectal carcinoid tumors. Gastrointest. Radiol. 9:23, 1984.
32. Ioachim, H.L., Weinstein, M.A., Robbins, R.D., et al.: Primary anorectal lymphoma. Cancer 60:1449, 1987.
33. Marshak, R.H., and Lindner, A.E.: Leiomyosarcoma of the colon. Am. J. Gastroenterol. 54:155, 1970.
34. Ioachim, H.L., Weinstein, M.A., Robbins, R.D., et al.: Primary anorectal lymphoma: A new manifestation of the acquired immune deficiency syndrome (AIDS). Cancer 60:1449, 1987.
35. Pantongrag-Brown, L., Nelson, A.M., Brown, A.E., et al.: Gastrointestinal manifestations of acquired immunodeficiency syndrome: Radiologic-pathologic correlation. RadioGraphics 15:1155, 1995.
36. Levine, M.S., Rubesin, S.E., Pantongrag-Brown, L., et al.: Non-Hodgkin's lymphoma of the gastrointestinal tract: Radiographic findings. AJR Am. J. Roentgenol. 168:165, 1997.
37. Fennessy, J.J., Sparberg, M., and Kirsner, J.B.: Early roentgen manifestations of mild ulcerative colitis and proctitis. Radiology 87:848, 1966.
38. Laufer, I.: The radiologic demonstration of early changes in ulcerative colitis by double contrast technique. J. Can. Assoc. Radiol. 26:116, 1975.
39. Laufer, I., and Hamilton, J.D.: The radiologic differentiation between ulcerative and granulomatous colitis by double contrast radiology. Am. J. Gastroenterol. 66:259, 1976.
40. Korelitz, B.I., and Sommers, S.C.: Differential diagnosis of ulcerative and granulomatous colitis by sigmoidoscopy, rectal biopsy and cell counts of rectal mucosa. Am. J. Gastroenterol. 61:460, 1974.
41. Laufer, I., and Costopoulos, L.: Early lesions of Crohn's disease. AJR Am. J. Roentgenol. 130:307, 1978.
42. DuBrow, R.A., and Frank, P.H.: Barium evaluation of anal canal in patients with inflammatory bowel disease. AJR Am. J. Roentgenol. 140:1151, 1983.
43. Devroede, G.J.: Differential diagnosis of colitis. Can. J. Surg. 17:369, 1974.
44. Quinn, T.C., Corey, L., Chaffee, R.G., et al.: The etiology of anorectal infections in homosexual men. Am. J. Med. 71:395, 1981.
45. Goodman, K.J.: Radiologic findings in anorectal gonorrhea. Gastrointest. Radiol. 3:223, 1978.
46. Sider, L., Mintzer, R.A., Mendelson, E.B., et al.: Radiographic findings of infectious proctitis in homosexual men. AJR Am. J. Roentgenol. 139:667, 1982.
47. Shah, S.J., and Scholz, F.J.: Anorectal herpes: Radiographic findings. Radiology 147:81, 1983.
48. Annamunthodo, H., and Marryatt, J.: Barium studies in intestinal lymphogranuloma venereum. Br. J. Radiol. 34:53, 1961.
49. Meyer, J.E.: Radiography of the distal colon and rectum after irradiation of carcinoma of the cervix. AJR Am. J. Roentgenol. 136:691, 1981.
50. Gelfand, M.D., Tepper, M., Katz, L.A., et al.: Acute irradiation proctitis in man. Gastroenterology 54:401, 1968.
51. Kilpatrick, Z.M., Farman, J., Yesner, R., et al.: Ischemic proctitis. JAMA 205:74, 1968.
52. Hing, M.C., Goldschmidt, C., Mathijs, J.M., et al.: Chronic colitis associated with human immunodeficiency virus infection. Med. J. Aust. 156:683, 1992.
53. Solomon, J.A., Levine, M.S., O'Brien, C., et al.: HIV colitis: Clinical and radiographic findings. AJR Am. J. Roentgenol. 168:681, 1997.
54. Flejou, J.F., Potet, F., Bogomeletz, W.V., et al.: Lymphoid follicular proctitis: A condition different from ulcerative proctitis? Dig. Dis. Sci. 33:314, 1988.
55. Rutter, K.R., and Riddell, R.H.: The solitary ulcer syndrome of the rectum. Clin. Gastroenterol. 4:505, 1975.
56. Feczko, P.J., O'Connell, D.J., Riddell, R.H., et al.: Solitary rectal ulcer syndrome: Radiologic manifestations. AJR Am. J. Roentgenol. 135:499, 1980.
57. Levine, M.S., Piccolello, M.L., Sollenberger, L.C., et al.: Solitary rectal ulcer syndrome: A radiologic diagnosis? Gastrointest. Radiol. 11:187, 1986.
58. Rosengren, J.E., Hildell, J., Lindstrom, C.G., et al.: Localized colitis cystica profunda. Gastrointest. Radiol. 7:79, 1982.

59. Miller, D.L.G., O'Malley, B.P., and Richmond, H.: Colitis cystica profunda. J. Can. Assoc. Radiol. *34*:70, 1983.

60. Schulman, A., and Fataar, S.: Extrinsic stretching, narrowing, and anterior indentation of the rectosigmoid junction. Clin. Radiol. *30*:163, 1979.

61. Farman, J., Faegenburg, D., Dallemand, S., et al.: Pelvic lipomatosis. Am. J. Gastroenterol. *60*:640, 1973.

62. Gedgaudas, R.K., Kelvin, F.M., Thompson, W.M., et al.: The value of the preoperative barium-enema examination in the assessment of pelvic masses. Radiology *116*:600, 1000.

63. Meyers, M.A.: Distribution of intra-abdominal malignant seeding: Dependency on dynamics of flow of ascitic fluid. AJR Am. J. Roentgenol. *119*:198, 1973.

64. Meyers, M.A.: Intraperitoneal spread of malignancies and its effect on the bowel. Clin. Radiol. *32*:129, 1981.

65. Fagan, C.F.: Endometriosis: Clinical and roentgenographic manifestations. Radiol. Clin. North Am. *12*:109, 1974.

66. Gordon, R.L., Evers, K., Kressel, H.Y., et al.: Double-contrast enema in pelvic endometriosis. AJR Am. J. Roentgenol. *138*:549, 1982.

67. Rubesin, S.E., Levine, M.S., Bezzi, M., et al.: Rectal involvement by prostatic carcinoma: Barium enema findings. AJR Am. J. Roentgenol. *152*:53, 1989.

Index

Note: Page numbers in *italics* refer to illustrations; page numbers followed by t refer to tables.

ISBN 0-7216-8211-1

90038

9 780721 682112